Nancy Caroline's
Emergency
Care in the Streets

Student Workbook

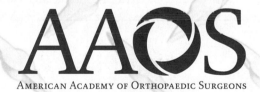

AMERICAN ACADEMY OF ORTHOPAEDIC SURGEONS

Author:

Nancy L. Caroline, MD

Editor:

Bob Elling, MPA, NREMT-P

JONES AND BARTLETT PUBLISHERS

Sudbury, Massachusetts

BOSTON   TORONTO   LONDON   SINGAPORE

Jones and Bartlett Publishers

World Headquarters
Jones and Bartlett Publishers
40 Tall Pine Drive
Sudbury, MA 01776
978-443-5000
info@jbpub.com
www.EMSzone.com

Jones and Bartlett Publishers Canada
6339 Ormindale Way
Mississauga, Ontario L5V 1J2
Canada

Jones and Bartlett Publishers International
Barb House, Barb Mews
London W6 7PA
United Kingdom

AAOS
AMERICAN ACADEMY OF ORTHOPAEDIC SURGEONS

American Academy of Orthopaedic Surgeons

Chief Executive Officer: Mark W. Wieting
Director, Department of Publications: Marilyn L. Fox, PhD
Managing Editor: Barbara A. Scotese

Jones and Bartlett's books and products are available through most bookstores and online booksellers. To contact Jones and Bartlett Publishers directly, call 800-832-0034, fax 978-443-8000, or visit our website www.jbpub.com.

Production Credits

Publisher—Public Safety Group: Kimberly Brophy
Managing Editor: Carol Guerrero
Associate Managing Editor: Amanda Green
Production Supervisor: Jenny L. Corriveau
Production Editor: Karen C. Ferreira
Editorial Assistant: Amanda Brandt
Interior Design: Anne Spencer
Manufacturing Buyer: Therese Connell
Interactive Technology Manager: Dawn Mahon Priest
Reprints Coordinator: Amy Browning
Composition: Omegatype Typography, Inc.
Cover Design: Kristin E. Ohlin
Associate Photo Researcher and Photographer: Christine McKeen
Printing and Binding: Courier Stoughton
Cover Printing: Courier Stoughton

Contributors

Deanna M. Leaver, NREMT-P
Hugh R. Skerker, BS, EMT-P
Andrew W. Stern, NREMT-P, MPA, MA

6048
Printed in the United States of America
11 10 09 08   10 9 8 7 6 5 4 3 2 1

CONTENTS

Section 4: Trauma

Section 5: Medical

Section 6: Special Considerations

CHAPTER

1 EMS Systems, Roles, and Responsibilities

Chapter Review

The following exercises provide an opportunity to test your knowledge of this chapter.

Matching

Match each of the definitions in the left column to the appropriate term in the right column.

_____ **1.** Outline the type of individual(s) who is(are) appropriate for the study.

_____ **2.** Statistics that can be performed in either a quantitative or qualitative style.

_____ **3.** A computer-generated list of subjects or groups.

_____ **4.** When the participants in the research study are advised of all aspects of the project.

_____ **5.** A final summary of information gained in a research project, after you have outlined the introduction, methods, results, and discussion sections.

_____ **6.** The findings of the project.

_____ **7.** A brief background of the research, along with previous studies, reason for the study, and a hypothesis of the project.

_____ **8.** A constructive discussion done after a call by the members of your team.

_____ **9.** A key role in EMS, person who receives information and then relays it to the appropriate resources.

_____ **10.** Granting certification to a provider from another state.

A. Systematic sampling
B. Results
C. Parameter
D. Inferential
E. Dispatcher
F. Unblinded study
G. Conclusion
H. Peer review
I. Introduction
J. Reciprocity

Multiple Choice

Read each item carefully, and then select the best response.

_____ **1.** In what year did the National Academy of Science and the National Research Council release the white paper entitled "Accidental Death and Disability: The Neglected Disease of Modern Society"?
  A. 1966
  B. 1967
  C. 1968
  D. 1969

_____ **2.** Which of the following is NOT an EMS system element?
  A. Resource management
  B. Public information and education
  C. Driving courses
  D. Medical direction

_____ **3.** What does EMD stand for?
  A. Emergency medical defibrillator
  B. Emergency medical doctor
  C. Emergency management director
  D. Emergency medical dispatch

_____ **4.** Which of the following may involve telemetry transmission during patient care?

  A. Off-line medical control   **C.** Protocols

  B. Online medical control   **D.** Standing orders

_____ **5.** What type of research is considered a basic observation only and no alterations occur?

  A. Experimental   **C.** Cross-sectional

  B. Descriptive   **D.** Qualitative

_____ **6.** Attributes of professionalism include all of the following, EXCEPT:

  A. Communication   **C.** Empathy

  B. Patient advocacy   **D.** Reciprocity

_____ **7.** Which of the following is required in most states before beginning a paramedic program?

  A. Advanced airway training   **C.** EMT basic certification

  B. Intravenous fluid therapy training   **D.** College-level anatomy and physiology

_____ **8.** Who is considered the father of paramedicine?

  A. Dr. David Boyd   **C.** Dr. Jean Larrey

  B. Dr. Eugene Nagel   **D.** Dr. Rob Puls

_____ **9.** Who is usually the first EMS person the public deals with?

  A. EMT-Basic   **C.** Dispatcher

  B. Law enforcement   **D.** Paramedic

_____ **10.** In 1999, which level of EMS saw a large change from the 1985 curriculum?

  A. Medical dispatchers   **C.** EMT-Intermediate

  B. EMT-Basic   **D.** EMT-Paramedic

Fill-in-the-Blank

Read each item carefully, and then complete the statement by filling in the missing word(s).

1. In the early 1960s during the war in Vietnam, the _____ _____ _____ _____ were staffed by specially trained physicians.

2. The _____ receives and enters all information on the call, interprets the information received, and relays it to the appropriate resources.

3. When your state grants certification (or licensure) to a provider from another state, it is known as _____.

4. The paramedic who can demonstrate to the patient, the patient's family members, and other health care providers the ability to identify and understand their feelings is known as _____.

5. During scene management, ensuring your own safety and the safety of your crew is your _____ _____.

6. The tool often used to continually evaluate your care is called _____ _____ _____.

7. _____ research is based on a clearly defined problem or question.

Ambulance Calls

The following case scenarios provide an opportunity to explore the concerns associated with patient management and paramedic care. Read each scenario, and then answer each question.

1. You are exiting a theater after watching a movie, when suddenly the woman in front of you falls down, landing on her knees and hands. She apparently has tripped in the dark on the steps. As you help her up, you find that she is not responding to you as she should. She says she feels very faint, and so you lower her back to the ground. She then loses consciousness, and you lower her all the way to the floor and make sure that her airway is open and she is breathing. You ask your spouse to find the management, call 9-1-1, and bring up the theater lights. Your patient is a 60-year-old woman who wakes up again and says she is all right and doesn't want anyone making a fuss over her. She just wants to go home.

a. What is some information you should give your spouse to tell the dispatcher?

_____

_____

_____

b. What are some reasons this patient should go to the hospital to get checked out?

_____

_____

_____

2. Wow, what an evening at the theater! After your patient has left in an ambulance, you head out the door to go home. Just as you are getting into your vehicle you hear a woman scream. It seems that she has been hit by a small pickup truck that was backing up to get a good parking spot. You run over to find a 40-year-old woman who is conscious and alert. She is sprawled out on the ground. She is screaming about her left leg, which is where the bumper of the pickup impacted her leg. She was knocked to the pavement. The driver of the pickup stopped when he heard the impact, and then pulled forward, which caused no more injury to the woman. She has an obvious deformity midthigh on the left leg. An EMT-B comes running to help because several people have already called 9-1-1. Because you are first on scene and the more highly trained responder, you take charge of this patient.

a. What is the first thing you should do on this "scene"?

_____

_____

_____

b. What steps should you take in treating this patient before the ambulance arrives?

_____

_____

_____

True/False

If you believe the statement to be more true than false, write the letter "T" in the space provided. If you believe the statement to be more false than true, write the letter "F."

_____ **1.** The first documented ambulance service was started in 1869 in New York City.

_____ **2.** The white paper provided authority and financial support for the development of basic and advanced life support services.

_____ **3.** An emergency medical dispatcher can give simple medical instructions to the caller.

_____ **4.** The primary level in the EMS system is the first responder.

_____ **5.** In EMS, paramedics include the highest number of trained and certified individuals in the field.

_____ **6.** The first priority of the scene is assessment of the patient.

_____ **7.** Peer review is used as a means of continuous quality improvement.

_____ **8.** Cross-sectional research is based on a clearly defined problem or question.

_____ **9.** Only the emergency vehicle operator is responsible for restocking the unit after a call.

_____ **10.** Injury prevention in the home is an attribute the paramedic should be comfortable discussing with patients and bystanders.

Short Answer

Complete this section with short written answers using the space provided.

1. Pretend you are a fly on the wall during this scene: A team of paramedics arrives on scene for a routine geriatric call. The woman has fallen and has a broken hip. Her daughter has found her and called 9-1-1. List below the professional attributes the paramedics should demonstrate on this call.

   a. _____

   b. _____

   c. _____

   d. _____

   e. _____

   f. _____

   g. _____

   h. _____

2. Being a paramedic involves taking on a lot of new and serious responsibilities. List the eight roles and responsibilities of a paramedic.

   a. _____

   b. _____

   c. _____

   d. _____

   e. _____

   f. _____

   g. _____

   h. _____

3. No paramedic service in the United States can perform advanced life support procedures without medical control. What is medical control, and why is it necessary?

_____

_____

_____

4. In fact, medical control consists of several different parts. Give an example of each of the following:

a. Online medical control: _____

b. Protocols: _____

c. Standing orders: _____

Crossword Puzzle

Use the clues on the following page to complete the puzzle below.

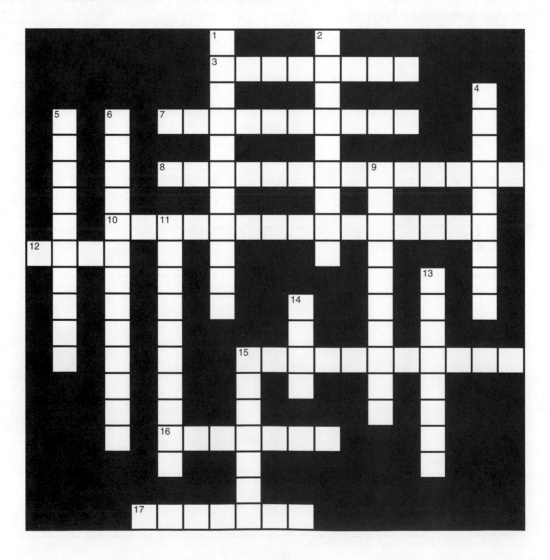

Across

3. The primary provider level in EMS
7. 1966 paper written by the National Academy of Science
8. A person trained in first aid and CPR
10. Physicians who serve as the "medical conscience" of the EMS system
12. The most common number in any given research project
15. Research that is a basic observation only
16. Identification with and understanding of your patient's feelings
17. The description of the findings of your project

Down

1. Granting certification to a provider from another state
2. The highest skill level you can achieve in EMS
4. Being open, honest, and truthful with your patient
5. The person whose work was the basis for the first paramedic curriculum
6. The legal record of what you did in the field
9. A review of calls, done by the people you work with
11. The person receiving and interpreting all the information of a call
13. A treatment plan for a specific illness
14. Mobile Army Surgical Hospital
15. Father of paramedicine

CHAPTER

2 The Well-Being of the Paramedic

Chapter Review

The following exercises provide an opportunity to test your knowledge of this chapter.

Matching

Stress is a major part of a paramedic's job. Match each of the sentences with the correct definition of stress.

A. Eustress   **B.** Distress

_____ **1.** You are running a 10K road race with your best friend. You have been training to beat her, and she is about 15 steps in front of you.

_____ **2.** You respond to a rollover collision and find out that the unrestrained driver of the vehicle is your 17-year-old son.

_____ **3.** You are assigned to work with Billy Bob for the next month. Billy Bob is not your favorite person and is always criticizing every move you make.

_____ **4.** You are taking your National Registry Paramedic exam next week, and you are studying in hopes of passing the test the first time.

_____ **5.** You find out the ambulance service that you work for is merging with a larger service. There is talk that your job will be eliminated.

_____ **6.** You are climbing Pikes Peak and you are about to make the summit (your lifelong dream), but you don't feel that you have enough energy left to climb the last 500 feet.

_____ **7.** Your spouse has left a letter explaining to you that he/she is divorcing you and that he/she has already cleaned out the bank accounts.

Match the correct stress response with the situation.

A. Alarm reaction   **B.** Alert response

_____ **1.** You hear gun shots as you pull up to a scene; your heart begins to race.

_____ **2.** You turn to find the source of the shots.

_____ **3.** After hearing a scream, you turn and run toward the sound.

Multiple Choice

Read each item carefully, and then select the best response.

_____ **1.** You respond to a 10-year-old boy who has been hit by a car. He is alert, but with a deformity to his lower left leg. The boy "baby talks" as he is answering your questions. This is a form of:

A. denial.   **C.** regression.

B. projection.   **D.** displacement.

_____ **2.** You respond to a multiple-casualty incident (MCI) involving a collision of a charter bus of gambling seniors and a car with four teenagers. At the scene, you find one teen with a broken arm who is cracking off-color jokes about the seniors. He is moving from one person to another making fun of their clothing, hairstyles, and anything else he notices about them. He might be suffering from:

- **A.** conversion hysteria.
- **B.** blind panic.
- **C.** depression.
- **D.** overreaction.

_____ **3.** Which of the following would NOT be a reason for a critical incident stress debriefing/defusing?

- **A.** A rollover with four people, resulting in minor injuries
- **B.** Death of a 3-month-old girl, as a result of child abuse
- **C.** A train derailment with 77 injured people and 22 deaths
- **D.** Your partner's suicide, with you as the responding paramedic

_____ **4.** As a result of the careless nature of your partner, you have been stuck by a needle that was used to start an IV on your patient. Which of the following should be done immediately?

- **A.** Get a medical evaluation from the ED physician.
- **B.** Document the negligence of your partner.
- **C.** Wash the area of the exposure with soap and water.
- **D.** Get a booster shot for all of your immunizations.

_____ **5.** Your service has just started a rotating shift. Which of the following will disturb your circadian rhythms the most?

- **A.** Eating healthy meals
- **B.** Drinking a lot of soda and coffee to keep you awake at work
- **C.** Lying down to sleep at the same time every day
- **D.** Keeping the room dark if you are sleeping during the day

_____ **6.** You are on your first "code." As you arrive on scene, you feel stressed. Which of the following management techniques would NOT help you during this call?

- **A.** Reframing
- **B.** Controlled breathing
- **C.** Progressive relaxation
- **D.** Regression

_____ **7.** You are on the scene of a major car crash. Your patient is an elderly gentleman who has now accepted the fact that he is really hurt and could be in the hospital for a long time. Which of the following reactions might the patient experience?

- **A.** Depression
- **B.** Fear
- **C.** Anger
- **D.** All of the above

_____ **8.** At a vehicle crash, you believe that you have everyone accounted for and taken care of. Suddenly you hear a baby crying and realize there is a child that you have not found yet. Your heart begins to race; this is an example of a/an:

- **A.** acute stress.
- **B.** alert response.
- **C.** alarm reaction.
- **D.** fight-or-flight response.

_____ **9.** After being told she might be suffering from a heart attack, an elderly woman hits the paramedic in anger and tells the paramedic he doesn't know what he is talking about. Which defense mechanism relates to this statement?

- **A.** Displacement
- **B.** Projection
- **C.** Alarm reaction
- **D.** Denial

_____ **10.** A paramedic who has been on duty for 6 months (without an extra day off) begins to show signs of physical and emotional breakdown. He is cynical and doesn't seem to be able to sleep. These are signs of:

- **A.** eustress.
- **B.** burnout.
- **C.** anxiety.
- **D.** alert response.

Fill-in-the-Blank

Read each item carefully, and then complete the statement by filling in the missing word(s).

1. The following paragraphs describe behaviors of different individuals under stress. For each description, fill in the defense mechanism that the individual is apparently using.

   a. Your partner has been irritable and ill-tempered ever since he arrived at work today. You are doing your best to keep a low profile and not to annoy him further, but nonetheless he snaps at you, "You sure are in a lousy mood today." Your partner is showing the mechanism of defense known as _____.

   b. You are called by a very distraught woman to tend to her husband, who has been having chest pain. When you reach the patient's house, he says, "I can't understand why my wife called for an ambulance; I'm just having a little indigestion, that's all." His face is gray, and he is sweating profusely. He is using the psychological defense mechanism known as _____.

   c. An 18-year-old woman is extricated from a wrecked automobile in which her boyfriend remains trapped. She says she has lost all sensation in her hands and feet. She does not appear terribly upset about that fact, and you cannot find any signs of injury on her body. She is using the psychological defense mechanism known as _____.

   d. At the scene of a car crash, you are trying to extricate an entrapped front-seat passenger who is seriously injured. The driver, who has not suffered any apparent injury, is giving you a hard time. "Be careful, will you! #&!@ Don't drop her! Watch what you're doing, you idiot!" He is very aggressive toward you, but you realize that his behavior is simply a _____ of the anger he feels toward himself for having caused the injury to his passenger.

2. Being a paramedic is a stressful job. For some, the stresses are too much and burnout can occur. The time to start thinking about burnout—and about how to prevent it—is now, during your training. Now is the time to develop strategies that will keep burnout from happening to you. Describe some of the steps you plan to take to keep from burning out as a paramedic.

   a. _____

   b. _____

   c. _____

   d. _____

   e. _____

   f. _____

   g. _____

   h. _____

Identify

In the following case study, list the six pertinent negatives with regard to Billy Bob's well-being. Also, identify two stress reactions of the patient.

It is midnight, and Billy Bob is still up watching a horror movie on TV and drinking his last soda out of the six-pack that he bought today. You're both on a 24-hour shift today, and he has just been laying around the TV room when he is not out on a call. He skipped his workout today so he could watch his favorite soap opera. He is bummed out that he is out of cigarettes and searching the kitchen for yet another bag of popcorn when the tones go off, indicating another call.

As you head from the bunk room to the ambulance, Billy Bob is yelling that it is all your fault there is another call, "If you wouldn't have gone to bed, we wouldn't have had another call tonight," he grumbles.

Once you arrive at the patient, you find an elderly woman who has fallen and possibly broken her hip. As you begin your treatment phase, the patient begins to blame you for all of her problems. As you load her into the ambulance, the patient reaches out and pinches your arm as hard as she can.

After you deliver your patient to the hospital, Billy Bob stops off to grab another pack of smokes and a bean burrito. As you pull into the bay, Billy Bob tells you to restock because he wants to watch the end of the movie. As he heads into the TV room he tells you his stomach is killing him and he might be your next patient.

1. Pertinent Negatives

a. _____

b. _____

c. _____

d. _____

e. _____

f. _____

2. Stress Reactions

a. _____

b. _____

Ambulance Calls

The following case scenarios provide an opportunity to explore the concerns associated with patient management and paramedic care. Read each scenario, and then answer each question.

1. Your unit responds to a call for a 3-month-old boy not breathing. When you enter the house you find a mother holding the boy, who is not breathing and is very pale. You and your partner John begin working the code. You start the steps of CPR while gathering as much information as possible about what has happened. As you arrive at the hospital with the infant, you know in your heart that the child is dead. The code team works further on the child, and finally the doctor calls for the time of death. John storms out of the room and out to the unit to begin cleanup. John begins to yell about the fact the child died, and how if he hadn't missed the first IV on the child he might still be alive. You finish your paperwork and then head back to the station. At the station, John refuses to talk about the call and says he wants to be alone. He ends up sitting at the table just staring off into space for the rest of the afternoon. At the next shift, John is very negative and flies off the handle at everyone that day. After the shift is over, John heads for the local bar instead of going home to his wife and 2-month-old son. Two weeks later, John is put on mandatory leave for his mental well-being.

   a. Explain how this one incident could have triggered John's decline.

   _____

   _____

   b. What are some steps that EVERY PARAMEDIC can take to reduce stress on the job?

   _____

   _____

   _____

   _____

2. A call comes in for a motor vehicle crash involving a pickup truck and a semi truck. It was a head-on collision with both vehicles going 60 mph. Your patient is a 56-year-old man. He was not wearing his seat belt when the crash occurred. He has multiple breaks of both arms and legs. He has a huge cut on his forehead that is bleeding profusely. You begin a rapid trauma assessment on him after doing a rapid extrication to a long backboard. In the back of the ambulance, you begin treatment by applying oxygen and starting two large-bore IVs. The patient is alert and is able to respond to you correctly. His blood pressure is 74/30 mm Hg, and respirations are 32 breaths/min and shallow. Skin is cool and clammy, and you have no pulses in the wrists or the feet. The cardiac monitor is showing sinus tachycardia with multifocal PVCs that are becoming very frequent. You don't hear good lung sounds and prepare for needle decompression of the right chest. You know that this patient is approaching death and is more than likely going to turn into a trauma code.

a. Your patient looks up at you and asks you if he is going to make it. How do you respond to him?

_____

_____

_____

b. What are the five stages that you might witness in this patient and how will the patient act during these stages?

1. _____

2. _____

3. _____

4. _____

5. _____

True/False

If you believe the statement to be more true than false, write the letter "T" in the space provided. If you believe the statement to be more false than true, write the letter "F."

_____ **1.** The USDA Food Pyramid contains eight different food groups.

_____ **2.** You should avoid caffeine and keep a regular sleep schedule.

_____ **3.** When lifting, you should use your back, so you don't injure your knees.

_____ **4.** Eustress is a negative type of stress.

_____ **5.** Initial management of stress is to control your breathing.

_____ **6.** Anger is a defense mechanism.

_____ **7.** Blind panic is when a patient will convert anxiety to a bodily dysfunction, such as a paralyzed extremity.

_____ **8.** Burnout is a consequence of chronic, unrelieved stress.

_____ **9.** The stages of death and dying are denial, anger, bargaining, depression, and anxiety.

_____ **10.** Gloves are the absolute essential of every EMS call.

_____ **11.** Gloves are the only PPE needed when suctioning a patient.

_____ **12.** A mask worn by you can protect the patient from your germs.

_____ **13.** Your safety is your number one priority.

_____ **14.** The first stage of the stress response is the "alert response."

Short Answer

Complete this section with short written answers using the space provided.

1. When faced with a perceived threat, the body reacts with a fight-or-flight response. From your own experience, list four signs or symptoms of the fight-or-flight response.

   a. _____

   b. _____

   c. _____

   d. _____

2. At times, you are the person that will be dealing with a grieving family. List the six guidelines for helping the family begin the process of dealing with their loss.

   a. _____

   b. _____

   c. _____

   d. _____

   e. _____

   f. _____

3. The way a person reacts to illness or injury is largely determined by the mechanisms that person has developed over the years for dealing with stressful situations. List five common reactions to illness and injury.

   a. _____

   b. _____

   c. _____

   d. _____

   e. _____

Word Find

Hidden in the following grid are 30 words or phrases related to what you have studied in this chapter. Find the hidden words in the grid below. Then use the words from the grid to answer the following questions (some words may be used to answer more than one question).

```
O M D F T A C O E T F D I P J E Y A Z
V X E E H N G Y U G I A R A C A I N O
E U M O P Y E O N S A O T N E R G O B
R U O W P R N M P I J I A I E Q J I G
E N T Z X R E L E E C T R T G O S T B
A O I J U A A S C R P I S R B U S C H
T I O B R C L T S E I Y S L A X E A A
I S N A E X I A C I H T O M G M R E S
N U S M C O C C R N O S E V F C T R S
G F E Q N X A Z O M S N D R W K S R L
Y N A L E R T I N G R E S P O N S E E
T O H D E S S E N S S E L P L E H V S
E C D G B R K U H E A D A C H E S O A
I L N M E A I N M O S N I C D W N N T
X A K V B A R G A I N I N G T Z Q E W
N X N O I S S E R G E R F K Z I M A O
A O D I V O R C E L A I N E D F O K R
C W C S C O V A R D E A T H A O C N K
B O I R N N L S N M V Z Z S O R Q Q B
```

1. The redirection of an emotion from the original object to a more acceptable object is _____.

2. Attributing your own feelings to someone else is _____.

3. Reaction of the body to any agent or situation is _____.

4. Reaction in which a startled animal stops all activity and turns toward the stimulus that startled it is

   _____ _____.

5. A way of dealing with unwanted data by ignoring it is _____.

6. The first stage of an acute stress response is _____ _____.

7. Return to an earlier mode of behavior is _____.

8. Exhaustion of physical or emotional strength from chronic stress is _____.

9. Unconscious translation of an emotional conflict into a physical symptom is _____

   _____.

10. Among the words or phrases hidden in the grid are six things that can TRIGGER STRESS in many individuals.

    List those six potential stress triggers.

    a. _____

    b. _____

    c. _____

    d. _____

    e. _____

    f. _____

11. List five situations, not included in the grid, that you personally find stressful.

    a. _____

    b. _____

    c. _____

    d. _____

    e. _____

12. Among the words or phrases hidden in the grid are six potential *reactions* of patients or others *to illness or injury*. List the reactions you found in the grid.

    a. _____

    b. _____

    c. _____

d. _____

e. _____

f. _____

13. People dealing with loss usually proceed through five *stages of grief*, which are all named in the grid. List them.

a. _____

b. _____

c. _____

d. _____

e. _____

14. The grid contains six *symptoms of impending burnout*. List them.

a. _____

b. _____

c. _____

d. _____

e. _____

f. _____

15. List two more symptoms of impending burnout that were not mentioned in the grid.

a. _____

b. _____

Problem Solving

Calculate the maximum heart rate and target heart rate for a person with a resting heart rate of 76 beats/min and an age of 46 years.

    a. Resting heart rate _____

    b. 220 – _____ (age) = _____ (Maximum heart rate)

    c. _____ (Maximum heart rate) – _____ (Resting heart rate) = _____ × 0.7 = _____ (round up)

    d. _____ (Total) + _____ (Resting heart rate) = _____ (Target heart rate)

CHAPTER

3 Illness and Injury Prevention

Chapter Review

The following exercises provide an opportunity to test your knowledge of this chapter.

Matching

Match each of the items in the right column to the appropriate sentence in the left column.

_____ 1. The road has had new guardrails installed in the area because a lot of crashes have occurred there.

_____ 2. The EMS agency is holding a free "Learn CPR Day" for residents of the town.

_____ 3. An insurance company offers a discount rate to 16-year-olds for taking driver's education.

_____ 4. The police are stopping students on the way to school and handing out coupons for a free hamburger to the students that are wearing their seat belts.

_____ 5. The car dealership is offering a free child car seat check this weekend.

_____ 6. My son was stopped for speeding and given a ticket that cost him $150.00.

_____ 7. The new car seats available have a five-point harness system instead of a bar that holds the child in the seat.

_____ 8. The ambulance crew will do an inspection of any elderly person's home to determine any potential risk areas. This service is provided free of charge.

_____ 9. Because of the law, all poisons must be listed on the front of every container that contains products that can cause poisoning.

_____ 10. We receive a discount on our home insurance because we have a smoke alarm on every floor of the house.

A. Education
B. Enforcement
C. Engineering/ environment
D. Economic incentives

Multiple Choice

Read each item carefully, and then select the best response.

_____ 1. Fred is up on the roof trying to fix the cable during the big game. He falls off and hurts his back. This is considered a/an _____ injury.

    A. intentional   **C.** secondary

    B. unintentional   **D.** environmental

_____ 2. Which of the following is NOT an intentional injury?

    A. Rape   **C.** Suicide

    B. Motor vehicle crash   **D.** Elder abuse

_____ **3.** When choosing objectives as you build an implementation plan, the _S_ in SMART stands for:

        A. signs.   **C.** simple.

        B swelling.   **D.** success.

_____ **4.** Which of the following patients could benefit from a "teachable moment"?

        A. An 18-year-old not wearing his seat belt who received cuts and bruises as a result of a motor vehicle collision

        B. A 3-year-old drowning patient

        C. An elderly person suffering from dementia

        D. A 45-year-old woman with a dog bite

_____ **5.** Which of the following is not a primary injury prevention measure?

        A. Wearing your seat belt   **C.** Smoking a pack a day

        B. Using safe lifting techniques   **D.** Wearing gloves at the scene of a crash

_____ **6.** When developing a prevention program, what is the second step out of the five steps discussed in the text?

        A. Plan and test interventions.   **C.** Set goals and objectives.

        B. Conduct a community assessment.   **D.** Define the injury problem.

_____ **7.** According to the Centers for Disease Control and Prevention (CDC), home injuries to children are most frequently caused by:

        A. abuse.   **C.** filled bathtubs.

        B. small toys.   **D.** cribs.

_____ **8.** What is the primary focus for an EMS provider when dealing with prevention?

        A. Primary injury prevention   **C.** Illness prevention

        B. Secondary injury prevention   **D.** Intervention research

_____ **9.** Which of the following is NOT a reason EMS should be involved in the prevention field?

        A. EMS providers reflect the composition of the community.

        B. EMS providers are high-profile role models.

        C. EMS personnel are contacted by auto makers for safety recommendations.

        D. EMS providers are welcomed by school systems.

_____ **10.** What is the leading killer among ages 1 year to 44 years?

        A. Heart disease and congenital defects of the heart

        B. Diabetes

        C. Influenza and pneumonia

        D. Unintentional injuries

Fill-in-the-Blank

Read each item carefully, and then complete the statement by filling in the missing word(s).

1. A/an _____ is a specific prevention measure that increases positive safety and health outcomes.

2. Abuse, suicide, and rape are defined as a/an _____ _____.

3. The four Es of prevention are _____, _____, _____/_____, and _____

         _____ .

4. The toy manufacturer no longer sews buttons on the teddy bears for eyes; instead it paints on the eyes with nontoxic paint.

   This is an automatic protection for our children, and it is known as _____ _____.

5. The public health model identifies three factors: they are the _____, the _____, and the _____.

6. When developing a prevention program, the type of objective that declares that all mobile homes will be provided with a smoke alarm is known as a/an _____ _____.

7. Specific, nonjudgmental advice given on a scene to a patient that is receptive to the message is called a _____ _____.

Identify

In the following case study, list the pertinent negatives that can lead to injury.

Mrs. M is so tired; she is 6 months pregnant with Katie's new brother. She works a night shift and takes care of curious 3-year-old Katie during the day. Their day starts with a bath for Katie. Mrs. M takes her out and dries her off and gets her dressed but forgets to pull the plug in the tub because the phone is ringing. Katie runs off to get some breakfast in the kitchen where she finds a pot of hot water for oatmeal boiling on the stove. Meanwhile, Mrs. M is still on the phone with her overbearing mother. Because Katie can't find anything to eat, she decides to go outside and play on the trampoline. Mr. M didn't get the safety net up last night when he put it together. Mrs. M finally gets off the phone with her mother and has a hard time finding Katie. Later on in the day, Mrs. M sneaks a nap while Katie is playing on the floor. Katie decides she wants to play sewing like her mommy and finds the knitting needles and scissors in mommy's bag beside the chair. Luckily, Katie decides to play barbershop instead of doctor on her mommy. When Mrs. M wakes up she is horrified to find lots of her own hair on the chair. Mrs. M. decides it would be better to take Katie to day care in the mornings while she catches up on her sleep!

Pertinent Negatives

1. _____

2. _____

3. _____

4. _____

Ambulance Calls

The following case scenarios provide an opportunity to explore the concerns associated with patient management and paramedic care. Read each scenario, and then answer each question.

1. Missy and Jake are on duty when the tones go off for a man down. As they respond to the call, they radio dispatch for more information. Dispatch tells them that this is a life line call, and they are unable to get any response when they call the residence. Not knowing what they will encounter, Missy and Jake radio for law enforcement backup. When they arrive at the residence and first knock on the door, they can hear shouts for help from inside the house. A police officer shows up to help, and they determine that all doors and windows are locked and there is no way into the house. The officer determines the basement window is the best one to break. Because Missy is the smallest person there, she is chosen to crawl through the basement window. She enters the house and finds an elderly man on the bathroom floor. After checking on the patient, she goes to unlock the front door. Missy and Jake determine that the man just fell trying to get from the toilet back to his wheelchair. He has no injuries and doesn't want to go to the hospital. He just needs a hand up. After calling a friend to come stay with the gentleman until his caregiver gets home, they load up and head back.

   a. Why is it a good idea that Missy and Jake call for an officer before they get to the scene?

   _____

   _____

   _____

b. What equipment should Missy have taken with her when she entered the home through the basement window?

_____

_____

_____

c. During this call, Missy and Jake can apply the teachable moment. What are some things they can teach their patient?

_____

_____

_____

2. Courtney and Larry have been called by the local elementary school to do a program for the third and fourth grades. They decide to educate the children on how and why to call 9-1-1. They arrive with a homemade videotape of a dispatcher taking a "call" from a child. The video shows all the steps of how and when to call, what the dispatcher will say, and how the ambulance will respond to them. Their tape shows a child calling 9-1-1 after she finds Grandpa asleep and is unable to wake him up. Three days later, when they are on shift again, Courtney and Larry get a call for a woman that won't wake up. The dispatcher has the woman's 8-year-old son on the phone. When they arrive, they find a woman who won't wake up on the couch and a very upset little boy. With a few good questions, they determine the mom is a diabetic. After getting a low reading on the glucometer, they start an IV and give her D_{50}. The woman wakes up, and after eating a sandwich, her glucose level stabilizes. They stay a little longer to make sure everything is going well before they allow her to sign off and not be transported. During this time, they find out the boy, Ryan, was at their demonstration a few days ago.

a. When Larry and Courtney created an implementation plan for their program, they developed their objective with the SMART plan. What does the SMART plan stand for?

S _____

M _____

A _____

R _____

T _____

b. How did their program help Ryan decide to get help for his mother?

_____

_____

_____

_____

_____

True/False

If you believe the statement to be more true than false, write the letter "T" in the space provided. If you believe the statement to be more false than true, write the letter "F."

_____ **1.** Tertiary prevention is defined as reducing the effects of an injury that has already happened.

_____ **2.** Unintentional injuries are the leading cause of death for people between 1 and 44 years of age.

_____ **3.** The three factors used in making a public health model are: the host, the event, and the postevent.

_____ **4.** The collection, analysis, and interpretation of injury data are called injury surveillance.

_____ **5.** A risk factor for an intentional injury would be not wearing your seat belt.

_____ **6.** In creating an implementation plan, you need a realistic timeline to complete your project.

_____ **7.** Two of the five steps in developing a prevention plan include conducting a community assessment and setting goals and objectives.

_____ **8.** When using SMART to meet your objectives, the *R* stands for risk.

_____ **9.** Funding for a prevention program can include donations from local media, grants, and sponsorships from different organizations.

_____ **10.** Every EMS call includes a teachable moment.

Short Answer

Complete this section with short written answers using the space provided.

1. What is the difference between primary injury prevention and secondary injury prevention? Give an example of each.

Primary injury prevention:

_____

_____

_____

Example:

_____

_____

_____

Secondary injury prevention:

_____

_____

_____

Example:

_____

_____

_____

2. Give three examples of why EMS providers should be active in the prevention field.

   a. _____

   b. _____

   c. _____

3. List the four Es of prevention and explain each one.

   a. _____

   b. _____

   c. _____

   d. _____

4. A public health model will help to identify a problem and how to approach the problem. Use this approach to list the three key factors involved in the problem of children and swimming pool drowning deaths.

   a. _____

   b. _____

   c. _____

5. Discuss three of the six risk factors connected with intentional violence.

   a. _____

   b. _____

   c. _____

Crossword Puzzle

Use the clues in the columns to complete the puzzle.

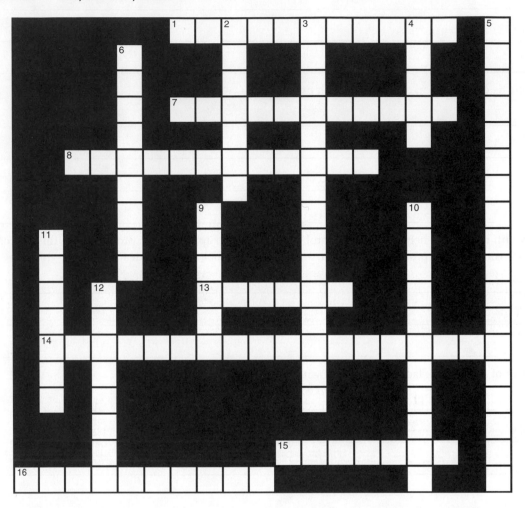

Across

1. The assault of a woman by another person, resulting in an injury, is known as a/an_____ injury.
7. Behavior that is forced to change by law is called _____.
8. _____ _____ was the number one cause of death in 2002.
13. The physician that created a matrix of injury prevention.
14. The ongoing collection and interpretation of injury data.
15. _____ injury prevention begins at home.
16. The *M* in SMART when dealing with goals and objectives in an implementation plan stands for _____.

Down

2. _____ accidents account for the most unintentional deaths.
3. When people are receptive to accepting advice from an EMS provider, it is considered a _____ _____.

4. The three factors in a public health model are host, _____, and the environment.
5. An effort to rehabilitate a person who has survived an injury.
6. The _____ _____ effect benefits other family members with messages of safety.
9. Very few calls actually require the use of _____ and sirens when responding.
10. Being male, with a history of alcohol abuse, mental illness, and poverty are all _____ _____ for intentional violence.
11. _____ interventions are those without any conscious change of behavior by an individual.
12. _____ are intentional or unintentional damage to a person.

Fill-in-the-Table

Fill in the missing parts of the table.

What were the top 10 causes of death (in 2002)?
1.
2.
3.
4. Chronic, lower respiratory disease
5.
6.
7. Influenza and pneumonia
8. Alzheimer's disease
9.
10.

CHAPTER

4 Medical and Legal Issues

Chapter Review

The following exercises provide an opportunity to test your knowledge of this chapter.

Matching

Match each of the numbered items to the appropriate sentence. For questions 1 to 6, indicate whether:

A. You may treat the patient without obtaining the patient's expressed consent.

B. You may NOT treat the patient without obtaining the patient's expressed consent.

_____ **1.** A 9-year-old child is struck by a car. He is bleeding profusely. His parents cannot be located.

_____ **2.** A 42-year-old man is injured in an automobile collision in which his car was totally demolished. He has bruises on his forehead. He seems confused. He says, "I'm all right. Let me alone. Just call me a taxi."

_____ **3.** A 58-year-old man has chest pain. His wife phoned for an ambulance. The man says, "It's nothing, just indigestion." He refuses to be examined or treated.

_____ **4.** A 30-year-old woman is pulled from the beach surf in cardiac arrest.

_____ **5.** A 25-year-old man is injured in a barroom altercation. He is bleeding profusely from his nose and mouth. He smells strongly of alcohol. He is very belligerent and shouts at you, "Leave me alone, you creeps. If you come any closer, I'll knock your teeth in."

_____ **6.** An 80-year-old woman has fainted at home. Her son found her on the floor and called for an ambulance. She is conscious when you arrive. She says to you, "You are all very sweet, but one can't live forever, you know, and I don't fancy hospitals."

For questions 7 to 10, match the following words to the correct situation.

A. Slander   **C.** Battery

B. Defamation   **D.** Assault

_____ **7.** The reporting paramedic wrote in his report that Mr. P was obviously drunk. The paramedic made that statement because he has a long-running feud with Mr. P and thought this was a great way to pay him back.

_____ **8.** Mrs. O'Malley told the EMT-B not to touch her. She did not want any help. The EMT-B went ahead and tried to grab Mrs. O'Malley and put her on the cot.

_____ **9.** Mitch is taking a patient into the hospital. The patient asks about the doctor on staff. Mitch tells the patient, "Sorry, buddy, but I wouldn't want that witch doctor treating me. Good luck, partner."

_____ **10.** Ryan is in the back of the ambulance with his patient Jake, who is 16 years old and has just rolled his car. Jake is really wound up and wants out of the ambulance. Ryan tells Jake that if he doesn't calm down, he is going to strap him down and give him a shot.

Multiple Choice

Read each item carefully, and then select the best response.

_____ 1. You have responded to a fender bender, where your patient is conscious and alert. The patient is able to answer all questions correctly, and the person declines treatment. Your overzealous partner starts to put a C-collar on the patient. What could he be charged with?

A. Assault

B. Battery

C. False imprisonment

D. Libel

_____ 2. You are on a volunteer squad, in a small town. At the grocery store, your neighbor starts asking you what happened the night before. You proceed to tell her that the local dentist was hitting his wife and you had to take her up to the hospital for a broken jaw. Along the way, you let slide a few of your own opinions about the dentist. Soon the story is all over town. The dentist is pretty upset and contacts a lawyer to initiate a lawsuit against you. What will you be charged with?

A. Defamation

B. Libel

C. Slander

D. Assault

_____ 3. What does HIPAA guarantee the patient?

A. The hospital cannot transfer a mother in labor.

B. The paramedic can treat the patient without consent if the paramedic feels the patient has a life-threatening problem.

C. The paramedic meets minimum qualifications.

D. That the patient's medical information will remain confidential at all times.

_____ 4. Which of the following is NOT needed to prove negligence of the paramedic?

A. The paramedic treated an unconscious patient.

C. The paramedic breached his or her duty.

B. The paramedic had a legal duty to act.

D. The patient was harmed by the paramedic.

_____ 5. You arrive at the ED with a patient with chest pain as your pager goes off for the next call of the night. In your hurry to get out of the hospital, you hand off your patient to the ward clerk, knowing that an RN will be coming soon to take over. You are guilty of:

A. proximate cause.

B. ordinary negligence.

C. gross negligence.

D. abandonment.

_____ 6. You are called to the local elementary school for a child who has fallen from the top of the slide. The child is not making any sense and is vomiting. The school is unable to reach her parents. Under what type of consent can you treat and transport this child?

A. Informed

B. Implied

C. Expressed

D. Involuntary

_____ 7. You respond to a man down. You find a homeless person in an alley. Which of the following findings would allow you to take the man to the hospital under implied consent?

A. He has not eaten for at least 6 hours.

C. His oxygen level is 82%.

B. He is not clean.

D. His blood glucose level is normal.

_____ 8. After transferring care to the nurse on the homeless man in the preceding question, which of the following does NOT belong in your written report?

A. The patient was unkempt and stunk badly.

C. The patient has not had anything to eat.

B. The patient had an oxygen level of 82%.

D. The patient's blood glucose was at a normal level.

_____ **9.** Which of the following patients must be reported?

A. A 16-year-old girl who refuses to eat
B. A new mother who is feeling very depressed

C. A 10-year-old boy who was bitten by a dog
D. A 25-year-old man who was binge drinking

_____ **10.** How are most civil cases resolved?

A. A settlement process
B. A trial by a judge

C. A trial by jury
D. None of the above

Fill-in-the-Blank

Read each item carefully, and then complete the statement by filling in the missing word(s).

1. Failure to obtain consent before providing medical treatment might give rise to charges of technical assault and battery. What are the requirements for obtaining consent to treat the following?

a. From a conscious, mentally competent adult, consent must be _____.

b. To treat a child, consent must be obtained from the _____ _____ or _____

   _____.

2. The patient is claiming that he was harmed by the paramedic's actions. In a lawsuit, the patient will be the _____,

and the paramedic will be the _____.

3. The paramedic is permitted by the medical director to carry out certain treatments. This is known as the paramedic's

_____ _____ _____.

4. A document that expresses the patient's wants, needs, and desires in relation to the patient's future medical care is known as

a/an _____ _____.

5. A minor who has been _____ is a minor under legal age, but because of marriage, pregnancy, or active military

service is treated as an adult.

6. When determining if your patient is mentally competent, you will ask a series of questions to make sure the patient is

orientated to _____, _____, and _____.

7. List the six characteristics of an effective patient care report (PCR):

a. _____

b. _____

c. _____

d. _____

e. _____

f. _____

Identify

In the following case study, list the chief complaint, vital signs, and pertinent negatives.

You are called to respond to the local bar and grill for a man not feeling well. When you arrive, you are confronted by a 34-year-old man who is acting very strange. He is yelling that he doesn't need anyone's help and just to leave him alone. All he wants is a sandwich and a beer. The patient refuses any type of help and correctly answers all of your questions. Once again, he says he wants to be left alone. Without consent and with a cranky patient you don't feel you can treat this patient. As you are ready to leave, the man falls off of the bar stool unconscious. You begin treatment by opening his airway and checking for breathing. He is breathing 20 breaths/min with an oxygen saturation level of 97%. The patient moans but makes no other noises. Your partner notices a medical ID bracelet stating the man is a diabetic. You take a blood glucose reading and find it to be 42 mg/dL. Your partner applies oxygen by a nonrebreathing mask and starts an IV on the patient. Vital signs on this patient are a blood pressure of 132/70 mm Hg, a pulse of 96 beats/min, lung sounds clear bilaterally, skin is cool, and pupils are a bit sluggish. You give 25 g of D_{50} by IV. Your patient begins to wake up very quickly and asks what is going on. He tells you he had taken his sugar reading earlier and realized he needed to eat so he stopped for food. He now is competent and does not want to be transported to the ED. After making sure his vital signs are in normal ranges and his blood glucose level has come up to a reading of 122 mg/dL, you discontinue the IV. Your partner writes up a report, and once again you check all of the patient's vital signs and find them normal. The patient again refuses transport after you have determined that he is competent. You have the patient sign off, and you return to your squad to prepare for the next call.

1. Chief Complaint

_____

_____

_____

2. Vital Signs

_____

_____

_____

3. Pertinent Negatives

_____

_____

_____

Ambulance Calls

The following case scenarios provide an opportunity to explore the concerns associated with patient management and paramedic care. Read each scenario, and then answer each question.

1. Described below are six emergency calls. Circle the letter beside those calls in which it is permissible for a paramedic to give treatment without obtaining expressed consent from the patient. In those cases in which you may *not* treat the patient without expressed consent, describe what *action you would take.*

   a. A 12-year-old boy has fallen at school and sprained his ankle. The school authorities have so far been unable to reach the boy's parents.

   _____

   _____

b. A middle-aged woman is found in cardiac arrest.

_____

_____

c. A young man called for an ambulance after his 19-year-old girlfriend swallowed a large number of sleeping pills. She is awake and refuses treatment. She says, "Go away and let me die."

_____

_____

d. A 20-year-old man has taken PCP (a psychedelic drug that often induces violent behavior) and has tried to gouge out his eyes. He is bleeding profusely from the face and screaming, "Don't come near me."

_____

_____

e. A 14-year-old boy was knocked from his bicycle and run over by a truck. He is unconscious and bleeding. Both legs appear fractured. Bystanders do not know the boy or his parents.

_____

_____

f. A 43-year-old man has crushing chest pain. His wife called for the ambulance. The man says he doesn't need an ambulance, he just has indigestion. His face is gray, and he is sweating profusely.

_____

_____

2. You are called to the scene of a crash in which a pedestrian has been struck by a car. The driver of the car says the pedestrian staggered out into the street in front of him. The pedestrian is now sitting on the curb. He has an obvious bruise on his head. He is unkempt and smells strongly of alcohol. He tells you that he doesn't want to go to the hospital. You suspect that the patient might not be competent to make that decision. List three things you can check to assess his mental competence.

a. _____

b. _____

c. _____

True/False

If you believe the statement to be more true than false, write the letter "T" in the space provided. If you believe the statement to be more false than true, write the letter "F."

_____ **1.** You can be sued for slander when you write a false statement in your report.

_____ **2.** The discovery period during a lawsuit can take anywhere from a few months to more than 2 years.

_____ **3.** You should contact medical control in the case of a physician's orders on a scene if the orders do not fit the emergency situation.

_____ **4.** HIPAA protects the patient's right to confidentiality.

_____ **5.** Good Samaritan laws are designed to protect all paramedics from lawsuits.

_____ **6.** To prove negligence on the part of the paramedic, the plaintiff must prove legal duty, breach of duty, failure to act, and harm.

_____ **7.** A DNR order is not considered an advance directive.

_____ **8.** You must gain informed consent from every competent adult before beginning treatment.

_____ **9.** You must have parental consent even for an emancipated minor.

_____ **10.** The paramedic's best defense in a lawsuit is his/her written report on the patient.

Short Answer

Complete this section with short written answers using the space provided.

1. Every state in the United States defines certain cases as "coroner's cases," that is, cases of death that you are obliged to report to law enforcement authorities. Although regulations vary somewhat from state to state, there are certain categories of cases that are nearly universally regarded as coroner's cases. List three such categories.

   a. _____

   b. _____

   c. _____

2. Good Samaritan legislation was written to stop any lawsuits being brought against people that tried to assist at an emergency scene. Explain why the Good Samaritan laws would not be a good defense for a paramedic who has a lawsuit brought against him or her.

   _____

   _____

   _____

3. If legal action is taken against a paramedic, the charge most likely to be brought is that of professional negligence, or "malpractice." To prove that the paramedic was negligent, the plaintiff must demonstrate four things. List the four elements required to prove negligence.

   a. _____

   b. _____

   c. _____

   d. _____

4. When legal questions arise regarding the care given to a patient, the paramedic's best protection is a legible, thorough, accurate medical record (PCR). That record should include at least the following:

   a. _____

   b. _____

   c. _____

   d. _____

   e. _____

   f. _____

5. List at least four types of cases that paramedics or other health care professionals in your state are required to report to the appropriate authorities.

   a. _____

   b. _____

   c. _____

   d. _____

6. Special precautions need to be observed in coroner's cases, lest you disturb evidence important to law enforcement officials. List four types of cases that are designated as coroner's cases in your state.

a. _____

b. _____

c. _____

d. _____

Word Find

Hidden in the following grid are 21 words or phrases related to what you have studied in this chapter. Find the hidden words in the grid below. Then use the words from the grid to answer the following questions (some words may be used to answer more than one of the questions).

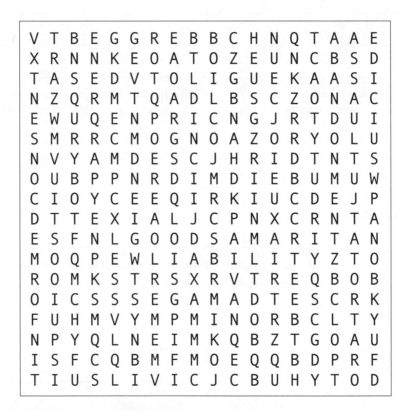

```
V T B E G G R E B B C H N Q T A A E
X R N N K E O A T O Z E U N C B S D
T A S E D V T O L I G U E K A A S I
N Z Q R M T Q A D L B S C Z O N A C
E W U Q E N P R I C N G J R T D U I
S M R R C M O G N O A Z O R Y O L U
N V Y A M D E S C J H R I D T N T S
O U B P P N R D I M D I E B U M U W
C I O Y C E E Q I R K I U C D E J P
D T T E X I A L J C P N X C R N T A
E S F N L G O O D S A M A R I T A N
M O Q P E W L I A B I L I T Y Z T O
R O M K S T R S X R V T R E Q B O B
O I C S S E G A M A D T E S C R K
F U H M V Y M P M I N O R B C L T Y
N P Y Q L N E I M K Q B Z T G O A U
I S F C Q B M F M O E Q Q B D P R F
T I U S L I V I C J C B U H Y T O D
```

1. The intentional and unjustified detention of a person against his or her will: _____ _____

2. An action instituted by a private individual against another private individual: _____ _____

3. Compensation for injury: _____

4. Assumption on behalf of a person unable to give permission for treatment that he or she would have done:

_____ _____

5. Act providing limited immunity from liability to persons who stop and help at the scene of an emergency:

_____ _____

6. A patient's voluntary agreement to be treated, after being told about the risks and benefits of the proposed treatment:

_____ _____. To give that agreement, a person must be conscious and mentally _____.

7. A finding in civil cases that the balance of evidence shows the defendant was responsible for the plaintiff's injuries: _____

8. To create in another person a fear of immediate bodily harm: _____

9. Wrongful act that gives rise to a civil action: _____

10. Abrupt termination of contact with the patient without giving him or her sufficient opportunity to find another equally qualified health professional to take over care: _____

11. Legal obligation of public ambulance services to respond to a call for help in their jurisdiction: _____

_____ _____

12. Any act of touching another person without that person's permission: _____

13. An act of omission or commission that results in injury to a patient: _____

14. Two examples of reportable cases: _____ and _____

15. Two examples of coroner's cases: _____ and _____

16. Permission from the parent or legal guardian is required to treat a _____.

17. The paramedic's best defense if he or she does have to go to court as a witness or defendant: _____ _____

18. The paramedic's best defense against being sued: _____ _____

Secret Message

Identify the following terms from the clues provided, and then use the letters to decode the secret message!

a. Termination of contact with the patient before the patient has time to arrange other care: _ _ _ _ _ _ _ _ M _ _ _ _
　　　　　　5　8　19　33　1　39　26　　22　40　11

b. Obligation to respond to a call in your jurisdiction: _ _ _ _　_ _ _　_ C _
　　　　　　27　30　6　28　24　36　25　　15

c. Official written procedure for diagnosis, treatment, etc: _ _ _ _ _ _ C _ L
　　　　　　18　38　2　34　13　　29

d. If a patient refuses treatment, the patient and a _ _ _ _ _ _ _ _ should sign the trip sheet.
　　　　　　3　21　20　23　9　7　10

e. Reflex that occurs when you touch the back of someone's throat: _ A _
　　　　　　35　　41

f. World Health Organization: _ _ _
　　　　　　37　4　32

g. Rhesus (as in a factor in the blood): _ _
　　　　　　14　16

h. Opposite of many: _ _ _
　　　　　　12　17　31

Secret Message:

_ _　_ _ _ _　_ _ _　_ _ _　_ _ _ _ _ _　_ _ _　_ _ _ _　_ _　_ _ _ _ _ _.
1　2　　3　4　5　6　7　　8　9　10　11　　12　13　14　　15　16　17　　18　19　20　21　22　23　24　　25　26　27　　28　29　30　　31　32　33　34　　35　36　　37　38　39　40　41

CHAPTER

5 Ethical Issues

Chapter Review

The following exercises provide an opportunity to test your knowledge of this chapter.

Matching

Match each of the items below to the appropriate sentence.

E = Ethical   M = Moral   UE = Unethical practice

_____ **1.** The patient's religion determines that no matter how sick the person is, the person will not seek medical attention.

_____ **2.** Our physician feels that Mother is terminal, but he wants to try at least one more medication to see if it can help her.

_____ **3.** My patient has overdosed on crack cocaine, so he is not worth working on.

_____ **4.** Even though my patient, who was drinking and driving, has just killed a family of four in a car crash, I will do my best to provide medical attention to him.

_____ **5.** A 42-year-old woman has tried to commit suicide by overdosing; if she wants to die, let's give her that wish by working this as a "slow code."

_____ **6.** The patient does not want any pain medication because he feels that those medications are considered "drugs".

_____ **7.** This patient obviously doesn't have the money for this ED visit; let's wait till all of the other patients have been taken care of before we work on this welfare case.

_____ **8.** Mark intentionally left out the fact that he gave the wrong drug dose on the PCR.

_____ **9.** After helping give birth to a premature stillborn child, the paramedic blessed the infant because the mother requested the child be blessed.

_____ **10.** The paramedic gave the drunk 18-year-old patient Lasix on the long transport to the hospital. He wanted to teach the patient a lesson. He thought that if the patient wet himself, it would be funny.

Multiple Choice

Read each item carefully, and then select the best response.

_____ **1.** What is the paramedic's best protection in court?

    A. A voice recording of every call

    B. A complete and accurate patient care report (PCR)

    C. Rewriting the PCR at a later date or time

    D. Video cameras in the back of the units

_____ **2.** In which of the following situations would you work "the code"?

    A. A woman who was found in rigor mortis in her bathroom

    B. A patient that was decapitated in a car wreck

    C. A 6-year-old child that was under the ice for 20 minutes

    D. A 56-year-old man who has had a tractor crush his chest area and has been trapped for 40 minutes

_____ **3.** What is the person (or procedure) called when one adult has the legal authority to make the health care decisions for another?

    A. Power of attorney   **C.** Surrogate decision maker

    B. Parents   **D.** None of the above

_____ **4.** Which of the following is NOT an advance directive?

    A. The doctors recommendations   **C.** A living will

    B. DNR order   **D.** A health care power of attorney

_____ **5.** In the NAEMT *Code of Ethics for Emergency Medical Technicians,* which of the following is NOT a fundamental responsibility?

    A. Alleviating suffering   **C.** Conserving life

    B. Promoting health   **D.** Providing moral support

_____ **6.** What is another name for medical ethics?

    A. Morality   **C.** Biotechnology

    B. Bioethics   **D.** Moral ethics

_____ **7.** Patient autonomy means that the patient has:

    A. to keep the same doctor always.   **C.** the right to confidentiality.

    B. the right to sue the doctor.   **D.** the right to decide about his or her own medical care.

_____ **8.** Which of the following provides access to vital information about a patient, including important medical conditions and possible DNR orders?

    A. Advance directives   **C.** Medical ID bracelet

    B. The patient's eyes   **D.** Power of attorney

_____ **9.** Which of the following are paramedics NOT obligated to report?

    A. Misconduct among colleagues

    B. Paramedics who strive to become an advocate for their community

    C. Medical errors made by oneself

    D. Medical errors witnessed

_____ **10.** Advance directives are executed while the patient:

    A. is unconscious.   **C.** is missing.

    B. is dead.   **D.** has decision-making capacity.

Fill-in-the-Blank

Read each item carefully, and then complete the statement by filling in the missing word(s).

1. The code of conduct that works off of the principles of religion, society, or a person and that affects a person's character and conduct is known as _____.

2. _____ _____ is the patient's right to direct his or her own medical care.

3. If you believe the physician has made a mistake in an order, you should ask the physician to _____

_____ _____.

4. A _____ _____ _____ _____ is a document that gives

specific instructions about resuscitation.

5. Some states have programs for _____ _____ printed on the back of a persons driver's

license.

6. When you witness misconduct of another EMS provider, you should report it to the appropriate _____

_____ _____.

7. As a new paramedic, you should choose a _____ to emulate.

Ambulance Calls

The following case scenario provides an opportunity to explore the concerns associated with patient management and paramedic care. Read the scenario, and then answer each question.

Martin and Linda begin their shift for the day at the doughnut shop. The first call comes in for a possible suicide. Martin tells Linda that because it sounds like a suicide, they might as well finish their doughnuts and coffee before they leave. Once in the squad, they respond to find an 18-year-old woman who has swallowed some sleeping pills. She is conscious and begins to vomit. Martin, who doesn't do well with vomit, tells Linda this one is all hers because he doesn't feel up to "babysitting." Linda gets baseline vital signs, starts an IV (she uses a 14-gauge needle to make sure the patient remembers it), and administers activated charcoal per protocol. En route to the hospital, Linda takes a SAMPLE history and tries to find out a little bit about why the patient was trying to commit suicide. Linda calls into the hospital to give her radio report. In the report, Linda refers to the patient as a "crazy, 18-year-old, who just got dumped by her boyfriend and was trying to get some attention by swallowing a bunch of pills." Because they have another 10 minutes to the hospital, Linda tries to fill the time by chatting with her patient. Linda, who is not happy about being thrown up on, starts to yell at the patient about being stupid and attempting this stunt. She informs her that no man is worth this and goes on to tell the patient about her own stupid husband. Linda continues to scold the patient about her "behavior" and tells her she is lucky she is not unconscious because Linda needs to practice intubating. Finally, as they pull into the hospital, Martin again lets a comment slide about "babysitting" before they give their report and hand off the patient. As they return to their squad, Martin and Linda are laughing and joking in the hallway of the ED about the patient and playing rock, paper, scissors to determine who is going to clean up the back of the squad.

1. When Martin and Linda delayed their response, was that a moral or an ethical problem? _____.

2. List the unethical and immoral treatments that Linda and Martin performed.

a. _____

b. _____

c. _____

d. _____

e. _____

f. _____

g. _____

h. _____

i. _____

j. _____

True/False

If you believe the statement to be more true than false, write the letter "T" in the space provided. If you believe the statement to be more false than true, write the letter "F."

_____ **1.** Ethics is a code of conduct that is defined by society and religion along with a person's conscience.

_____ **2.** The Code of Ethics for EMTs states that EMTs should adhere to standards of personal ethics that reflect credit upon the profession.

_____ **3.** You should always place the welfare of your patient ahead of any personal considerations, except for your own safety.

_____ **4.** Patient autonomy is the power of attorney making medical decisions for the patient.

_____ **5.** A DNR order can be printed on a medical ID bracelet.

_____ **6.** Advance directives are usually made once the patient can no longer make the decisions for his or her own health care.

_____ **7.** A person who makes health care decisions for another or carries the power of attorney is called a surrogate decision maker.

_____ **8.** Your general focus during resuscitation should be to provide at least an hour of your best efforts.

_____ **9.** If you witness misconduct by another EMS provider, you should report that person immediately to the chain of command.

_____ **10.** You should always work on a SIDS baby even if the baby is in rigor mortis.

Short Answer

Complete this section with short written answers using the space provided.

1. Ethics is the rules of right and wrong that we live by. Medial ethics is rules of right and wrong that guide behavior of health care professionals. State in one or two sentences what you regard as the guiding principle of your work as a paramedic.

_____

_____

_____

_____

_____

2. How would you handle a senior paramedic who continually makes racist remarks about your patients?

_____

_____

_____

_____

_____

3. Explain the things you would look for in a DNR order when you arrive on scene to find the patient in cardiac arrest.

_____

_____

_____

_____

Word Find

Hidden in the following grid are 19 words or phrases related to what you have studied in this chapter. Find the hidden words in the grid below. Then use the words from the grid to answer the following questions (some words may be used to answer more than one question).

```
G W I C L R Y G A C T Z U L M O R A L S G U M T S
S U R R O G A T E D E C I S I O N M A K E R S I E
E E Q N R K I I N K V V R I I E R U Q C N T W G X
D S V Q S O M D D E I A S Z A R A Q R Z R G R W U
D C U B Q A R T G N M L N U G F H F L O N Y T P A
V I S B N G F T G F D S B C C S K K F D W G D G L
Q H P Q A Z S W K I I S S M E B K F X A F S Y P M
D T K R W E I M A S J C U A R D E A Z C A C O I I
K E L J O L C J B J U K E P R E I W I E L W A E S
N O C S L F I N Z T D T M A L A K R O Y E E L M C
O I N C Q U E E A N N L N I Q M H N E R J A W H O
I B R Q P R A S B T R B T I G D S R O C O N X M N
T D B Y T Q Y I S O S U I S P K G F P R T T U O D
A P U W J L P M Q I F B W M I T A T A G Z I G A U
N J I L G S F X P U O Y U E N T A P T J U U V T C
O Z A E M B A N P R U N R S T Y L N I Y G L W E T
D Z B L R E X G T Z R F A O U Y P K E Z N U L I S
N J U B R X W V O C V S R L W K T R N A B L R C D
A S Y M O N O T U A T N E I T A P T T C L Z I Y G
G N E M J C Z H S A E W T S J H M C A W O H Y F W
R T B A G J F R I Y L F F C E D E J B B T D L O K
O S T O O R S S A R G N R L J B C O U E I P E S J
H A Q B T B O J D J K V X T N C N U S U Z X V I W
M E D I C A L E R R O R S D U Z O E E Q R B F Z J
Y Y X T S D X Y N T L P B V I A Y A P V X F S O U
```

1. As a paramedic, you would report _____ _____, _____,

   _____ _____, _____ _____, and _____

   _____ to your medical director.

2. A _____ and a _____ _____ are forms of _____

   _____.

3. A _____ _____ _____ and a _____

   _____ _____ are two forms of a person who will make medical decisions for you.

4. People can sign the back of their driver's license if they wish to participate in _____ _____

   in the event of their death.

5. EMS uses _____ _____ efforts to confirm the effectiveness of its procedures.

6. A paramedic should always act _____.

7. _____ is the philosophy of right and wrong, whereas _____ is a code of conduct.

8. Sometimes medical ethics is called _____.

9. When working a _____, you should realize that at some point you will face _____

   _____.

10. People work on the principle of _____ _____ when deciding what they want in their

    _____ _____.

CHAPTER

6 Pathophysiology

Chapter Review

The following exercises provide an opportunity to test your knowledge of this chapter.

Matching

Match the cell adaptations to the appropriate definitions.

_____ **1.** An alteration in the size, shape, and organization of cells

_____ **2.** An increase in the size of cells caused by synthesis of more subcellular components, which in turn leads to an increase in tissue and organ size

_____ **3.** A decrease in cell size caused by a loss of subcellular components, which in turn leads to a decrease in tissue and organ size

_____ **4.** Reversible, cellular adaptation in which one adult cell type is replaced by another adult cell type

_____ **5.** An increase in the actual number of cells in an organ or tissue, usually resulting in an increase in size of organ or tissue

A. Atrophy
B. Hypertrophy
C. Hyperplasia
D. Dysplasia
E. Metaplasia

Match the types of shock to the appropriate definitions.

_____ **6.** The result of widespread infection

_____ **7.** Occurs when blood flow becomes blocked in the heart or great vessels

_____ **8.** The result of spinal cord injury

_____ **9.** Occurs when histamine and other vasodilator proteins are released upon exposure to an allergen

_____ **10.** Occurs when the heart cannot circulate enough blood to maintain adequate peripheral oxygen delivery

_____ **11.** Occurs when there is widespread dilation of the resistance vessels, the capacitance vessels, or both

_____ **12.** Occurs when the circulating blood volume is unable to deliver adequate oxygen and nutrients to the body

A. Cardiogenic shock
B. Obstructive shock
C. Hypovolemic shock
D. Distributive shock
E. Anaphylactic shock
F. Septic shock
G. Neurogenic shock

Multiple Choice

Read each item carefully, and then select the best response.

_____ 1. The part of the cell that produces adenosine triphosphate (ATP), the major energy source of the body, is called:

A. endoplasmic reticulum.

B. golgi complex.

C. mitochondria.

D. lysosomes.

_____ 2. An increase in the size of cells caused by synthesis of more subcellular components, which in turn leads to an increase in tissue and organ size, is called:

A. hypertrophy.

B. hyperplasia.

C. dysplasia.

D. metaplasia.

_____ 3. The movement of a solvent from an area of low solute concentration to one of high concentration through a permeable membrane to equalize concentrations on both sides of the membrane is called:

A. diffusion.

B. active transport.

C. filtration.

D. osmosis.

_____ 4. When examining rates of disease, what term refers to the number of cases in a particular population?

A. Incidence

B. Prevalence

C. Distribution

D. Tendency

_____ 5. What term describes the type of derived necrosis that manifests as the loss of all features of the tissue and cells so that they come to resemble cheese when viewed through a microscope?

A. Liquefaction necrosis

B. Fat necrosis

C. Dry gangrene

D. Caseation necrosis

_____ 6. Which of the following is caused by an autosomal dominant inheritance (where a person needs to inherit only one copy of the particular form of the gene to show the trait)?

A. Sickle cell anemia

B. Attached earlobe

C. Tay-Sachs disease

D. Freckles

_____ 7. Individuals who suffer from long QT syndrome are at risk of all of the following EXCEPT:

A. ventricular arrhythmias.

B. palpitations.

C. torsades de pointes.

D. atrial fibrillation.

_____ 8. Clinical manifestation of Alzheimer's disease occurs in how many distinct stage(s)?

A. Four

B. Three

C. Two

D. One

_____ 9. Central shock consists of what two types of shock?

A. Hypovolemic and distributive

B. Cardiogenic and distributive

C. Cardiogenic and obstructive

D. Hypovolemic and obstructive

_____ 10. The most abundant type of white blood cells are called:

A. neutrophils.

B. eosinophils.

C. basophils.

D. monocytes.

Labeling

Label the following diagrams with the correct terms.

1. Label the components of the organelles of a cell.

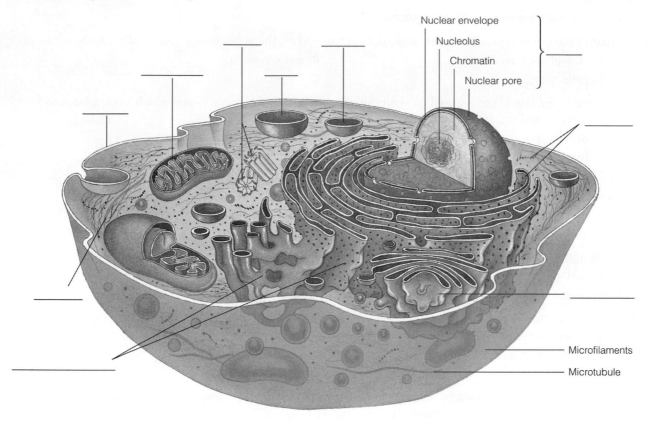

Nuclear envelope

Nucleolus

Chromatin

Nuclear pore

Microfilaments

Microtubule

A. Nucleus

B. Ribosome

C. Golgi complex

D. Lysosome

E. Vacuole

F. Plasma membrane

G. Cytoplasm

H. Endoplasmic reticulum

I. Centriole

J. Mitochondrion

2. Fill in the missing words that describe a type I allergic reaction.

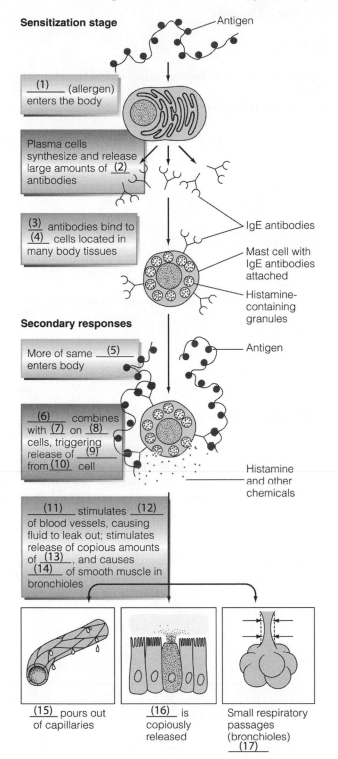

Sensitization stage

Antigen

_____(1)_____ (allergen) enters the body

Plasma cells synthesize and release large amounts of _____(2)_____ antibodies

_____(3)_____ antibodies bind to _____(4)_____ cells located in many body tissues

IgE antibodies

Mast cell with IgE antibodies attached

Histamine-containing granules

Secondary responses

More of same _____(5)_____ enters body

Antigen

_____(6)_____ combines with _____(7)_____ on _____(8)_____ cells, triggering release of _____(9)_____ from _____(10)_____ cell

Histamine and other chemicals

_____(11)_____ stimulates _____(12)_____ of blood vessels, causing fluid to leak out; stimulates release of copious amounts of _____(13)_____, and causes _____(14)_____ of smooth muscle in bronchioles

_____(15)_____ pours out of capillaries

_____(16)_____ is copiously released

Small respiratory passages (bronchioles) _____(17)_____

1. _____

2. _____

3. _____

4. _____

5. _____

6. _____

7. _____

8. _____

9. _____

10. _____

11. _____

12. _____

13. _____

14. _____

15. _____

16. _____

17. _____

Fill-in-the-Blank

Read each item carefully, and then complete the statement by filling in the missing word(s).

1. The dynamic process, also called the dynamic steady state, is known as _____.

2. _____ _____ is a special type of connective tissue that contains large amounts of lipids.

3. _____ is an increase in the actual number of cells in an organ or tissue.

4. _____ are found primarily in the carotid artery, aorta, and kidneys and are sensitive to changes in blood pressure.

5. A decrease in urine output is called _____.

6. _____ is an elevated potassium level.

7. The molecules that modulate the changes in pH are called _____.

8. Normal cell death is called _____.

9. _____ _____ _____ _____ is a progressive condition usually characterized by concurrent failure of several organs, such as the lungs, liver, and kidneys.

10. _____ is a protein produced by cells when they are invaded by a virus.

Identify

In the following case study, list the chief complaint, vital signs, and pertinent patient history.

You respond to a call to a nursing home for a 78-year-old man who is having difficulty breathing. Upon arrival, you find your patient sitting up in a lounge chair looking distressed. You walk into the room, introduce yourself, and ask what's wrong. The patient responds, with what appears to be great difficulty, "Can't breathe." Your partner starts to obtain vital signs as you place the patient on a nonrebreathing mask. You obtain the following history between the patient and staff. The symptoms started about 30 minutes ago with shortness of breath and coughing. The night nurse tells you the patient said he was chilled, sweaty, and felt warm. His temperature was taken before your arrival and was recorded on the chart as 102.5°F. The medical record states he has chronic obstructive pulmonary disease (COPD) with a 40-year history of two packs of cigarettes a day. Your partner tells you that respirations are 28 breaths/min and shallow, the pulse is 90 beats/min with occasional irregular beats, blood pressure is 160/90 mm Hg, and oxygen saturation is 90%. You and your partner decide to place the patient on constant positive airway pressure (CPAP) to assist. Just before placing the mask, the patient starts to cough and brings up blood-tinged sputum. You prepare the patient and transport. He is hospitalized for a week with a diagnosis of pneumonia before returning to the nursing home.

1. Chief Complaint

_____

_____

_____

2. Vital Signs

_____

_____

_____

3. Pertinent Patient History

_____

_____

_____

Ambulance Calls

The following case scenarios provide an opportunity to explore the concerns associated with patient management and paramedic care. Read each scenario, and then answer each question.

1. While on a chest pain call you are taking the SAMPLE history, and the patient tells you he is taking an angiotensin-converting enzyme (ACE) inhibitor for high blood pressure. Your partner has placed the patient on the monitor and informs you that there is a peaked T wave and a wide QRS complex with tachycardia.

    a. What do you suspect is the life-threatening emergency that is being identified on the echocardiogram (ECG)?

    _____

    _____

    b. What drug should be considered as the first-line medication for this condition?

    _____

    _____

2. Approximately a half million people living in the United States are believed to have Crohn's disease. When a person has an acute episode, he or she may call emergency medical services (EMS).

    a. Crohn's disease is a disorder of which body system?

    _____

    _____

    b. What symptoms would you expect a Crohn's patient to have?

    _____

    _____

3. It is not uncommon to encounter an elderly patient who has Alzheimer's disease as an underlying problem. What are some of the factors that might affect your ability to get a good SAMPLE history and provide care for an Alzheimer's patient?

    _____

    _____

True/False

If you believe the statement to be more true than false, write the letter "T" in the space provided. If you believe the statement to be more false than true, write the letter "F."

_____ **1.** Epithelium covers the external surfaces of the body.

_____ **2.** Dendrites receive electrical impulses from axons of other nerve cells and conduct the impulses toward the body cell.

_____ **3.** Metaplasia is an alteration in the size, shape, and organization of cells.

_____ **4.** Tonicity refers to the tension exerted on a cell caused by water movement across the cell membrane.

_____ **5.** A blood pH of less than 7.35 is called alkalosis.

_____ **6.** With autosomal-recessive inheritance, a person must inherit only one copy of a particular form of a gene to show that trait.

_____ **7.** Distributive shock occurs when blood flow becomes blocked in the great vessels.

_____ **8.** Acquired immunity is a highly specific, inducible, discriminatory, and unforgetting method by which armies of cells respond to an immune stimulant.

_____ **9.** Interferon is a synthetic fatty substance produced by cells when invaded by bacteria.

_____ **10.** Rh factor is an antigen that is present in the erythrocytes of about 85% of the population and is of key importance in blood typing.

Short Answer

Complete this section with short written answers using the space provided.

1. The body loses water in a number of ways. What are the four major ways in which water is lost from the body?

a. _____

b. _____

c. _____

d. _____

2. What are the four forces that control the equilibrium between the capillary and the interstitial space?

a. _____

b. _____

c. _____

d. _____

3. Metabolic acidosis is an accumulation of abnormal acids in the blood. List three conditions that can cause this.

a. _____

b. _____

c. _____

4. Cellular injury can result from various causes. List five causes.

a. _____

b. _____

c. _____

d. _____

e. _____

5. List six respiratory diseases that may be caused by environmental pollutants, viruses, or bacteria.

a. _____

b. _____

c. _____

d. _____

e. _____

f. _____

6. List four conditions for which you should always consider syncope to be caused by a life-threatening arrhythmia until proved otherwise.

a. _____

b. _____

c. _____

d. _____

7. Clinical manifestation of Alzheimer's disease occurs in three distinct stages. Give a short overview (summary) of each stage.

Stage 1: _____

Stage 2: _____

Stage 3: _____

8. List the five general types of leukocytes.

a. _____   d. _____

b. _____   e. _____

c. _____

9. The goal of the cellular component of acute inflammatory response is for the inflammatory cells (polymorphonuclear neutrophils) to arrive at the site in the tissue where they are needed. The process involves two major stages: intravascular and extravascular phases. During the later phase, leukocytes travel to the inflammation site and kill organisms. Name the five events in this sequence.

a. _____

b. _____

c. _____

d. _____

e. _____

10. What are the three stages of *general adaptation syndrome*?

a. _____   b. _____   c. _____

Crossword Puzzle

Use the clues in the column to complete the puzzle.

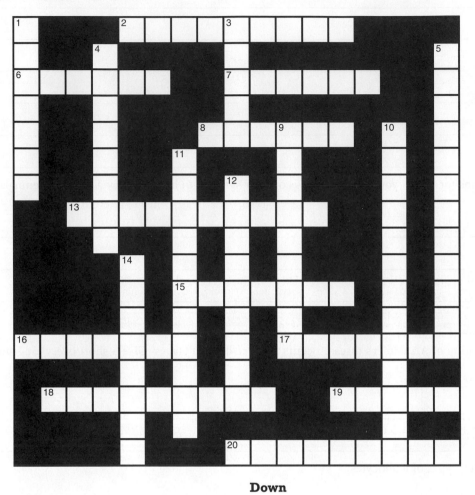

Across

2. The _____ is the number of deaths from a disease in a given population.

6. _____ is the protein that polymerizes (bonds) to form the fibrous component of a blood clot.

7. _____ is a chronic inflammation condition resulting in intermittent wheezing and excess mucus production.

8. The _____ system includes all structures and processes associated with the body's defense against foreign substances and disease-causing agents.

13. _____ is an inherited disorder characterized by excessive bleeding.

15. Hypersensitivity reaction to the presence of an agent (allergen) is called a/an _____.

16. _____ tissue is a special type of connective tissue that contains large amounts of lipids.

17. _____ is a decrease in cell size due to a loss of subcellular components.

18. _____ are products of cells that affect the function of other cells.

19. _____ typically conduct electrical impulses away from the cell body.

20. _____ is normal cell death.

Down

1. _____ are molecules that modulate changes in pH.

3. The first of the three stages of general adaptation syndrome is called _____.

4. Permanent aggregation of melanin in the skin is called _____.

5. The _____ response is a response of the tissues of the body to irritation or injury characterized by pain, swelling, redness, and heat.

9. Multiple small, raised areas on the skin, also known as hives, that may be one of the warning signs of impending anaphylaxis is called _____.

10. _____ are found primarily in the carotid artery, aorta, and kidneys, and are sensitive to changes in blood pressure.

11. _____ is defined as a decreased serum potassium level.

12. _____ measures the disease-causing ability of a microorganism.

14. Determining the cause of disease is called _____.

Fill-in-the-Table

Fill in the missing parts of the table.

1. Identify the signs and symptoms of compensated and decompensated hypoperfusion.

Signs and Symptoms in the Phases of Hypoperfusion	
Compensated	**Decompensated**
■ Agitation, anxiety, restlessness	■ Altered mental status (verbal to unresponsive)
■	■
■	■ Labored or irregular breathing
■	
■ Pallor with cyanotic lips	■
■	
■	■
■ Delayed capillary refill in infants and children	
■	■ Dilated pupils
■	■
	■

CHAPTER
7 Pharmacology

Chapter Review

The following exercises provide an opportunity to test your knowledge of this chapter.

Matching

Listed here are some of the routes by which a medication can be administered. Arrange the list in order, according to the speed of absorption into the body, starting with the route by which medications are absorbed the fastest.

_____ **1.** Fastest route	**A.** Subcutaneous injection
_____ **2.**	**B.** Endotracheal spray
_____ **3.**	**C.** Topical application
_____ **4.**	**D.** Intravenous injection
_____ **5.**	**E.** Sublingual tablet
_____ **6.**	**F.** Oral (swallowed)
_____ **7.**	**G.** Intracardiac injection
_____ **8.**	**H.** Rectal (suppository)
_____ **9.** Slowest route	**I.** Intramuscular injection

Multiple Choice

Read each item carefully, and then select the best response.

_____ **1.** The nonproprietary name is a general name for a drug and is not manufacturer specific. What is another name for nonproprietary drugs?

    A. Chemical   **C.** Trade

    B. Generic   **D.** Official

_____ **2.** What was the first US federal law, legislated in 1906, aimed at protecting the public from mislabeled and harmful drugs?

    A. Food, Drug, and Cosmetic Act   **C.** Pure Food Act

    B. Harrison Narcotic Act   **D.** Narcotic Control Act

_____ **3.** Which US government agency has jurisdiction over monitoring drug advertising and ensuring that it is not misleading?

      A. Food and Drug Administration   **C.** Drug Enforcement Administration

      B. Centers for Disease Control and Prevention   **D.** Federal Trade Commission

_____ **4.** The part of the nervous system that sends sensory impulses from internal structures (such as the vessels, heart, and abdomen) through afferent autonomic nerves to the brain is considered:

      A. autonomic.   **C.** sympathetic.

      B. peripheral.   **D.** parasympathetic.

_____ **5.** The process of chemical signaling between cells is:

      A. adrenergic.   **C.** ganglionic.

      B. synaptic.   **D.** neurotransmission.

_____ **6.** What is a liquid containing one or more chemical substances entirely dissolved, usually in water, called?

      A. Suspension   **C.** Emulsion

      B. Syrup   **D.** Solution

_____ **7.** What is the name given to a concentrated preparation of a drug made by putting the drug into solution and evaporating the excess solvent until the concentration reaches a prescribed standard?

      A. Tablet   **C.** Pill

      B. Extract   **D.** Pulvule

_____ **8.** Which of the following is NOT a parenteral route of medication administration?

      A. Intraosseous   **C.** Subcutaneous

      B. Enteral   **D.** Intramuscular

_____ **9.** What is the name given to the active transport process in which medications are bound to specific transporters, aiding in their elimination?

      A. Glomerular filtration   **C.** Tubular secretion

      B. Biotransformation   **D.** Partial reabsorption

_____ **10.** A unique response that is specific to a person and is not seen in other patients is known as:

      A. idiosyncrasy.   **C.** cross-tolerance.

      B. iatrogenic reaction.   **D.** tachyphylaxis.

Labeling

Label the following diagrams with the correct terms.

1. Organization of the Nervous System

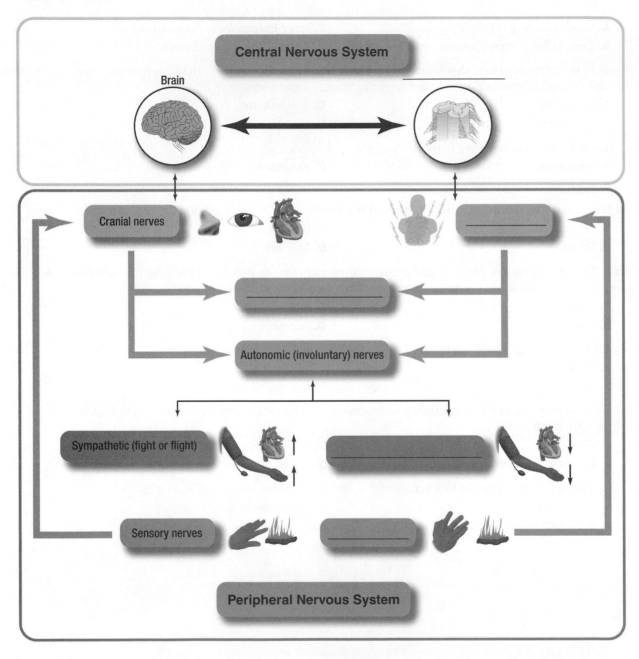

2. Label the photos with the four principal sources that drugs are derived from.

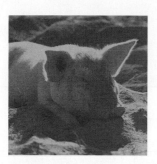 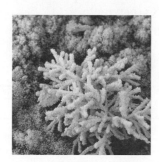 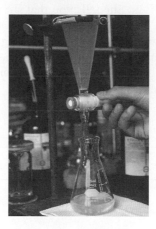 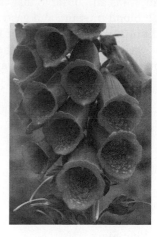

_____   _____   _____   _____

Fill-in-the-Blank

Read each item carefully, and then complete the statement by filling in the missing word(s).

1. A medication's _____ are the reasons or conditions for which the medication is given.

2. There are conditions under which it is inappropriate to administer a particular medication. These are referred to as the

_____.

3. Opioid _____ reverse the effects of opioid drugs.

4. When excessive cholinergics, such as a nerve agent, are present, a patient may exhibit signs that can be remembered by using

the mnemonic SLUDGE, which stands for **S**_____, **L**_____, **U**_____, **D**_____,

G_____, and **E**_____.

5. The adrenergic that produces peripheral vasoconstriction and mild bronchoconstriction is called a/an _____

receptor.

6. The adrenergic that stimulates vasodilation and bronchodilation is called a/an _____ receptor.

7. _____ medications cause the kidneys to remove excess amounts of salt and water from the body.

8. Medications that affect heart rate are said to have a/an _____ effect.

9. _____ effects are changes in the force of the heart's contractions.

10. When a drug alters the velocity of the conduction of electricity through the heart, it has a/an _____ effect.

Identify

In the following case study, list the chief complaint, vital signs, and pertinent negatives.

You are called to a private residence for a 65-year-old woman who has general body weakness. Upon arrival, you find a woman sitting on a couch in the living room. When you ask what the problem is, she tells you that she has heart palpatations. She appears not to be in any distress. Her husband tells you she went to the doctor's yesterday, and she seems to be doing okay because it was just a checkup. You check vital signs and find the pulse is 60 beats/min, regular and weak, respirations are slightly labored at 22 breaths/min, and the blood pressure is 90/60 mm Hg. While your partner starts an IV, you get a SAMPLE history. You know the symptoms and observe that the patient seems pale. She tells you she has no pain, no nausea, and that she is on medication for high blood pressure and gastric reflux. She tells you that she was put on a new medication yesterday for her gastric reflux and an additional medication for her high blood pressure. She has had no hospitalizations and has been in relatively good health. The patient was watching TV when her symptoms started. According to her husband, it is time for the patient's afternoon medications, but you think that she should wait until she gets to the hospital, a 15-minute transport time, and discuss them with the doctor before taking. You transport and obtain a 12-lead echocardiogram (ECG) en route.

1. Chief Complaint

_____

_____

_____

2. Vital Signs

_____

_____

_____

3. Pertinent Negatives

_____

_____

_____

Ambulance Calls

The following case scenarios provide an opportunity to explore the concerns associated with patient management and paramedic care. Read each scenario, and then answer each question.

1. You are on the scene for a 55-year-old man who is reporting an 8 on 10 chest pain that came on while he was shoveling snow. You have placed the patient on supplemental oxygen, given aspirin and nitroglycerin, and your partner is starting an IV and is obtaining a 12-lead ECG. The nitroglycerin has had no effect, and the patient is reporting 10 on 10 for pain. After obtaining vital signs and finding his blood pressure to be 160/100 mm Hg, you decide to give morphine. The six rights for medication administration run through your head as you prepare the drug for administration. What are the six rights and how do they apply?

a. _____

b. _____

c. _____

d. _____

e. _____

f. _____

2. Advanced Cardiac Life Support (ACLS) protocols require numerous medications to be administered during a cardiac arrest scenario. The pharmacokinetics on a body in cardiac arrest affect absorption (transfer of a medication from its administration site to specific organs and tissues). As a paramedic, what factors can potentially affect absorption and can be profound in a cardiac arrest situation?

a. _____

b. _____

c. _____

d. _____

e. _____

3. The young and old potentially present factors that can affect the actions of medications that are administered in the prehospital setting. What are eight factors that the paramedic should consider when providing care to the young and old, including additional factors that may need to be considered if the patient has underlying medical conditions?

a. _____

b. _____

c. _____

d. _____

e. _____

f. _____

g. _____

h. _____

True/False

If you believe the statement to be more true than false, write the letter "T" in the space provided. If you believe the statement to be more false than true, write the letter "F."

_____ **1.** The general, nonproprietary name for a drug is its official name.

_____ **2.** Schedule V drugs have the highest abuse potential and a propensity for severe dependency.

_____ **3.** The changes in pharmacokinetics in geriatric patients are comparable to those observed in young children.

_____ **4.** Infants do not achieve the same level of hepatic function as adults until they reach 6 months of age.

_____ **5.** Afferent nerves carry messages from the brain to the muscles and all of the other organs of the body.

_____ **6.** The peripheral nervous system consists of all nervous tissue outside the brain and spinal cord and is separated into two divisions.

_____ **7.** The attraction between a medication and its receptors is referred to as an agonist.

_____ **8.** Idiosyncrasy is an abnormal reaction by a person to a medication to which most other people do not react.

_____ **9.** Percutaneous route is generally performed by placing medication directly onto the patient's skin.

_____ **10.** Parenteral routes include those in which medications are administered via any route other than the alimentary canal.

Short Answer

Complete this section with short written answers using the space provided.

1. The medical director of your organization announces that a new medication will be introduced into the protocols. As part of an in-service to learn about this new drug you are given the pharmaceutical company's profile. What are the four different names that will be listed on this literature?

   a. _____

   b. _____

   c. _____

   d. _____

2. What are the components of a drug profile?

   a. _____

   b. _____

   c. _____

   d. _____

   e. _____

   f. _____

   g. _____

   h. _____

   i. _____

   j. _____

   k. _____

3. In excretion, the body eliminates the remnants of the drug. List the three mechanisms of excretion through the kidneys.

   a. _____

   b. _____

   c. _____

4. Unanticipated adverse reactions are known as iatrogenic responses. Name at least six of these responses.

   a. _____

   b. _____

   c. _____

   d. _____

   e. _____

   f. _____

5. Adrenergic receptors are targeted by numerous drugs given in the prehospital setting. List the four adrenergic receptors and their effects.

a. _____

b. _____

c. _____

d. _____

Word Find

Hidden in the following grid are 23 words or phrases related to what you have studied in this chapter. Find the hidden words in the grid below. Then use the words from the grid to answer the following questions (some words may be used to answer more than one question).

```
A G X T S E C Q T F P N N A M
E I E Y N A L I N A O O U M J
S L R N P E R U R L I I X P D
K U I S E I M E V S I T Z U J
P L U X P R N I L L S O T L I
V L I S I T I U N L U L S E S
E D Q M E R M C U I M P U L O
E D Z R M E L I N P L O S E L
E M A N E D A R T A N G P R U
J L T C A R T X E G M H E U T
S U P P O S I T O R Y E N T I
H C T A P T A B L E T L S C O
O I N T M E N T Y N A S I N N
M W C Z I N P E L I N K O I R
S O A B H F I K V N U V N T I
```

1. Preparation of a drug for external use, usually to relieve some discomfort: a/an _____ or _____

2. Aqueous suspension of an insoluble drug: _____

3. Preparation of a volatile substance dissolved in alcohol: _____

4. Dilute alcoholic extract of a drug: _____

5. A drug suspended in sugar and water: _____

6. Oil distributed in small globules in water: _____

7. A drug shaped into a ball or oval, often coated to disguise an unpleasant taste: _____

8. A cylindrical gelatin container enclosing a dose of medication: _____

9. Resembles question 8, but not made of gelatin and does not separate: _____

10. A powdered drug that has been molded or compressed into a small disk: _____

11. A drug mixed in a firm base that melts at body temperature: _____

12. A medication impregnated in adhesive that is applied to the surface of the skin: _____

13. A semisolid preparation for external application, usually containing a medicinal substance: _____

14. A drug suspended in alcohol and flavoring: _____

15. A concentrated preparation of a drug made by putting the drug into solution and evaporating off the excess solvent to a prescribed standard: _____

16. A liquid containing one or more chemical substances *entirely dissolved,* usually in water: _____. That liquid may be supplied as a single dose in a sealed glass container, called a/an _____, or in a multidose _____ with a rubber stopper.

17. A preparation of a finely divided drug whose ingredients separate out on standing: _____

18. Any route of administration other than through the digestive tract: _____

19. Lasix is the _____ _____ of the drug whose _____ name is furosemide.

Fill-in-the-Table
Fill in the missing parts of the tables.

1. Fill in the rates of absorption by the different routes indicated.

Rates of Absorption by Different Routes	
Route of Administration	**Time Until Drug Takes Effect***
Topical	
Oral	
Rectal	
SC injection	15–30 min
IM injection	
Sublingual tablet	
Sublingual injection	3 min
Inhalation	3 min
Endotracheal	
IO	
IV	
Intracardiac	15 s
In a healthy person with normal perfusion.	

2. List the components of a drug profile.

Component of Drug Profile	Description
	Chemical, generic, and trade names with graphic representation
	How the medication causes the intended effect
	Reason or condition for which medication is given
	How the medication is absorbed or distributed
	Undesired effects from the medication
	All the routes by which the drug can be administered
	Profiles the various forms and concentration of how the drug is made available for clinical use
	Amount of drug that should be administered for a particular condition
	Conditions under which it is inappropriate to administer a particular medication
	Contains all the information necessary to safely and effectively administer the medication to pediatric, geriatric, or pregnant patients

CHAPTER

8 Vascular Access and Medication Administration

Chapter Review

The following exercises provide an opportunity to test your knowledge of this chapter.

Matching

In choosing an intravenous fluid for any given patient, it is important to know what effects that fluid will have on the patient's overall fluid balance. Some fluids tend to remain within the vascular space, whereas others move quickly out of the vascular space and into the interstitial or intracellular compartment. For each of the following situations, indicate whether the intravenous fluid preferred initially would be:

A. Lactated Ringer's   **B.** Normal saline

_____ **1.** A 30-year-old man is injured in a car crash. He is confused and disoriented. His skin is cold and clammy. His pulse is 128 beats/min, respirations 24 breaths/min and shallow, and blood pressure is palpable at 80 mm Hg.

_____ **2.** A 28-year-old construction worker collapsed at the work site on a very hot day. His skin is cool and sweaty, pulse is 100 beats/min, and a blood pressure of 100/60 mm Hg.

_____ **3.** A 22-year-old woman is rescued from a structural fire with burns over 45% of her body. Current vital signs are a pulse 88 beats/min, respirations 20 breaths/min and labored, and blood pressure of 110/80 mm Hg.

_____ **4.** A 48-year-old man has crushing chest pain. He has a pulse of 100 beats/min and irregular, respirations 18 breaths/min, and a blood pressure of 180/100 mm Hg.

_____ **5.** A 30-year-old man complaining of very severe abdominal pain. His abdomen is very tender, and he winces every time the ambulance goes over a bump. His pulse is 110 beats/min and regular, respirations 24 breaths/min and shallow, and a blood pressure of 100/70 mm Hg.

_____ **6.** A 16-year-old boy has had 3 days of severe diarrhea. His skin "tents" when you pinch it. His pulse is 120 beats/min, respirations 22 breaths/min, and a blood pressure of 100/60 mm Hg.

Match the correct word to the definition.

_____ **1.** Carrier for red and white blood cells

_____ **2.** Inorganic molecules that do not contain carbon

_____ **3.** The fluid that dissolves components

_____ **4.** Forty-five percent of body weight, the water that is inside the cells

A. Intracellular fluid
B. Electrolytes
C. Intravascular fluid
D. Solvent

Multiple Choice

Read each item carefully, and then select the best response.

_____ **1.** Interstitial fluid is fluid that is:
- **A.** contained inside the cells.
- **B.** the water within the blood.
- **C.** the water that bathes the cells.
- **D.** all the water in the body.

_____ **2.** When hypocalcemia occurs in your patient, which of the following signs and symptoms would you expect to see?
- **A.** Muscle cramps, hypotension, carpopedal spasms
- **B.** Muscle weakness, lethargy, and hot flushed skin
- **C.** Cardiac arrest, hyperstimulation of the nerve cells
- **D.** Shortness of breath, heart arrhythmias

_____ **3.** Which of the following solutions is the best choice for administration, in the prehospital setting, when the patient needs to have body fluids replaced?
- **A.** Hypertonic
- **B.** Hypotonic
- **C.** Colloid
- **D.** Crystalloid

_____ **4.** Which administration set will allow for 60 gtts per milliliter?
- **A.** Blood tubing
- **B.** Microdrip set
- **C.** Macrodrip set
- **D.** Volutrol administration set

_____ **5.** When inserting an IV catheter, the bevel should be:
- **A.** facing down.
- **B.** facing up.
- **C.** pointed to the side.
- **D.** rolled as you insert it.

_____ **6.** After starting an IV on a patient, which of the following is not necessary to document?
- **A.** The site of the IV
- **B.** The gauge of the needle you used
- **C.** The patient's pain scale when you started the IV
- **D.** The type of fluid you are using

_____ **7.** There are many complications with an IV site; _____ means there is an inflammation of the vein.
- **A.** Thrombophlebitis
- **B.** Hematoma
- **C.** Occlusion
- **D.** Vein irritation

_____ **8.** Which of the following is NOT a sign of an allergic reaction to IV therapy?
- **A.** Urticaria
- **B.** Shortness of breath
- **C.** Bradycardia
- **D.** Edema of the face

_____ **9.** When taking a blood sample in the field, what is the green top tube used for?
- **A.** Determining the patient's blood type
- **B.** Checking glucose and electrolyte levels
- **C.** Determining how long it takes for the patient's blood to clot
- **D.** Checking for alcohol and drugs in the blood system

_____ **10.** Which of the following is an example of an antiseptic?
- **A.** Virex
- **B.** Iodine
- **C.** Cidex
- **D.** Microcide

_____ **11.** Which parenteral medication route is usually the fastest and most commonly used in the prehospital setting?
- **A.** Intradermal
- **B.** Subcutaneous
- **C.** Intramuscular
- **D.** Intravenous

_____ **12.** A/an _____ is a breakable sterile glass container that carries a single dose of medication.
- **A.** vial
- **B.** ampule
- **C.** mix-o-vial
- **D.** prefill

_____ **13.** A/an _____ injection is given at a 90° angle.

    A. Subcutaneous   **C.** Intramuscular

    B. Intravascular   **D.** Bolus

_____ **14.** Which of the following medications can be given down the ET tube?

    A. Atropine   **C.** Nitroglycerin

    B. Adenosine   **D.** Lasix

_____ **15.** How much normal saline should you use as a flush after administering a medication through a gastric tube?

    A. 15 to 30 mL   **C.** 60 to 75 mL

    B. 30 to 60 mL   **D.** You do not use normal saline for a flush.

Labeling

Label the common sites for intramuscular injections.

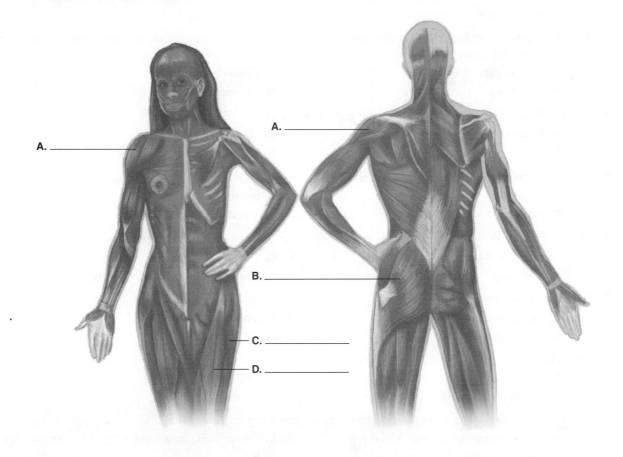

A. _____

A. _____

B. _____

C. _____

D. _____

Fill-in-the-Blank

Read each item carefully, and then complete the statement by filling in the missing word(s).

1. Intravenous solution containing large molecules such as proteins: _____.

2. Intravenous solution that does *not* contain large molecules such as proteins: _____. One example of such a solution

is normal _____.

3. When two solutions of different solute concentration are placed on either side of a semipermeable membrane, the *more*

concentrated solution is said to be _____ with respect to the less concentrated solution. Conversely, the *less* concentrated solution is considered _____ with respect to the more concentrated solution. If the two solutions have the *same* concentration, they are said to be _____. Thus, for example, 4% saline is _____ with respect to serum; Ringer's solution is _____ with respect to serum; and half normal saline (0.45% NaCl) is _____ with respect to serum.

4. When two solutions of different solute concentrations are placed on either side of a semipermeable membrane, water will move *from* the solution of _____ (higher or lower?) solute concentration *to* the solution of _____ (higher or lower?) solute concentration. The process by which water migrates in that fashion is called _____.

5. The cardinal sign of *over*hydration is _____.

Ambulance Calls

All of the patients described in the following scenarios are experiencing one or another problem related to their intravenous therapy. Identify the problem in each case, and explain what you will do to manage it.

1. The patient is a 59-year-old man with severe chest pain on whom you have started a "keep-open" IV. It is a long way to the hospital, and about 10 minutes into the transport, he starts complaining of breathing difficulty. You notice that his respirations have become more rapid, and when you listen to his chest, you can hear bubbly noises. Meanwhile, you suddenly notice that the liter bag of IV fluid is empty.
   a. What is the patient's problem?

   _____

   _____

   b. What are you going to do about it?

   _____

   _____

2. You have started an IV on a frail old woman. After a few minutes, you notice that the IV is infusing more and more slowly. You open the clamp wide, but that doesn't help. You lower the IV bag below the stretcher; there is no blood return into the tubing. Then you check the IV site. There seems to be a lump in the skin, and the skin feels quite cool.
   a. What is the patient's problem?

   _____

   _____

   b. What are you going to do about it?

   _____

   _____

   c. What other things might cause an IV to slow down or stop?

   _____

   _____

3. You are starting an IV near the wrist of a petite young woman. When the IV catheter enters the vessel, bright red blood comes spurting back in your face.

a. What is the patient's problem?

_____

_____

b. What are you going to do about it?

_____

_____

4. You are transporting a patient between hospitals. The patient has an IV already running (it was started earlier in the day by the paramedics who brought the patient to the first hospital). The patient complains of pain at the IV site, and you notice that it is red, hot, and swollen.

a. What is the patient's problem?

_____

_____

b. What are you going to do about it?

_____

_____

c. How could this problem have been prevented?

(1) _____

(2) _____

(3) _____

(4) _____

5. A driver is found conscious but very restless. He keeps asking you, "Can't you give me some water? I'm so thirsty—please give me something to drink." His skin is cold and sweaty. You do not see any external signs of serious injury.

a. Do you think this patient has been seriously injured? _____ Explain the reasons for your answer.

_____

_____

b. You decide to start an IV with lactated Ringer's, which is a _____ (colloid or crystalloid?) solution. Your protocol calls for administering 200 mL/h in these circumstances. You have an administration set that delivers 10 drops per milliliter. At how many drops per minute will you have to set the infusion rate to deliver 200 mL/h? _____ gtt/min (Show your calculations.)

c. A few minutes after you adjust the IV rate, you notice that the IV has slowed down to the point that it is hardly flowing at all. List the five steps you would take to try to identify and solve the problem with the IV.

(1) _____

(2)_____

(3)_____

(4)_____

(5)_____

True/False

If you believe the statement to be more true than false, write the letter "T" in the space provided. If you believe the statement to be more false than true, write the letter "F."

_____ **1.** An ion with a negative charge is called a cation.

_____ **2.** "Where sodium goes, water follows."

_____ **3.** Calcium is the primary buffer in body fluids.

_____ **4.** The normal concentration of glucose in the body is 50 to 100 milligrams per 100 milliliters.

_____ **5.** The process of moving from a higher concentration to a lower concentration is called diffusion.

_____ **6.** Tonicity is the concentration of calcium inside and outside the cell.

_____ **7.** A healthy person will lose up to 1 liter of fluid a day as a result of urine output and exhalation.

_____ **8.** Lactated Ringer's is used for patients who have lost a large amount of blood in the field.

_____ **9.** A crystalloid solution can carry oxygen to the cells.

_____ **10.** A macrodrip administration set delivers 10 or 15 gtt/mL.

_____ **11.** A good thing to do when starting an IV is to work down, in case you miss the first attempt.

_____ **12.** A butterfly catheter has a Teflon catheter over the hollow needle.

_____ **13.** You should always have the bevel to the side when starting an IV.

_____ **14.** When changing an IV bag, you must start all over with the process and restart your IV.

_____ **15.** When an IV infiltrates, you will notice edema at the catheter site.

_____ **16.** When you have cannulated an artery, you must pull the catheter out and apply direct pressure for at least 5 minutes.

_____ **17.** A healthy adult can handle only 1 to 2 extra liters of fluid.

_____ **18.** A red top tube is used to determine the blood type of a patient.

_____ **19.** An IO infusion is easier to use, so it should be used as much as possible for the pediatric patient.

_____ **20.** When placing an IO needle, you should feel two "pops."

_____ **21.** The basic unit of weight in the metric system is the gram.

_____ **22.** One pound is equal to 2.2 kilograms.

_____ **23.** The desired dose is what is ordered to give to the patient.

_____ **24.** Dopamine is delivered to the patient in micrograms.

_____ **25.** There are six "rights" of drug administration.

Short Answer

Complete this section with short written answers using the space provided.

1. Name three ways to make the vein "stand up" so it is easier to see it.

a. _____

b. _____

c. _____

2. List the four things that are a MUST when documenting the IV.

a. _____

b. _____

c. _____

d. _____

3. There are six local reactions that can happen when starting an IV. List three complications and their signs and symptoms.

a. _____

b. _____

c. _____

4. List the six points of information you should document when you administer a medication to a patient.

a. _____

b. _____

c. _____

d. _____

e. _____

f. _____

Crossword Puzzle

Use the clues in the column to complete the puzzle.

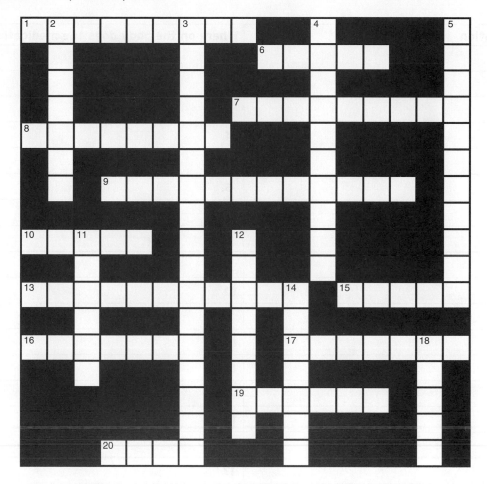

Across

1. The physical blockage of the vein or the catheter.
6. When starting an IV, avoid an area where the vein crosses over a/an _____.
7. A/an _____ catheter has a hollow needle and two plastic wings.
8. A microdrip set that allows only 100 or 200 mL of fluid to be given.
9. When IV fluid escapes from the vein into the surrounding tissue.
10. The _____ chamber is the area of an IV catheter that fills with blood to help indicate when a vein is cannulated.
13. Low potassium levels.
15. The color of the blood tube that is used to evaluate electrolytes and glucose levels.
16. The fluid that does the dissolving, or the solution that contains the dissolved components.
17. The route where medication is absorbed through some portion of the gastrointestinal tract.
19. The type of math that is used in pharmacology.
20. Another word for electrolytes.

Down

2. A solution that contains molecules (usually proteins) that are too large to pass out of the capillary membranes and, therefore, remain in the vascular compartment.
3. Fluid with almost the same osmolarity as serum and other bodily fluids.
4. _____ is a type of diffusion used by the kidneys to clean the blood.
5. Inadequate total system fluid volume.
11. Breakable sterile glass container that holds a single dose of medication.
12. The accumulation of blood in the tissue surrounding the IV site.
14. A method of cleansing used to prevent contamination of a site when performing an invasive procedure (such as starting an IV) is called _____ technique.
18. The constricting band should be _____ the IV site.

Fill-in-the-Table

Fill in the missing parts of the table.

Route of Administration	Where on the body does the medication go?
Enteral route	1.
Oral	2.
Intradermal	3.
Percutaneous	4.
Sublingual	5.
Endotracheal	6.
Buccal	7.
Transdermal	8.
Intramuscular	9.
Rectal	10.
Parenteral	11.
Subcutaneous	12.
Intravascular	13.
Ocular	14.
Aural	15.
Inhalation	16.
Intranasal	17.

Problem Solving

Practice your calculation skills by solving the following math problems.

1. You have started an IV on a bakery worker suffering from heat exhaustion. Your physician instructs you to run normal saline by IV at 200 mL/h. Your bag of saline is a 1,000-mL bag. Your administration set delivers 10 gtt/mL. At what rate (how many drops per minute) do you have to run the infusion to give 200 mL/h? (Show your calculations.)

2. You have started a "keep-open" IV with a microdrip infusion set (which delivers 60 gtt/mL). Your instructions are to run the IV at 30 mL/h. At what rate (how many drops per minute) should you set the flow? (Show your calculations.)

3. You are ordered to give a lidocaine drip at a rate of 2 mg/min. You have on hand:
   - A vial containing 50 mL of 4% lidocaine
   - A 500-mL bag of D_5W
   - A microdrip administration set that delivers 60 gtt/mL

a. How many *grams* of lidocaine are in the vial? _____ g (Show your calculations.)

b. When you add the contents of the vial to the IV bag, what will be the concentration of lidocaine in the IV bag? _____ g/mL (Show your calculations.)

c. How many milliliters per minute (mL/min) will the patient have to receive to get the dosage ordered (2 mg/min)? _____ mL/min (Show your calculations.)

d. How many *drops* per minute (gtt/min) is that equivalent to? _____ gtt/min (Show your calculations.)

4. Convert 12 grams to milligrams: 12 g × _____ = _____ mg

5. Convert 156 pounds to kilograms: 156 lb ÷ _____ = _____ kg (round up)

6. Now use the second method to estimate the patient's weight in kilograms.

The patient weighs 135 lb.

Step 1: Divide the patient's weight by 2: _____ ÷ 2 =_____

Step 2: Take the total from above and multiply it by 10%: _____ × .10 = _____ (round up)

*Remember to round the percentage number for easier subtraction. _____

Step 3: Take the total of step 1 and subtract the rounded percentage.

_____ – _____ = _____ patient's weight in kilograms; once again you may need to round up to

_____ . What weight would you use for the patient? _____ kg

7. You are ordered to give a patient 6 mg of morphine. The morphine comes in 10 mg/mL. How much will you give?

_____ mL

8. You are ordered to give 2 mg of Valium. Your vial contains 20 mg in 10 mL. What is the concentration on hand?

_____ mg/mL   How many mL will you give? _____ mL

9. You are ordered to deliver 10 µg/kg/min of dopamine for an 80-kg patient. You have mixed 800 mg of dopamine into a 500-mL bag of normal saline. Show your calculations for the following.

a. What is your desired dose?_____ µg/min

b. Determine your dose on hand._____ mg/mL

c. Convert the mg from answer B to µg. _____ µg/mL

d. Determine the amount of volume to infuse per minute. Use your desired dose to calculate this. _____ mL/min

e. Determine how many drops/min will deliver your desired dose, using a microdrip set (60 gtt/mL). _____ gtt/min

10. Fill in the tables below so that each row will contain four ways of representing the same values.

Microgram (μg)	Milligram (mg)	Gram (g)	Kilogram (kg)
500	0.5	0.0005	0.0000005
		1.0	
			1.0
	1.0		
1.0			
	800.0		
15.0			

Milliliter (mL)	Deciliter (dL)	Liter (L)
5,000.0	50	5.0
1.0		
	0.1	
		1.0
250.0		0.25

11. Fill in the blanks in the calculations below changing your patient's weight from pounds to kilograms using the "10% trick". Compare your answers using the formula:

patient's weight (lb) ÷ 2.2 = patient's weight (kg)

Patient's weight in pounds (lb)	Patient's weight (lb) ÷ 2	Weight (lb) ÷ 2 × 10% (move the decimal one place to the left)	Subtract your 10% from the weight ÷ 2	Patient's weight in kilograms (kg)	Patient's weight in lb ÷ 2.2 = patient's weight kilograms (kg)
60 lb	60 ÷ 2 = 30	30 × 10% = 3	30 − 3 = 27	27 kg	27.27 kg
16					
138					
8					
250					
36					
82					
180					
330					

12. Volume conversions

Fill in the blanks below indicating the amount of medication found in each bag of normal saline (NS) assuming the *concentration* is the same in each bag. Follow the example in the table below:

1,000 mL NS	500 mL NS	250 mL NS	100 mL NS	50 mL NS
100 g	50 g	25 g	10 g	5 g
	800 g			
		250 g		
			4 g	
	50 g			

13. Determine the number of milliliters (mL) of fluid infused over 1 minute to your patient by filling in the blanks below.

a. 60 gtt admin set infused 120 gtt/min = _____ mL/min

b. 15 gtt admin set infused 120 gtt/min = _____ mL/min

c. 30 gtt admin set infused 120 gtt/min = _____ mL/min

14. Convert the following temperatures from Fahrenheit (F) to Celsius (C) by completing the table below. Follow the example in the first row.

This table is based on the formula $(F - 32) \times 0.555 = C$

Temp in degrees F	Degrees F - 32	Degrees F - 32 × 0.555	Temp in degrees C
32 F			
95			
98.6	98.6 - 32 = 66.6	66.6 × 0.555 = 36.96	36.96 (approx 37)
101			
104			

15. Determine how much medication is prescribed for your patient by body weight by filling in the table below.

Desired dose	Patient's weight in pounds (lb)	Patient's weight in kilograms (kg)	Medication administered
1 mg/kg lidocaine	90	90 ÷ 2.2 = 40.9 kg (≈ 41 kg)	41 kg × 1 mg lidocaine = 41 mg lidocaine to administer
0.2 mg/kg atropine	30		
0.05 mg/kg lorezapam	180		
30 mg/kg methylprednisolone	220		
15 mg/kg phenobarbitol	12		

16. Calculate the volume of normal saline needed to administer to the following trauma patients. Base your calculations on volumes replaced at 20 mL/kg of patient body weight.

Patient's weight in pounds (lb)	Patient's weight in kilograms Weight in lb ÷ 2.2 = wt kg or use the "10% trick"	Volume to be infused with first bolus @ 20 mL/kg
60		
80		
100		
125		
150		
175		
190		
220		
300		

17. Find the weight of the following medications in 1 mL of solution:

a. 100 mg/10 mL lidocaine = _____ mg/1 mL lidocaine

b. 1 mg/10 mL epinephrine = _____ mg/1 mL epinephrine

c. 40 mg/14 mL furosemide = _____ mg/1 mL furosemide

d. 6 mg/2 mL adenosine = _____ mg/1 mL adenosine

e. 20 mg/5 mL diazepam = _____ mg/1 mL diazepam

f. 10 mg/5 mL naloxone = _____ mg/1 mL naloxone

g. 2 mg/5 mL albuterol = _____ mg/1 mL albuterol

h. 150 mg/3 mL amiodarone = _____ mg/1 mL amiodarone

i. 25 g/125 mL activated charcoal = _____ g/1 mL activated charcoal = _____ mg/1 mL activated charcoal

18. Find the weight of the following medications in 1 mL of solution:
Follow the example below.
50% dextrose = 50 g/100 mL = 0.5 g/1 mL
a. 1% xylocaine

b. 10% dextrose

c. 0.5% albuterol

   d. 10% calcium chloride

   e. 50% magnesium sulfate

   f. 5% alupent

   g. 0.9% sodium chloride

19. Determine the amount of dopamine in <u>micrograms</u> (µg) per milliliter when 800 <u>milligrams</u> (mg) of dopamine are added to the following bags of normal saline (NS). (Note: 1 mg = 1,000 µg)

   a. 800 mg dopamine is added to a 500-mL bag NS = _____ µg/mL

   b. 800 mg dopamine is added to a 250-mL bag NS = _____ µg/mL

   c. 800 mg dopamine is added to a 1,000-mL bag NS = _____ µg/mL

   d. 800 mg dopamine is added to a 100-mL bag NS = _____ µg/mL

20. Medical control has directed you to administer the correct dosage of medication for your patient (desired dose). The concentration available to you is listed for each calculation. Determine the volume of medication you will administer for each order.

   Desired dose in mg ÷ concentration in mg/mL = volume to administer

   a. You are ordered to give 15 mg labetolol. You have a vial with 100 mg/20 mL solution in stock.

   b. You are ordered to give 3 mg halperidol. You have a 1-mL ampule containing 5 mg of medication.

   c. You are directed to administer 750 mg calcium chloride. You have a bottle containing 1,000 mg of medication in 10 mL of solution.

Skill Drills

Test your knowledge of skill drills by placing the following photos in the correct order. Number the first step with a "1," the second step with a "2," etc.

1. *Drawing Medication From an Ampule*

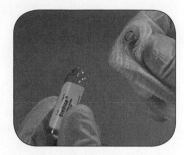

Grip the neck of the ampule using a 4" × 4" gauze pad, and snap the neck off.

_____

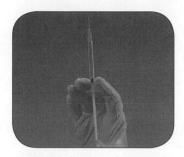

Gently press on the plunger to dispel any air bubbles, and recap the needle using the one-handed method.

_____

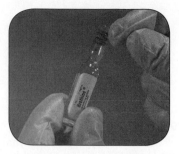

Gently tap the stem of the ampule to shake medication into the base.

_____

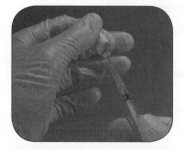

Without touching the outer sides of the ampule, insert the needle into the medication in the ampule, and draw the solution into the syringe.

_____

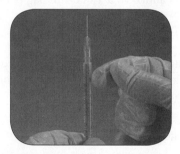

Holding the syringe with the needle pointing up, gently tap the barrel to loosen air trapped inside.

_____

2. *Administering a Medication via Small-Volume Nebulizer*

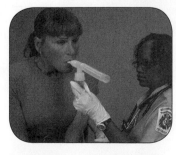

Instruct the patient to breathe as deeply as possible and hold his or her breath for 3 to 5 seconds before exhaling. Monitor the patient for effects.

_____

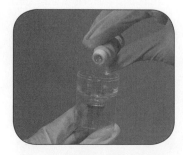

Add premixed medication to the bowl of the nebulizer.

_____

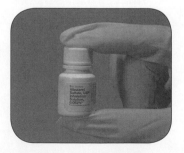

Check the medication and the expiration date.

_____

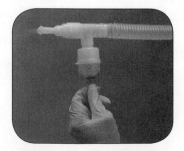

Connect the T piece with the mouthpiece to the top of the bowl, connect it to the oxygen tubing, and set the flowmeter at 6 L/min.

_____

Test your knowledge of this skill drill by filling in the correct words in the photo captions.

3. *Drawing Medication From a Vial*

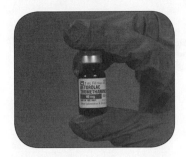

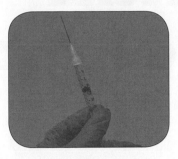

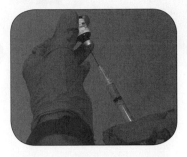

Step 1: Check the medication and its _____ date.

Step 2: Determine the amount of medication needed, and draw that amount of _____ into the syringe.

Step 3: Invert the _____, and insert the needle through the rubber stopper. Expel the air in the syringe to the vial, and then withdraw the amount of medication needed.

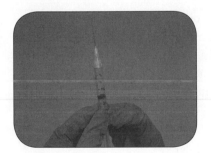

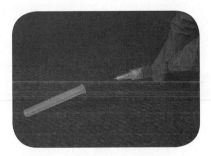

Step 4: Withdraw the _____, and expel any air in the syringe.

Step 5: Recap the needle using the _____-_____ method.

CHAPTER

9 Human Development

Chapter Review

The following exercises provide an opportunity to test your knowledge of this chapter.

Matching

Match each of the terms in the right column to the appropriate description in the left column.

_____ **1.** Person who is 1 month to 1 year of age   **A.** Adolescent

_____ **2.** Person who is 0 to 1 month of age   **B.** Early adult

_____ **3.** Person who is 3 to 6 years of age   **C.** Infant

_____ **4.** Person who is 19 to 40 years of age   **D.** Late adult

_____ **5.** Person who is 41 to 60 years of age   **E.** Middle adult

_____ **6.** Life expectancy   **F.** Preschooler

_____ **7.** Person who is 12 to 18 years of age   **G.** School age

_____ **8.** Person who is 61 years of age or older   **H.** Toddler

_____ **9.** Person who is 6 to 12 years of age   **I.** Newborn

_____ **10.** Person who is 1 to 3 years of age   **J.** Average number of years one is predicted to live

Multiple Choice

Read each item carefully, and then select the best response.

_____ **1.** When a newborn's cheek is touched, he or she turns toward the touch. This is called the _____ reflex.

    A. Moro   **C.** Sucking

    B. Palmar   **D.** Rooting

_____ **2.** The tidal volume of an infant starts at _____ mL/kg.

    A. 4 to 6   **C.** 8 to 12

    B. 6 to 8   **D.** 12 to 14

_____ **3.** Which of the infant's fontanelles can be used as a possible indicator of dehydration if sunken?

    A. Posterior   **C.** Sphenoidal

    B. Mastoid   **D.** Anterior

_____ **4.** At approximately what age does an infant start to become afraid of strangers?

    A. 1 to 2 months   **C.** 9 to 10 months

    B. 6 to 7 months   **D.** 1 year old

_____ **5.** The filtration function of the kidneys declines by about _____ percent between 20 and 90 years of age.

    A. < 25   **C.** 50

    B. 25   **D.** 75

_____ **6.** Bleeding can empty into voids in the older adult brain, resulting in what type of hemorrhage?

    A. Meningeal   **C.** Ventricular

    B. Epidural   **D.** Subdural

_____ **7.** In the 5 years preceding death, mental function is presumed to decline, a theory referred to as the:

    A. terminal drop hypothesis.   **C.** geriatric shrinkage syndrome.

    B. organic dementia hypothesis.   **D.** end-of-life physiopsych decline.

_____ **8.** In late adults, vital capacity of the lungs decreases and residual volume increases. The effect can produce which of the following conditions?

    A. Hypercarbia   **C.** Hypoxia

    B. Hypocarbia   **D.** Hyperoxygenation

_____ **9.** Which one of the following is NOT a usual response of the cardiovascular system with late adults?

    A. Decrease in heart rate   **C.** Increase in systolic blood pressure

    B. Cardiac output matches demand   **D.** Partial blockage of blood flow

_____ **10.** School-age children learn various types of reasoning in their development. Which of the following is a type of reasoning they learn?

    A. Cognitive   **C.** Conventional

    B. Distributive   **D.** Affective

Labeling

Label the four fontanelles of the infant's head.

Front

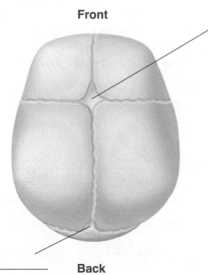

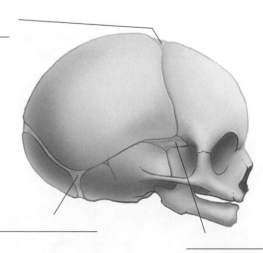

Back

Fill-in-the-Blank

Read each item carefully, and then complete the statement by filling in the missing word(s).

1. Just after birth, the ductus venosus constricts and closes. As a consequence, the infant's blood pressure changes, and the

_____ _____, an opening in the septum of the heart, closes.

2. A/an _____ _____ occurs when an object is placed in the infant's palm.

3. An infant's _____ allow the head to be molded when the newborn passes through the birth canal.

4. _____ _____, located on either end of the infant's bones, aid in the lengthening of a child's bones.

5. _____, or the formation of a close, personal relationship, is usually based on a secure attachment.

6. _____ and _____ refer to a stage of development from birth to about 18 months of age. Most infants

desire that their world be planned, organized, and _____.

7. Atherosclerosis can contribute to the development of a/an _____, or weakening and bulging of a blood vessel wall.

8. In late adults, blood flow in the _____ (membranes that connect organs to the abdominal wall) may drop by as

much as 50%.

9. In the 5 years preceding death, mental function is presumed to decline. This is a theory referred to as the _____

_____ _____.

10. In late adults, the size of the airway _____ and the surface areas of the alveoli _____.

Identify

In the following case study, list the chief complaint, vital signs, and SAMPLE history.

A call to an assisted living facility brings you to a 75-year-old woman who, while walking from the living room to the kitchen, tripped on a chair and fell. When you enter the apartment, the patient tells you she fell and has a great deal of pain in her hip. You gently palpate the injured area and the patient yells. You take a set of vital signs and find a pulse of 90 beats/min and thready, respirations of 24 breaths/min and shallow, and the blood pressure is 100/70 mm Hg. The SAMPLE history identifies an externally rotated foot and discoloration of the hip on the same side. The patient reports no allergies and is on several medications for congestive heart failure. She had a heart attack last year and she has a two-pack-a-day history of smoking for more than 30 years but stopped smoking about 5 years ago. She ate breakfast 3 hours ago. You place the patient on an ECG monitor, establish an IV, and package her for transport.

1. Chief Complaint

_____

_____

_____

2. Vital Signs

_____

_____

_____

3. SAMPLE History

_____

_____

_____

_____

_____

Ambulance Calls

The following case scenarios provide an opportunity to explore the concerns associated with patient management and paramedic care. Read each scenario, and then answer each question.

1. Your unit is dispatched to a call for an infant with a seizure. The response time is 5 minutes, and when you enter the residence you find a distraught mother who is very anxious. The seizure seems to have stopped, but you understand the importance of an immediate initial assessment (the MS–ABC Priority Plan). You immediately notice the child has good color except for a little cyanosis of the fingers. The child is actively breathing, and the rate is adequate. Your partner starts to administer blow-by oxygen, and you examine the child quickly from head to toe to make sure there is no external bleeding or signs of trauma. The child is starting to respond and become more active. You prepare for transport and decide the child is stable and alert enough so that the neurologic status can be assessed. What reflexes would you check and how would you test them? What are considered to be the appropriate response(s) from the infant? Fill in the following grid.

Reflex	How to Test	Appropriate Response
a.		
b.		
c.		
d.		

2. A call to an assisted living facility finds a 75-year-old woman sitting with her partner and complaining of general body weakness. You approach the patient but have trouble communicating with her, and while doing the SAMPLE history you have trouble getting necessary information from her. You decide that when asking about her past medical history you should ask about individual body systems because this might help to identify the current problem.

a. What are some of the communication issues that you might have encountered while taking the history of this patient?

_____

_____

_____

b. What are some possible concerns that you are thinking of while attempting to obtain the past medical history and ask the rest of the SAMPLE questions?

_____

_____

_____

3. You receive a call to a residence of a 16-year-old young woman with a chief complaint of abdominal pain. The young woman is lying on the couch in the living room and her mother and a girlfriend are also in the room. Your partner is a male who is taking the lead on the assessment and SAMPLE history. While doing the SAMPLE history, he asks the patient if there is a possibility she is pregnant. She immediately and emphatically answers no. He then decides that he should palpate the abdomen and immediately proceeds to do so with little explanation. The patient seems embarrassed. You realize that you need to package the patient and transport.

a. What consideration should your partner have taken into account before questioning this patient about the possibility of pregnancy?

_____

_____

_____

b. Is there a more appropriate way to handle the physical exam of the abdomen?

_____

_____

_____

True/False

If you believe the statement to be more true than false, write the letter "T" in the space provided. If you believe the statement to be more false than true, write the letter "F."

_____ **1.** An infant's ventilations that are too forceful can result in barotrauma.

_____ **2.** The rooting reflex occurs when an infant's lips are stroked.

_____ **3.** If the posterior fontanelle is sunken, the infant is most likely dehydrated.

_____ **4.** Anxious avoidant attachment is observed in infants who are repeatedly rejected.

_____ **5.** A toddler is at the critical age in human development to learn various types of reasoning.

_____ **6.** Cardiac function declines with age consequent to anatomic and physiologic changes largely related to atherosclerosis.

_____ **7.** In late adults, vital capacity of the lungs decreases and stagnant air remains in the alveoli and hampers gas exchange, which can produce hypercarbia.

_____ **8.** In late adults, there is a surge of increased mental functioning in the last few years of life.

_____ **9.** Age-related shrinkage creates a void between the brain and outermost layer of the meninges.

_____ **10.** The number of nephrons in the kidneys increases between ages 30 and 80 years.

Short Answer

Complete this section with short written answers using the space provided.

1. Infants are born with certain reflexes and responses that can assist you in the neurologic assessment of an infant. Name four of these reflexes.

   a. _____

   b. _____

   c. _____

   d. _____

2. Cardiac function declines with age largely as a result of atherosclerosis. This disorder, which commonly affects coronary vessels, results from the formation of plaque. What two substances are responsible for the buildup of plaque?

   a. _____

   b. _____

3. Loss of what mechanisms in the respiratory system of the late adult makes aspiration and obstruction more likely?

   a. _____

   b. _____

   c. _____

   d. _____

   e. _____

4. Late adults have sensory changes that can affect mobility and safety. What sensory changes occur in this age group?

   a. _____

   b. _____

   c. _____

   d. _____

   e. _____

5. Colds often develop and may manifest as what types of infections?

   a. _____

   b. _____

6. Playing games is the way that toddlers learn. What can a child of this age learn from play?

   a. _____

   b. _____

   c. _____

7. In the late elderly, vital capacity of the lungs decreases. Name three factors that contribute to this decline.

a. _____

b. _____

c. _____

Crossword Puzzle

Use the clues in the column to complete the puzzle.

Across

3. _____ adults are ages 41 to 60 years of age.

5. Ventilations to infants that are too forcefully applied when using a bag-valve device can result in trauma from pressure called _____.

8. _____ plates, located on either side of an infant's bones, aid in lengthening a child's bones.

9. With infants, _____, or the formation of a close, personal relationship, is usually based on secure attachments.

10. Membranes that connect organs to the abdominal wall are called _____.

11. _____ and mistrust refer to a stage of development from birth to about 18 months of age.

14. The _____ ovale is an opening in the newborn's heart that closes shortly after birth.

15. An age-related change seen in late adults is that the heart rate _____.

Down

1. A swelling or enlargement of part of a blood vessel, resulting from weakening of the vessel wall is called a/an _____.

2. School-age is the time in development when various types of _____ start to develop.

3. A/an _____ reflex is sometimes called a startle reflex and happens when an infant is caught off guard and opens his/her arms wide and spreads the fingers.

4. The _____ is an opening in the skull of an infant that, if sunken in, means the infant is most likely dehydrated.

6. Anxious _____ attachment is observed with an infant who is repeatedly rejected.

7. The brain _____ may shrink 10% to 20% by 80 years of age.

8. A palmer _____ is when an object is placed into an infant's palm.

12. Rooting _____ occurs when something touches an infant's cheek, and the infant instinctively turns his or her head toward the touch.

13. Three words that best describe an early adult's world: work, family, and _____.

Fill-in-the-Table

Fill in the missing parts of the tables.

1. Subtle changes occur during adolescence; one change is the development of secondary sexual characteristics. Fill in the table with these characteristics.

Male Characteristics	Female Characteristics

2. Fill in the table with the appropriate respiratory rates for the various ages listed to the left.

Vital Signs at Various Ages				
Age	Pulse Rate (beats/min)	Respirations (breaths/min)	Blood Pressure (mm Hg)	Temperature (°F)
Newborn (0 to 1 month)	90 to 180		50 to 70	98 to 100
Infant (1 month to 1 year)	100 to 160		70 to 95	96.8 to 99.6
Toddler (1 to 3 years)	90 to 150		80 to 100	96.8 to 99.6
Preschool age (3 to 6 years)	80 to 140		80 to 100	98.6
School age (6 to 12 years)	70 to 120		80 to 110	98.6
Adolescent (12 to 18 years)	60 to 100		90 to 110	98.6
Early adult (19 to 40 years)	70		90 to 140	98.6
Middle adult (41 to 60 years)	70		90 to 140	98.6
Late adult (61 and older)	Depends on health		Depends on health	98.6

CHAPTER

10 Patient Communication

Chapter Review

The following exercises provide an opportunity to test your knowledge of this chapter.

Matching

For each of the following questions from a patient interview, indicate whether it is:

  O = an open-ended question

  C = a closed-ended question

_____ **1.** What happened today?

_____ **2.** Do you remember the collision?

_____ **3.** What is a normal blood pressure for you?

_____ **4.** Are you pregnant?

_____ **5.** Have you been sick in the last few weeks?

_____ **6.** Do you have asthma?

_____ **7.** What medications do you take?

_____ **8.** What does the pain feel like to you?

_____ **9.** Do you wear contact lenses?

_____ **10.** How much do you weigh?

Multiple Choice

Read each item carefully, and then select the best response.

_____ **1.** Which of the following is a way to communicate with your patient?

  A. Verbal communication   **C.** Listening to the patient

  B. Body language   **D.** All of the above

_____ **2.** What is the best way to develop rapport with your patient?

  A. Have genuine concern for your patient.   **C.** Hug your patient.

  B. Always call the patient by a pet name.   **D.** Always use medical terminology.

_____ **3.** Which of the following would suggest a mental impairment when first addressing your patient?

  A. The patient responds with a coherent speech pattern.

  B. The patient does not turn and look at you when you speak.

  C. The patient waits a second before answering your question.

  D. The patient has a meaningful response to your greeting.

_____ **4.** When dealing with a fearful patient, which of the following will not be useful?

      A. Showing concern for the patient   **C.** Acting like a professional

      B. Standing with your arms crossed   **D.** Telling the patient about his ECG rhythm

_____ **5.** Which of the following strategies will help you get a useful response from your patient?

      A. Asking questions with specific medical terms   **C.** Being quiet and letting the patient talk

      B. Talking constantly with your patient   **D.** Asking the patient to write down her feelings

_____ **6.** If you don't understand what the patient is trying to say to you, you should:

      A. just nod and say, "I understand."

      B. let the patient continue until you do catch something you understand.

      C. ask the patient to explain in more detail.

      D. ask the patient a closed-ended question.

_____ **7.** What is the best way to convey honesty to your patient?

      A. By using frequent and direct eye contact   **C.** Kneeling on the floor in front of the patient

      B. Patting the patient on the arm   **D.** Always having a smile on your face

_____ **8.** When assessing a patient's memory, which of the following is NOT a useful tool?

      A. Asking the patient's name

      B. Asking the patient what he or she had for breakfast the day before

      C. Asking the patient where he is

      D. Asking the patient what happened to her

_____ **9.** Which of the following cultures consider direct eye contact rude?

      A. Islamic   **C.** Brazilian

      B. French   **D.** Asian

_____ **10.** When treating a patient from another culture, what is a good rule of thumb?

      A. Always use hand gestures.

      B. Never use hand gestures.

      C. Always use medical terms.

      D. Use pet names for the patient because it makes the patient feel you like him or her.

Fill-in-the-Blank

Read each item carefully, and then complete the statement by filling in the missing word(s).

1. The "S" in EMS stands for _____.

2. The act of transmitting information to another person is called _____.

3. When dealing with a crisis, your challenge is to remain _____.

4. Voice _____ is just as important as the words that you say.

5. When addressing your patient and waiting for the patient's response, you are actually assessing _____

pairs of the cranial nerves.

6. A/an _____-_____ _____ is a question that does not have a yes or

no answer.

7. When using touch to assure your patient, you should touch a _____ part of the patient's body.

8. If your patient is hostile, and you are unable to diffuse the patient's anger, you may need to call the

_____.

9. When treating a child, _____ are useful tools for bridging the emotional gap with the child.

10. The best offense when dealing with a cross-culture patient is _____.

Identify

In the following case study, list the chief complaint, vital signs, and pertinent negatives.

You are called to a 66-year-old woman with cancer. Upon arrival you note the patient is in a hospital bed in the living room. She is lying down and is visibly having trouble breathing. Her spouse is present and presents a DNR order. The order is the original and is current with all the appropriate signatures. By checking her driver's license you verify that the patient is the patient on the order. The husband has called because he cannot wake her. You cannot get any response from the patient, and she does not respond to a sternal rub. She still has a gag reflex. You take vital signs on the patient, which include blood pressure (you hear one thump at 46 mm Hg), respirations are 30 breaths/min and are shallow and irregular, oxygen saturation is 80% on room air, and lung sounds are hard to hear. Her pulse is very irregular and you note that it is about 32 beats/min. She is cool to the touch and you note some mottling. At this time, the hospice nurse arrives for her morning check on the patient. She explains to the spouse that there is nothing your team can do, and the end of the patient's life is nearing. You clean up your equipment and tell the husband that you are sorry and ask him if there is anything you can do for him. He thanks you and says no, that the hospice nurse has made all the arrangements. After talking to your supervisor, you return to your unit to service for the next call.

1. Chief Complaint

_____

_____

_____

2. Vital Signs

_____

_____

_____

3. Pertinent Negatives

_____

_____

_____

Ambulance Calls

The following case scenarios provide an opportunity to explore the concerns associated with patient management and paramedic care. Read each scenario, and then answer each question.

1. You are called to the scene of a bad road collision in which a semitrailer plowed head-on into a passenger car. The driver of the car is pinned inside his vehicle, very seriously injured. You manage to gain access to the patient and start tending to him while you await help in what will be a lengthy extrication procedure. The patient is still conscious, and he asks you, "Am I going to die?" There is, in fact, a high probability that he *will* die. Describe how you would reply to this patient's question.

_____

_____

_____

_____

_____

_____

2. You are called to a suburban neighborhood where a 22-year-old diabetic patient is having some problems with her glucose levels. Your assessment determines that you need to start an IV and give the patient D_{50}. How would you explain to your patient what you are about to do?

_____

_____

_____

_____

_____

_____

3. You are dispatched to a call for chest pain. The scene is a large farm in the rural Midwest. Upon your arrival, a man in a pickup truck meets you at the front gate. He waves for you to follow him. He leads you to a large area on the farm where many camper-trailers are parked. As you get out of your ambulance, the driver of the truck approaches you. He introduces himself as the owner of the farm, and tells you that the grandmother of his harvest foreman is experiencing chest pain. He also explains that the foreman and his family are migrant farm workers, who speak mostly Spanish.

As you enter a camper, a worried Hispanic gentleman meets you, and the farmer introduces you as "el paramedico." The man extends his hand to you to shake it, and says, "Gracias, gracias, señor," and gestures for you follow him. You are led to a cramped bedroom, where an elderly Hispanic woman is lying on a bed, propped up with several blankets. There are several Catholic icons on the wall, as well as a statue of the Virgin Mary at the bedside. The woman has a string of beads in her hand. You notice several small candles burning on a dresser next to the bed. The man gestures toward her and says,

"Mi abuela." The woman presents with pale complexion, diaphoresis, obvious dyspnea, and has a facial grimace that you associate with severe pain. You have an EMT-B partner and an EMT-B student intern riding with you, so you direct your partner to start setting up the ECG monitor, and the student to take vital signs. The excited student says, "Yo," and starts to work. Knowing the patient needs oxygen, you bend over and blow out the candles, not wanting the hazard of open flame around the oxygen. This action really seems to upset the woman, who lets out a little cry. You don't speak any Spanish, so you kneel beside the bed, and very slowly ask, "What . . . is . . . your . . . name?" The woman looks in confusion to her grandson, who says "nombre." The woman tells you, very proudly, "Mi nombre es Señora Talia Elizabet Cordoba de Castille." You feel around your uniform for your pen to write it down, and realize you left it in the ambulance. You find the red pen you have been using to correct the student's reports, and begin to write down her name. The woman lets out a hysterical shriek, and tries to back away from you on the bed. There is suddenly much excited confusion in the room, and the grandson is trying desperately to calm his grandmother. The woman is very agitated, and the ECG monitor shows you a sinus tachycardia with several PVCs. You tell the EMT-B student to run and get the cot. He responds with another "yo" and makes the "rock on" sign with his left hand. The woman's eyes get wide and she shrieks again, only this time she faints. The grandson cries out, "Abuela!" and then tearfully asks you to perform last rites. You inform the grandson that his grandmother is not dead, but needs to be transported immediately. You really don't like the way this call is progressing and just want to get back in the ambulance.

In the preceding scenario, you not only have a language barrier, but a religious one as well. Hispanic families are very close-knit, and older Hispanics are generally very religious, especially those who have come from the "old country." The majority practice Roman Catholicism and may also be very superstitious. Old World beliefs in the forces of good and evil may be very prevalent, and traditional religious practices may also be interspersed with additional spiritual beliefs. Some of these may include Candomble, which is a mixture of Roman Catholicism and African Voodoo, practiced predominately in the Pan-Caribbean regions and South America; Santeria, which is popular in Cuba, the Caribbean, and South America; espiritismo, which is practiced in Puerto Rico and Central America predominately; and curanderismo, which is found in Mexico, the American Southwest, and still exists in "Old Spain."

In some of these traditions, the color yellow is associated with death, the color red with witchcraft, and white with resisting evil spells. Thus, writing a person's name in red ink may be perceived as an attempt to "cast a spell" and gain power over the individual.

Hispanics generally use two surnames. The first surname listed is from the father, and the second surname listed is from the mother. When speaking to someone, use his or her father's surname. A married woman may attach her husband's surname to the end of hers with a "de." A widower may indicate her widowed status by including "vda" (widow of) in her name as well. Hispanics are very proud of their family names, and a good name is often more important than wealth or status. They also expect to be treated with dignity and respect (familiar theme, no?) and will reciprocate the same. It is very important in the paramedic–patient relationship to treat the Hispanic patient with polite formality and address them by title (Mr., Mrs., Señor, Señora). Once rapport is established, the paramedic can gain valuable inroads in the trust factor by politely asking about family members or loved ones. Hispanics, especially older Hispanics, base clinical trust on *individual* perception, not an institutional one.

a. What should you have asked the farmer before you entered the residence?

_____

_____

_____

_____

b. Upon seeing all the religious symbols in the room, what should you have done before blowing out the candles?

_____

_____

_____

_____

c. Why did the student intern upset the woman?

_____

_____

_____

_____

_____

_____

d. Why is a translator so important at this scene?

_____

_____

_____

_____

True/False

If you believe the statement to be more true than false, write the letter "T" in the space provided. If you believe the statement to be more false than true, write the letter "F."

_____   **1.** Active listening begins with repeating the key parts of the patient's responses to questions.

_____   **2.** During a loud scene, the best thing to do is shout.

_____   **3.** People in a crisis could care less about your nonverbal communications.

_____   **4.** It is okay to use pet names with your patients.

_____   **5.** One of the most important treatments you can provide is reassurance.

_____   **6.** Your morals must always take a back seat to your professional ethics.

_____   **7.** A "payoff" question may provide you with hidden reasons for the patient's illness.

_____   **8.** You should always provide false hope for a patient who is facing death.

_____   **9.** When your patient is afraid, you should act like a law enforcement officer because it provides assurance to your patient.

_____   **10.** You should involve the parents when you are assessing a small child.

Short Answer

Complete this section with short written answers using the space provided.

1. Describe the three types of questions/techniques that can make your questioning more productive during an interview with your patient.

   a. _____

   b. _____

   c. _____

2. List three nonverbal communication skills that you think you will use the most as a paramedic.

   a. _____

   b. _____

   c. _____

3. You respond to a very hostile patient who appears to be having a psychiatric problem. He is pacing back and forth and is yelling words that are not making sense. What would you do in this situation?

   _____

   _____

   _____

   _____

   _____

   _____

Crossword Puzzle

Use the clues in the column to complete the puzzle.

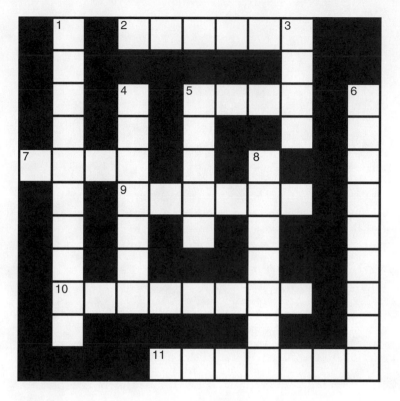

Across

2. Adolescents can be very _____ when it comes to examining their bodies.
5. _____ language is a form of communication.
7. Use the patient's name like a _____.
9. A/an _____-ended question will give you a yes or no answer.
10. A form of aggressive body language might be a _____ fist.
11. When touching your patient to convey assurance, you should touch them in a _____ spot.

Down

1. Direct _____ _____ conveys honesty to your patients.
3. _____ are useful when dealing with a scared child.
4. When a patient thanks you, you should say you're _____.
5. When assessing a pediatric patient, you should be at or _____ their eye level.
6. Touching your patient is a _____ communication skill.
8. One word that will help you deal with all patients is _____.

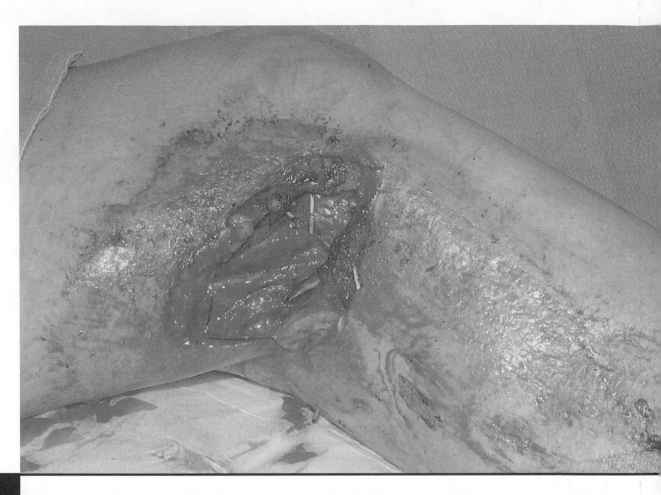

50-Year-Old Male with Severe External Bleeding

You are dispatched to a residence at 325 West San Saba for a 50-year-old male involved in a chainsaw accident. Dispatch advises you that the caller was panicked, stating that the patient was "bleeding to death." The time of call is 9:30 AM, and your response time to the scene is less than 3 minutes.

You arrive at the scene to find the patient sitting in his front yard. He is screaming in pain while attempting to stop the bleeding from a severe avulsion injury behind his right knee. The patient's wife tells you that her husband was cutting wood with a chainsaw. Evidently, the chainsaw slipped and swung around behind him, striking him behind the knee. You perform an initial assessment while your partner begins immediate treatment.

Initial Assessment

Mechanism of Injury	Chainsaw injury to the leg
Level of Consciousness	Conscious and alert, restless
Chief Complaint	Severe avulsion injury behind the right knee
Airway and Breathing	Airway is patent; respirations, increased with adequate tidal volume
Circulation	Pulse is weak and rapid; skin is cool, clammy, and pale; bright red blood is spurting from the injury behind his knee

1. What is the appropriate order of initial management for this patient?

_____

_____

_____

_____

The appropriate initial management has been provided for the patient. Because the patient is experiencing signs of shock, you perform a rapid trauma assessment. Your partner quickly retrieves the stretcher from the ambulance.

Rapid Trauma Assessment

Head	No obvious trauma
Neck	Trachea is midline; jugular veins, normal; no cervical spine deformities.
Chest	No obvious trauma; chest wall, stable and symmetrical; breath sounds, clear and equal bilaterally to auscultation
Abdomen/Pelvis	Abdomen, soft and nontender; pelvis, stable
Lower Extremities	Large avulsion behind right knee (bandaged); pedal pulses, bilaterally absent; sensory and motor functions, grossly intact
Upper Extremities	No obvious trauma; radial pulses, present and weak; sensory and motor functions; grossly intact
Posterior	No obvious trauma

After placing the patient onto the stretcher, he is quickly loaded into the ambulance. While you are setting up your IV lines, your partner notices that blood is soaking through the dressing covering the patient's wound.

2. How will you manage the continued bleeding from the patient's injury?

_____

_____

_____

_____

Additional measures have controlled the bleeding from the patient's injury. While you are preparing to start two large-bore IV lines, your partner obtains baseline vital signs and a SAMPLE history. A cardiac monitor is applied and reveals a sinus tachycardia at 130 beats/min.

Baseline Vital Signs and SAMPLE History

Blood Pressure	84/54 mm Hg
Pulse	132 beats/min, weak and regular
Respirations	24 breaths/min, adequate tidal volume
Oxygen Saturation	96% (on 100% oxygen)
Signs and Symptoms	Avulsion injury with severe bleeding (controlled), signs of shock
Allergies	Demerol, Amoxicillin
Medications	Lotrel
Pertinent Past History	Hypertension
Last Oral Intake	Breakfast, 3 hours ago
Events Leading to the Injury	"I was cutting wood with a chainsaw, when it slipped."

You depart the scene for a trauma center located approximately 25 miles away. Two large-bore IV lines have been successfully established, and you adjust the flow rates accordingly. The patient remains conscious; however, he is increasingly restless.

3. What is the appropriate IV fluid resuscitation regimen for this patient?

4. What is the difference between crystalloid and colloid solutions?

After infusing the appropriate volume of normal saline, the patient's condition has improved. He is less restless, and his blood pressure is now 96/60 mm Hg. After reassessing the bandaged wound and noting that the bleeding remains controlled, you perform a detailed physical examination.

Detailed Physical Examination

Head and Face	No obvious trauma to the scalp; ears, nose, and mouth are clear; pupils are midpoint, equal, and reactive to light.
Neck	Trachea is midline; jugular veins, normal; no cervical spine deformities.
Chest	No obvious trauma; chest wall, stable and symmetrical; breath sounds, clear and equal bilaterally to auscultation
Abdomen/Pelvis	Abdomen, soft and nontender; pelvis, stable
Lower Extremities	Large avulsion behind right knee (bandaged); pedal pulses, bilaterally absent; sensory and motor functions, grossly intact
Upper Extremities	No obvious trauma; radial pulses, present and stronger; sensory and motor functions, grossly intact
Posterior	No obvious trauma

5. What is the purpose of performing a detailed physical examination?

_____

_____

_____

_____

The patient's condition continues to improve with your treatment. He remains conscious and alert; however, he is still slightly restless. The cardiac monitor displays a sinus tachycardia at 100 beats/min. With an estimated time of arrival at the trauma center of 10 minutes, you perform an ongoing assessment and then call your radio report to the receiving facility.

Ongoing Assessment

Level of Consciousness	Conscious and alert to person, place, and time; slightly restless
Airway and Breathing	Airway remains patent; respirations, 18 breaths/min with adequate tidal volume
Oxygen Saturation	98% (on 100% oxygen)
Blood Pressure	108/70 mm Hg
Pulse	100 beats/min, stronger and regular
ECG	Sinus tachycardia

Upon arriving at the trauma center, you are greeted by the attending physician. After further stabilization in the emergency department, the patient is taken to surgery where a partially severed popliteal artery was found and successfully repaired. Following a brief stay in the hospital, the patient was discharged home.

CHAPTER

11 Airway Management and Ventilation

Chapter Review

The following exercises provide an opportunity to test your knowledge of this chapter.

Matching

For each of the patients described here, indicate which of the following is the best method for opening the airway.

A. Head tilt–chin lift   **B.** Jaw-thrust maneuver

_____ **1.** A construction worker found unconscious on the ground after falling 30 feet from scaffolding.

_____ **2.** A 35-year-old man found unconscious from a drug overdose; he is breathing spontaneously.

_____ **3.** A 45-year-old man in cardiac arrest from a probable heart attack. You have arrived at his side without any ancillary equipment.

_____ **4.** A 15-year-old boy who dove into a shallow pool and struck his head on the bottom. Bystanders removed him from the pool before you arrived. He is unconscious but breathing spontaneously (and noisily) when you arrive.

Nasotracheal intubation is an excellent technique for establishing control over the airway under selected circumstances. In other circumstances, it is preferable to insert the tracheal tube through the mouth; and in yet other circumstances, it may be necessary to establish an airway surgically, by cricothyrotomy. For each of the following patients indicate which of the following intubation method is preferred:

N Blind nasotracheal intubation is the preferred technique.

T Tracheal intubation is the preferred technique.

C Cricothyrotomy is the preferred technique.

_____ **5.** A 60-year-old man in cardiac arrest.

_____ **6.** A 22-year-old woman with complete airway obstruction from laryngeal edema.

_____ **7.** A 26-year-old collision victim with clear fluid draining from his nose and left ear.

_____ **8.** An 18-year-old man in a coma from a drug overdose.

_____ **9.** A 42-year-old woman extricated from a wrecked car; she is unconscious and has a depressed skull fracture at the back of her head.

_____ **10.** A 58-year-old man with pulmonary edema; he has been taking warfarin (Coumadin; an anticoagulant drug) ever since his heart attack last year.

_____ **11.** A 6-year-old boy who choked on a piece of meat.

_____ **12.** A 50-year-old man who was given succinylcholine (a paralyzing drug) prior to an intubation attempt; the attempt failed, and afterward it became impossible to maintain his airway by manual methods.

For each of the following patients, indicate the most appropriate device for administering supplemental oxygen. You may choose among the following. (*Note:* You may use any of the items once, more than once, or not at all.)

A. Nasal cannula

B. Nonrebreathing mask

C. Pocket mask with added oxygen

D. Bag-mask device with an oxygen reservoir

E. Flow-restricted, oxygen-powered ventilation device

_____ **13.** A 60-year-old man in severe respiratory distress from pulmonary edema.

_____ **14.** A 52-year-old man complaining of crushing chest pain.

_____ **15.** A car crash victim in cardiac arrest; you are doing one-rescuer cardiopulmonary resuscitation (CPR) because your partner is busy with another casualty.

_____ **16.** An 81-year-old woman who suddenly stopped speaking this morning and cannot move her left arm or left leg.

_____ **17.** A 22-year-old man who has overdosed on heroin; he is unconscious and breathing shallowly 6 breaths/min.

_____ **18.** A 32-year-old car crash victim who was thrown forward against the steering wheel; he is coughing up blood, and his lips look rather blue.

_____ **19.** A middle-aged man who collapsed in the street; he is in cardiac arrest by the time you arrive.

_____ **20.** An unconscious child rescued from a house fire.

Multiple Choice

Read each item carefully, and then select the best response.

_____ **1.** What is the leaf-shaped structure that prevents food and liquid from getting into the larynx during swallowing?

A. Vallecula **C.** Epiglottis

B. Uvula **D.** Pharynx

_____ **2.** What is the most common airway obstruction?

A. The tongue **C.** Blood

B. Food **D.** Vomitus

_____ **3.** What is the preferred device to deliver supplemental oxygen to the patient who is breathing?

A. Nasal cannula **C.** Simple face mask

B. Bag-mask device **D.** Nonrebreathing mask

_____ **4.** What is the most definite way to control the airway in an unconscious patient?

A. Bag-mask device **C.** Oral airway adjunct

B. Endotracheal tube **D.** Head tilt–chin lift

_____ **5.** In what position should the patient's head be placed when preparing to intubate with a Combitube?

A. Flexed forward **C.** Hyperextended back

B. Neutral position **D.** Slightly to the right

_____ **6.** What medication is the only depolarizing neuromuscular blocking agent that is used in the field?

A. Vecuronium **C.** Norcuron

B. Pancuronium **D.** Succinylcholine

_____ **7.** How much sterile saline should you have ready when you are performing a needle cricothyrotomy?

A. 3 mL **C.** 7 mL

B. 5 mL **D.** 10 mL

_____ **8.** How much alveolar volume does the typical adult have?

        A. 150 mL   **C.** 500 mL

        B. 350 mL   **D.** 3,000 mL

_____ **9.** The diaphragm is innervated by which of the following nerves?

        A. Intercostal nerves   **C.** Phrenic nerves

        B. Vagus nerve   **D.** Diaphragmatic nerve

_____ **10.** Which abnormal respiratory pattern do you see in the patient with ketoacidosis?

        A. Cheyne-Stokes   **C.** Biots

        B. Agonal   **D.** Kussmaul

_____ **11.** What is the major advantage of a multilumen airway device?

        A. It fits all patients from pediatric to adult.   **C.** It cannot be placed improperly.

        B. It prevents all aspiration.   **D.** It always provides 100% oxygen to the patient.

_____ **12.** Which of the following is *not* a complication of placing a multilumen airway device?

        A. Vomiting   **C.** Esophageal trauma

        B. Unrecognized displacement of the tube   **D.** Hyperventilation

_____ **13.** How much air should inflate the proximal balloon on the Combitube?

        A. 15 mL   **C.** 100 mL

        B. 25 mL   **D.** 150 mL

_____ **14.** When should you use a laryngeal mask airway (LMA) in the field?

        A. When the patient cannot be intubated as an alternative to the bag-mask device (alone)

        B. When the patient is morbidly obese and has a difficult airway

        C. When the patient has coronary heart failure (CHF) and is unconscious

        D. When the patient is under 5 feet tall and needs attention to the airway

_____ **15.** How many sizes does the LMA come in?

        A. 3   **C.** 7

        B. 5   **D.** 10

Labeling

Label the following diagrams with the correct terms.

    1. Parts of the larynx

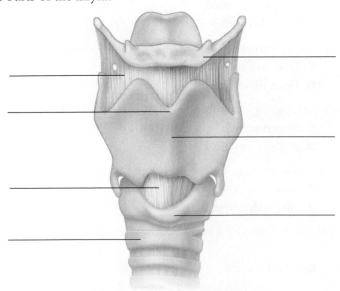

2. The child's epiglottis and surrounding structures.

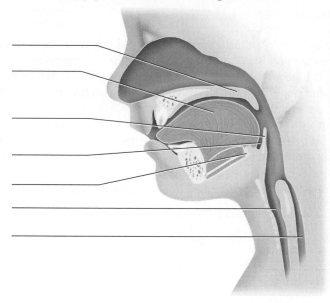

Fill-in-the-Blank

Read each item carefully, and then complete the statement by filling in the missing word(s).

1. The principal *hazard* associated with intubation is _____. That hazard can be minimized by _____.

2. For tracheal intubation to proceed smoothly, it is essential to position the patient correctly to bring the trachea into alignment with the mouth and pharynx. To do so, you need to place the patient in the _____ position.

3. An intubation attempt should take no longer than _____ seconds.

4. Breathing is normally controlled by a respiratory center in the brain stem. In a healthy person, the primary stimulus to breathe is a _____ (rise or fall) in the level of _____ (oxygen or carbon dioxide) in the blood. In some patients with chronic obstructive pulmonary disease, that mechanism is no longer fully operative, and *their* principal stimulus to breathe is a _____ (rise or fall) in the level of _____ (oxygen or carbon dioxide) in the blood.

5. Foreign body airway obstructions are sometimes the result of decreased airway reflexes. These are caused by _____ and _____ _____.

6. When you suction the airway, a nonrigid catheter is called a _____-_____, but the rigid tip is called a _____-_____ catheter.

7. When you insert an oral airway into a pediatric patient, the airway device is inserted with the tip _____ _____ _____ _____ _____ _____.

8. You should always adequately _____ a patient before you intubate.

Identify

In the following case study, list the chief complaint, vital signs, and pertinent negatives.

You are called to the high school for a teenager choking. When you arrive, you are directed to a 14-year-old boy who was walking down the hallway when someone scared him from behind. He was chewing on a small cap of a pen when this happened and has sucked the cap into his airway. He is seated in the tripod position and is blue around the lips. You immediately assess that he is breathing because with each breath he makes a whistling noise. A teacher performed the Heimlich maneuver on him in the hallway initially, and he can at least draw a small breath in. Your partner applies a nonrebreathing mask at 15 L/min. The patient is breathing 28 breaths/min and shallow. He has decreased lung sounds on the right side and clear sounds on the left. His heart rate is 98 beats/min and regular and his blood pressure is 128/86 mm Hg. His skin is blue tinged in the face and fingertips and is cool. His oxygen saturation is 88%, and he is a little confused. Because the patient is conscious and you know the cap is in the lungs, and because of the sounds in the lung fields, you position the boy on the cot sitting up with oxygen running and take off for the hospital. You run code 3 (lights and siren) into the emergency department (ED). Later, you learn the patient had to be taken into surgery to remove the cap.

1. Chief Complaint

_____

_____

_____

2. Vital Signs

_____

_____

_____

3. Pertinent Negatives

_____

_____

_____

Ambulance Calls

The following case scenarios provide an opportunity to explore the concerns associated with patient management and paramedic care. Read each scenario, and then answer each question.

1. You finish a call and return to Joe's Steak 'n Lobster Shack where you were having dinner when a previous emergency arose. You hope that they haven't already fed your sirloin to the dog. Happily, Joe has kept your steak waiting for you, and he whips it into the microwave to rewarm it. At last, the steak is back in front of you, along with a generous order of french fries. You lift your knife and fork to dig in when out of the corner of your eye you see a strange pantomime occurring two tables away. A middle-aged man in a business suit suddenly pushes himself away from the table, clutches his neck, and lurches to his feet. He staggers a few paces, and then pitches to the floor—all in complete silence.

   a. The man is showing signs of:

      (1) food poisoning.

      (2) choking.

      (3) strep throat.

      (4) anaphylaxis.

      (5) hysteria.

b. What treatment is needed?

        (1) Pump out his stomach.

        (2) Give him manual thrusts.

        (3) Have him gargle with salt water.

        (4) Give epinephrine 1:1,000, 0.5 mL SQ.

        (5) Give diazepam (Valium), 10 mg IM.

2. You are having a barbecue in the backyard one Sunday. The beer has been flowing freely, and everyone is in a jolly mood. You tell a funny story, and everyone present starts laughing uproariously, including one of your friends who had just taken a big bite out of his hot dog. Suddenly, he starts coughing violently. His face gets very red.

  a. At that point, you should do which of the following actions?

        (1) Tilt his head back and attempt to ventilate.

        (2) Perform a quick finger sweep to remove accessible obstructing material.

        (3) Give manual thrusts.

        (4) Reach into his throat with the barbecue tongs and try to snare the hot dog.

        (5) Encourage him to keep coughing.

  b. That course of action does not seem to help. Your friend becomes completely silent, and his face turns a dusky gray as he struggles to breathe. What should you do now?

        (1) Tilt his head back and attempt to ventilate.

        (2) Perform a quick finger sweep to remove accessible obstructing material.

        (3) Do the Heimlich maneuver.

        (4) Reach into his throat with the barbecue tongs and try to snare the hot dog.

        (5) Encourage him to keep coughing.

  c. Your friend collapses unconscious to the ground. List the next four steps you would take.

    (1) _____

    (2) _____

    (3) _____

    (4) _____

  d. Meanwhile an ambulance has arrived (someone had the sense to phone 9-1-1!), and a couple of paramedics come stampeding through your flower garden carrying what looks like all the equipment from their rig. Now that you have equipment available, what steps will be taken?

    (1) _____

    (2) _____

    (3) _____

3. You are struggling to intubate a 30-year-old body builder who collapsed while working out at the local health club. You found him in cardiac arrest. Despite the fact that you have positioned him just as the textbook instructs, you can't seem to bring his vocal cords into view; they remain hidden just above your laryngoscope blade.

  a. To bring the cords into view, you ask your partner to _____ _____ _____

    _____ _____ _____ _____ .

b. That maneuver also accomplishes another useful thing, namely, it helps prevent _____ _____ with aspiration during positive-pressure ventilation.

c. You manage at last to insert the endotracheal tube. Now you need to make sure that the tube is really in the trachea. List two of the many ways of verifying that the endotracheal tube is in the right place.

(1) _____

(2) _____

4. You are attempting a blind nasotracheal intubation on a 60-kg 24-year-old individual who took an overdose of sleeping pills. You have succeeded in advancing the tip of the endotracheal tube just beyond the oropharynx.

a. As you continue to advance the tube, how can you tell whether the tip is moving toward the glottis (as opposed to the esophagus)?

(1) _____

(2) _____

b. As you are advancing the tube, you become aware that the bleeps from the cardiac monitor are getting farther apart. What has happened?

_____

_____

c. What should you do about it?

(1) _____

(2) _____

(3) _____

d. As you try again to advance the tube, you notice gastric contents creeping up the back of the patient's throat, a process

called _____.

e. What is the danger associated with that process?

_____

_____

f. What should you do about it?

_____

_____

g. The tip of the tracheal tube is finally just where you want it—poised above the vocal cords awaiting the final push into the trachea. At what point in the respiratory cycle will you give the tube that final push?

_____

_____

5. You are involved in a search-and-rescue mission to find a middle-aged hiker lost in the woods. At last you find him, sitting down propped against a tree. He tells you that he experienced severe chest pain and could not go on. Because there is a strong possibility that he is experiencing an acute myocardial infarction (heart attack), you and your partner will have to carry him back to the ambulance, about a 40-minute walk. You hook the patient to supplemental oxygen via nasal cannula at a flow rate of 5 L/min. You notice that the pressure gauge on your E cylinder is reading 800 psi.

a. How long is the oxygen in the E cylinder going to last?

_____

_____

b. Is that going to be long enough to get the patient back to the ambulance? (Show your calculations.)

_____

_____

6. You are sitting at the movies on your night off when you notice someone a few rows ahead of you suddenly slump over. You leap like a gazelle over several rows of seats to reach the person's side, and you discover that he has stopped breathing. You drag him into an aisle and start mouth-to-mouth ventilation. How can you tell if you are actually getting air into his lungs?

(1) _____

(2) _____

(3) _____

7. As you continue mouth-to-mouth ventilation on the patient described in question 6, you reflect that you would like to avoid causing gastric distention because you would prefer not to deal with the mess that might follow.

a. What can you do to minimize gastric distention during artificial ventilation?

(1) _____

(2) _____

(3) _____

b. Despite your best efforts, however, you notice the man's belly is starting to get enlarged. What should you do?

_____

_____

c. After about another 3 or 4 minutes, his belly is *much* larger, and you are finding it very hard to ventilate him. What should you do now?

_____

_____

8. After your experience in the movie theater, you promise yourself that you will never go *anywhere* without a pocket mask in your pocket, not only to make things more pleasant for yourself, but also because the pocket mask has several advantages over other methods of giving artificial ventilation. List four advantages of a pocket mask.

(1) _____

(2) _____

(3) _____

(4) _____

9. A 53-year-old man calls for an ambulance because of shortness of breath. You find him in severe respiratory distress, with foam bubbling out of his mouth. Your examination reveals signs of congestive heart failure (a condition in which fluid backs up into the lungs and interferes with gas exchange).

a. The patient's pulse oximeter reading when you first arrive shows an oxygen saturation (SaO_2) of 86%. That reading is (Circle the best answer):

       (1) normal for the patient's age.   **(3)** abnormally low.

       (2) abnormally high.   **(4)** probably an artifact.

b. What measure should you take immediately?

_____

_____

c. You treat the patient according to your protocol for congestive heart failure (we'll learn more about all that in Chapter 27), and his condition improves markedly. Now the oxygen saturation reading is 96%. You move the patient to a stretcher and bring him out to the ambulance for transport. When you have him loaded in the ambulance, you notice that the oxygen saturation is now reading 85%. The patient, however, still looks comfortable and is not in any respiratory distress, so you conclude that the reading on the pulse oximeter must be an error. List three of the possible causes of the erroneous reading in this patient:

(1) _____

(2) _____

(3) _____

10. You are attempting a blind nasotracheal intubation on an unconscious patient who took an overdose of sleeping pills. When you think you have the tracheal tube in place, you check out the end-tidal carbon dioxide monitor that you've snapped onto the tracheal tube. Its color is purple, indicating that the air being exhaled through the tube contains less than 0.5% carbon dioxide.

a. What can you conclude from that reading?

_____

_____

b. What actions should you take?

_____

_____

11. A passenger riding in a car is breathing quietly at 12 breaths/min, taking in 500 mL of air with each breath.

a. What is his minute volume? _____ mL per minute

b. The car is struck by a semitrailer. The passenger receives an injury to his cervical spine, which paralyzes him from the neck down (his intercostal muscles are also affected). His respiratory rate increases to 20 breaths/min, but his tidal volume falls to 200 mL. What is his minute volume now? _____ mL/min

c. What effect do you expect that change in minute volume to have on the patient's arterial PCO_2?

_____

_____

d. That, in turn, will cause the patient's pH to _____ (rise or fall).

e. The resulting derangement in his acid–base balance is called a _____ (respiratory or metabolic)

_____ (acidosis or alkalosis).

f. What treatment is required?

_____

_____

12. Now it's on to a cardiac arrest in a fourth-floor walk-up apartment. You grab the jump kit and the handiest D cylinder from the ambulance, while your partner takes the drug box and defibrillator, and you sprint up the four flights of stairs to the patient's apartment. While your partner starts CPR, you "crack" the oxygen cylinder, hook up the oxygen to a bag-mask device, and open the flow control to 10 L/min. As you do so, you notice the reading on the pressure gauge is 900 psi. How much time do you have before you need to switch to a fresh cylinder?

_____ minutes (The cylinder constant for a D cylinder is 0.16. Show your calculations.)

_____

_____

13. A 34-year-old man has been injured in a road collision in which his head apparently struck the windshield with some force. When you first reach the scene, the patient is unconscious. He is breathing 8 breaths/min, inhaling approximately 500 mL of air with each breath.

a. What is his minute volume? _____ per minute

b. Is that volume greater or less than normal? _____

c. Therefore, we can conclude that the patient's arterial PCO_2 will tend to _____ (increase or decrease), so his

pH will _____ (increase or decrease). The net effect will be an acid–base disorder called a _____

(respiratory or metabolic) _____ (acidosis or alkalosis). The way you can help correct that abnormality

is to _____.

14. You are doing a shift in the emergency department, and the laboratory calls down with a blood gas report. You notice that the PCO_2 reported is quite high (hypercarbia)—about 55 mm Hg.

a. Hypercarbia can be caused by:

(1) _____

(2) _____

(3) _____

(4) _____

b. What can be done to normalize the patient's PCO_2?

_____

_____

15. The laboratory calls down another blood gas report. "You'd better check on this guy," the lab technician says. "His PO_2 is only 48 mm Hg." As you sprint off to alert the doctor about the blood gas results, you review in your mind the conditions that can cause hypoxemia.

a. List six conditions that can cause hypoxemia.

(1) _____

(2) _____

(3) _____

(4) _____

(5) _____

(6) _____

b. What is the treatment for hypoxemia?

_____

_____

c. A compound whose pH is *less* than 7.0 is called a/an _____, whereas a compound whose pH is *greater* than 7.0 is called a/an _____.

d. A/an _____ is a substance that dissociates into charged components in water. A positively charged molecule, such as Na^+, is a/an _____, whereas a negatively charged molecule, such as Cl^-, is called a/an

_____.

e. The most important component of the red blood cell, or _____, is an iron-containing protein called

_____, which binds oxygen in the lungs and releases oxygen in the tissues. When that protein is not saturated with oxygen, it imparts a bluish color to the blood, which is reflected in a bluish color of the skin called _____.

f. When there is failure of tissue perfusion for any reason, the resulting state is called _____. One way that state can come about is if there is cardiac standstill or _____. However that state of inadequate tissue perfusion occurs, one of the immediate results is that the body cells, unable to obtain enough oxygen, switch to _____ metabolism.

True/False

If you believe the statement to be more true than false, write the letter "T" in the space provided. If you believe the statement to be more false than true, write the letter "F."

_____ **1.** Any patient who is to be suctioned should first be preoxygenated.

_____ **2.** You should not suction while inserting the catheter.

_____ **3.** Suction for only 2 minutes at a time.

_____ **4.** A tonsil-tip catheter is a good choice for suctioning the oropharynx.

_____ **5.** Once a patient is intubated, suction through the tracheal tube every 5 to 10 minutes to keep the tube free of secretions.

Short Answer

Complete this section with short written answers using the space provided.

1. Obstruction of the upper airway is an immediate threat to life. The upper airway may become obstructed in several ways. List four causes of upper airway obstruction, and put an asterisk beside the most common cause.

a. _____

b. _____

c. _____

d. _____

2. Tracheal intubation has several advantages over other methods of airway control. List three advantages of endotracheal intubation.

a. _____

b. _____

c. _____

3. Despite all its advantages, endotracheal intubation is not for all patients. Like every other medical procedure, it has specific indications. List three indications for endotracheal intubation.

a. _____

b. _____

c. _____

4. Endotracheal intubation is not without potential complications. The most serious acute complications can, however, be avoided by meticulous attention to correct technique.

a. List a potential complication of endotracheal intubation.

_____

b. How can it be avoided?

(1) _____

(2) _____

(3) _____

c. How can it be detected and corrected if it does occur?

(1) _____

(2) _____

(3) _____

d. List another potential complication of endotracheal intubation.

_____

e. How can it be avoided?

_____

f. How can it be detected and corrected if it does occur?

_____

_____

5. In some emergency medical services (EMS) systems, paramedics are authorized to use paralyzing drugs to facilitate tracheal intubation. Although such drugs undoubtedly make life easier for the paramedic, they may make life quite precarious for the _patient_! What is the principal hazard of administering a neuromuscular blocking agent to a patient who needs to be intubated?

_____

_____

_____

_____

6. A person is breathing quietly at 12 breaths/min with a tidal volume of 500 mL.
   a. Calculate his _minute volume_.

_____

   b. List two things that could cause his minute volume to _decrease_.

   (1) _____

   (2) _____

   c. If the person's minute volume does decrease, what change will you see in his arterial blood gases?

_____

_____

7. Oxygen is a drug, and like any other drug, it should be given when there are indications for its use. List six indications for administering supplemental oxygen to a patient.

   a. _____

   b. _____

   c. _____

   d. _____

   e. _____

   f. _____

8. Sometimes the patient himself will "tell" you, through his symptoms and signs, that either his oxygenation, his ventilation, or both are insufficient—that he is suffering from acute respiratory insufficiency. List four signs of acute respiratory insufficiency.

a. _____

b. _____

c. _____

d. _____

9. Oxygen is stored in cylinders at pressures up to 2,000 psi, which means that oxygen cylinders have to be treated with respect! List six safety precautions that should be observed when using or storing oxygen cylinders.

a. _____

b. _____

c. _____

d. _____

e. _____

f. _____

10. Respiratory arrest occurs quite a way down the pathway from life to death. List six things that can cause a person to stop breathing.

a. _____

b. _____

c. _____

d. _____

e. _____

f. _____

11. List three ways of identifying someone in respiratory arrest.

a. _____

b. _____

c. _____

12. A person who has suffered respiratory arrest will need _____ (controlled or assisted) ventilation.

13. What is the difference between controlled and assisted ventilation?

_____

_____

_____

14. What is the objective of *any* form of artificial ventilation?

_____

_____

_____

15. List three situations in which information from pulse oximetry could be helpful to you in the field.

a. _____

b. _____

c. _____

16. A car crash victim who has sustained injury to the cervical spinal cord may develop weakness or paralysis of his respiratory muscles. If so, such a patient may not have the strength to inhale as deeply as he otherwise would. Thus, his minute volume will _____ (increase or decrease), leading to a/an _____ in his arterial PCO_2.

17. It is critically important to recognize a person who is choking so that appropriate measures can be taken quickly enough to prevent that person from dying from hypoxemia.

   a. List three signs of choking.

   (1) _____

   (2) _____

   (3) _____

   b. List the steps in treating a conscious, choking victim (assume that you have with you any equipment you might need).

   (1) _____

   (2) _____

   (3) _____

18. List eight indications for administering supplemental oxygen.

   a. _____

   b. _____

   c. _____

   d. _____

   e. _____

   f. _____

   g. _____

   h. _____

19. List four signs of respiratory distress.

a. _____

b. _____

c. _____

d. _____

20. List three indications for endotracheal intubation in the prehospital setting.

a. _____

b. _____

c. _____

21. What treatment would you give a patient found in respiratory acidosis?

_____

_____

_____

Word Find

Hidden in the following grid are 35 words or phrases related to what you have studied in this chapter. Find the hidden words in the grid below. Then use the words from the grid to answer the following questions (some words may be used to answer more than one of the questions).

```
A R E S P I R A T I O N J H W H K
A N Q S I N G U L T U S S Y Y E G
N A I C I T A I B R A C O P Y H A
C R E R A E J X S A O B E O L L B
B E M O A R B A U C R R V V V R G
A S U F T C B R H H V R K E O A D
R Y L S E O T O C E A D O N H I E
U W O V L S H H N A A L C T G M A
E E V G E T G T O D U H O I U E D
L T E L C A I O R S I X F L O X S
P E T O T L R M B O Y O O A C O P
H Z U T A S L U L G A V X T X P A
A G N T S R R E E E L W Z I U Y C
R I I I I P S N N A J L V O D H E
Y O M S S G Y P D L A R Y N X E V
N I E A D A A I B R A C R E P Y H
X S S H U N T D I A P H R A G M S
```

1. Imagine you are an oxygen molecule floating past someone's face, minding your own business, just as that person is starting to take a deep breath. As his _____ and _____ contract, the volume of his chest increases, so that the pressure inside the chest (intrathoracic pressure) decreases. As a consequence, air is sucked in through the _____, and you are swept along with it.

After having a shower and completing a security check in the nasal hairs, you enter the _____. You then proceed down the _____, through the _____, and into the _____. (Had you gone down the esophagus instead, you would eventually have been expelled from the stomach as part of a/an _____.) Moving a little farther, you find yourself at a crossroads, called the _____, where you can either take a left turn into the left _____ or a right turn into the right _____. You choose the straighter, shorter path, to the _____. The airway in which you are traveling branches many times into smaller and smaller _____, until finally you reach a tiny sac at the end of the road, a/an _____. There you find the first opportunity to cross a membrane into a capillary and board a red blood cell for the journey to peripheral tissues. (Up to this point in your journey, you have been traveling only in _____, that is, the part of the airway where gas exchange does not take place.)

Some of your friends who started the journey with you did not make it as far as you did. One of them accidentally tickled the throat on his way down the airway and got expelled with gale force by a/an _____, which is the airway's most powerful mechanism for eliminating foreign material. Another of your colleagues found himself recruited into a hiccup, also known as _____.

Yet another friend of yours made the journey all the way down the airway only to find the air spaces at the end of the line collapsed, a situation called _____. It had come about when a little bleb on the surface of the lung ruptured, allowing air to enter the space between the visceral and parietal _____, and thereby creating a small _____. The net effect was that blood reaching the collapsed alveoli could not pick up any _____ like yourself, but rather had to return to the left heart as if it had never passed through the lungs at all, a situation called _____. If a very large proportion of alveoli are nonfunctional (eg, collapsed, filled with fluids), a large part of the blood circulating through the lungs will be similarly affected, and the person's arterial PCO_2 will fall below normal (ie, below about 60 mm Hg), a condition known as _____.

Sometimes scattered alveoli collapse simply because a person doesn't take deep enough breaths to keep all his alveoli inflated. The body therefore has a mechanism to help periodically pop open collapsed alveoli, and that is to _____. Do so now, before you proceed to the next question.

2. The exchange of gases among the tissues, lungs, and atmosphere is called _____. The movement of air in and out of the lungs (more specifically, the flushing of _____ out of the lungs by breathing) is called _____, and it is inhaled or exhaled each minute, that is, the _____ (= respiratory rate × _____). If that volume of air inhaled each minute is *less* than normal, the arterial PCO_2 _____ (falls or rises), and the blood gases show _____ (excess CO_2 in the blood). We call that situation _____, that is, breathing that is insufficient to remove excess CO_2 from the body. The most extreme example occurs when a person is not breathing at all (respiratory arrest, or _____).

On the other hand, when someone breathes very deeply or very rapidly (or both), his PCO_2 will fall; that is, he will develop _____. We refer to that situation—when excessive breathing lowers the PCO_2 below about 35 mm Hg—as _____.

Fill-in-the-Table

Fill in the missing parts of the table.

1. In mastering the use of any given piece of equipment, it is essential to learn not only *how* to use the equipment but also *when* to use it (and when *not* to use it). Artificial airways can be enormously helpful when applied in the appropriate circumstances; they can be downright dangerous when used in inappropriate circumstances. Fill in the following table to summarize the indications and contraindications for the oropharyngeal airway (OPA) and the nasopharyngeal airway (NPA).

	Oropharyngeal Airway	Nasopharyngeal Airway
Use for		
Do not use for		

2. Oxygen-Delivery Devices

Device	Flow Rate	Oxygen Delivered
Nasal cannula		
Nonrebreathing mask		
Bag-mask device with reservoir		

3. Airway adjuncts can be very helpful in ensuring a patent air passage, but one needs to use the right adjunct in the right situation. Fill in the following table to remind yourself what to use (and not to use) when.

Adjunct	Indicated for	Do not use in
Oropharyngeal airway		
Combitube		
LMA		
Endotracheal intubation		

Skill Drills

Test your knowledge of skill drills by placing the following photos in the correct order. Number the first step with a "1," the second step with a "2," and so forth.

1. *Nasogastric Tube Insertion in a Conscious Patient*

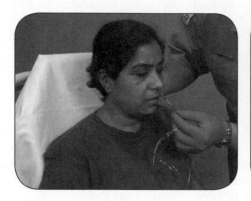

Advance the tube gently along the nasal floor.

_____

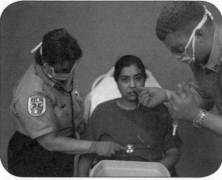

Confirm proper placement: auscultate over the epigastrium while injecting 30 to 50 mL of air and/or observe for gastric contents in the tube. There should be no reflux around the tube.

_____

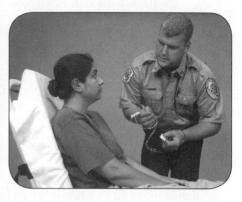

Explain the procedure to the patient, and oxygenate the patient if necessary. Ensure that the patient's head is in a neutral position and suppress the gag reflex with a topical anesthetic spray.

_____

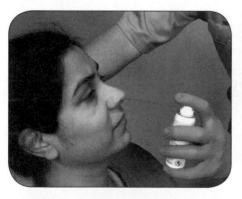

Constrict the blood vessels in the nares with a topical alpha agonist.

_____

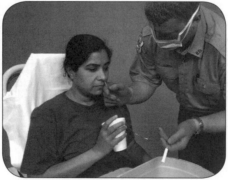

Encourage the patient to swallow or drink to facilitate passage of the tube.

_____

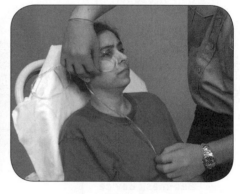

Measure the tube for the correct depth of insertion (nose to ear to xiphoid process).

_____

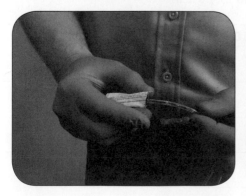

Lubricate the tube with a water-soluble gel.

_____

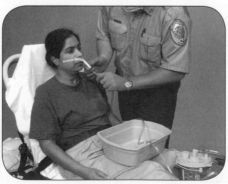

Apply suction to the tube to aspirate the gastric contents, and secure the tube in place.

_____

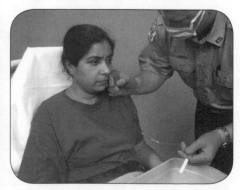

Advance the tube into the stomach.

_____

2. *Using Colorimetric Capnography for Carbon Dioxide Detection*

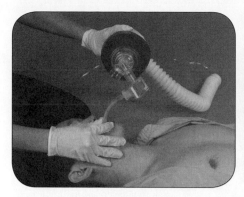

Monitor the device for appropriate reading (appropriate color change or digital reading).

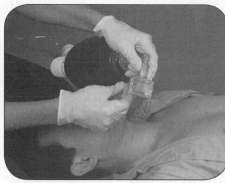

Reattach the ventilation device to the ET tube, and resume ventilations.

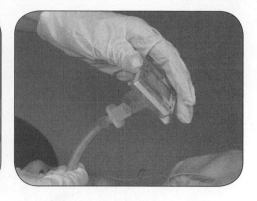

Attach an in-line colorimetric capnographer or capnometer to the proximal adapter of the ET tube.

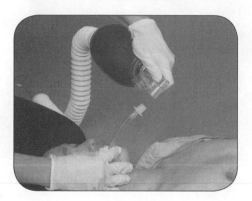

Detach the ventilation device from the ET tube.

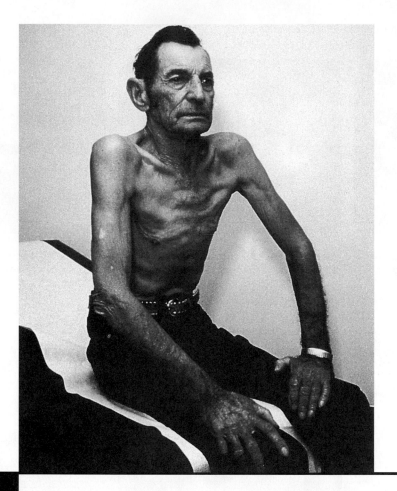

62-Year-Old Male in Respiratory Distress

At 11:55 am, your unit is dispatched to a local urgent care clinic at 321 S Main St for a 62-year-old male with respiratory distress. Your response time to the scene is approximately 3 minutes.

You arrive at the clinic at 11:58 and are directed to one of the treatment rooms by a nurse. You find the patient sitting in a tripod position in obvious respiratory distress. You introduce yourself to the patient, who speaks to you in broken sentences. As your partner opens the jump kit, you perform an initial assessment.

Initial Assessment

Level of consciousness	The patient is slow to answer questions, and states in broken sentences, "I am having more trouble breathing than I usually do."
Chief complaint	Conscious, but confused
Airway and breathing	Airway patent; respirations, rapid and labored
Circulation	Radial pulse, increased, weak, and irregular; perioral cyanosis present

The clinic nurse tells you that she attempted to place the patient on oxygen, but he kept removing the mask from his face. She tried applying a nasal cannula, which the patient also refused.

1. What initial management is indicated for this patient?

_____

_____

_____

_____

With the assistance of the clinic nurse, your partner initiates the appropriate airway management. The nurse tells you that the patient's condition has worsened since he first arrived at the clinic. She provides you with his presenting information as you perform a focused history and physical examination.

Focused History and Physical Examination

Onset	"The patient told me that he recently had 'flu-like symptoms', which were followed by a sudden worsening of the respiratory distress that he normally has."
Provocation/palliation	"He said that it was a little easier to breathe when he leans forward."
Quality	"He was able to speak in full sentences initially, but now he can barely get two words out."
Radiation/referred pain	"He did not complain of any pain."
Severity	"Compared to his initial presentation, his breathing is much worse now."
Time	"He told me that this began yesterday afternoon."
Interventions prior to EMS arrival	"I tried to give him oxygen, but he would not allow it, either by face mask or nasal cannula."
Chest exam	Chest is barrel-shaped; intercostal retractions and use of accessory muscles are noted.
Breath sounds	Breath sounds are diminished bilaterally; expiratory wheezing and rhonchi are heard in all lung fields.
Oxygen saturation	83% (ventilated with 100% oxygen)
Temperature	101.5° F

The patient was placed on a cardiac monitor prior to your arrival. You run a 6-second strip and analyze his cardiac rhythm (**Figure 2-1**).

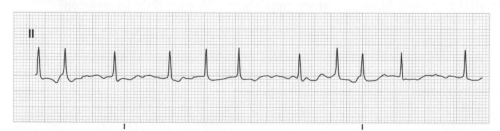

■ **Figure 2-1** Your patient's cardiac rhythm.

2. What is your interpretation of this cardiac rhythm?

_____

_____

_____

_____

You obtain baseline vital signs and a SAMPLE history. A receptionist hands you the patient's medical records, from which you obtain his medical history.

Baseline Vital Signs and SAMPLE History	
Blood pressure	148/88 mm Hg
Pulse	110 beats/min, weak and irregular
Respirations	32 breaths/min, labored (baseline); ventilation rate, 15 breaths/min
Oxygen saturation	81% (ventilated with 100% oxygen)
Signs and symptoms	Recent cold symptoms, severe respiratory distress, retractions, cyanosis, confusion
Allergies	Penicillin, aspirin, Demerol
Medications	Albuterol, Lanoxin, warfarin, Aldomet
Pertinent past history	Emphysema, hypertension, atrial fibrillation, long history of smoking
Last oral intake	According to the nurse, "His last meal was the previous night. He could not remember the exact time."
Events leading to present illness	Recent cold symptoms

3. What is your field impression of this patient?

_____

_____

_____

As your partner continues to manage the patient's airway, you quickly establish an IV line of normal saline and set the flow rate to keep the vein open.

4. Are the patient's vital signs and SAMPLE history consistent with your field impression?

_____

_____

_____

Despite positive pressure ventilation with the bag-valve-mask (BVM) device, the patient's oxygen saturation continues to fall. Additionally, his mental status has markedly diminished. Your partner states that he is meeting significant resistance when ventilating.

5. What specific treatment is required for this patient's condition?

_____

_____

_____

Your partner has definitively secured the patient's airway, and the appropriate medications have been administered. Following these interventions, a quick reassessment of the patient shows marked improvement in oxygen saturation. You place him onto the stretcher, load him into the ambulance, and begin transport to a hospital that is 7 miles away. En route, you connect the patient to an automatic transport ventilator (ATV), perform an ongoing assessment, and then call your radio report to the receiving hospital.

Ongoing Assessment	
Level of consciousness	Improved, becoming resistant to ventilatory support
Airway and breathing	Intubated and ventilated at a rate of 15 breaths/min
Oxygen saturation	92% (ventilated with 100% oxygen)
Blood pressure	138/80 mm Hg
Pulse	96 beats/min, strong and irregular
Chest exam	Minimal intercostal retractions
Breath sounds	Widespread rales and a few wheezes, otherwise equal bilaterally

6. Is further treatment required for this patient?

_____

_____

_____

7. Are there any special considerations for this patient?

_____

_____

_____

The patient is delivered to the emergency department. His condition has improved significantly following your treatment. You give your verbal report to the attending physician, who orders a stat portable chest radiograph and an arterial blood gas analysis.

Following additional assessment and management in the emergency department, the patient is diagnosed with acute chronic obstructive pulmonary disease (COPD) exacerbation secondary to pneumonia.

He is given additional medications, including antibiotics, and is admitted to the medical intensive care unit. Following a 10-day stay in the hospital, the patient is discharged home.

CHAPTER

12 Patient History

Chapter Review

The following exercises provide an opportunity to test your knowledge of this chapter.

Matching

For each of the following questions from a patient interview, indicate whether it is:

A. A well-phrased question   **B.** A poorly phrased question

_____ **1.** What seems to be the problem?

_____ **2.** When did all this start?

_____ **3.** Did the pain start when you were exerting yourself?

_____ **4.** What is the pain like?

_____ **5.** Is the pain sharp or dull?

_____ **6.** Do you get short of breath when the pain comes on?

_____ **7.** Has the pain gotten worse since it started?

_____ **8.** How has the pain changed since it started?

_____ **9.** What were you doing when the pain started?

_____ **10.** Have you ever had pain like this before?

_____ **11.** What medications do you take regularly?

_____ **12.** Are you allergic to any medications?

_____ **13.** What else is bothering you, besides the pain?

Multiple Choice

Read each item carefully, and then select the best response.

_____ **1.** When responding to a call, a paramedic's demeanor and appearance should be all of the following except:

    A. clean.   **C.** positive.

    B. overbearing.   **D.** efficient.

_____ **2.** Which of the following statements/questions would be considered a facilitating communication technique?

    A. That's all the information I need.

    B. You don't have to tell me if you don't want to.

    C. Can you think of anything else about his medical history?

    D. Can you narrow down his history to just the past few months?

_____ **3.** Which communication technique is not helpful in a stressful situation?

    A. Confrontation   **C.** Empathetic response

    B. Facilitation   **D.** Clarification

_____ **4.** What should the thinking paramedic do when faced with a possible physical abuse situation?

    A. Document.   **C.** Accuse the abuser to try and get the real story.

    B. Gather evidence in a paper bag.   **D.** Call for law enforcement before leaving the scene.

_____ **5.** When a patient has a period of silence during a call, it should make you:

    A. begin to ask more questions.

    B. realize the patient may not trust you and respect the silence.

    C. look for a reason the patient is not talking such as a change in condition.

    D. look for a weapon on the patient.

_____ **6.** Your patient will not quit talking! Which of the following reasons is *not* a reason for chattiness?

    A. The patient is on meth.   **C.** The patient has had several cups of coffee.

    B. The patient is very nervous.   **D.** All of the above.

_____ **7.** You are dealing with a very angry young man who is being arrested for DWI. He has a broken leg and arm, and you are transporting him to the hospital. What is the best way to treat this situation?

    A. Make sure you strap him down tight to the backboard so he can't get away.

    B. Tell him if he doesn't calm down you will give him some Valium and calm him down yourself.

    C. Treat him as you would any patient and keep your anger and smart comments to yourself.

    D. Yell back at him and let him know that you are the boss and will not tolerate this in the back of your squad.

_____ **8.** Which statement is false when dealing with a blind person?

    A. Always put things back exactly where you picked them up from.

    B. Speak slowly and clearly.

    C. Announce your identity and reason for being there.

    D. Let the person know where you are and where you are going to at all times during transport.

_____ **9.** Which of the following signs and symptoms are *not* a sign of depression?

    A. Feeling of high energy   **C.** Eating disruptions

    B. Irritability   **D.** Pain with no source

_____ **10.** What is a good thing to remember when asking for history from family members?

    A. They will always know the patient's history.

    B. They will be aware of drug or alcohol use.

    C. You are not at liberty to share the patient's condition with them.

    D. You will be able to give them an update on the patient once they reach the hospital.

Labeling

Place the letter S for sick (life-threatening) or the letters NS for not sick next to each person according to the signs and symptoms.

_____   **1.** 18-month-old boy who is limp and dusky blue in the face

_____   **2.** 54-year-old woman with diffuse abdominal pain

_____   **3.** 43-year-old man with confusion, sweating, and left arm pain

_____   **4.** 22-year-old woman with rapid breathing, tingling in arms and feet

_____   **5.** 4-year-old girl who is crying and has pain in her ear

_____ **6.** 75-year-old man who is unable to speak or answer questions

_____ **7.** 66-year-old woman who is unresponsive and breathing deeply and rapidly

_____ **8.** 36-year-old woman who is depressed and doesn't want to talk

Fill-in-the-Blank

Read each item carefully, and then complete the statement by filling in the missing word(s).

1. You will make your _____ _____ based on the patient's chief complaint, vital signs, and history.

2. The first step in making an approach to a patient is to _____ _____.

3. Once you have established the patient's chief complaint, you will want to check into the history of the _____ _____.

4. Always try to position yourself at the patient's _____ _____ when you are asking questions.

5. You respond to a patient that is deaf. When communicating with the patient, you should be _____ _____ _____ with him or her.

6. _____ is described as one step above sympathy.

7. When talking with a patient, you repeat back to the patient a short synopsis of what he or she has told you; this technique is known as _____.

8. _____ governs the disclosure of patient information.

9. Always review transfer information before transferring a patient to a new facility so you know the patient's _____ _____.

10. When you are gathering information, you must be _____ and _____.

Ambulance Calls

The following case scenarios provide an opportunity to explore the concerns associated with patient management and paramedic care. Read each scenario, and then answer each question.

1. You are called to the crash scene pictured on the following page.

    a. List four potential sources of information about what happened to the patient or about his medical background.

        (1) _____

        (2) _____

        (3) _____

        (4) _____

    b. List five pieces of information you can derive simply from observing the scene.

        (1) _____

        (2) _____

        (3) _____

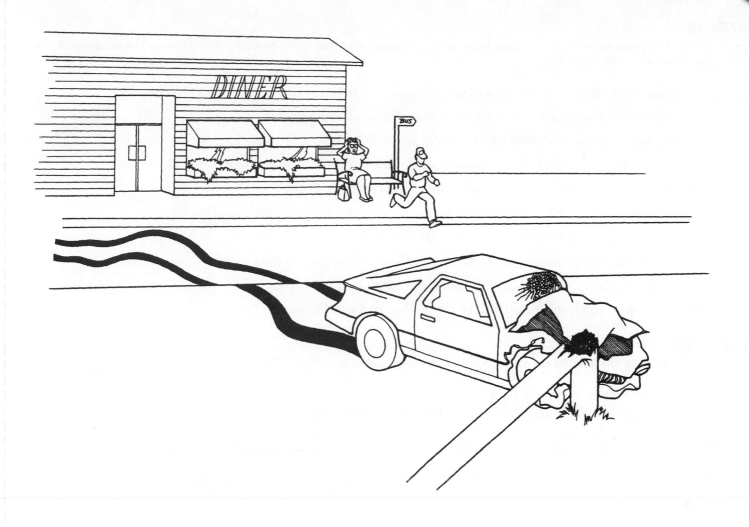

(4) _____

(5) _____

c. List four reasons why it is necessary to take a history from the driver of the car.

(1) _____

(2) _____

(3) _____

(4) _____

d. Before you start taking the history, however, you need to take some preliminary steps. List them.

(1) _____

(2) _____

(3) _____

(4) _____

(5) _____

True/False

If you believe the statement to be more true than false, write the letter "T" in the space provided. If you believe the statement to be more false than true, write the letter "F."

_____ **1.** Being able to think and perform well under pressure is a big part of being able to be a good paramedic.

_____ **2.** Patients will always be honest when it comes to their sexual history.

_____ **3.** You will always be able to tell who is a heavy user of alcohol.

_____ **4.** Patients sometimes need a few seconds to gather their thoughts and answer your questions.

_____ **5.** Law enforcement should be called for EVERY hostile patient.

_____ **6.** You should always check blood glucose on every patient that has an altered mental status.

_____ **7.** Patients may suffer trauma because of a medical problem.

_____ **8.** You should be able to make your field diagnosis based on the patient's chief complaint.

_____ **9.** Using "pet names" with a patient will put the person at ease.

_____ **10.** Clarification technique is used when trying to clear up a vague history.

Short Answer

Complete this section with short written answers using the space provided.

1. A patient's chief complaint is "pain in my gut."

   a. List six questions you would ask in eliciting the *history of the present illness*.

      (1) _____

      (2) _____

      (3) _____

      (4) _____

      (5) _____

      (6) _____

   b. List four questions you would ask about his *other medical history*.

      (1) _____

      (2) _____

      (3) _____

      (4) _____

2. Taking the history of a patient with a head injury may provide important clues to the nature of the injury and its potential seriousness. List five questions that need to be answered in taking the history of a patient with a head injury:

   a. _____

   b. _____

   c. _____

d. _____

e. _____

3. You are called to the scene of a multi-vehicle crash on the interstate highway. As you approach the scene, you begin making your size-up of the scene. List four questions you need to answer in making your size-up of the collision scene.

a. _____

b. _____

c. _____

d. _____

4. Patient assessment consists largely of detective work—searching for and interpreting clues to form a picture of the patient's problem. At the scene of an incident or, for that matter, in the patient's home, there may be several sources of information about the patient. List four potential sources of information about the patient and what has happened to him or her.

a. _____

b. _____

c. _____

d. _____

Word Find

Hidden in the following grid are 17 signs and 17 symptoms related to what you have studied in this chapter. Find the hidden words in the grid below. Then use the words from the grid and categorize each word as a sign or a symptom.

```
S E P S C T R G Y D Y N A B J T R H N P H
B L D S S Y N Q F X O H S A R G E T A R Z
H C I R O I A E N I W L L H E B G I O U A
M N I P L R U N S I C R A M P S N Y F B E
S H I L U G E N O W U L S I T C U I E H N
T H E A I P E T H S I A E N P Y H C A T P
E W A T P T D E H T I E Y E K C A L B N S
S A A L O T E E O R O S Z G I H P U F A Y
L F R P B Z S S T P O X C D N P N Q V U D
R I Y A I E I E A A W A Y D D F E U R S R
F H I N C S H L H O L O T N I X A M N E V
P E G I R H L T J C C I L R Z Z I J O A G
F D V X B O E N A W P M D U Z D U D I K D
W U A E R E S I U R B P Q B Y G K I T D V
U I B R R P D P N L S J Z T S M K W S R Z
H E A D A C H E D H I F R R P D Q H E Q D
O D Q O E Y P W I W C D L A E I T Y G V Y
S T O M A C H A C H E T M E L A C A I E M
S T R I D O R F E L V A I H L J T R D L O
S N I E V K C E N D E D N E T S I D N C B
G L Q J V L A L H F H X G I Y B M A I I W
```

Signs

1. _____
2. _____
3. _____
4. _____
5. _____
6. _____
7. _____
8. _____
9. _____
10. _____
11. _____
12. _____
13. _____
14. _____
15. _____
16. _____
17. _____

Symptoms

1. _____
2. _____
3. _____
4. _____
5. _____
6. _____
7. _____
8. _____
9. _____
10. _____
11. _____
12. _____
13. _____
14. _____
15. _____
16. _____
17. _____

Fill-in-the-Table

Fill in the EMS lingo for the following clues that were provided by your patient:

Layman's Lingo	EMS Lingo
My sugars	
Fell out	
Has the fits	
Water pills	

CHAPTER

13 Physical Examination

Chapter Review

The following exercises provide an opportunity to test your knowledge of this chapter.

Matching

Match each of the conditions in the right column to the appropriate skin description in the left column.

_____	**1.** Hot, red, dry	**A.**	Shock
_____	**2.** Hot, red, wet	**B.**	Heat stroke
_____	**3.** Cold, white, dry	**C.**	Cold exposure
_____	**4.** Cold, pale, clammy	**D.**	Fever

Match each of the following abnormal respiratory noises with the description that best fits.

_____ **1.** Fine, crackling sounds produced by airways popping open   **A.** Snoring

_____ **2.** High-pitched, whistling sounds produced by air moving through narrowed small airways (bronchioles)   **B.** Gurgling

    C. Stridor

_____ **3.** Rasping sound that signals partial upper airway obstruction by the tongue   **D.** Crackles

    E. Wheezes

_____ **4.** Sound made by fluid in the pharynx or larynx

_____ **5.** Harsh inspiratory squeak produced by severe narrowing of the upper airway, as in laryngeal edema

Match each of the signs listed to the right with the phrase that best describes its possible diagnostic significance. (Note: More than one sign may have the same diagnostic significance.)

_____ **1.** Narcotics overdose

_____ **2.** Cardiac arrest

_____ **3.** Heart failure

_____ **4.** Skull fracture

_____ **5.** Stroke

_____ **6.** Hypoxemia

_____ **7.** Respiratory distress

_____ **8.** Shock

_____ **9.** Diabetic ketoacidosis

_____ **10.** Spinal cord injury

_____ **11.** Increased right ventricular pressure

_____ **12.** Laryngeal edema

_____ **13.** Pelvic fracture

_____ **14.** Fluid/blood in the pericardium

_____ **15.** Intra-abdominal bleeding

_____ **16.** Peritonitis

_____ **17.** Fracture of the orbit (eye socket in the skull)

_____ **18.** Pneumothorax

A. Ecchymosis around the eyes

B. Fruity odor to the breath

C. Stridor

D. Pitting edema of both ankles

E. Paralysis of upward gaze

F. Muffled heart sounds

G. Battle's sign

H. Patient lies very still; cries out when stretcher is jarred

I. Pinpoint pupils

J. Cyanosis of the lips

K. Capillary refill takes 5 seconds

L. Restlessness

M. Absent pulse

N. Retraction of the suprasternal muscles

O. Jugular veins distended to 10 cm with the patient sitting

P. Crackling sensation in the skin over the chest

Q. Distended, bruised abdomen in trauma victim

R. Pain on compression of the iliac crests

S. Priapism

T. No movement or sensation in the right arm or leg

U. S_3 gallop

V. Clear fluid draining from the ear

Multiple Choice

Read each item carefully, and then select the best response.

_____ **1.** While assessing a trauma patient, you press down lightly on the abdomen. This technique is called:

    A. inspection.

    B. percussion.

    C. auscultation.

    D. palpation.

_____ **2.** When using a pulse oximeter, which of the following statements is NOT true?

    A. It measures only the percentage of hemoglobin saturation.

    B. It can help determine the patient's heart rhythm.

    C. A cold person can have a false reading.

    D. A hypotensive patient can have a false reading.

_____ **3.** What is essential in getting an accurate blood pressure reading?

    A. Using the right size cuff

    B. Not having any clothing on the arm

    C. Having the arm perfectly straight

    D. The age of the patient

_____ **4.** When assessing a patient's mental status, _P_ on the AVPU scale stands for which of the following?

    A. Pupil size

    B. Pallor of the skin

    C. Painful stimuli

    D. Presence

_____ **5.** Clubbing of the fingertips is possibly caused by which of the following conditions?

     A. Bacterial endocarditis   **C.** Chronic respiratory disease

     B. Systemic illness   **D.** Cirrhosis of the liver

_____ **6.** An elderly woman who was walking across the living room reports that she felt and heard a "pop" in her hip and she fell down. You think that there is a possibility she has a broken hip. What process has happened to create this injury?

     A. Pathologic fracture   **C.** Psychogenic fracture

     B. Physiologic fracture   **D.** Psychical fracture

_____ **7.** In assessing a spine, you find an exaggerated inward curve of the lumbar area. This is known as:

     A. kyphosis.   **C.** Cullen's sign.

     B. lordosis.   **D.** dislocation of the lumbar spine.

_____ **8.** You are auscultating the carotid arteries and you hear a "whooshing." You are hearing bruit, and this indicates:

     A. a heart murmur.

     B. turbulent blood flow around a cardiac valve.

     C. turbulent blood flow in the carotid arteries.

     D. turbulent blood flow around a cardiac valve.

_____ **9.** When checking the cranial nerve IV, you will be checking for which of the following?

     A. Hearing and balance   **C.** Visual acuity

     B. Smell   **D.** Eye movements

_____ **10.** You are assessing a patient and notice cyanotic patches on the lower extremities. This is known as _____, and it is seen in severe states of shock and hypoperfusion.

     A. tenting   **C.** mottling

     B. turgor   **D.** crepitus

Labeling

Label the following diagrams with the missing terms.

1. Nine Regions of the Abdomen

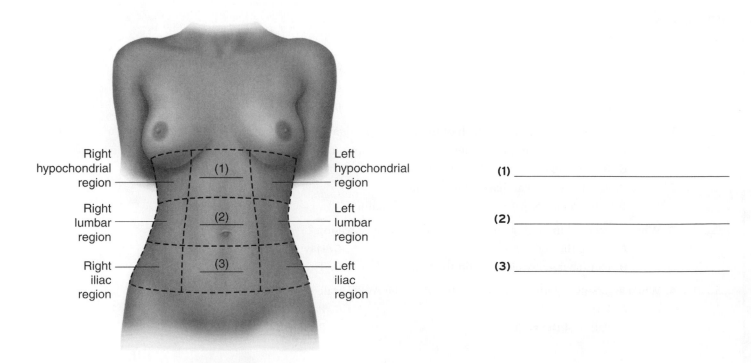

(1) _____

(2) _____

(3) _____

2. Lymphatic System

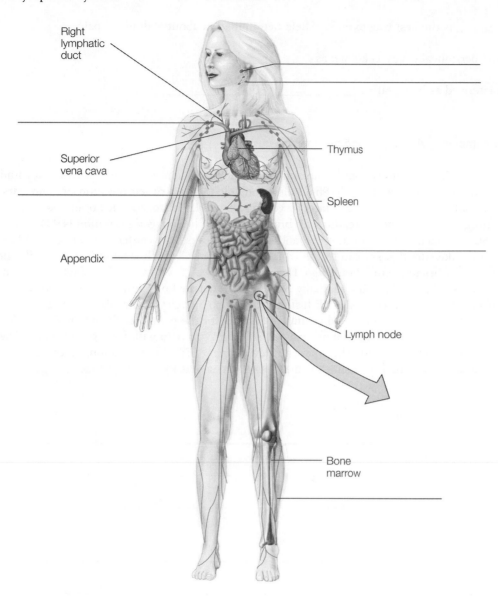

Right
lymphatic
duct

Superior
vena cava

Thymus

Spleen

Appendix

Lymph node

Bone
marrow

Fill-in-the-Blank

Read each item carefully, and then complete the statement by filling in the missing word(s).

1. _____ _____ are the most basic, objective data when determining patient status.

2. The _____ allows you to look inside a patient's eyes and assess the retina.

3. The largest organ system in the body is the _____.

4. In normal room light, pupils will appear to be _____, with less light they will _____, and with high

levels of light the pupils will _____.

5. In the second phase of a chest exam, the _____ _____ is conducted.

6. Rhonchi sounds are _____ _____ in the base of the lungs.

7. Filling and contraction of the heart produces _____, and _____ happens during cardiac relaxation.

8. A/an _____ _____ is the best way to make a field determination about abdominal pain.

9. A collection of fluid buildup in the peritoneal cavity is known as _____.

10. Abdominal organs are often characterized as being either _____ or _____.

Identify

In the following case study, list the chief complaint, vital signs, and pertinent negatives.

Chuck and Susan are called to a residence for a 28-year-old woman complaining of abdominal pain. Upon their arrival, they find the patient, Lori, on the couch with her knees drawn up to her stomach. She is alert and able to answer their questions, but appears to be in a lot of distress. Her skin is pale and cool to the touch. Chuck starts by getting a SAMPLE history while Susan takes the vital signs. Her respirations are even, and the lungs are clear. She is breathing 20 breaths/min and her oxygen saturation is 98%. Lori's blood pressure is low, at 100/78 mm Hg. Susan attaches the heart monitor, and it shows a sinus tachycardia with a rate of 112 beats/min. Susan also takes the pulse manually to make sure that she can feel the quality of the pulse, which is bounding. Lori rates her pain at an 8 on a scale of 1 to 10 and says that it began about 3 hours ago. Her last period was 5 weeks ago, but she has been late before and doesn't think that she is pregnant. She has no bleeding vaginally. Susan does a detailed physical exam on Lori's abdomen, finding severe pain and rigidity in the lower left quadrant. Her SAMPLE history showed no allergies or medications. She does have two children, and both were normal births. She had lunch and has no trauma to account for the pain. Chuck and Susan both feel this could be an ectopic pregnancy. They place Lori on supplemental oxygen and start an IV to help with the signs of shock. They place her on the cot in a position of comfort and transport her to the emergency department (ED) for evaluation. Later, they learn Lori did have an ectopic pregnancy and had to go into surgery to stop the bleeding and take out the fallopian tube.

1. Chief Complaint

_____

_____

_____

2. Vital Signs

_____

_____

_____

3. Pertinent Negatives

_____

_____

_____

Ambulance Calls

The following case scenarios provide an opportunity to explore the concerns associated with patient management and paramedic care. Read each scenario, and then answer each question.

1. Cory and Jake decide to build a tree house. Of course, Jake, being an anxious 10-year-old, wants a double-decker house. He climbs higher in the tree, and then loses his footing. His fall is broken by the girding of the structure, and he continues to fall through it until hitting the ground. Jake has fallen a total of 17 feet but is conscious as his dad calls 9-1-1. When the crew arrives, they find Jake in the position he fell. The scene is safe and Cory and Jake's dad are there to answer questions about the incident.

a. What questions would you ask Cory or Jake's dad?

(1) _____

(2) _____

(3) _____

(4) _____

(5) _____

(6) _____

Manual stabilization is taken of Jake's head while a rapid trauma assessment is begun. Jake is answering questions correctly, but he is in a lot of pain. There are no life-threatening wounds; however, he has a small amount of blood in his nose and mouth. He is having problems spitting it out.

b. What would you do at this point?

_____

_____

_____

During the rapid trauma assessment, you find that Jake's left arm is deformed between the shoulder and the elbow. He also has pain and tenderness in the upper quadrants of his stomach. On visual inspection you note redness and realize that a two-by-four broke the boy's fall out of the tree. You and your partner agree that this is a load-and-go patient. You quickly apply the appropriate collar and log roll Jake onto a backboard. As you check the posterior portion of his back, you find a small nail impaled to its head in Jake's upper back below the scapula.

c. Would you splint Jake's arm en route?

_____

_____

_____

d. How would you deal with the nail?

_____

_____

_____

e. What type of injury could this cause Jake?

_____

_____

_____

En route, you take baseline vital signs, establish IVs, and begin a detailed physical exam on Jake.

f. Why would you do a detailed physical exam?

_____

You arrive at a trauma center and give a full report to the physician. You have discovered the beginning of bruising behind Jake's left ear. His pupils are unequal. He has several small cuts on his face and head. He has decreased lung sounds around the region of the impaled nail. Both upper quadrants are showing bruising, tenderness, and some rigidity. He has several deep scratches and cuts on his legs that you managed en route. His vital signs are acceptable, but are showing signs of shock. After a few hours in surgery, Jake will recover fully. His dad, however, decides the tree house should have railings around the edge to prevent any more falls.

g. What injuries would you consider to be life threatening (relating to Jake's incident)?

_____

_____

_____

True/False

If you believe the statement to be more true than false, write the letter "T" in the space provided. If you believe the statement to be more false than true, write the letter "F."

_____   **1.** Children do not dehydrate as fast as adults do.

_____   **2.** Delirium is associated with an acute sudden change in mental status.

_____   **3.** Aphasia is difficulty speaking.

_____   **4.** Babinski reflex is a normal finding in an older adult.

_____   **5.** When assessing a limb for ischemia, you should use the five Ps of acute arterial insufficiency.

_____   **6.** You should always assess a pulse in three different places on the foot.

_____   **7.** To assess a shoulder dislocation, you should be in front of the patient and looking down at both shoulders.

_____   **8.** Female and male genitalia should be assessed in a limited and discreet fashion.

_____   **9.** Jugular venous distention is commonly caused by right-sided heart failure.

_____   **10.** You must have a stethoscope for evaluating blood pressure.

Short Answer

Complete this section with short written answers using the space provided.

1. By the time you have finished describing the patient's general appearance, even in only a sentence or two, the physician at the other end of the radio should already have a good general picture of the patient and of the urgency of the patient's situation. What parameters are included in the description of a patient's "general appearance"?

a. _____

b. _____

c. _____

d. _____

e. _____

2. You are called to the scene of a road incident in which a car plowed into a utility pole. The driver of the car is sitting on the grass beside his wrecked vehicle, looking dazed and confused. What parameters would you use to assess his level of consciousness, and how would you report your findings?

_____

_____

_____

_____

_____

3. Measure the vital signs of a classmate or family member.

   a. Describe your findings.

     Temperature: _____

     Pulse: _____

     Respirations: _____

     Blood pressure: _____

   b. If the room had been very noisy, what alternative method could you have used for measuring the systolic blood pressure?

_____

_____

_____

   c. Why is it customary to keep one's hand on the pulse when measuring the respiratory rate?

_____

_____

_____

For each of the following sets of vital signs taken in adults, indicate whether the vital signs are within the range of normal. If they are not, indicate in what way they are abnormal and what underlying condition they may suggest to you from your experience as an EMT-B or from what you have learned so far in this text.

4. Pulse = 120 beats/min, thready, and regular
Respirations = 20 breaths/min, shallow, slightly labored
Blood pressure = 72 mm Hg systolic (by palpation)

   a. These vital signs are _____ (normal or abnormal).

   b. If they are abnormal, what is abnormal about them?

_____

_____

_____

c. If they are abnormal, what do they suggest to you about what might be wrong with the patient?

_____

_____

_____

5. Pulse = 72 beats/min, full, and regular
   Respirations = 4 breaths/min and snoring
   Blood pressure = 110/70 mm Hg

   a. These vital signs are _____ (normal or abnormal).

   b. If they are abnormal, what is abnormal about them?

   _____

   _____

   _____

   c. If they are abnormal, what do they suggest to you about what might be wrong with the patient?

   _____

   _____

   _____

   d. Suppose you had the additional information that the patient's pupils were extremely constricted. Would that help you interpret the vital signs? How?

   _____

   _____

   _____

6. Pulse = 60 beats/min, full, and slightly irregular
   Respirations = 30 breaths/min and deep; no unusual odors on the breath
   Blood pressure = 200/140 mm Hg

   a. These vital signs are _____ (normal or abnormal).

   b. If they are abnormal, what is abnormal about them?

   _____

   _____

   _____

   c. If they are abnormal, what do they suggest to you about what might be wrong with the patient?

   _____

   _____

   _____

d. Suppose you had the additional information that the patient's pupils were unequal—one was midposition, the other widely dilated. Would that help you interpret the vital signs? How?

_____

_____

_____

7. Pulse = 56 beats/min, full, and regular
   Respirations = 12 breaths/min and unlabored
   Blood pressure = 120/65 mm Hg

   a. These vital signs are _____ (normal or abnormal).

   b. If they are abnormal, what is abnormal about them?

   _____

   _____

   _____

   c. If they are abnormal, what do they suggest to you about what might be wrong with the patient?

   _____

   _____

   _____

8. The head-to-toe exam may also provide evidence of significant head injury. List three signs that would suggest the presence of a skull fracture.

   a. _____

   b. _____

   c. _____

   d. _____

Crossword Puzzles

Use the clues below to complete the puzzle.

Across

1. Distinct areas of skin that correspond to nerves
5. There are _____ lobes in the lungs
6. The conduit for respiration and digestion
8. Mnemonic for exam of the head and related structures
10. Striking the body surface, creating sounds
12. Another name for crackles in the lungs
13. Artery in which we palpate an infant's pulse
14. Sound that can come from the heart or lungs
15. As you approach the scene you form a _____ impression

Down

2. Involuntary motor responses due to stimuli
3. Measurements of pulse, respirations, and blood pressure
4. A sunken _____ in a child represents dehydration
7. Weakened abdominal wall musculature
9. Contraction of the abdominal muscles due to pain
11. Classic sign of inflammation, redness

Fill-in-the-Table

Fill in the missing parts of the tables.

1. In examining a person who has been injured ("trauma patient"), you look for different signs than you would if you were examining an ill person ("medical patient"). Fill in the following table to indicate what you would look for in particular when examining the different body regions of a trauma patient and a medical patient.

Body Region	Trauma Patient	Medical Patient
Head		
Neck		
Chest		
Abdomen		
Back		
Extremities		

2. In the rapid trauma assessment/exam or detailed physical exam of a multitrauma patient, you must look for very specific clues to specific injuries. Fill in the following table to indicate what you will be looking for in particular as you examine each part of the body.

Body Region	What I Will Be Looking for in Particular
Head	
Neck	
Chest	
Abdomen	
Extremities	
Back/buttocks	

Skill Drills

Test your knowledge of skill drills by placing the following photos in the correct order. Number the first step with a "1," the second step with a "2," and so forth.

1. *Examining the Nervous System*

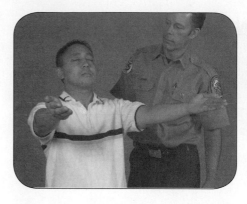

Perform the pronator drift test by asking the patient to close his or her eyes and hold both arms out in front of the body.

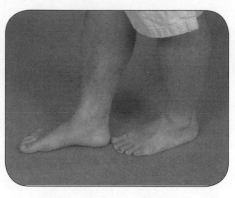

If appropriate, test the patient's gait and balance by having the patient walk heel-to-toe or perform the heel-to-shin stance.

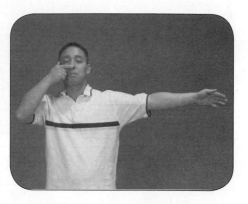

Evaluate the patient's coordination by performing the finger-to-nose test using alternating hands.

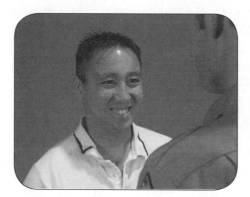

Evaluate cranial nerve function.

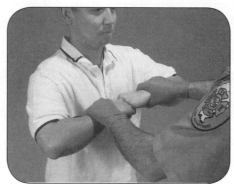

Evaluate the patient's neuromuscular status by checking muscle strength against resistance.

2. Examining the Chest

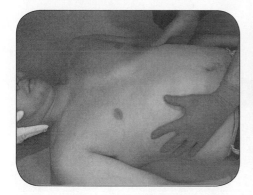

Note the shape of the chest.

_____

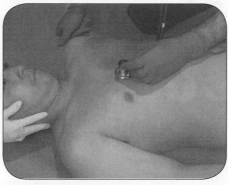

Auscultate the lung fields, noting any abnormal lung sounds.

_____

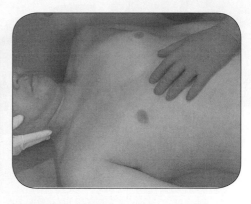

Inspect the chest for any obvious DCAP-BTLS.

_____

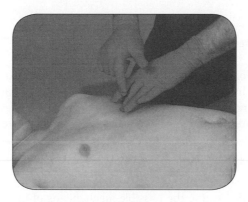

Percuss the chest to detect any abnormalities.

_____

CHAPTER

14 Patient Assessment

Chapter Review

The following exercises provide an opportunity to test your knowledge of this chapter.

Matching

Order each of the items in the correct sequence.

1. You are called to the scene of a road crash in which a semitrailer jackknifed off the road into a ravine. The bystander who reported the collision from a highway telephone was too agitated to give much information, but he did mention that a passenger was lying on the ground beside the truck and "not moving at all." When you reach the scene, you will perform all of the following actions. Arrange the actions in the sequence in which you will carry them out.

A. Check the passenger for a pulse; if he has no pulse, start external chest compressions.

B. Stabilize any fractures among the casualties.

C. Determine whether you need backup support.

D. Examine the scene closely to determine the possible mechanisms of injury (MOI).

E. Determine whether there are any hazards to the rescuers.

F. Determine whether the passenger is breathing; if not, start artificial ventilation.

G. Do a head-to-toe physical examination of each casualty.

H. Package the casualties for transport.

I. Determine whether you will need special equipment to gain access to the driver of the truck.

J. Make sure the passenger has an open airway.

K. Control any bleeding you detect in the passenger.

L. Take a focused history from the driver.

(1) _____   (5) _____   (9) _____

(2) _____   (6) _____   (10) _____

(3) _____   (7) _____   (11) _____

(4) _____   (8) _____   (12) _____

2. A gas leak in the downtown area led to a large explosion. You are called to the scene of the explosion where several people were injured by flying glass and debris. There is a great deal of noise and confusion at the scene. A middle-aged woman is lying unconscious on the sidewalk. She is covered with blood. Arrange the following steps of her management in the correct sequence.

A. Determine if she has a pulse; if not, start external chest compressions.

B. Find the source of bleeding, and control the bleeding.

C. Open her airway.

D. Cover any wounds with sterile dressings.

E. Determine if she is breathing; if not, start artificial ventilation.

(1) _____   (3) _____   (5) _____

(2) _____   (4) _____

Multiple Choice

Read each item carefully, and then select the best response.

_____ **1.** The scene size-up component of the patient assessment includes all of the following, EXCEPT:

    A. focused assessment.   **C.** requesting additional resources.

    B. mechanism of injury (MOI).   **D.** scene safety.

_____ **2.** During the initial assessment, the paramedic must:

    A. treat medical and trauma patients differently.   **C.** identify priority patients.

    B. determine the SAMPLE history.   **D.** obtain baseline vital signs.

_____ **3.** Which of the following BSI precautions may be appropriate during the scene size-up and a patient examination?

    A. Gloves   **C.** N-95 masks

    B. Gowns   **D.** All of the above

_____ **4.** When on a scene where people act aggressively, or appear to be threatening, it is best for the paramedic to:

    A. consider retreating to the rig until the scene is secure.

    B. explain that you are there to help and do not intend any harm to the patient.

    C. explain that you are not law enforcement.

    D. begin acting authoritarian and aggressive toward the instigators.

_____ **5.** The most time-sensitive and important aspect of the patient assessment where life threats are detected and quickly treated is considered the:

    A. primary assessment.   **C.** initial assessment.

    B. expanded primary assessment.   **D.** general impression.

_____ **6.** Which of the following is considered a "priority patient"?

    A. A pregnant patient involved in a minor motor vehicle crash without any complications

    B. A large multiple-casualty incident with a patient in cardiac arrest

    C. A patient who does not pass the "look test," giving a poor general impression

    D. A bystander who witnessed the event and is traumatized by what he saw

_____ **7.** Evaluating an unresponsive medical patient requires you, the paramedic, to rely on:

    A. a head-to-toe physical exam.   **C.** the bystander or family information.

    B. the presence of a MedicAlert® tag.   **D.** all of the above.

_____ **8.** The rapid trauma assessment is generally completed when:

    A. on all entrapped patients.

    B. on any patient who doesn't have a readily identifiable medical problem.

    C. before all life threats have been identified and treated.

    D. after the initial assessment and prior to the focused physical exam.

_____ **9.** Which of the following patients typically requires a detailed physical exam?

    A. A man with a minor laceration obtained while cutting vegetables in the kitchen

    B. An athlete who was kicked in the shin while playing soccer

    C. An intoxicated bar patron who fell off a stool and struck his head

    D. A baseball catcher struck in the face while wearing his protective mask

_____ **10.** When assessing a patient's airway status, it is often helpful to do which of the following?

    A. Think from the simple to the complex.

    B. Intubate the patient quickly to manage the airway definitively.

    C. Alter your assessment based on the patient's age.

    D. Always open an unconscious patient's airway with a head tilt–chin lift.

Labeling

Indicate the steps you would take for the circumstances provided

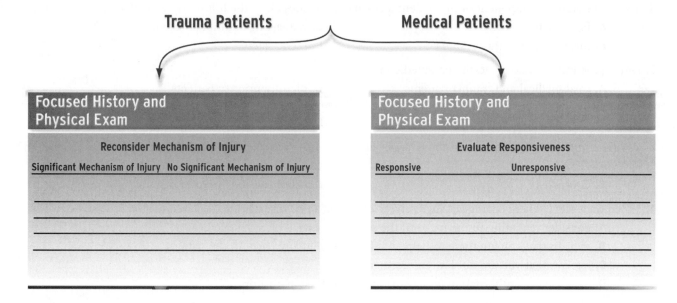

Fill-in-the-Blank

Read each item carefully, and then complete the statement by filling in the missing word(s).

1. Your first and foremost concern on any call is ensuring your own _____ and the safety of the other emergency

medical services (EMS) _____ _____.

2. Paramedics find patients fueled by methamphetamines to be _____ and _____ _____.

Sometimes they are _____ with weapons.

3. Assessing and evaluating the MOI can help you _____ the likelihood of certain _____ having occurred

and estimate their _____.

4. The information gleaned from the _____ _____ is crucial to the overall outcome for your patient.

Treat _____ _____ as you find them.

5. Components of the past medical history include the patient's general state of _____, _____ and

_____ diseases, _____, and _____.

6. For patients with _____ complaints, assess breath sounds _____ and _____.

7. _____ vital signs and the "tilt test" are measurements of a patient's _____ _____ and pulse

that are taken in the _____ and _____ or standing positions.

8. Crash and rescue scenes often include _____ risks, such as unstable _____, moving _____,

jagged metal and broken glass, fire or explosion hazards, downed power lines, and, possibly, _____ materials.

Identify

In the following case studies, determine if the chief complaint is a medical or trauma patient. If the patient is a trauma patient, indicate the mechanism of injury (MOI), your transport decision, and why. If the patient is a medical patient, indicate the level of consciousness, your transport decision, and why.

1. It's high school prom night. Despite all the warnings and education someone always seems to make a bad decision. Tonight is no exception. You've responded to a single-car crash into a very large oak tree. The car is split down the middle. The apparent driver is missing and can't be located. The passenger wasn't wearing a seat belt and was ejected. On arrival he is covered in blood and has a Glasgow Coma score of <8.

_____

_____

_____

_____

_____

_____

2. It's another routine night shift. You arrive on scene to find an elderly woman who has fallen down two or three stairs. She is conscious, but not alert to the precipitating events leading to her fall. She has a large hematoma above her right eye. She appears to have left-sided hemiparesis and is slurring her words. She has what appears to be a facial droop. Family members state that she has a history of atrial fibrillation and takes medication for that arrhythmia.

_____

_____

_____

_____

_____

3. You are dispatched to a well-known residential location. You've treated this patient many times in the past. You arrive on scene to discover that it's the same old story. The patient is unconscious with snoring respirations. He just doesn't take very good care of himself. You begin the task of assessing him and notice that his blood glucose level is 48 mg/dL. You place him on a nonrebreathing mask and begin to treat him.

_____

_____

_____

_____

_____

Ambulance Calls

The following case scenarios provide an opportunity to explore the concerns associated with patient management and paramedic care. Read each scenario, and then answer each question.

1. A middle-aged man was the driver of a car that ran head-on into a truck parked on the opposite side of the road. You find the driver of the car unconscious in his wrecked vehicle.

   a. Describe how you would open and maintain the patient's airway.

_____

_____

_____

_____

   b. Continuing with the initial assessment, you note that the patient's respirations are very shallow; he seems to be breathing mostly with his abdominal muscles. What further steps are needed at this point?

_____

_____

_____

_____

   c. Proceeding with your assessment, you find that the patient's skin is warm and dry. His pulse is 72 beats/min and regular, respirations are 24 breaths/min and shallow, and blood pressure is 70 systolic. What is the most likely explanation of those findings?

_____

_____

_____

_____

   d. What further steps do you now need to take in managing this patient?

     (1) _____

     (2) _____

2. A 62-year-old driver of a car is hit from the side. The door on the driver's side is smashed in. The patient is conscious and in respiratory distress. The left chest is bruised, tender, and does not move symmetrically on respiration. Her skin is warm. Her pulse is 92 beats/min and slightly irregular, respirations are 30 breaths/min and shallow, and blood pressure is 136/82 mm Hg.

a. Indicate whether the patient is

       C In critical condition (the "load-and-go" category)

       N Not in critical condition

_____

b. What steps would you take at the scene?

   (1) _____

   (2) _____

   (3 _____

   (4) _____

   (5) _____

c. What steps would you take during transport?

   (1) _____

   (2) _____

   (3 _____

   (4) _____

3. You are called late one night for a "man down" in a somewhat seedy section of the city. Arriving at the scene, you find a shabbily dressed man of middle age slumped unconscious in an alley. He is not carrying any wallet or identification. The police say they have no idea how long he has been there. On examination, the man is unresponsive to painful stimulus. His skin is cool and dry. Vital signs are a pulse of 53 beats/min and regular, respirations of 32 breaths/min and deep, and a blood pressure of 200/120 mm Hg. The lighting isn't good enough to allow an assessment for Battle's sign or raccoon's eyes, but you can determine that there is no blood or fluid coming from the ears or nose. The left pupil is dilated and does not react to light. His breath smells of alcohol. The chest is clear. The abdomen is soft. His legs appear somewhat stiff, and it's hard to flex them.

a. List five causes of unconsciousness, and put an asterisk beside the one you think is the most likely cause in this case.

   (1) _____

   (2) _____

   (3) _____

   (4) _____

   (5) _____

b. List the steps you would take in treating this patient.

   (1) _____

   (2) _____

   (3) _____

   (4) _____

   (5) _____

(6) _____

(7) _____

True/False

If you believe the statement to be more true than false, write the letter "T" in the space provided. If you believe the statement to be more false than true, write the letter "F."

_____ **1.** Patient assessment is a complex skill made up of four primary components: information gathering, physical examination, vital signs, and previous medical history.

_____ **2.** Smoke is the byproduct of incomplete combustion and can contain many toxins, pathogens, and carcinogens.

_____ **3.** Establishing a perimeter around an emergency scene is rarely required.

_____ **4.** The nature of illness is the general type of illness a patient is experiencing.

_____ **5.** Changes in the state of consciousness may provide the first clue to an alteration in the patient's condition.

_____ **6.** Anatomic differences between age groups are not relevant when performing the head tilt–chin lift maneuver.

_____ **7.** An irregular pulse can indicate a serious condition. As such, consider all patients with an irregular pulse at risk until proven otherwise.

_____ **8.** The past medical history is infrequently linked to the patient's current problem.

_____ **9.** Referred pain has its origin in a particular organ but is described by the patient as pain in a different location.

_____ **10.** A tilt test or orthostatic change is considered positive when the patient's blood pressure shows a decrease in systolic pressure (up to 20 mm Hg), an increase in diastolic pressure of 10 mm Hg (a narrowing pulse pressure), and an increase in heart rate by 20 beats/min.

_____ **11.** The detailed cardiac exam can be stressful and produce anxiety in patients because you are asking them to divulge personal information to a paramedic they have known for only 10 minutes.

_____ **12.** The ongoing assessment represents a continuous, yet cyclic, process that you perform throughout transport, right up to the time you turn patient care over to the emergency department staff.

Short Answer

Complete this section with short written answers using the space provided.

1. Before performing a rapid trauma assessment or even taking the vital signs, it is customary to make a quick check for obvious injuries. Why not simply wait until those injuries are detected during the focused physical exam?

_____

_____

_____

_____

2. In responding to emergencies outside the hospital, the paramedic must always proceed according to a standard set of priorities. Why is that list of priorities necessary in emergency care in general and in emergency care in the prehospital setting in particular?

_____

_____

_____

_____

Crossword

Use the clues below to complete the puzzle.

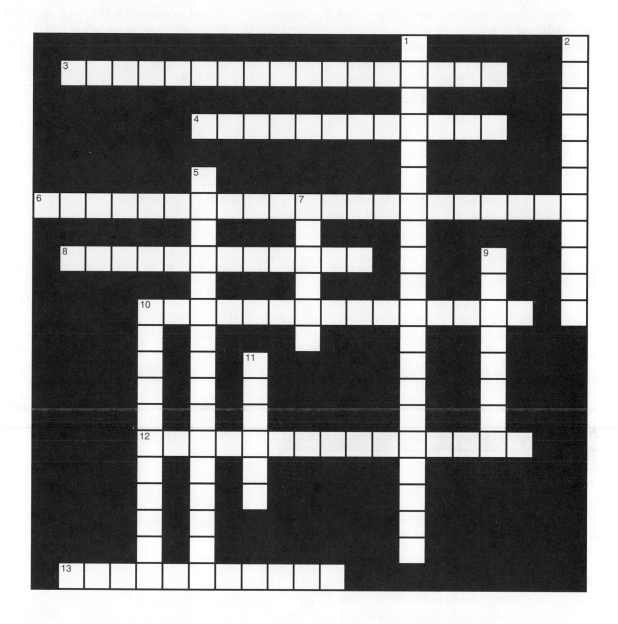

Across

3. Involves five separate mini-assessments: mental status, motor response, cranial nerve function, reflexes, and sensory response

4. AVPU

6. This assessment is usually performed on patients with any significant mechanism of injury (MOI)

8. Diminished or absent breath sounds, JVD, and progressive dyspnea

10. If they are improperly installed or positioned in the vehicle, they can be rendered useless as a safety device

12. The general type of illness a patient is experiencing

13. First step of the patient assessment process

Down

1. Done on a trauma patient en route when you have extended transport time

2. The patient's blood pressure shows a decrease in systolic pressure (up to 20 mm Hg), an increase in diastolic pressure of 10 mm Hg, and an increase in heart rate by 20 beats/min

5. Patients who will benefit from limited time at the scene and rapid transport

7. Secondary restraint system that has saved countless lives

9. Mnemonic for rapid trauma assessment

10. Indication of intraperitoneal hemorrhage

11. History of present illness

Fill-in-the-Table

Fill in the missing parts of the table.

1. Whether a patient has an injury or a medical problem, the objective of the initial assessment is the same: to detect life-threatening conditions. For a trauma patient, however, the particular details you are looking for in the initial assessment are different from those you seek in the medical patient. Fill in the following table to indicate what you would look for at each step of the initial assessment of an injured patient found unconscious.

Step	What I Would Look for at This Step
Mental status	
Airway	
Breathing	
Circulation	
Transport decision	

2. Skin color can indicate a particular condition or emergency. Fill in the possible causes for red, white, blue, or mottled skin.

Inspection of the Skin	
Skin Color	**Possible Cause**
Red	Fever Hypertension _____ _____
White (pallor)	Excessive blood loss _____
Blue (cyanosis)	Hypoxemia _____
Mottled	_____

Skill Drills

Test your knowledge of skill drills by placing the following photos in the correct order. Number the first step with a "1," the second step with a "2," and so forth.

The Rapid Trauma Assessment

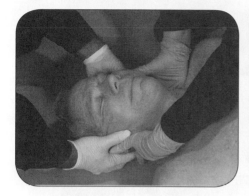

Palpate down the posterior cervical spine.

_____

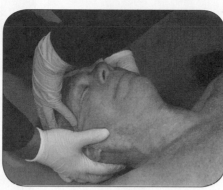

Inspect and palpate the skull.

_____

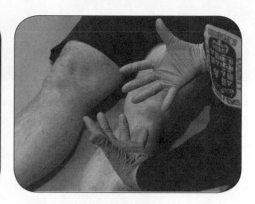

Check your gloves for blood.

_____

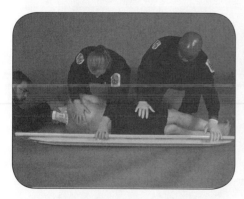

If you log roll the patient to a backboard, examine and palpate the thoracic and lumbar spine.

_____

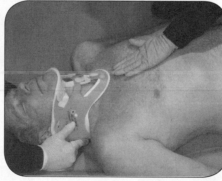

Assess for a flail chest or fractured sternum.

_____

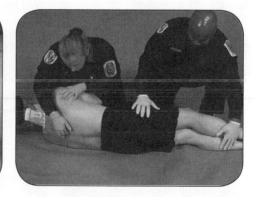

Inspect and palpate the back.

_____

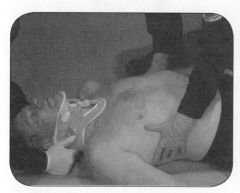

Assess for fractured ribs or a flail chest.

_____

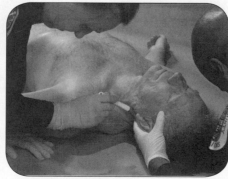

Look in and behind the patient's ears.

_____

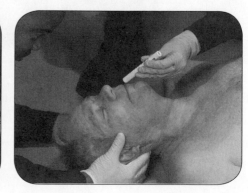

Inspect the nose.

_____

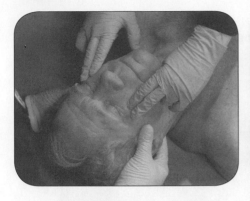

Check the pupils, and quickly palpate the orbits.

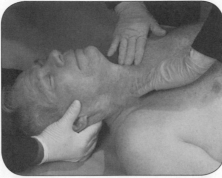

Assess the neck.

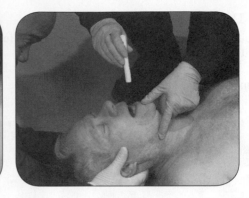

Assess the mouth.

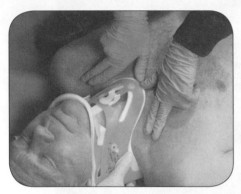

Inspect and palpate the chest.

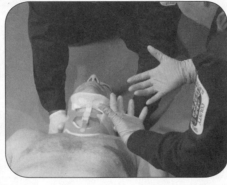

Check your gloves for any signs of bleeding. Place a properly sized rigid cervical collar.

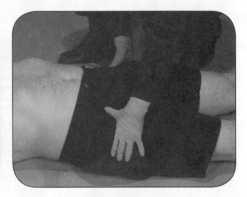

Assess the pelvic girdle.

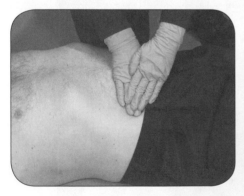

Inspect and palpate all four quadrants of the abdomen.

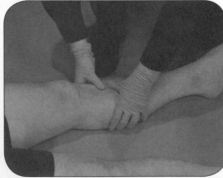

Inspect and palpate both lower extremities from hip to ankle.

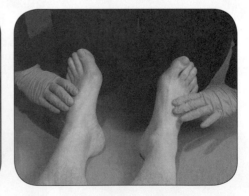

Simultaneously assess pedal pulses.

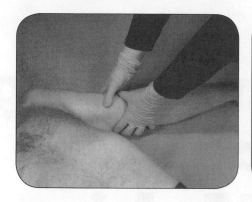

Inspect and palpate the arms, and assess pulse, motor function, and sensation.

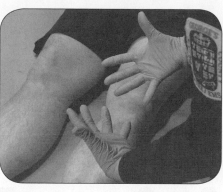

Check your gloves for blood.

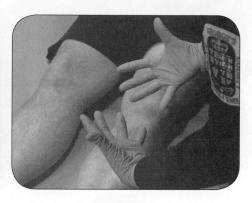

Check your gloves for blood.

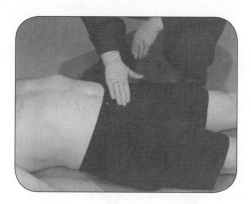

Palpate over the bladder.

CHAPTER

15 Critical Thinking and Clinical Decision Making

Chapter Review

The following exercises provide an opportunity to test your knowledge of this chapter.

Matching

For each sentence listed below, decide if you would:

A. Follow protocols

B. Use independent decisions

_____ **1.** An 86-year-old woman with facial droop and slurred speech

_____ **2.** A 14-year-old boy, unconscious, who is trapped in a drain pipe

_____ **3.** A diabetic woman with low blood sugar

_____ **4.** A 47-year-old man with "classic ischemic" chest pain

_____ **5.** A crop duster crash with a conscious pilot who is yelling for help

_____ **6.** A school where a person has shot several students

_____ **7.** An allergic reaction to a bee sting on a 12-year-old girl

_____ **8.** A motor vehicle crash where the car is smoking and appears to be on fire

_____ **9.** A 20-year-old basketball player in cardiac arrest during a game

_____ **10.** A man stuck inside a grain elevator, and he is being pulled under the grain

Multiple Choice

Read each item carefully, and then select the best response.

_____ **1.** _____ is processing the information presented by the patient you are treating.

    A. Gathering   **C.** Synthesizing

    B. Evaluating   **D.** Thinking

_____ **2.** Which of the following items is NOT included in the concept formation process?

    A. Smell   **C.** Hearing

    B. Sample history   **D.** Seeing

_____ **3.** What is the second stage of critical thinking?

    A. Application of principle   **C.** Concept formation

    B. Reflection in action   **D.** Data interpretation

_____ **4.** What does "reflection in action" mean?
      A. A call review of the run you just completed
      B. Checking your interventions as you apply them to your patient
      C. Stopping before you apply the intervention to make sure you are doing the right thing
      D. Checking the protocols prior to doing anything

_____ **5.** Which of the following does not belong to the "Six Rs" that were discussed in the chapter?
      A. Read the scene   **C.** Read the patient
      B. Read the protocols   **D.** React

_____ **6.** You respond to a patient's home for chest pain. You are determining the chief complaint and taking the baseline vital signs. In which of the "Six Rs" are you working right now?
      A. Reading the scene   **C.** Reevaluating
      B. Reacting   **D.** Reading the patient

_____ **7.** When responding to a critical patient, it is best to use a mental checklist for what reason?
      A. So you don't forget to take vital signs
      B. So you always follow your protocols
      C. To facilitate better thinking on the scene
      D. So you will never be sued

_____ **8.** Which of the following is NOT used to synthesize your patient's information?
      A. Patient history   **C.** Current complaints
      B. Patient allergies   **D.** Previous diseases

_____ **9.** Which of the following adult patients would be considered to have a serious condition?
      A. Acute presentation of a first-time event
      B. Acute presentation of a chronic event
      C. Patient with small lacerations
      D. Partial thickness burns to an extremity with less than 5% BSA

_____ **10.** What is the "third" cornerstone of effective paramedic practice?
      A. Development and implementation of a patient care plan
      B. Having the ability to think and work under pressure
      C. Having the ability of judgment and making independent decisions
      D. Having the ability to gather, evaluate, and synthesize information

Fill-in-the-Blank

Read each item carefully, and then complete the statement by filling in the missing word(s).

1. By taking a sample history and baseline vital signs, you are _____ information about your patient.

2. Your care plan for your patient is almost always defined by your _____.

3. Your final cornerstone of practicing as a paramedic is to _____ and _____ under pressure.

4. The process of gathering information by smell, sight, hearing, and touch is known as _____ _____.

5. Patients with major multi-system trauma, acute chronic conditions, and devastating single-system trauma would be examples

of patients with _____ _____ _____ .

6. Once you have assessed your patient and you begin treatment, you are using a _____

_____ .

7. When responding to a scene, you have to consider the _____ when managing the patients on the

scene.

8. When dealing with a critical patient, you take vitals signs three or more times. The readings allow you to assess

_____ .

Identify

In the following case study, list the chief complaint, vital signs, and any pertinent negatives.

It is 4:00 pm and you have been called to a residence for a woman who is not feeling well. When you arrive, you find a 56-year-old woman with a general feeling of malaise. You begin talking with her to gather some information while your partner takes baseline vital signs. During your SAMPLE history, you find out that she is a diabetic. Your partner tests her blood glucose level and it is 110 mg/dL. She states she is very careful because of her illness. Her blood pressure is 160/100 mm Hg, pulse is 92 beats/min and regular with normal sinus rhythm showing on the ECG monitor, but she is showing a little ST-segment depression. You ask her if she has ever had a heart attack and she says no. Her oxygen saturation on room air is 97%, all lung fields are clear, and she is breathing at 18 breaths/min. She is warm and dry and her pupils are PEARRL (Pupils Equal And Round, Regular in size, react to Light). She says she has been feeling this way for a few days and is so tired she hasn't been able to do anything. She was afraid that something major might be wrong with her, so she decided to give 9-1-1 a call. You tell the woman that she might have had a cardiac event and you want to take her in. You apply oxygen by nonrebreathing mask at 15 L/min, start an IV, and give her some nitroglycerin paste to bring down the blood pressure en route. With the nitroglycerin, oxygen, and the IV in a TKO drip, you take a 12-lead ECG en route and transport her to the local ED. The nitroglycerin brings the blood pressure down to 120/70 mm Hg. All other vitals stay the same. Later you learn she has had a small MI but because of her diabetes she never had the classic signs.

1. Chief Complaint

_____

_____

_____

2. Vital Signs

_____

_____

_____

3. Pertinent Negatives

_____

_____

_____

Ambulance Calls

The following case scenario provides an opportunity to explore the concerns associated with patient management and paramedic care. Read the scenario, and then answer each question.

1. You are on a rural squad, with no regional trauma center nearby. You are dispatched to a grade school for a child who has fallen out of a tree. The school is reporting that the child is still on the ground outside on the playground. When you arrive, you find a 9-year-old girl sitting up. You ask your partner to take C-spine precautions while you start your initial assessment. The teacher says she was approximately 15 feet up when she fell. You note a large broken branch about 7 feet off the ground and the teacher says she hit that branch on the way down on her left side and then landed on her head, on the hard dirt. The child is unable to tell you her name and is confused about where she is and the day of the week. After finding no obvious life threats during the initial assessment you proceed with a rapid trauma assessment because of the significant MOI. You decide she is a critical patient because of the MOI, and call for Life Flight to take her to the regional trauma center. Your partner applies a C-collar and you carefully place her onto a long backboard. You apply supplemental oxygen by nonrebreathing mask at 15 L/min. Your partner takes baseline vital signs that reveal: blood pressure 120/80 mm Hg, pulse 52 beats/min, and respirations 6 breaths/min. Lung sounds are clear. She responds only to painful stimuli at this point, and her oxygen saturation is at 88%. Her pupils are unequal with the left much larger than the right pupil. The patient begins to gag and vomit. You suction all secretions, place an oral airway, and start to assist her ventilations with the bag mask device. Your partner gets an IV started as the helicopter is landing. The patient no longer has a gag reflex, so the flight medics insert an advanced airway. The Life Flight crew load her and take off for the regional trauma center. Later you learn the girl died as a result of massive head injury.

   a. What is your first clue that this patient should be treated as a critical patient?

   _____

   _____

   _____

   _____

   _____

   b. Under what consent can you transport this child without her parents' permission?

   _____

   _____

   _____

   _____

   _____

   c. What do your baseline vital signs suggest on this patient?

   _____

   _____

   _____

   _____

   _____

d. What is your first concern with the patient, and how can you manage that concern?

_____

_____

_____

_____

2. You are traveling home to Grandma's house for a wonderful Thanksgiving dinner. Traffic slows and comes to a stop. Knowing what you do about traffic and collisions, you pull out your jump kit and head up the road. A mini van loaded down with people has crossed the center line and hit a car with another family in it. There are people everywhere, some trying to help patients from the vehicles and others just standing around. The 9-1-1 system has already been called, but you can't hear any sirens yet because you are about 20 miles from any town. You realize that there are critical patients in the van and the Jaws of Life will be needed to extricate those patients.

a. How are you going to identify yourself and gain control of this scene?

_____

_____

_____

_____

b. What type of equipment are you going to need at this scene?

_____

_____

_____

_____

c. Are you going to begin any type of treatment before help arrives?

_____

_____

_____

_____

True/False

If you believe the statement to be more true than false, write the letter "T" in the space provided. If you believe the statement to be more false than true, write the letter "F" in the space provided.

_____ **1.** The first cornerstone of your practice is having the ability to gather, evaluate, and synthesize information on the scene.

_____ **2.** Once you have evaluated the information you obtained from the scene, the patient, or a bystander, and determined which information is valid or invalid, you need to process—or synthesize—this information.

_____ **3.** Protocols, standing orders, and patient care algorithms will address every patient for the paramedic and give a clear defined path to treatment.

_____ **4.** The patient that presents with an acute presentation of a new medical condition is considered a patient with a critical life threat.

_____ **5.** The second stage of critical thinking is concept formation.

_____ **6.** Reflection in action is the process of reassessing your patient.

_____ **7.** When you identify a patient with medical ambiguity, it means that you have pinpointed the cause of the patient's medical problem.

_____ **8.** When "reading the scene," you are looking for information that is available only at the scene.

Short Answer

Complete this section with short written answers using the space provided.

1. Discuss the use of the "Six Rs" when responding to a routine call.

   a. Read the scene: _____

   _____

   b. Read the patient: _____

   _____

   c. React: _____

   _____

   d. Reevaluate: _____

   _____

   e. Revise the plan: _____

   _____

   f. Review your performance: _____

   _____

2. When using the cornerstone principles of critical thinking, discuss the differences in gathering information, evaluating information, and synthesizing.

   _____

   _____

   _____

   _____

   _____

   _____

   _____

Word Find

Hidden in the following grid are 19 words or phrases related to what you have studied in this chapter. Find the hidden words in the grid below. Then use the words from the grid to answer the following questions (some words may be used to answer more than one question).

```
S T E P U A F M V H J E K T S Y M G
V A R V O D J R A R B Y N N K N N V
E R P I A A Z I I C G E V Q K I N E
S J E P L L N E O O M B M M K X O R
O U D J L X U N T E D N J N W N I V
B D M E D I C A L A M B I G U I T Y
S G T Z D E C P T T H P D Y P C B
E M J C P A M A C E T L X O E S A A
R E F T E I T A T L C C U R F X N E
V N S N Z L E A A I O R F C X S B T
A T O K A R F C F G O O F F S X Q A
T X V H U O I E N J R N J R A U R U
I G V O K T N Z R M S C E N E J A L
O M U S I O B T A I N I N G Q J M A
N B L R M Q G N Y F I T N E D I E V
O V C X C Q C E Z I S E H T N Y S E
I I D T R E K Y Q H J S J C V J I E
R I P X R K M E H M N I O S X E V R
```

1. Upon arriving at a _____, the paramedic begins to _____ what is happening.

2. During the second stage of the _____ _____ process, you must evaluate all of the information you have

   gathered.

3. After _____ has been collected and _____ have been formed, the paramedic is ready for a/an _____ plan.

4. After a call has been completed, the paramedics will _____ on their _____ at the call.

5. When _____ lung sounds, you will use a stethoscope to _____ the patient's lungs.

6. Once you have gathered information, you need to process or _____ this information.

7. A paramedic must learn to _____ the chief complaint of a patient. This is not easy when the patient's signs and

   symptoms lead to _____ _____.

8. When at a scene, you must be able to _____ to the scene and _____ your patient when your treatment plan is not working.

9. One of the most important _____ you need to judge is your patient's affect.

10. You must be able to _____ your treatment plan based on your _____.

11. Your working diagnosis must always have a practical _____, to suit each patient.

CHAPTER

16 Communications and Documentation

Chapter Review

The following exercises provide an opportunity to test your knowledge of this chapter.

Matching

It does little good to take a careful history and conduct a thorough physical examination if you cannot communicate your findings to others. To do so, you need to know how to organize those findings in such a way that other medical professionals will really hear what you have to say.

To begin with, you need to know which information belongs in the patient's history and which should be reported as part of the physical examination on your PCR. Label each of the following statements to indicate which part of the PCR pertains to each item:

_____ 1. There was no pedal edema (edema of the ankles).

_____ 2. The patient is allergic to penicillin.

_____ 3. The pain came on while he was watching television.

_____ 4. The blood pressure was 190/110 mm Hg.

_____ 5. He was administered supplemental oxygen by nasal cannula at 4 L/min.

_____ 6. The patient is a 51-year-old man with chest pain.

_____ 7. The chest was clear.

_____ 8. His skin was pale, cold, and sweaty (diaphoretic).

_____ 9. The patient was transported in a semi-Fowler's position.

_____ 10. Nothing seemed to make the pain better or worse.

_____ 11. The pulse was 52 beats/min and full, with an occasional premature beat.

_____ 12. The neck veins were not distended.

_____ 13. There was no cyanosis of the lips.

_____ 14. The patient takes Maalox (alumina/magnesia) and cimetidine (Tagamet) regularly.

_____ 15. He also felt nauseated.

_____ 16. His abdomen was soft and nontender.

_____ 17. His respirations were 20 breaths/min and unlabored.

_____ 18. He was sitting in a chair and appeared to be frightened.

_____ 19. He is under the care of Dr. Tums for an ulcer.

_____ 20. He was alert and oriented to person, place, and day.

_____ 21. He denies any shortness of breath.

A. The chief complaint

B. Part of the history of the present illness

C. Part of the patient's other medical history

D. Part of the description of the patient's general appearance

E. Part of the vital signs

F. Part of the head-to-toe physical examination

G. Part of the treatment

H. Part of the patient's condition during transport

_____ **22.** An IV was started with D_5W to a KVO rate.

_____ **23.** The pain radiates down his left arm.

_____ **24.** The blood pressure came down to 170/90 mm Hg during transport.

_____ **25.** He describes the pain as squeezing.

_____ **26.** Lung sounds were clear.

27. Now, rearrange the preceding statements into the order in which they should be presented.

(1) _____   (10) _____   (19) _____

(2) _____   (11) _____   (20) _____

(3) _____   (12) _____   (21) _____

(4) _____   (13) _____   (22) _____

(5) _____   (14) _____   (23) _____

(6) _____   (15) _____   (24) _____

(7) _____   (16) _____   (25) _____

(8) _____   (17) _____   (26) _____

(9) _____   (18) _____

Now try the same exercise with a patient who has been injured. Keeping in mind what you will need to document on your PCR, label each of the following statements to indicate which part of the PCR pertains to each item:

_____ **28.** The right leg was severely angulated at the mid-femur.

_____ **29.** The pulse was 92 beats/min, somewhat weak, and regular.

_____ **30.** Bystanders say that the car that hit him was traveling very fast.

_____ **31.** He has a MedicAlert bracelet that says he is a diabetic.

_____ **32.** There is a bruise on the left forehead.

_____ **33.** His skin is pale, cool, and moist.

_____ **34.** He was secured to a long backboard.

_____ **35.** The patient is a middle-aged man who was struck by a car while crossing the street.

_____ **36.** Respirations were 30 breaths/min, deep, and noisy; blood pressure was 160/100 mm Hg.

_____ **37.** The patient was unconscious and did not withdraw from painful stimuli.

_____ **38.** An oropharyngeal airway was inserted, and supplementary oxygen was given by nasal cannula at 4 L/min.

_____ **39.** He apparently staggered into the street without looking, as if he were drunk.

_____ **40.** The chest wall was stable, and breath sounds were equal bilaterally.

_____ **41.** We put the right leg in a traction splint.

_____ **42.** The pupils were equal, midposition, and reactive to light.

_____ **43.** There was no change in his condition during transport.

_____ **44.** There was no blood or fluid draining from his nose or ears.

A. The chief complaint

B. Part of the history of the present illness

C. Part of the patient's other medical history

D. Part of the description of the patient's general appearance

E. Part of the vital signs

F. Part of the head-to-toe physical examination

G. Part of the treatment

H. Part of the patient's condition during transport

_____ **45.** His abdomen was soft.

_____ **46.** The dorsalis pedis pulses were equal.

47. Now, arrange the preceding statements in the correct order for presentation.

(1) _____   (8) _____   (15) _____

(2) _____   (9) _____   (16) _____

(3) _____   (10) _____   (17) _____

(4) _____   (11) _____   (18) _____

(5) _____   (12) _____   (19) _____

(6) _____   (13) _____

(7) _____   (14) _____

For each of the following statements, indicate whether the statement is most applicable to VHF radio, UHF radio, or cellular telephone:

_____ **48.** Best means for calling the base from skyscraper row downtown

_____ **49.** Best means for calling the base from a rural, wooded area

_____ **50.** Best means for sending a 12-lead ECG to medical command

_____ **51.** Best means for calling a patient's family doctor

_____ **52.** FCC-preferred for routine voice communications

_____ **53.** FCC-approved for one-lead ECG transmission

_____ **54.** Can be monitored by someone with a scanner

V VHF radio

U UHF radio

C Cellular telephone

55. The following statements come from a patient's case history. Arrange them in the correct order for transmission by radio to medical command.

A. Pulse is 50 beats/min and regular, respirations are 36 breaths/min and deep, and blood pressure is 180/126 mm Hg.

B. The patient has a history of high blood pressure.

C. The deep tendon reflexes are hyperactive.

D. Her daughter says the patient complained of a severe headache before she collapsed.

E. The patient was still conscious when we arrived, but she rapidly lost consciousness.

F. The patient is a 60-year-old woman who collapsed in the bathroom while sitting on the toilet.

G. We are administering supplemental oxygen at 4 L/min by nasal cannula.

H. The patient's medications include nitroglycerin and Aldomet (methyldopa).

I. Her left pupil is larger than the right and does not react to light.

J. She was apparently well until this morning.

K. Her neck is somewhat stiff.

L. She was hospitalized 6 years ago for an AMI.

(1) _____   (5) _____   (9) _____

(2) _____   (6) _____   (10) _____

(3) _____   (7) _____   (11) _____

(4) _____   (8) _____   (12) _____

Multiple Choice

Read each item carefully, and then select the best response.

_____ **1.** Which of the following best describes the use of slang terms?
  A. Helpful when communicating with the hospital because of patient confidentiality.
  B. Breaks up the stress of the job by interjecting "dark humor."
  C. Unprofessional and disrespectful.
  D. Helpful when communicating with other paramedics.

_____ **2.** EMS systems require a large number of personnel to work and communicate together. All of the following are part of this communication, EXCEPT:
  A. Emergency medical dispatcher (EMD)   **C.** Computer-aided dispatch (CAD)
  B. A citizen notifier   **D.** Online medical control with base station physician

_____ **3.** Federal oversight of emergency medical communication is accomplished by:
  A. civil defense.   **C.** Federal Emergency Management Agency (FEMA).
  B. the Department of Homeland Security.   **D.** Federal Communications Commission (FCC).

_____ **4.** The transmission of ECGs to hospital base stations is an important component in the evolution of modern-day paramedicine. All of the following can cause a distortion of the signals, EXCEPT:
  A. Loose ECG electrodes   **C.** Ventricular fibrillation
  B. 60-cycle interference   **D.** Weak batteries, geographic factors

_____ **5.** What is the mode of two-way radio transmission called that allows the ability to talk and listen simultaneously by using two separate radio frequencies at once?
  A. Multiplex   **C.** Duplex
  B. Stereoflex   **D.** Simplex

_____ **6.** Proper documentation is an essential job function of a paramedic. This formal written report is referred to as a:
  A. trip sheet.   **C.** call sheet.
  B. patient care report.   **D.** All of the above.

_____ **7.** PCRs may be used as all of the following, EXCEPT:
  A. A patient description for the media   **C.** Quality assurance reviews
  B. Legal documents   **D.** Billing documents

_____ **8.** Different EMS systems might use a variety of report-writing formats. Which of the following is an example of a report-writing format?
  A. HEARSAY   **C.** SOAP
  B. TALK   **D.** SAMPLE

_____ **9.** Patients may have the ability and right to refuse medical care. Which of the following patients would be appropriate for refusing?
  A. A 10-year-old boy injured in a skateboard crash
  B. A 28-year-old woman who fell off of a bar stool and struck her head
  C. An 18-year-old woman who is conscious and alert
  D. An elderly man who called for assistance and was found shivering in an unheated house

_____ **10.** When a paramedic discovers that he or she has made a documentation error on a PCR, it is okay for the paramedic to do which of the following actions?
  A. Erase or "white out" the mistake
  B. Destroy the original report and rewrite the report without the error
  C. Draw a single line through the error, initial it, and insert the corrected information next to it
  D. Have the paramedic's partner write an addendum

Fill-in-the-Blank

You have just been appointed Communications Director for your regional EMS operation, and you have been asked to draw up plans for an EMS communications system. To do so, you have to figure out who needs to communicate with whom in such a system and what is the best technical means (pager, radio, landline, or cellular phone) to achieve each link in the communications chain. Fill in the following blanks with the answers you have come up with.

1. _____ needs to be able to talk with _____. The best technical means of establishing that link is _____.

2. _____ needs to be able to talk with _____. The best technical means of establishing that link is _____.

3. _____ needs to be able to talk with _____. The best technical means of establishing that link is _____.

4. _____ needs to be able to talk with _____. The best technical means of establishing that link is _____.

5. _____ needs to be able to talk with _____. The best technical means of establishing that link is _____.

6. _____ needs to be able to talk with _____. The best technical means of establishing that link is _____.

Identify

After reading the following case history, fill in the information in the blanks below.

The patient is a 49-year-old man who called for an ambulance because of chest pain. The pain was "squeezing" in character, radiated to the left shoulder and jaw, and had been present for 2 hours. The pain was accompanied by increasing difficulty in breathing, relieved somewhat by sitting upright. The patient denied nausea, vomiting, sweating, or palpitations. He is known to be a heart patient and takes nitroglycerin at home; he took two nitroglycerin today, without relief. He denies any history of hypertension or diabetes. He has been treated for peptic ulcer in the past.

On physical examination, the patient was sitting bolt upright; he appeared alert and apprehensive and was in moderate respiratory distress, breathing shallowly 30 breaths/min. Pulse was 130 beats/min, weak and regular, and blood pressure was 200/90 mm Hg. His neck veins were distended to the angle of the jaw at 45°. Wet crackles were heard at both lung bases, and auscultation of the heart revealed a gallop rhythm. The abdomen was not distended. There was 1+ presacral and ankle edema.

The patient was given supplemental oxygen by nasal cannula at 6 L/min and transported to Mount Fiore Hospital in a semi-Fowler's position. His vital signs remained stable throughout transport.

1. Chief Complaint

_____

_____

_____

2. History of the Present Illness

_____

_____

_____

_____

3. Other Medical History

_____

_____

_____

_____

4. General Appearance

_____

_____

_____

5. Vital Signs

_____

_____

_____

6. Head-to-Toe Exam

_____

_____

_____

7. Treatment Given

_____

_____

_____

8. Pertinent Negatives

_____

_____

_____

Ambulance Calls

The following case scenarios provide an opportunity to explore the concerns associated with patient management and paramedic care. Read each scenario, and then answer each question.

1. Following is a transcript of a transmission between a paramedic unit in the field and a local hospital. The transmission does *not* follow the guidelines for good radio communications. Read through the transmission, and then list all the errors in it that you can find.

   AMBULANCE: Medic 12 to County Hospital.

   HOSPITAL: Who's calling County Hospital?

   AMBULANCE: This is Medic 12.

   HOSPITAL: Go ahead, Medic 12.

   AMBULANCE: Be advised that we are en route to your location with Maggie Jones, a lady well endowed with adipose tissue who's complaining of SOB.

   HOSPITAL: Could you please 10–9 that chief complaint?

   AMBULANCE: What's the matter, are you deaf or something? S. O. B. S as in silly, O as in old, B as in bag. Stand by for the ECG. [Pause.]

   AMBULANCE: Medic 12 to County Hospital. Did you get the strip?

   HOSPITAL: Yes.

   AMBULANCE: Say again.

   HOSPITAL: Yes, we received the strip. The doctor wants to know how old the patient is.

   AMBULANCE: She's 58.

   HOSPITAL: And does she have any medical history?

   AMBULANCE: Yeah, she's a cardiac patient and takes digitalis, atenolol, potassium chloride, chlorothiazide, and a whole bunch of other stuff here.

   HOSPITAL: Did you get any vitals?

   AMBULANCE: That's affirmative. The blood pressure is 180/120 mm Hg, the pulse is 44 beats/min, and the respirations are, let's see, here it is, the respirations are 30 breaths/min.

   HOSPITAL: Doctor's orders are to give 1 mg of atropine IV.

   AMBULANCE: That's a 10–4. Will do.

   HOSPITAL: What's your ETA?

   AMBULANCE: About 10 minutes.

   HOSPITAL: We'll see you then.

   AMBULANCE: Roger. Pop a few doughnuts into the microwave for us, will you?

   What's wrong with this transmission?

   a. _____

   _____

   b. _____

   _____

c. _____
_____

d. _____
_____

e. _____
_____

f. _____
_____

g. _____
_____

h. _____
_____

2. You are covering for the dispatcher during his lunch break. ("Don't worry about a thing," you tell him as he heads out the door. "This job's a piece of cake.") The dispatcher has no sooner departed than the telephone rings. You answer on the first ring, and a caller blurts out, "There's been a terrible accident. Oh my God, it's terrible, it's terrible," and he starts sobbing. List the questions you will ask this caller, and indicate at what point you will dispatch an ambulance.

_____
_____
_____
_____
_____
_____
_____
_____
_____
_____

_____

_____

_____

_____

True/False

If you believe the statement to be more true than false, write the letter "T" in the space provided. If you believe the statement to be more false than true, write the letter "F."

_____ **1.** Times used to document actions on a PCR generally use Greenwich Mean Time (GMT).

_____ **2.** To accurately document time, paramedics should "synchronize" their watches with the Public Safety Access Point (PSAP).

_____ **3.** Accurate documentation depends on all information being provided, including times, narrative, and check boxes.

_____ **4.** EMS may use VHF, UHF, and "trunking systems."

_____ **5.** Paramedics skilled in arrhythmia recognition don't rely heavily on ECG telemetry.

_____ **6.** An EMS base station consisting of a transmitter, receiver, and antenna is usually mounted in the front console of an ambulance for emergency communications.

_____ **7.** To have clarity of transmission there must be a sender, a clear message, a receiver, and a feedback loop.

_____ **8.** HIPAA doesn't need to be a concern to paramedics when they communicate patient information via radio.

_____ **9.** Sometimes it might be more practical to step out of the patient exam room or to speak in a softer tone to provide the history and transfer information to the receiving medical practitioner.

_____ **10.** An EMD is nothing more than a "call taker" that relays the initial dispatch information.

Short Answer

Complete this section with short written answers using the space provided.

1. An ambulance run report, or trip sheet, must also contain other information besides that contained in a traditional medical history. List at least one other item of information that needs to be recorded on a trip sheet, and explain why that information is important.

a. Information that should be recorded:

_____

_____

b. Why that information is important:

_____

_____

2. Give two reasons why you should make certain that your trip sheet (PCR) is as accurate and complete as possible.

a. _____

b. _____

3. You are planning a radio system for your ambulance service, which consists of six vehicles serving an area of 150 square miles. List the components you will need, and state the function of each component.

Component	Function

4. To the paramedic knee-deep in mud trying to extricate the patient involved in a road traffic collision, the dispatcher's job looks pretty easy. In fact, the job is not easy at all. List four tasks the dispatcher has to perform to ensure that the EMS system operates as it should.

a. _____

b. _____

c. _____

d. _____

5. According to the dictionary, communication is a process by which information is exchanged. In EMS, information must go back and forth in several different channels. Suppose you had to design the communications network for *your* EMS system. Who needs to be connected to whom? Draw a diagram to show those connections or describe who should be in contact with one another.

6. Create a sample radio report for this patient scenario. Be sure to include all findings, care provided, and status of improvement of the patient. Then, write a mock patient care report for this call, including all information provided, history obtained, and care provided.

You are en route to the hospital with a conscious, alert 58-year-old man that appears to be having an acute MI. The ETA is about 20 minutes. With the patient's consent you have mutually decided that the most appropriate facility to treat him has a 24-hour interventional cardiac catheter lab.

   The patient's chief complaint is substernal chest pressure that was radiating down his left arm. It began after he started shoveling snow. He describes the pain initially to be 10 on 10, with 10 being the worst pain he ever felt. He also states feeling nauseated and appears to be anxious and sweaty.

   His previous medical history includes hypertension and hypercholesterolemia. The patient states that he believes that his father had a heart attack when he was in his 40s. The patient is allergic to Novocain (procaine; causes nausea). He takes 325 mg of aspirin daily PO. He also takes atorvastatin (Lipitor). The patient ate lunch 3 hours ago and was directed to self-administer 162 mg of aspirin by the EMD.

The patient's exam includes bilateral crackles in the bases, pulse of 110 beats/min, and a blood pressure of 146/82 mm Hg. His SaO_2 is 96% on high-flow supplemental oxygen via nonrebreathing face mask. The ECG indicates a sinus tachycardia and elevations in V_3 and V_4.

The patient has been treated with morphine oxygen, nitroglycerin, and the self-administered aspirin.

_____

_____

_____

_____

_____

_____

_____

_____

_____

_____

_____

_____

_____

_____

_____

_____

_____

_____

_____

Secret Message

Identify the following terms from the clues provided, and then use the letters to decode the secret message!

The secret message is something to keep in mind every time you pick up the radio microphone.

a. Radio system on two frequencies: _ _ _ _ _ X
                                      30 9 16 52 36

b. Channel with a lot of interference: _ _ _ _ _
                                          45 23 58 10 49

c. Transmission of physiologic data by radio: _ _ _ _ _ L _ _ _ _ _ _
                                                  50 20 44 14 39   6 37 56 25 28 7

d. Miniature transmitter for rebroadcasting signals: _ _ P _ _ _ _ R
                                                         13 27   51 48 55 17

e. One cps: _ _ _ _ Z
              26 34 40 11

f. Portion of the radio frequency spectrum: _ _ _ D
                                               38 41 21

g. Sound of a telephone: _ _ _ _
                            33 53 24 60

h. Best way to find out a patient's chief complaint: _ _ _
                                                        29 54 19

i. Letter *N* in international phonetic alphabet: _ _ V _ _ _ _ _
                                                     59 8   2 35 1 46 5

j. Errors: _ _ _ _ _
             22 32 4 3 15

k. Principal: _ _ _ _
                 47 12 31 42

l. Which patient needs TLC: _ _ _
                               18 57 43

Secret Message

_ _ _ _ _ _ _ _ _ _ _
1 2 3 4 5 6 7 8 9 10 11 12 13 14 15 16 17 18 19 20 21 22 23 24 25 26 27 28 29 30 31 32

_ _ _ _ _ _ _ _ _ _ _ _ _ _ _ _ _ _ _ _ _ _ _ _ _ .
33 34 35 36 37 38 39 40 41 42 43 44 45 46 47 48 49 50 51 52 53 54 55 56 57 58 59 60

Fill-in-the-Table

Fill in the table with the International Phonetic Alphabet.

A		J		S	
B		K		T	
C		L		U	
D		M		V	
E		N		W	
F		O		X	
G		P		Y	
H		Q		Z	
I		R			

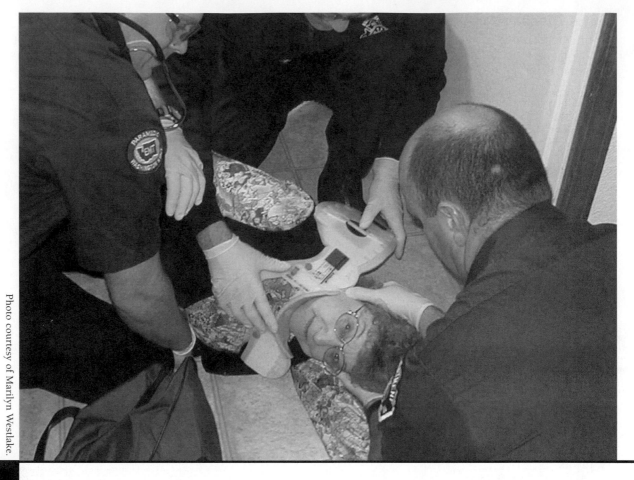

SECTION 3 CASE STUDY

70-Year-Old Female with a Hip Fracture

At 9:20 AM, you are dispatched to 517 West Graham Street for a 70-year-old female who has fallen. The patient's neighbor, who checks in on her from time to time, discovered the woman after she did not answer her phone. Your response time to the scene is approximately 10 minutes.

You arrive at the scene at 9:30 AM. Upon entering the residence, you find the patient lying on her left side in her living room. She tells you that she fell the prior day, but cannot remember the exact time. Your partner provides manual inline stabilization of the patient's head while you perform an initial assessment.

Initial Assessment	
Mechanism of Injury	Fall
Level of Consciousness	Conscious, but confused
Chief Complaint	"My left hip hurts."
Airway and Breathing	Airway is patent; respirations, normal rate and quality.
Circulation	Radial pulse, normal rate and regular; no gross bleeding

1. What are common contributing factors to falls in the elderly?

_____

_____

_____

_____

Because of her confusion, you place the patient on supplemental oxygen. You perform a focused physical examination while your partner maintains manual stabilization of the patient's head. The neighbor goes into the kitchen to retrieve the patient's medications.

Focused Physical Examination	
Inspection	Lateral rotation of the left foot, left leg appears shorter than the right
Palpation	Pain to left hip upon palpation and with movement of the left leg; no crepitus noted
Neurovascular	Pedal pulses are present bilaterally; gross sensory and motor functions appear intact bilaterally.
Time of Injury	"Yesterday, but I cannot remember the exact time."

Further examination of the patient reveals the presence of severe kyphosis. Because of the mechanism of injury, you apply a cervical collar and prepare to immobilize the patient's spine. According to the neighbor, the patient is usually well oriented and not confused.

2. What are some common causes of altered mental status in the elderly?

_____

_____

_____

_____

3. What is kyphosis? How will you immobilize this patient's spine and hip?

_____

_____

_____

_____

After immobilizing the patient's spine and injured hip, your partner obtains the patient's blood glucose reading, which is 50 mg/dL. After initiating an IV line of normal saline and administering 25 grams of glucose, the patient's mental status markedly improves. You apply a cardiac monitor, assess the patient's cardiac rhythm **(Figure 3-1)**, and then obtain baseline vital signs and a SAMPLE history. The neighbor returns with the patient's medications.

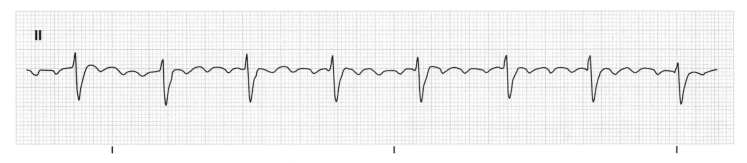

■ **Figure 3-1** Your patient's cardiac rhythm.

Baseline Vital Signs and SAMPLE History	
Blood Pressure	150/90 mm Hg
Pulse	66 beats/min, strong and regular
Respirations	22 breaths/min, adequate tidal volume
Oxygen Saturation	95% (on 100% oxygen)
Signs and Symptoms	Pain to left hip, confusion (resolved)
Allergies	Sulfonamides, Demerol, penicillin
Medications	Vasotec, Calan, Diuril, K-Dur
Pertinent Past History	Atrial flutter, hypertension
Last Oral Intake	"I ate yesterday morning, shortly before I fell."
Events Leading to the Injury	"I slipped on a throw rug while walking into my living room."

The patient is loaded into the ambulance and transport to a local hospital is initiated. Repeat blood glucose analysis reveals a reading of 101 mg/dL. While en route, you talk to the patient and monitor her for signs of deterioration.

4. How does aging affect the body's ability to compensate for shock?

_____

_____

_____

_____

The patient's condition remains stable throughout transport. With an estimated time of arrival at the hospital of 5 minutes, you perform an ongoing assessment and then call your report to the receiving facility.

Ongoing Assessment

Level of Consciousness	Conscious and alert to person, place, and time
Airway and Breathing	Airway remains patent; respirations, 20 breaths/min with adequate tidal volume.
Oxygen Saturation	95% (on 100% oxygen)
Blood Pressure	148/86 mm Hg
Pulse	68 beats/min, strong and regular
ECG	Atrial flutter with 4:1 conduction

The patient is delivered to the hospital without incident. Radiographic evaluation confirms a fracture of the left hip. Further examination by the physician reveals no other injuries or illnesses. The patient is admitted to the orthopaedic ward, and, after three days, is transferred to a rehabilitation facility.

CASE STUDY

CHAPTER

17 Trauma Systems and Mechanism of Injury

Chapter Review

The following exercises provide an opportunity to test your knowledge of this chapter.

Matching

For each of the injuries listed below, indicate which incident it is likely to be associated with. (*Note:* Some injuries may be associated with more than one type of mechanism.)

_____ 1. "Whiplash" injury

_____ 2. Lateral rib fractures

_____ 3. Fracture of the tibia/fibula

_____ 4. Fracture of the patella

_____ 5. Fracture of the humerus

_____ 6. Skull fracture

_____ 7. Laryngeal fracture

_____ 8. Flail chest

_____ 9. Pelvic fracture

_____ 10. Cervical spine injury

A. Head-on collision (unrestrained driver)

B. Lateral impact (unrestrained front seat passenger)

C. Rear-impact collision (unrestrained driver)

D. Pedestrian struck by an oncoming car

Multiple Choice

Read each item carefully, and then select the best response.

_____ 1. Which of the following is not a criterion for referral to a regional trauma center?

   A. 45-year-old patient restrained in a low-speed auto crash

   B. Pelvic fracture

   C. Motorcycle crash >20 mph

   D. A pregnant patient

_____ 2. The "Platinum Ten Minutes" refers to the:

   A. amount of time taken to extricate a patient from a motor vehicle crash.

   B. total response time to a traumatic incident.

   C. goal of the maximum time spent at a scene for a critical trauma patient.

   D. time deciding on your "transport decision."

_____ **3.** Which of the following is not considered a "type" of trauma?

    A. Deceleration   **C.** Motor vehicle collision

    B. Acute respiratory distress syndrome (ARDS)   **D.** Bruises

_____ **4.** Pediatric pedestrian injuries are different from adult pedestrian injuries because:

    A. the skulls of children are not fused, which allows for energy absorption.

    B. children are shorter, so the vehicle will "ride over" them.

    C. children are more likely to "fly over" the vehicle.

    D. the bumper is more likely to strike the femur rather than the lower extremities.

_____ **5.** The following is important information to provide to the trauma team EXCEPT:

    A. the name of the street gang.   **C.** the kind of bullet or projectile.

    B. the range at which the firearm was fired.   **D.** the type of weapon used.

_____ **6.** Blast injuries may also be seen in which of the following scenarios?

    A. Mining mishaps   **C.** Terrorist activities

    B. Chemical plants   **D.** All of the above.

_____ **7.** The following are factors in the seriousness of firearms injuries EXCEPT:

    A. the type of tissue injured.   **C.** fragmentation.

    B. missile velocity.   **D.** firearm manufacturer.

_____ **8.** All of the following are examples of mechanical energy EXCEPT:

    A. mechanical energy.   **C.** electrical energy.

    B. kinetic energy.   **D.** chemical energy.

_____ **9.** The following should be used in the transport decisions EXCEPT:

    A. mechanism of injury (MOI).   **C.** proximity to designated trauma facilities.

    B. patient severity of injury.   **D.** insurance coverage.

_____ **10.** Facial injuries, pulmonary contusion, flail chest, ruptured aorta, and fractured sternum are examples of which of the following?

    A. "Ring" of chest injuries   **C.** Head-on crashes

    B. Lateral impacts   **D.** "Down and under pathway"

Labeling

Label the following diagram with the correct mechanisms of blast injuries.

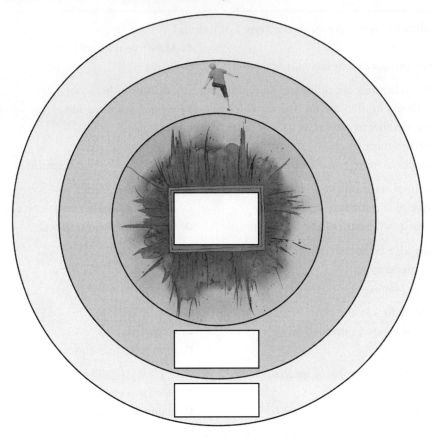

Fill-in-the-Blank

Read each item carefully, and then complete the statement by filling in the missing word(s).

1. Increased morbidity and mortality, especially chest trauma, are more common in _____ _____, particularly rib and sternal fractures.

2. The severity of a stab wound depends on the _____ area involved, depth of _____, blade length, and angle of

penetration.

3. _____ _____ _____ is one of the most concerning of pulmonary blast injuries.

4. Severity of injuries in falls from heights depends on the following factors:

  a. _____

  b. _____

  c. _____

  d. _____

  e. _____

5. Specific injuries associated with seat belt use include _____ fractures and _____ sprains.

Identify

In the following case studies, list the mechanism of injury (MOI), chief complaint, vital signs, and pertinent negatives.

1. You receive a call while working in a paramedic first response vehicle for a motor vehicle crash. On arrival you find two patients who are out of the vehicle and are standing along the roadside. You notice that the vehicle appears to have rolled over onto its side. No other patients are involved, and the scene is deemed safe for patient contact and treatment. One occupant denies any complaint and doesn't want anything to do with EMS. The other patient is holding his right forearm and complains of neck pain. The injured occupant states that he had his seat belt on. You notice that the airbag was deployed. The injured man denies loss of consciousness, shortness of breath, or other complaints. Your physical exam indicates that the patient is slightly ashen and has an obvious bruising and deformity to his right midshaft radius/ulna. He has positive distal pulses, motor and sensory function (PMS), and the following findings: pulse is 110 beats/min and regular, respirations are 16 breaths/min and unlabored, blood pressure is 106/96 mm Hg. The patient denies significant previous medical history.

a. Mechanism of Injury

_____

_____

_____

b. Chief Complaint

_____

_____

_____

c. Vital Signs

_____

_____

_____

d. Pertinent Negatives

_____

_____

_____

2. Today you are assigned to work on an advanced life support ambulance. Your response area includes many high-speed interstate highways. It's toward the end of your shift and, until now, the day has been uneventful. Medcom dispatches you, priority one, to a reported motorcycle crash with one critical injury. On arrival you notice a long line of stopped traffic and concerned bystanders. They are frantically waving you toward the injured patient. You notice a one-vehicle, motorcycle vs. guardrail collision. The patient appears to be talking, but you notice a pool of blood alongside him as well as a cracked helmet. He has a badly deformed lower leg that you quickly conclude is fractured or dislocated. The patient is in obvious pain and is able to communicate that he "hurts all over." You quickly begin to assess the patient, and he appears agitated, ashen, diaphoretic, and slightly short of breath. He has delayed (>2-second) capillary refill, and he has diminished left side breath sounds and no tracheal deviation. His pulse is 120 beats/min, respiratory rate is 28 breaths/min, and blood pressure is unobtainable. You note that the patient has a palpable femoral pulse but no radial or brachial pulse.

a. Mechanism of Injury

_____

_____

_____

b. Chief Complaint

_____

_____

_____

c. Vital Signs

_____

_____

_____

d. Pertinent Negatives

_____

_____

_____

3. You respond to a "routine" call at an adult care facility for a "fall." Your patient is an 82-year-old woman who is laying on a carpeted floor with a walker positioned beside her. She appears conscious but slightly confused. She doesn't really know why she fell or how she ended up on the ground. She asks you to help her up. You begin your initial assessment of the patient when she denies any knowledge of the incident. During the rapid trauma assessment, she denies any chest discomfort, shortness of breath, neck or back pain. You note some deformity and rotation to her right lower extremity. On palpation it is tender to the touch. The patient is confused regarding her previous medical history. The staff tells you that she has a history of TIAs and heart problems. She is on multiple medications and is allergic to morphine sulfate. Her abdomen is soft and nontender. Her vital signs are pulse 58 beats/min and irregular, blood pressure 158/110 mm Hg, and the skin is pale, cool, and dry.

a. Mechanism of Injury

_____

_____

_____

b. Chief Complaint

_____

_____

_____

c. Vital Signs

_____

_____

_____

d. Pertinent Negatives

_____

_____

_____

Ambulance Calls

The following case scenarios provide an opportunity to explore the concerns associated with mechanism of care and trauma systems. Read each scenario, and then answer each question.

1. You are called to the scene of a back-road single-vehicle collision in which a car plowed into a utility pole. The driver of the car is sitting on the grass beside his wrecked vehicle looking dazed and confused. What parameters would you use to assess the mechanism of injury (MOI) and suspected injuries and/or injury patterns?

   a. _____

   b. _____

   c. _____

   d. _____

   e. _____

   f. _____

2. You are summoned to the scene of a smoky apartment-house fire. When you arrive, one of the firefighters directs you to a casualty who has been carried to a spot just beyond the fire lines. The firefighter tells you that the man jumped from a window.

   a. What further information do you need to obtain about this patient to evaluate the potential seriousness of the injuries he might have sustained making that jump?

   _____

   _____

   _____

   b. Assuming that he landed on his feet, what injuries might you expect him to have suffered?

   _____

   _____

   _____

3. On your very next call, you are summoned to a housing project where a 2-year-old child managed to crawl over the edge of a second-story balcony and fall into the playground below. What sort of injuries would this child most likely have sustained, and why?

   _____

   _____

   _____

   _____

4. You are called to a somewhat disreputable downtown area for a "man shot." You arrive on the scene to see the patient lying on the ground in the center of a small group of men, some of them apparently intoxicated and all of them talking at once.

   a. What is the *first* action you will take before entering the scene?

   _____

   _____

b. What information do you need to obtain regarding the shooting incident?

(1) _____

(2) _____

(3) _____

(4) _____

(5) _____

5. A fire at a warehouse of a large construction company ignites the stock of dynamite and produces an explosion that shatters windows for blocks around. As you respond to the scene, you review in your mind the different kinds of injuries you might soon have to deal with. List the four *mechanisms* of injuries that can be produced by an explosion and describe each one.

a. _____

_____

_____

b. _____

_____

_____

c. _____

_____

_____

d. _____

_____

_____

6. Among the patients you treat at the scene of the explosion is a young man who had been taking a walk about half a block from the construction company when the explosion occurred. The man states that the blast "knocked me clear off my feet." He complains of a "tight feeling in my chest" and blurry vision. On physical examination, he appears somewhat confused; he cannot tell you the date or what day of the week it is. His vital signs are pulse 100 beats/min, full and regular; respirations 30 breaths/min and somewhat shallow; blood pressure 120/80 mm Hg. His skin is warm and dry. Aside from a little dried blood in the left ear canal, there are no other physical findings. What tissues are at risk? What is the evidence for you thinking so?

Tissues at Risk	Evidence
1.	
2.	
3.	

True/False

If you believe the statement to be more true than false, write the letter "T" in the space provided. If you believe the statement to be more false than true, write the letter "F."

_____ **1.** One of the top five leading causes of traumatic death is drowning.

_____ **2.** A Level IV Trauma Center provides the most comprehensive trauma care possible.

_____ **3.** Transport considerations are not necessary if the patient is seriously hurt.

_____ **4.** Blunt trauma typically occurs in motor vehicle crashes.

_____ **5.** The "paper bag syndrome" can result in a pneumothorax.

_____ **6.** Small children should be seated in the front seats of motor vehicles to benefit from the protection offered by air bags.

_____ **7.** One of the earliest signs of hypovolemic shock is a fall in blood pressure.

_____ **8.** Patients in hypovolemic shock tend to suffer metabolic acidosis.

_____ **9.** The intravenous fluid of choice to provide volume to a patient in hypovolemic shock is 5% dextrose in water (D_5W).

_____ **10.** A patient may go into shock without losing any blood or fluid from the body.

Short Answer

Complete this section with short written answers using the space provided.

1. A 2,000-lb automobile is traveling at 20 mph when it strikes a pedestrian.

  a. What happens to the kinetic energy of the vehicle at the moment of impact?

  _____

  _____

  b. If the vehicle weighed 6,000 lb instead of 2,000 lb, what difference would that make in terms of its kinetic energy?

  _____

  _____

  c. If the vehicle was traveling at 60 mph rather than 20 mph, what difference would that make in terms of its kinetic energy?

  _____

  _____

2. A car traveling at 50 mph goes out of control and slams into a concrete wall. That sequence of events in fact produces three separate collisions, each involving a transfer of kinetic energy. What objects are involved in each of the three collisions, and what happens to the kinetic energy in each case?

  a. Collision 1: _____

  _____

  _____

  b. Collision 2: _____

  _____

  _____

  c. Collision 3: _____

  _____

  _____

3. Careful inspection of a wrecked vehicle can enable the rescuer to detect injuries among the patients that might not otherwise be obvious. For each of the vehicular findings mentioned in the following list, list the injuries that are likely to be associated.

   a. Deformed dashboard

     (1) _____

     (2) _____

     (3) _____

     (4) _____

     (5) _____

   b. Deformed steering column

     (1) _____

     (2) _____

     (3) _____

     (4) _____

     (5) _____

     (6) _____

   c. Cracked windshield

     (1) _____

     (2) _____

     (3) _____

     (4) _____

   d. Door smashed in

     (1) _____

     (2) _____

4. One of the most lethal objects in a motor vehicle is the steering wheel. Whenever you find structural damage to a steering wheel—indeed, whenever there is significant deformity to the front end of a car involved in a collision—you must be alert for the presence of the "ring of injuries" impact that the steering wheel may have produced in the driver of the car. List six injuries that may be associated with steering wheel trauma.

   a. _____

   b. _____

   c. _____

   d. _____

   e. _____

   f. _____

Word Find

Hidden in the following grid are 15 words or phrases related to what you have studied in this chapter. Find the hidden words in the grid below. Then use the words from the grid to answer the following questions (some words may be used to answer more than one question).

```
I G L U R X G S A K S Q D N D
M N A Z P I H R C H J E Z O I
P I T C A A J E E I N H W C C
L T E O Q F N A A I T N Y I F
O A R A U N R D A D A E N S F
S R A Y M I T R O N O A N J T
I T L J N U T B D V P N F I D
O E I G P S A U E M E K A T K
N N M O E B N R Y F C R Y Z F
A E P R P D A T T Q N D H B O
J P A D E N I A R T S E R N U
Z F C R U S Z F T H N J E Y A
N Y T L E N T R Y W O U N D G
V E L O C I T Y U J R I L O L
G N I S L U V A K M Z Z G B T
```

1. _____ of the aorta can result in rapid loss of all of the body's blood and death.

2. A tearing away of forcible separation is considered _____.

3. An impact on the body by objects that cause injury without penetrating soft tissues or internal organs or cavities is called

_____ _____.

4. _____ _____, "T-bone," and side collisions impart energy to the near-side occupant almost

directly to the pelvis and chest.

5. The occupant is pushed under the steering column; this is called the _____-_____-

_____ pathway.

6. The lead point is the head _____-_____-_____ pathway.

7. _____ victims have a 45% reduction in fatalities.

8. Rear-impact collisions cause _____ victims to be propelled into the back seat.

9. In a _____-_____ collision with two vehicles traveling in opposite directions along a

straight line, transferred energy is represented in part as the sum of both their speeds.

10. Injuries are described as consequences of blunt or _____ trauma.

11. The point at which a penetrating object enters the body is called a/an _____ _____.

12. A bursting inward is _____.

13. Knowledge of _____ can help one predict injury patterns found in a patient.

14. The eardrum is the _____ membrane.

15. _____ refers to how fast the patient was traveling.

Fill-in-the-Table

Fill in the missing parts of the table.

1. Key elements for trauma centers: Fill in the key elements for the corresponding definition.

Key Elements for Trauma Centers		
Level	**Definition**	**Key Elements**
Level I	A comprehensive regional resource that is a tertiary care facility. Capable of providing total care for every aspect of injury—from prevention through rehabilitation.	**1.** 24-hour in-house coverage by general surgeons **2.** Availability of care in specialties such as orthopaedic surgery, neurosurgery, anesthesiology, emergency medicine, radiology, internal medicine, and critical care **3.** **4.** Provides leadership in prevention, public education, and continuing education of trauma team members **5.**
Level II	Able to initiate definitive care for all injured patients.	**1.** 24-hour immediate coverage by general surgeons **2.** Availability of orthopaedic surgery, neurosurgery, anesthesiology, emergency medicine, radiology, and critical care **3.** **4.** **5.** Provides continued improvement in trauma care through a comprehensive quality assessment program
Level III	Has demonstrated the ability to provide prompt assessment, resuscitation, and stabilization of injured patients and emergency operations.	**1.** 24-hour immediate coverage by emergency medicine physicians and prompt availability of general surgeons and anesthesiologists **2.** Program dedicated to continued improvement in trauma care through a comprehensive quality assessment program **3.** **4.** **5.** **6.** Also dedicated to improving trauma care through a comprehensive quality assessment program
Level IV	Has demonstrated the ability to provide Advanced Trauma Life Support (ATLS) before transfer of patients to a higher level trauma center.	**1.** **2.** **3.** Committed to continued improvement of these trauma care activities through a formal quality assessment program **4.** Involved in prevention, outreach, and education within its community

2. List the "ring" of chest injuries from impacting the steering wheel or dashboard:

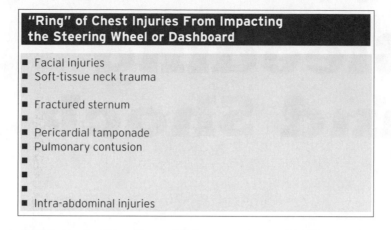

**"Ring" of Chest Injuries From Impacting
the Steering Wheel or Dashboard**

- Facial injuries
- Soft-tissue neck trauma
-
- Fractured sternum
-
- Pericardial tamponade
- Pulmonary contusion
-
-
-
- Intra-abdominal injuries

Problem Solving

Use the formula for kinetic energy to answer the following questions.

$$KE = \frac{M}{2} \times V^2$$

You have responded to a motor vehicle crash. This was a collision involving a car and a stationary bridge abutment. There are two patients. You note that your patient appears to be a 6-ft man who weighs approximately 200 lb. The patient is conscious and alert, and while talking to him you discover that he was not wearing a seat belt and he was traveling at 50 mph.

1. Use the formula for calculating kinetic energy (KE) to determine the KE units involved in this crash. The second passenger in the vehicle was also unbelted, and she weighs 120 lb.

2. How many KE units are involved with the second passenger?

CHAPTER

18 Bleeding and Shock

Chapter Review

The following exercises provide an opportunity to test your knowledge of this chapter.

Matching
Match each of the definitions in the left column to the appropriate terms in the right column.

_____ 1. The most common cause of shock

_____ 2. Protein that gives blood the red color

_____ 3. Dark, tarry stools that indicate bleeding in the lower gastrointestinal (GI) tract

_____ 4. Stools that are bright red in color

_____ 5. Bleeding from the nose

_____ 6. Usually the last measurable factor to change in shock

_____ 7. The early stage of shock in which the body can still compensate for blood loss

_____ 8. When blood is shunted away from the liver, kidneys, and lungs

_____ 9. Crystalloid solution that contains potassium and calcium

_____ 10. Crystalloid solution used for dehydrated patients

A. Compensated shock

B. Blood pressure

C. Lactated Ringer's

D. Hemoglobin

E. Normal saline

F. Hematochezia

G. Bleeding

H. Irreversible shock

I. Epistaxis

J. Melena

Multiple Choice
Read each item carefully, and then select the best response.

_____ 1. _____ is the pressure in the aorta against which the left ventricle must pump blood.

    A. Stroke volume

    B. Afterload

    C. Cardiac output

    D. Ejection fraction

_____ 2. Which of the following substances accounts for more than half of the body's blood volume?

    A. Erythrocytes

    B. Leukocytes

    C. Plasma

    D. Hemoglobin

_____ 3. On average, an arterial bleed takes how many minutes to clot with direct pressure?

    A. Two

    B. Three

    C. Five

    D. Seven

_____ **4.** The body cannot tolerate an acute blood loss of _____%. This loss will produce a significant change in vital signs of the adult patient.

        A. 5   **C.** 15

        B. 10   **D.** 20

_____ **5.** When you encounter a patient that is bleeding, the first thing you should do is:

        A. estimate the blood loss.   **C.** check for breathing.

        B. apply direct pressure.   **D.** don personal protective equipment (PPE).

_____ **6.** A stool that has bright red blood is called:

        A. hematochezia.   **C.** hematuria.

        B. melena.   **D.** epistaxis.

_____ **7.** Which of the following is considered a contraindication to using the pneumatic anti-shock garments (PASG/MAST)?

        A. Intraperitoneal bleeding

        B. Head injury with a blood pressure of 50 mm Hg systolic

        C. Intraperitoneal bleeding with a blood pressure of 50 mm Hg systolic

        D. Severe hypotension

_____ **8.** Widespread dilation of the resistance vessels leads to distributive shock. Which of the following is a common type of distributive shock?

        A. Cardiogenic shock   **C.** Septic shock

        B. Hypovolemic shock   **D.** Obstructive shock

_____ **9.** Which of the following statements about dextran is correct?

        A. You don't need to type or cross-match before using dextran.

        B. Dextran doesn't stay in the vascular space long.

        C. Dextran can help stop bleeding.

        D. Dextran can coat the red blood cells and interfere with clotting.

_____ **10.** During a time of inadequate perfusion, the kidneys can go as long as how many minutes before there is permanent damage?

        A. 30   **C.** 60

        B. 45   **D.** 90

Labeling

Label the following diagram with the correct terms.

1. Label the following parts of the cardiovascular system:

   - Superior vena cava
   - Aorta
   - Right atrium
   - Right ventricle

   - Inferior vena cava
   - (Lower) aorta
   - Left ventricle
   - Left atrium

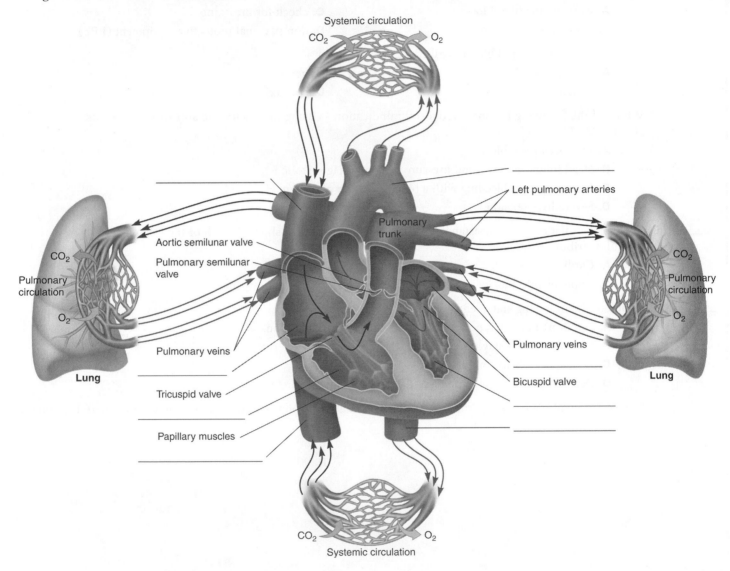

Fill-in-the-Blank

Read each item carefully, and then complete the statement by filling in the missing word(s).

1. A now somewhat controversial treatment for shock is the military anti-shock trousers, or _____, also known

   as the _____.

2. Red blood cells contain _____, a protein that gives blood its reddish color.

3. Blood circulation through an organ or tissue that meets the cells' current needs for oxygen, nutrients, and waste removal is

   known as _____.

4. _____ is the process in which platelets aggregate at the site, plugging the hole and sealing injured portions of the

   vessel.

5. A lower GI bleed is indicated with the passing of _____, which is a dark, tarry-looking stool.

6. _____ is bleeding from the nose.

7. _____ happens when the level of tissue perfusion drops below normal limits.

8. As blood pressure drops, _____, which are located in the carotid sinuses and the aortic arch, sense the lower

   pressure and activate the vasomotor center to constrict the vessels in the body.

9. The two types of shock in the Weil-Shubin classification are _____ shock and _____ shock.

10. A progressive condition of combined failure of several organs at the same time is known as _____-_____

    _____ _____.

11. _____ _____ is the difference between the systolic and diastolic pressures.

12. The three phases of shock are _____, _____, and _____ shock.

13. The intravenous (IV) fluid of choice when replacing lost blood volume is _____ _____.

14. Shock that is caused by an allergic reaction is _____ shock.

15. Solutions that do not contain proteins or any other large molecules are known as _____.

Identify

In the following case study, list the chief complaint, vital signs, and pertinent negatives.

You are called to the home of a 74-year-old man who is experiencing chest pain. Upon arrival, you begin your chest pain protocol. John, the patient, is experiencing tightness in his chest and left arm. You place John on high-flow supplemental oxygen and obtain a 12-lead echocardiogram (ECG). You determine that John's heart is in a sinus bradycardia with a rate of 52 beats/min. His lungs have some crackles at the base, he is breathing 24 breaths/min, and his room air saturation is 92%. He is slightly confused, but comes around with the oxygen and is able to answer all your questions. His pupils are equal and round, regular in size, and react to light (PEARRL). You are unable to feel a pulse in his wrist. His blood pressure is 80/56 mm Hg, and he is diaphoretic. You determine that the rate and strength of John's heart are causing the problem. You realize that John is in cardiogenic shock. You start an IV and a low-dose dopamine drip. You feel that John is a top priority and head to the hospital as quickly as possible.

1. Chief Complaint

_____

_____

_____

2. Vital Signs

_____

_____

_____

3. Pertinent Negatives

_____

_____

_____

Ambulance Calls

The following case scenarios provide an opportunity to explore the concerns associated with patient management and paramedic care. Read each scenario, and then answer each question.

1. A middle-aged man was struck by a car as he was crossing the street. You find him lying by the side of the road, complaining of severe pain in his abdomen, where the car hit him. You would like to make an assessment of his state of perfusion. How will you assess the following?

   a. His _peripheral_ perfusion:

   _____

   b. The perfusion to his _vital organs:_

   _____

2. You are called to a downtown bar in which firearms were deployed to settle a difference of opinion. You find a man lying on the floor of the bar, unconscious, his trouser leg soaked in blood. In the correct sequence, list the steps you would take in treating this patient.

   a. _____

   b. _____

   c. _____

   d. _____

   e. _____

   f. _____

3. One rainy day, a car bomb was detonated in front of a foreign consulate, and a number of bystanders were injured by flying debris, including jagged pieces of metal torn from the car's body. The first patient you come upon is bleeding from multiple sites, including a deep gash on the right side of the neck and a laceration that has partially severed the right leg at the groin. The leg laceration is gushing blood; it is too proximal to benefit from a tourniquet. It's hard to evaluate skin condition in the rain. Pulse is around 100 beats/min and somewhat weak; respirations are 30 breaths/min.

   a. What steps would you take at the scene?

   (1) _____

   (2) _____

   (3) _____

   (4) _____

   b. What steps would you take during transport?

   (1) _____

   (2) _____

   (3) _____

4. A second patient from the car bombing, a young man, was sideswiped by a piece of flying debris, which made a clean 14-inch incision straight across his abdomen. He is conscious and in moderate distress. Pulse is 104 beats/min and regular, respirations are 28 breaths/min and slightly labored, and blood pressure is 104/70 mm Hg. What looks to be a major portion of the patient's intestines are outside the abdomen.

   a. What steps would you take at the scene?

   (1) _____

   (2) _____

   (3) _____

   b. What steps would you take during transport?

   (1) _____

   (2) _____

   (3) _____

5. A third patient from the car bombing is another young man in considerable respiratory distress. There is a 2-inch wide hole in his right chest through which you can hear air being sucked on inhalation. His skin is warm. His pulse is 108 beats/min and regular; respirations are 30 breaths/min and gasping; blood pressure is 112/64 mm Hg.

   a. What steps would you take at the scene?

   (1) _____

   (2) _____

   (3) _____

b. What steps would you take during transport?

(1) _____

(2) _____

(3) _____

6. A 59-year-old man was the driver of a car that plowed into a bridge abutment in the early hours of the morning. The patient is conscious, but very restless. He is sweating profusely. His chest is stable (it's too dark to see whether there are bruises). He can move all his extremities. His pulse is 82 beats/min, respirations are 28 breaths/min, and blood pressure is 100/70 mm Hg.

a. What steps would you take at the scene?

(1) _____

(2) _____

(3) _____

(4) _____

(5) _____

b. What steps would you take during transport?

(1) _____

(2) _____

(3) _____

(4) _____

True/False

If you believe the statement to be more true than false, write the letter "T" in the space provided. If you believe the statement to be more false than true, write the letter "F."

_____ **1.** One of the earliest signs of hypovolemic shock is a fall in the blood pressure.

_____ **2.** Patients in hypovolemic shock tend to suffer metabolic acidosis.

_____ **3.** The intravenous fluid of choice to provide volume to a patient in hypovolemic shock is 5% dextrose in water (D_5W).

_____ **4.** A patient may go into shock without losing any blood or fluid from the body.

_____ **5.** The amount of blood pumped through the circulatory system in 1 minute is known as the cardiac output.

_____ **6.** The function of plasma is to produce red blood cells (RBCs) and white blood cells (WBCs).

_____ **7.** Nontraumatic internal bleeding usually happens in the gastrointestinal tract.

_____ **8.** A 1-year-old child has a blood volume of around 800 mL.

_____ **9.** You can use a wire, rope, or any narrow material as a tourniquet.

_____ **10.** Definitive management for internal hemorrhage is in the hospital.

Short Answer

Complete this section with short written answers using the space provided.

1. Three components are required for a functioning circulatory system. If any one of those components is impaired, shock may result. List the three necessary components.

   a. _____

   b. _____

   c. _____

2. The type of shock you will see most frequently in the prehospital setting is hemorrhagic shock. It is very important to detect hemorrhagic shock early and to start treatment early. To do so, you must have a high index of suspicion in assessing patients at risk of hemorrhagic shock, which means you must be aware of the situations in which hemorrhagic shock is likely to occur. List four causes of hemorrhagic shock.

   a. _____

   b. _____

   c. _____

   d. _____

3. It is easier to remember the signs and symptoms of shock if you understand the mechanisms by which those signs and symptoms occur. List four signs or symptoms of shock, and beside each, explain what change in the body causes that sign or symptom.

   Sign or Symptom   **Mechanism That Causes the Sign or Symptom**

   a. _____

   b. _____

   c. _____

   d. _____

4. It is not necessary in the field to make a specific diagnosis of a patient's abdominal pain, but it is necessary to be able to recognize when a potentially life-threatening situation exists. Any patient with abdominal pain showing symptoms or signs of shock must be considered to be in danger.

   To recognize that danger, you must be able to spot the symptoms and signs of shock. List six symptoms and signs of shock.

   a. _____

   b. _____

   c. _____

   d. _____

   e. _____

   f. _____

5. List six symptoms and signs of dehydration.

a. _____

b. _____

c. _____

d. _____

e. _____

f. _____

6. List five methods for the control of external hemorrhage.

a. _____

b. _____

c. _____

d. _____

e. _____

Word Find

Hidden in the following grid are 25 words or phrases related to what you have studied in this chapter. Find the hidden words in the grid below. Then use the words from the grid to answer the following questions (some words may be used to answer more than one question).

```
N D C E P I S T A X I S T E K G A
C O E I G C I T P E S N A R H E T
S I I C B A E B X Z I Q T Y Y R R
T C N T O O H P S O U S S T P U O
E E H E C M R R P I A D O H O S A
L N X I G A P E R M L C M R V S L
E T S T C O R E A O F U E O O E E
T R O I E U I F N N M P H C L R V
A A J R S R B D N S A E Q Y E P I
L L R S L P N Y R O A M H T M T T
P F E M Y R E A G A I T U E I C C
C R G P A S G S L T C T E S C E U
P E P I N E P H R I N E C D B R R
E V I T U B I R T S I D I E U I T
S E T Y C O K U E L X M Q M J D S
S E N S I T I Z A T I O N H E E B
E E K A M E D O I G N A N L V L O
```

1. Largest artery in the body: _____

2. Body's measure to pump the same amount of blood that is returned to the heart: _____ _____

3. White blood cells: _____

4. Red blood cells: _____

5. Cells responsible for clot formation: _____

6. Bleeding caused by a break in the skin: _____

7. Another word for bleeding: _____

8. You should always take these kinds of precautions: _____

9. Bleeding from the nose: _____

10. First step in controlling bleeding: _____ _____

11. Apply heavy pressure here to control severe bleeding: _____ _____

12. Apply at the end of a severed vessel to control bleeding: _____

13. Both names for an inflatable shock garment that surrounds the legs: _____ and _____

14. Shock caused by heart failure: _____

15. Hormone that increases pulse rate and strength: _____

16. Shock that occurs as a result of blood flow being blocked and not reaching the heart: _____

17. Shock caused by blood volume being too low to distribute oxygen and nutrients to the body: _____

18. Cardiogenic and obstructive shock both contribute to this kind of shock: _____

19. Widespread dilation of the capacitance or resistance vessels: _____

20. Shock caused by a systolic blood pressure of less than 90 mm Hg and the presence of sepsis syndrome: _____

21. Occurs as a result of widespread infection: _____

22. To develop a heightened reaction to a substance: _____

23. Large areas of subcutaneous edema with a sudden onset: _____

24. Metabolism without oxygen: _____

25. Another word for progressive shock: _____

Fill-in-the-Table

Fill in the missing parts of the table.

Compensated Versus Decompensated Hypoperfusion	
Compensated Hypoperfusion	**Decompensated Hypoperfusion**
■ Agitation, anxiety, restlessness	■ Altered mental status (verbal to unresponsive)
■ _____	■ _____
■ _____	■ Labored or irregular breathing
■ _____	■ Thready or absent peripheral pulses
■ _____	■ _____
■ Nausea, vomiting	_____
■ Delayed capillary refill in infants and children	■ _____
■ Thirst	■ _____
■ _____	_____
	■ Impending cardiac arrest

Skill Drills

Test your knowledge of skill drills by placing the following photos in the correct order. Number the first step with a "1," the second step with a "2," and so forth.

1. *Treating Shock*

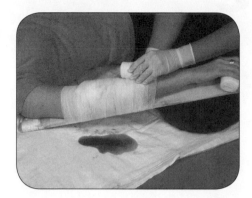

Splint broken bones or joint injuries.

_____

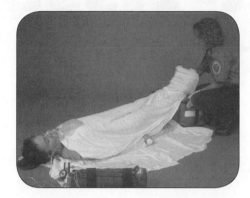

If no fractures are suspected, elevate the legs 12". Insert an IV line, and administer warm fluid en route to the ED. Insert an IV line at the scene only if transport of the patient is delayed (such as if the patient is pinned).

_____

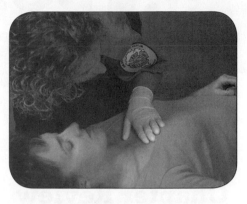

Keep the patient supine, open the airway, and check breathing and pulse. Give high-flow supplemental oxygen, and assist ventilations if needed.

_____

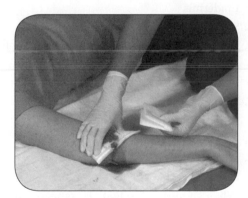

Control obvious external bleeding.

_____

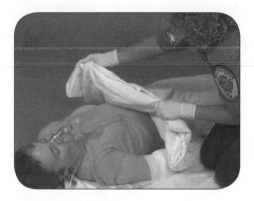

Place blankets under and over the patient.

_____

CHAPTER

19 Soft-Tissue Injury

Chapter Review

The following exercises provide an opportunity to test your knowledge of this chapter.

Matching

Match each of the items in the left column to the appropriate definition in the right column.

_____ 1. The largest organ of the body

_____ 2. Cravats

_____ 3. Phagocytosis

_____ 4. Compartment syndrome

_____ 5. Closed wound

_____ 6. Pressure injuries

_____ 7. Capillary bleeding

_____ 8. Underlying the epidermis

_____ 9. Crush syndrome

_____ 10. Pressure point

_____ 11. Process of new cells repairing a soft-tissue injury

_____ 12. Scene safety

_____ 13. Found in scar tissue, hair, bones, and connective tissue

_____ 14. Adipose tissue

_____ 15. Abrasion

_____ 16. Gangrene

_____ 17. Primary phase

_____ 18. Histamine

_____ 19. Laceration

_____ 20. Outermost layer of skin

A. Infection caused by *Clostridium perfringens*

B. Epidermis

C. Superficial wound caused by scraping

D. Cut inflicted by a sharp instrument; may be a clean or jagged incision

E. Subcutaneous layer

F. Triangular bandages

G. Causes dilation of blood vessels

H. First aspect to address in any scenario

I. Dermis

J. Dark red and oozing

K. When an area of the body is trapped longer than 4 hours

L. Skin

M. Damage to tissue below the epidermis; epidermis is intact

N. Brachial artery

O. Edema and swelling resulting in increased pressure within soft tissue

P. Occurs in bedridden patients

Q. Engulfment of bacteria

R. Rapidly developing pressure wave in an explosion

S. Collagen

T. Epithelialization

Multiple Choice

Read each item carefully, and then select the best response.

_____ 1. The condition that develops when edema and swelling result in increased pressure within soft tissues is called:
- **A.** crush syndrome.
- **B.** Volkmann contracture.
- **C.** compartment syndrome.
- **D.** rhabdomyolysis.

_____ 2. Blood vessels, nerves, tendons, muscles, and internal organs can all be damaged by:
- **A.** compartment syndrome.
- **B.** improperly applied dressings.
- **C.** use of a wet dressing instead of a dry dressing.
- **D.** application of a tourniquet.

_____ 3. When should impaled objects be removed?
- **A.** When the object affects packaging and transport.
- **B.** When the object affects the eye.
- **C.** When bleeding cannot be successfully controlled.
- **D.** The paramedic should never remove an impaled object.

_____ 4. Blast injuries can lead to which of the following conditions?
- **A.** Pulmonary edema
- **B.** Amputations
- **C.** Tympanic membrane rupture
- **D.** All of the above.

_____ 5. Patients with soft-tissue injuries:
- **A.** rarely have life-threatening injuries.
- **B.** should be "signed-off" to save EMS system resources.
- **C.** should be treated with aggressive ALS treatment in the event of unforeseen injury.
- **D.** have a high incidence of morbidity and mortality.

_____ 6. Many open wounds require surgical intervention for closure to bring the wound edges together to permit optimal healing. Of the following methods, which is *not* routinely used?
- **A.** Medical glue
- **B.** Staples
- **C.** Rope
- **D.** Sutures

_____ 7. There are numerous types of soft-tissue injuries. Many of them are relatively minor, but some have potentially serious outcomes. Which of the following injuries requires transportation?
- **A.** Abrasion
- **B.** Laceration
- **C.** Cosmetic complications
- **D.** Incision

_____ 8. Oftentimes soft-tissue injuries involve hemorrhaging. All of the following would be considered appropriate bleeding management EXCEPT:
- **A.** direct pressure with thick, bulky dressings.
- **B.** pressure with elastic bandages.
- **C.** "wet" dressings.
- **D.** elevation of the extremity and pressure points.

_____ 9. Soft-tissue injuries to the neck may lead to which of the following complications?
- **A.** Air embolism
- **B.** Spinal injury
- **C.** Airway disruption
- **D.** All of the above.

_____ 10. Which of the following can interfere with wound healing?
- **A.** An underlying cardiac history
- **B.** A seizure disorder
- **C.** Carpal tunnel syndrome
- **D.** A history of diabetes

Labeling

1. Label the components of the skin in the following diagram.

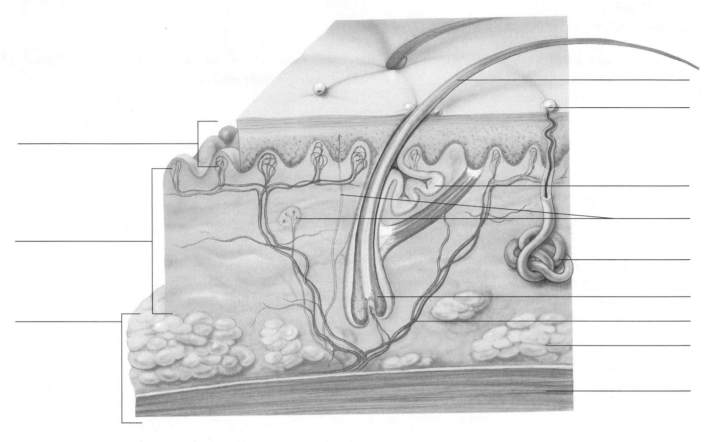

2. Determine which types of open wounds are shown in each of the following photos.

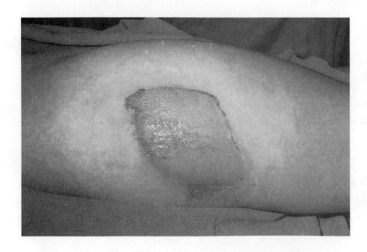

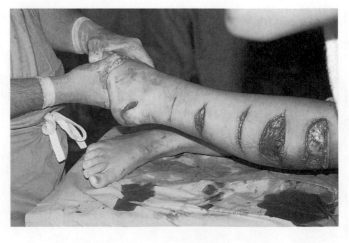

a. _____

b. _____

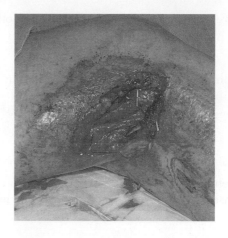

d. _____

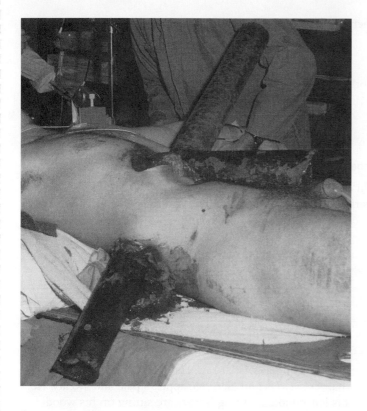

c. _____

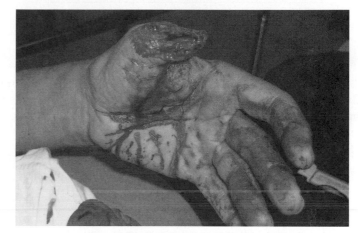

e. _____

Fill-in-the-Blank

Read each item carefully, and then complete the statement by filling in the missing word(s).

1. _____ injuries require substantial irrigation and _____ before closing by an emergency practitioner.

2. Visible clues of infection include _____, _____, _____, _____, and _____

_____.

3. *Clostridium tetani* causes the body to produce a potent _____, which results in painful muscle _____ that are

strong enough to fracture _____.

4. The seriousness of a laceration depends on its _____ and the _____ that have been damaged.

5. One of the body's first responses to a vessel injury is localized _____ that reduces the flow of blood.

6. When responding to a reported explosion, wait for _____ to secure the scene and declare it _____ before

you approach any victims. When a blast seems to be intentional, the paramedic should look for possible _____ devices. Responders have been injured and _____ by other explosive devices planted away from the original

detonation.

7. Because wet dressings provide a medium for _____ and other pathogens to grow, their use is _____ in the

field.

Identify

In the following case studies, identify the type of soft-tissue injury and the care that you would provide.

1. You are called to the scene of a local campsite where a 10-year-old boy was playing with his pocket knife, whittling some wood, when he cut himself. The injury is a jagged incision to his right forearm. There is moderate darkish-red blood oozing from the site.

_____

_____

_____

_____

2. A patient was working in his home shop when he became distracted while using a circular saw. He inadvertently cut the fingers on his left hand. When you arrive the patient is sitting in a chair conscious and alert. He appears pale and sweaty. He has several blood-soaked towels covering his hand. You notice that his left middle and ring fingers are sitting on his wood-crafting bench.

_____

_____

_____

_____

3. It's a busy shift. On this call you are dispatched to a bar fight. On arrival there is a crowd hovering around a woman who complains of pain in her right side and moderate shortness of breath. Her companion states that she was involved in a dispute and felt a sharp object impact her right side. The patient is somewhat angry and combative and wants to continue the dispute. As you examine the injury you notice a minimal amount of bleeding that appears to have stopped. The patient has a quarter-inch circular opening to her chest. There appears to be a small amount of swelling and a rush of air when she breathes.

_____

_____

_____

_____

Ambulance Calls

The following case scenarios provide an opportunity to explore the concerns associated with patient management and paramedic care. Read each scenario, and then answer each question.

1. You are summoned to Bugsy's Butcher Shop to tend to the proprietor, Bugsy Butterfingers, who dropped a meat cleaver on his left leg. There is a large gash in the left calf, and it is bleeding profusely.

a. List five methods you might use to try to control the bleeding, and put an asterisk next to the method likely to be the most effective. Please note that BSI precautions are being done appropriately.

(1) _____

(2) _____

(3) _____

(4) _____

(5) _____

b. Suppose Bugsy's wound had been on the forearm rather than on the leg. Which artery could you have compressed in that case to help control the bleeding?

_____

2. One of Bugsy's employees, Frank Fillet, becomes so distracted watching you care for his boss that he accidentally chops off two of his fingers while preparing an order of steaks.

a. How will you treat Frank's injury?

_____

_____

_____

b. What will you do with the two fingers lying on the chopping board?

_____

_____

_____

3. Yet another worker in the butcher shop, Hercules Hamburger, had been watching, slack-jawed and transfixed, as this drama was unfolding. So intent was he on the spectacle that he did not realize his right hand had entered the meat grinder—not until, that is, the hand became engaged in the grinding blades. Hearing his screams, a customer rushes over to where Hercules is standing and manages to shut off the meat grinder, but not before Hercules' hand and forearm have been badly mangled. You already have your hands full with Bugsy and Frank, so you instruct the "Good Samaritan" who shut off the meat grinder, "Have him lie down, and try to control the bleeding—I'll be with him in just a minute." Obligingly, the customer grabs a piece of rope that he finds behind the counter, winds it around Hercules' upper arm, and slips a ball-point pen into the knot to serve as tourniquet. He twists the rope as tight as he possibly can, secures the pen, and uses the butcher's apron to wrap the entire hand and arm.

Although the customer was trying to be helpful, in fact he made several very serious mistakes. List them here:

a. _____

b. _____

c. _____

d. _____

4. During deer-hunting season, two young backpackers were strolling through the woods when hunters, mistaking the pair for deer, discharged their crossbows at them. One arrow entered the eye of the first backpacker, while another arrow went straight through the cheek of the second backpacker.

   a. Describe the steps you would take in treating the backpacker with the arrow in his eye. Please note that BSI precautions are being done appropriately.

_____

_____

_____

_____

   b. Describe the steps you would take in treating the backpacker who has an arrow impaled in his cheek.

_____

_____

_____

_____

5. You're folding up your deck chair when you happen to see a jogger running erratically down the beach toward you. His shorts are torn, and there is blood trickling down one leg. "What happened to you?" you ask.

   "Some big Doberman tackled me as I was running. I figured the best thing to do was keep running to where I left my car." You note the tooth marks and a laceration on the runner's left leg.

   How would you manage this patient? Please note that BSI precautions are being done appropriately.

   a. _____

_____

   b. _____

_____

   c. _____

_____

   d. _____

_____

True/False

If you believe the statement to be more true than false, write the letter "T" in the space provided. If you believe the statement to be more false than true, write the letter "F."

_____ **1.** Amputation is a form of avulsion.

_____ **2.** Soft-tissue trauma is the leading form of injury.

_____ **3.** Sweating is regulated through the parasympathetic nervous system.

_____ **4.** Subcutaneous blood vessels have a crucial role in regulating body temperature.

_____ **5.** The precise function of sebum secreted by the sebaceous glands is not well known.

_____ **6.** Human bites carry a higher risk of infection than animal bites do.

_____ **7.** Keloid scars typically develop in areas of high tissue stress.

_____ **8.** Tetanus infection causes the body to produce a potent toxin that results in lockjaw.

_____ **9.** Explosion patients are more likely to be killed or permanently disabled by the fifth phase of the incident.

_____ **10.** Bleeding control is a key principle in treating open wounds.

Short Answer

Complete this section with short written answers using the space provided.

1. You can appreciate the possible consequences of injury to the skin if you understand what functions healthy, intact skin performs. List four functions performed by the skin in a healthy person.

a. _____

b. _____

c. _____

d. _____

2. Healing of wounds is a natural process that involves several overlapping stages. List the five stages of wound healing.

a. _____

b. _____

c. _____

d. _____

e. _____

3. Wounds are characterized as either closed or open. List the characteristics of closed wounds.

a. _____

b. _____

c. _____

4. Crush syndrome is a serious injury that can occur when an area of the body has been trapped for 4 hours or longer. List the progression of crush syndrome.

a. _____

b. _____

c. _____

d. _____

Word Find

Hidden in the following grid are 15 words or phrases related to what you have studied in this chapter. Find the hidden words in the grid below. Then use the words from the grid to answer the following questions (some words may be used to answer more than one question).

```
E T A X V D T C K S W E F A Q E F N S
C K Y C O T E C Q E C T M O T A E N U
C N L U L G O D E K L E K A S O G O O
H Y R W K Q A S M J H O L C V B I P E
Y U M F M O E P J T B U I A W B W V N
M G U N A A C F Y A N O S D L N E N A
O N X G N T X R U A T C D X S F K A T
S I B J N O E Z R O U J A E H C F V U
I V P G C V Z G M L J P E D L A A J C
S O L A O I E Y A Z F I Y T I A K R B
N L K N N D W R B M G F C V K P P I U
B G G O T Z I N O I S U T N O C O M S
E E A F R Z H O M E O S T A S I S S I
O D Z G A N G R E N E C S F Y R T V E
E X J T C J P S A N B B B J X M F S S
T Q I E T S I S Y L O Y M O D B A H R
K O S Y U X K P T H F N B E E C L C K
N J X Z R E D N S K G X N J M E D S I
C H V I E J V G L N M K T L K U M V P
```

1. In _____, new blood vessels form as the body attempts to bring oxygen and nutrients to the injured tissue.

2. A bruise is also known as a _____.

3. _____ is the second stage in the progression of crush syndrome.

4. Reddening of the skin is known as _____.

5. Physical injury will trigger mast cells to _____.

6. The unraveling of skin from the hand is _____.

7. Fat is _____ tissue.

8. _____ scars typically develop in people with darkly pigmented skin.

9. Three thousand cases of _____ occur in the United States each year.

10. A black and blue mark is also referred to as _____.

11. Maintaining the constancy of the internal environment is _____.

12. Do not remove an _____ _____ in the field.

13. The _____ layer lies beneath the dermis and contains adipose tissue.

14. An incision of the skin and underlying soft tissue with a scalpel is _____.

15. A deformity of the hand, fingers, and wrist resulting from damage to forearm muscles is a _____ _____.

Skill Drills

Test your knowledge of skill drills by placing the following photos in the correct order. Number the first step with a "1", the second step with a "2" etc.

1. *Controlling Bleeding from a Soft-Tissue Injury*

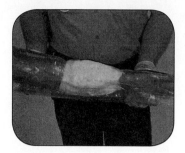 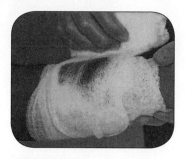 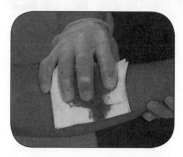 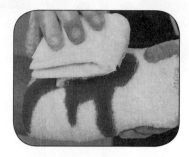

| Splint the extremity. | Maintain pressure with a roller bandage. | Apply direct pressure with a sterile bandage. | If bleeding continues, apply second dressing and roller bandage over the first. |

_____   _____   _____   _____

2. *Applying a Tourniquet*

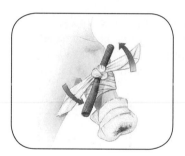 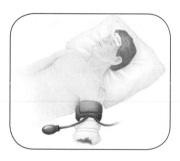 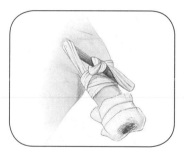

Twist the stick until the bleeding stops.

You can also use a blood pressure cuff as an effective tourniquet.

Secure the stick so that it will not unwind. Write "TK" and the exact time you applied the tourniquet on a piece of adhesive tape, fasten the tape to the patient's forehead, and notify hospital personnel on arrival.

_____   _____   _____

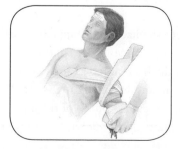 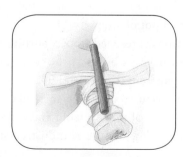

Create a 4", multilayered bandage. Wrap the bandage twice around the extremity, just above the bleeding site, and tie a half-knot.

Place a stick on top of the half-knot and tie a square knot over the stick.

_____   _____

CHAPTER

20 Burns

Chapter Review

The following exercises provide an opportunity to test your knowledge of this chapter.

Matching

Match each of the items with the appropriate treatment in question 1, and sequence in question 2.

1. In the course of a busy week, you are called on to treat eight burn victims in a variety of circumstances. In each case, you have to determine whether the patient has suffered a critical burn because, if so, he or she must be evacuated directly to the Regional Burn Center, which is 24 miles away; noncritical burns, on the other hand, can be managed by the community hospital right in town. Here is a description of the patients you saw. Beside each description, indicate whether:

   A. The patient has a critical burn and should be brought to a burn center.
   B. The patient does not have a critical burn and can be managed in the community hospital.

   _____ **(1)** A 2-year-old boy who overturned a pot of soup from the stovetop onto himself; both legs and the anterior trunk are burned.
   _____ **(2)** A 57-year-old diabetic woman with a scald burn of her left lower leg.
   _____ **(3)** A 28-year-old woman with a scald burn of her entire right arm.
   _____ **(4)** A lineman who suffered an electric shock. There is a small bull's-eye entrance wound on the left hand; you cannot find the exit wound. The lineman did not fall. His left leg feels rock hard.
   _____ **(5)** A 22-year-old short-order cook with partial-thickness (second-degree) burns over both anterior thighs, sustained when he spilled a pot of soup.
   _____ **(6)** A 34-year-old woman rescued from a burning building, where she had been trapped in her smoke-filled bedroom. She has partial-thickness burns of the right forearm. She is coughing up sooty sputum.
   _____ **(7)** A 25-year-old man who tripped and fell onto the hibachi on the back porch as he was preparing to barbecue some steaks. His hand went straight into the bed of red-hot charcoal, and his shirt caught fire. He has full-thickness (third-degree) burns of the left hand and forearm, and partial-thickness burns of the anterior chest.
   _____ **(8)** A plumber who spilled a bottle of industrial-strength liquid drain cleaner down the front of his trousers.

2. You are called to treat a patient who was in a tenement fire. He is a middle-aged man who apparently fell asleep in an armchair while holding a lit cigarette. You arrive at the scene just as he is being carried unconscious from the building and note that his clothes are still smoldering. Following, in random order, are the steps you will have to take in managing this patient. Arrange the steps in the correct sequence.

A. Administer supplemental oxygen.

B. Start an IV.

C. Open the airway manually.

D. Put out the fire.

E. Remove the patient's clothing.

F. Pass a nasogastric tube into his stomach.

G. Determine the extent and depth of the burn.

H. Intubate the trachea (if a BLS airway is not adequate).

I. Cover the burns with sterile dressings.

J. Obtain a set of baseline vital signs.

(1) _____   (6) _____

(2) _____   (7) _____

(3) _____   (8) _____

(4) _____   (9) _____

(5) _____   (10) _____

Multiple Choice

Read each item carefully, and then select the best response.

_____ **1.** What is the second "rule" when in a lightning storm?

    A. Take shelter in a structure.   **C.** Don't be the smallest conductor.

    B. Avoid touching a conductor.   **D.** Don't stand near the tallest conductor.

_____ **2.** When dealing with acute radiation syndrome, which of the following is not likely to happen to the patient?

    A. Central nervous system changes   **C.** Gastrointestinal changes

    B. Urinary changes   **D.** Hematologic changes

_____ **3.** There are three methods of calculating an area of burned skin. Which method is the most used?

    A. Rule of nines   **C.** Rule of palm

    B. The Lund and Browder Chart   **D.** A Broselow™ tape

_____ **4.** You have arrived on scene to find a 12-year-old girl who has been burnt by chicken noodle soup from the stove. She has blisters and redness on her chest. How would you classify this burn?

    A. It is a full-thickness burn.   **C.** It is a partial-thickness burn.

    B. It is a first-degree burn.   **D.** It is a superficial burn.

_____ **5.** An adult man's back is worth what percentage when using the rule of nines?

    A. 9%   **C.** 27%

    B. 18%   **D.** 36%

_____ **6.** What does *immediate management* mean when dealing with a burn?

    A. Managing the airway   **C.** Stopping the burning

    B. Scene safety   **D.** Keeping the patient warm

_____ **7.** The Parkland formula determines how much fluid a burn patient should receive when?

      A. During the first hour   **C.** During the first 12 hours

      B. During transport to the hospital   **D.** During the first 24 hours

_____ **8.** What is the best way to give pain medication to the burn patient?

      A. IV route   **C.** By mouth

      B. Subcutaneous injection   **D.** Intramuscular injection

_____ **9.** What should you do first when treating a patient with a chemical burn?

      A. Remove all the patient's clothing.   **C.** Brush the chemicals off of the skin.

      B. Begin flushing with copious amounts of water. **D.** Wait for a hazardous materials team to arrive.

_____ **10.** You arrive on scene to find a child engaged in an electrical outlet. The child is "held" by the electricity. What should you do?

      A. Use a wooden pole to push the child away from the source.

      B. Throw a rope to the child and pull him away from the source.

      C. Wait until someone shuts off the power to the source.

      D. Cut the wires inside the electrical box.

Labeling

Label the following diagrams with the correct terms.

    1. Label the components of the skin in the following diagram.

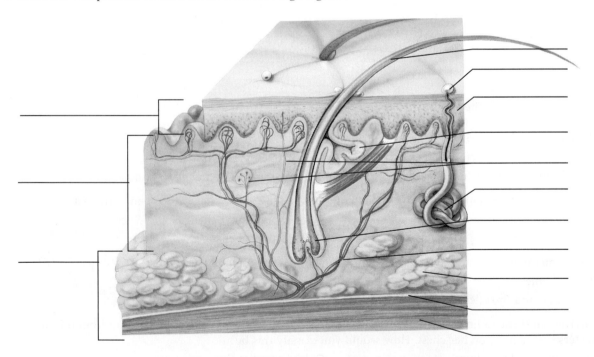

2. Classify the following as: superficial, partial-thickness, or full-thickness burns.

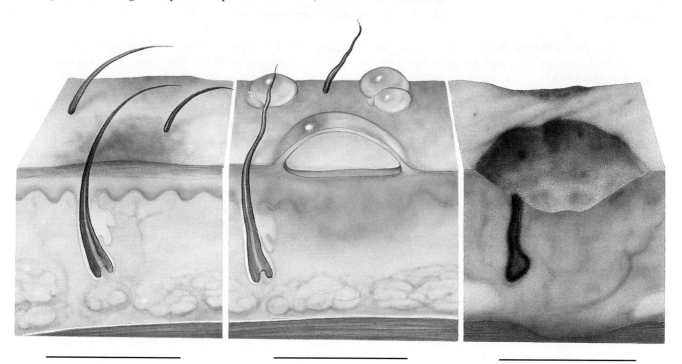

_____   _____   _____

Fill-in-the-Blank

Read each item carefully, and then complete the statement by filling in the missing word(s).

1. The _____ is the largest and one of the most complex organs in the body.

2. Sweat glands are found in the _____.

3. A _____ burn is most commonly seen in children.

4. Chemical burns can occur when the skin comes in contact with _____, _____, or _____, or other corrosive materials.

5. _____ happens when a chemical inserts oxygen, sulfur, or halogen atoms into the body's proteins.

6. You should always make sure the _____ _____ _____ before beginning any management of a patient struck by lightning.

7. There are three types of ionizing radiation: _____, _____, and _____.

8. The central area of a burn that has suffered the most damage is known as the _____ _____ _____.

9. When treating a full-thickness burn, you should apply a _____ _____ to the area that has been burned.

10. A patient with a radiation burn must be _____ before being transported to the emergency department (ED).

Identify

In the following case study, list the chief complaint, vital signs, and pertinent negatives.

Around noon you are called out to the local burger joint for a 56-year-old woman who has been burned by oil from a hot fryer. Upon arrival, you find her with holes in her jeans on the top of both thighs. She is crying and immediately rates her pain as unbearable. You cut the jeans away to find that there is an area covering most of the front of both thighs that is blistering and very red. She is breathing 22 breaths/min, her oxygen saturation is 97%, and lungs sounds are clear. You apply supplemental oxygen via a nonrebreathing mask at 15 L/min. You have your partner take the rest of the vital signs as you apply Water-Jel dressing to the burned areas. Her blood pressure is 150/100 mm Hg, her pulse is 114 beats/min, and her rhythm on the monitor is sinus tachycardia. You do catch a PVC on the monitor, but don't see another after watching for a full minute. She is cool to the touch and you feel she might be going into shock. You cover her with a blanket and start an IV of normal saline. She is able to answer all your questions, and she has no medical history or allergies. You find no other areas of burns as you do a rapid trauma assessment. She states she slipped on the floor when carrying the hot oil to the disposal. She splashed the oil on the front of her legs. She does rate her pain 10/10, and so you give her 5 mg of morphine for the pain en route to the hospital. When you arrive at the hospital, which is only 5 minutes from the burger joint, her pain has dropped to a 3/10.

1. Chief Complaint

_____

_____

_____

2. Vital Signs

_____

_____

_____

3. Pertinent Negatives

_____

_____

_____

Ambulance Calls

The following case scenarios provide an opportunity to explore the concerns associated with patient management and paramedic care. Read each scenario, and then answer each question.

1. You are called to the scene of a smoky apartment-house fire to treat a man who jumped from his bedroom window about 15 feet above the ground. What you observe at first glance is the following: He is now lying unconscious on the ground. His trousers are smoldering. His beard is partly burned off, and his lips are swollen. His left leg is splayed out at a peculiar angle. List in the correct sequence the steps you would take in managing this patient.

a. _____

b. _____

c. _____

d. _____

e. _____

f. _____

g. _____

h. _____

2. While you are securing the IV on the patient described in the previous question, firefighters lead the patient's wife over to you (they just rescued her from another room). A quick check does not reveal any injuries, but you give her supplemental oxygen by nasal cannula anyway because of her exposure to smoke. Meanwhile, you take advantage of the opportunity to get some information about her husband. List five questions you would ask this woman regarding her husband and what happened to him.

a. _____

b. _____

c. _____

d. _____

e. _____

3. Meanwhile, the firefighters bring you yet another victim of the fire, a college student who climbed down a fire escape in the back of the building. He has burns to the right side of his body and complains of severe pain in the right arm. On examination you find the following:

- The *right arm* is mottled red and exquisitely sensitive to the lightest touch (even the breeze blowing past it causes pain).
- The *right flank* is fiery red and also very painful.
- The *right lower leg* has a leathery appearance. In places, you can see thrombosed veins beneath the surface. When you touch the skin with a sterile needle, the patient does not feel the pinprick.

a. The burn on the right arm is probably a _____ burn.

The appropriate treatment for that burn is: _____

_____

_____

b. The burn on the flank is probably a _____ burn.

The appropriate treatment for that burn is: _____

_____

_____

c. The burn on the right leg is probably a _____ burn.

The appropriate treatment for that burn is: _____

_____

_____

4. You are called to a construction site 20 miles out of town for a "man electrocuted." According to the person who telephoned your dispatcher, one of the construction workers apparently bulldozed through a buried electric cable. He dismounted his bulldozer and picked up the cable to toss it aside, not realizing that it was live, and his hand "froze" to the cable.

a. En route to the call, you review in your mind the types of injuries that may occur in connection with electrocution. You remember that there may be three different types of burns.

(1) _____

(2) _____

(3) _____

b. You also recall that high-voltage electricity may cause a variety of nonburn injuries. List six possible injuries or abnormal conditions that you need to be alert for in this patient.

(1) _____

(2) _____

(3) _____

(4) _____

(5) _____

(6) _____

c. When you reach the construction site, you see a knot of agitated people over at one end of the site. One of them is holding a long two-by-four, with which he apparently jarred the victim loose from the cable. The victim is lying very still and appears to be unconscious. The free end of the cable is now arcing along the ground like an angry snake. List the steps you will take in dealing with this situation in the sequence in which you will perform them.

(1) _____

(2) _____

(3) _____

(4) _____

(5) _____

(6) _____

(7) _____

(8) _____

(9) _____

(10) _____

5. You are summoned to a house fire where the firefighters have just rescued a young man from a particularly smoky part of the building. He is unconscious, and you notice that his clothes are smoldering.

a. Whenever a person has been unconscious in a smoky environment, you have to worry about the possibility of respiratory injury. List six signs that should lead you to suspect the presence of respiratory injury in a burned patient.

(1) _____

(2) _____

(3) _____

(4) _____

(5) _____

(6) _____

b. What is the *first* step you should take in dealing with this patient?

_____

_____

c. In due course, you remove his clothing and examine him from head to toe to evaluate the depth and extent of the burn. You find the following:

- Full-thickness burns of the posterior surfaces of both legs, extending well into the buttocks and groin
- Partial-thickness burns of the entire left arm and a hand-sized patch of the left flank

(1) What percentage of the patient's body has been burned? _____%

(2) Does the patient have a critical burn? _____ If yes, according to what criteria?

(a) _____

(b) _____

(c) _____

d. Use the Parkland formula to calculate the rate at which you should run the patient's IV. Assume that he weighs 70 kg and that your infusion set delivers 10 gtt/mL. (Show your calculations.)

The IV should be run at _____ gtt/min.

_____

_____

e. After a few minutes of oxygen therapy, the patient regains consciousness and begins complaining of excruciating pain, especially in his groin and left arm. Medical control instructs you to administer morphine.

(1) What is the correct dosage of morphine for this patient? _____

(2) By what route should it be given? _____

(3) List three possible adverse side effects that you should be ready to deal with.

(a) _____

(b) _____

(c) _____

6. You are standing by at a three-alarm fire when a woman is brought down a ladder by firefighters and carried to your ambulance. "The whole apartment was full of smoke," one of the firefighters tells you, "everything smoldering—carpets, mattresses, furniture." The woman is conscious but confused. She complains of a severe headache. Her vital signs are a pulse of 120 beats/min and thready, respirations of 40 breaths/min and labored, and blood pressure is 160/90 mm Hg. You find no evidence of burns or other injury.

a. What is your major concern in this patient, given the history and her symptoms and signs?

_____

_____

_____

_____

b. List the steps you would take in managing this patient.

(1) _____

(2) _____

(3) _____

(4) _____

(5) _____

(6) _____

7. In examining a patient, you find that he has mixed partial- and full-thickness burns of his entire left leg and posterior right leg, extending into his groin. There are also partial-thickness burns over most of the left forearm.

a. What percentage of his body is burned? (Show your calculations.)   _____%

_____

_____

b. Does he have a critical burn?   _____   Explain the reason for your answer.

(1) _____

(2) _____

c. In doing the rapid trauma assessment, you are unable to detect either a dorsalis pedis or an anterior tibial pulse in the left foot. What do you think is the most likely reason?

_____

_____

d. What are you going to do about it?

_____

_____

True/False

If you believe the statement to be more true than false, write the letter "T" in the space provided. If you believe the statement to be more false than true, write the letter "F."

_____ **1.** If you know the identity of the chemical that caused the burn, it is preferable to start treatment with a chemical antidote (eg, to apply a weak acid to an alkali burn and vice versa).

_____ **2.** When a person has been burned by a chemical agent, the skin should be flushed for a minimum of 30 minutes with copious amounts of water.

_____ **3.** It is important to use only sterile water to flush a chemical burn, lest you contaminate the burn wound.

_____ **4.** In burns caused by hot tar, it is crucial to remove the tar from contact with the skin as quickly as possible to prevent systemic tar poisoning.

_____ **5.** If chemicals have splashed into someone's eyes, the eyes should be irrigated with a steady stream of water for at least 30 minutes.

_____ **6.** Burn shock occurs because of the fluid loss across the damaged skin and the volume shifts within the rest of the body.

_____ **7.** Most deaths occur during a fire because of the person actually being burnt.

_____ **8.** Carbon monoxide binds to the hemoglobin 500 times faster than oxygen does.

_____ **9.** Currents as small as 0.1 amp may cause ventricular fibrillation if the current passes through the heart.

_____ **10.** You should peel away clothing that has "melted" into the flesh of a burn patient.

Short Answer

Complete this section with short written answers using the space provided.

1. Discuss the four rules that can help you avoid being struck by lightning.

a. _____

b. _____

c. _____

d. _____

2. Suspect that a patient with flame burns has a respiratory injury if any of the following signs are present:

a. _____

b. _____

c. _____

d. _____

e. _____

f. _____

3. Injury from a high-voltage electric source or from lightning may produce any of the following:

a. _____

b. _____

c. _____

d. _____

e. _____

f. _____

g. _____

h. _____

i. _____

j. _____

Word Find

Hidden in the following grid are 23 words or phrases related to what you have studied in this chapter. Find the hidden words in the grid below. Then use the words from the grid to answer the following questions (some words may be used to answer more than one of the questions).

```
S P N E K D G K Y D V Y A Z U W S
U A O T N R E T C E W I I Q V S U
O R I Y Q T E S S O M E I T S P P
E K T O K F R I Q E H N E E Z I E
N L A C A B C A R U T S N K F A R
A A L S A A C E N E A K N L S M F
T N U K N T P P G C C M U R L K I
U D G T Y Y N U J I E S A F U G C
C N E J H G M O H K H I F T Q B I
R I R K O E N T C T I X E X I K A
S N O T N F L B R U S H O F F O L
N A M T P L E V I S S E R G G A N
S L R U U I N E G A L L O C E F X
E E E F B U R N S P E C I A L T Y
B M H A T R I A L U I F O E G N S
U R T C G X H E Q F D I C F G Y P
M V J B F Q H P Y K E I V Y L L F
```

1. The skin is also known as the _____.

2. Another word for temperature regulation preformed by the skin is _____.

3. A process in which the outer layer of nonliving cells is shed is called _____.

4. The darkness of a person's skin is a result of the amount of _____ present in the dermis.

5. _____ is a fibrous protein that gives the skin resistance to breakage.

6. _____ blood vessels also play a large role in thermoregulation.

7. An oily substance that is produced by the sebaceous gland in each hair follicle is known as _____.

8. When touching a hot stove, the patient ends up with a/an _____ burn.

9. Fluid volume shift and fluid loss across the damaged skin can result in _____ _____.

10. Mustard gas is classified as a/an _____.

11. A common arrhythmia that occurs with electrical injury is _____ fibrillation or flutter.

12. _____ is your primary concern when dealing with fire and electrical burns.

13. The least affected area of a burn is known as the zone of _____.

14. A third-degree burn is also known as a/an _____ - _____ burn.

15. A burn patient's care is measured in _____, not hours.

16. The _____ formula tells us how much fluid a burn patient should receive in the first 24 hours after the injury.

17. You should provide _____ pain management for the burn patient.

18. You can apply a cold compress to the patient with a/an _____ burn.

19. When you have a patient that is covered in dry lime, you should _____ _____ the patient first.

20. When a patient gets chemicals in the eyes, you should _____ the eyes.

21. Electrical burns can have a/an _____ and _____ wound.

22. A patient suffering from a full-thickness burn should be transferred to a/an _____ _____ center.

Fill-in-the-Table

Fill in the missing parts of the table.

Approximate the amount of fluid the burned patient will need by using the Parkland Formula. During the first 24 hours, the burned patient will need:

4 mL × body weight (in kg) × percentage of body surface burned

Parkland Formula Chart										
% Burn	**10 kg**	**20 kg**	**30 kg**	**40 kg**	**50 kg**	**60 kg**	**70 kg**	**80 kg**	**90 kg**	**100 kg**
10	25			100	125	150	175		225	250
20	50			200	250	300	350		450	500
30	75			300	375	450	525		675	750
40	100			400	500	600	700		900	1,000
50	125			500	625	750	875		1,125	1,250
60	150			600	750	900	1,050		1,350	1,500
70	175			700	875	1,050	1,225		1,575	1,750
80	200			800	1,000	1,200	1,400		1,800	2,000
90	225			900	1,125	1,350	1,575		2,025	2,250
20 mL/kg	200			800	1,000	1,200	1,400		1,800	2,000

This table represents the fluid recommended in the *first hour* (⅛ of the initial 8-hour dose) by the Parkland formula. The final row represents the amount of a 20-mL/kg bolus.

Problem Solving

Practice your calculation skills by solving the following math problems.

1. On examining the patient, you find burns covering the following areas:

   - The whole right leg (front and back)
   - The anterior left leg
   - The anterior trunk
   - The whole right arm

   a. Use the rule of nines to calculate what percentage of the patient's body surface area is burned: _____ %. (Show your calculations.)

   _____

   _____

   b. If the patient weighs 154 lb, at what rate should you run his IV? Use the Parkland formula to calculate the rate (and don't forget to convert his weight to kilograms first!). (Show your calculations.)

   IV rate = _____ mL/h

   _____

   _____

   c. If you have a standard infusion set that delivers 10 gtt/mL, at how many drops per minute do you have to run the IV to deliver the volume you calculated?

   IV rate = _____ gtt/min

   _____

   _____

   d. What intravenous fluid will you use?

   _____

   _____

CHAPTER

21 Head and Face Injuries

Chapter Review

The following exercises provide an opportunity to test your knowledge of this chapter.

Matching

Match each of the items in the left column to the appropriate injury in the right column.

_____ **1.** A 15-year-old skateboarder has hit the side of his head after a fall. He is initially unconscious, but regains consciousness only to lapse again about an hour later. His mother then cannot wake him up again.

_____ **2.** A football player comes off the field after a helmet-to-helmet hit. He is a little disoriented and cannot remember the play. The coach says he just got his bell rung. He shows no other signs later in the evening or the next day.

_____ **3.** The other football player also comes off the field. He is very confused. He loses consciousness in the locker room for about 3 minutes. He is confused for the next 2 days.

_____ **4.** A 40-year-old woman is scrubbing the floor, and as she rises up she hits the back of her head on the sink. At the time, she gets a slight headache. Later in the evening her speech becomes slightly slurred.

_____ **5.** A 12-year-old girl is hit on the head with a baseball bat by her brother. She is knocked out but wakes back up to tell her mom what happened. Her mother decides to have her checked out. On the way to the doctor's office, the girl appears to go to sleep, and when they arrive the mother cannot wake her.

_____ **6.** The patient was the driver of a vehicle that was struck from the left side by another car. The door on the driver's side is dented in. The patient is conscious, but witnesses say that he was "out cold" for a few minutes immediately after the collision. He complains of a headache and pins and needles in his left hip and left leg. His skull is tender to palpation in the area just superior to the left ear. While he is under your care, his level of consciousness deteriorates until he is unconscious altogether, and his respirations become very slow.

_____ **7.** The patient was a participant in a barroom brawl. This patient was "knocked out cold" for a few minutes. Now he seems alert, but he cannot remember what happened. He complains of a little dizziness. His vital signs are normal.

_____ **8.** The patient was a front-seat passenger in a car that careened into a utility pole. He is confused and sleepy when you find him. His speech is slurred, and there is weakness of the right leg. He becomes more and more lethargic while under your care and vomits twice. The left pupil seems to be getting larger than the right.

_____ **9.** The patient was an unrestrained front-seat passenger in a car involved in a head-on collision with another car. He apparently struck his head on the windshield because the windshield in front of the patient is cracked. The patient is

A. Cerebral concussion

B. Cerebral contusion

C. Epidural hematoma

D. Subdural hematoma

E. Intracerebral hematoma

F. Subarachnoid hemorrhage

found unconscious. His left pupil is larger than the right. His pulse is 56 beats/min, and his blood pressure is 190/90 mm Hg. Respirations are irregular.

_____ **10.** You are called to a 70-year-old woman with a terrible headache. She hit her head on the cupboard about 2 hours ago. She initially had a severe headache at the site of the injury, but now it has moved to a larger area of her head. She is only responsive to questions and begins to vomit while you are taking care of her. She rapidly moves to unresponsive and begins to have a seizure.

Multiple Choice

Read each item carefully, and then select the best response.

_____ **1.** The base of the skull has an opening that allows the spinal cord to connect to the brain. What is the opening called?
- **A.** Fontanelle
- **B.** Mastoid process
- **C.** Cribriform plate
- **D.** Foramen magnum

_____ **2.** The oculomotor nerve is the _____ cranial nerve.
- **A.** first
- **B.** second
- **C.** third
- **D.** fourth

_____ **3.** How many adult teeth should the normal adult have?
- **A.** 32
- **B.** 34
- **C.** 30
- **D.** 36

_____ **4.** The brain consumes what percentage of the body's total oxygen?
- **A.** 10%
- **B.** 20%
- **C.** 30%
- **D.** 40%

_____ **5.** Within the diencephalon there are several divisions. Which division processes sensory input, influences moods, and controls general body movements?
- **A.** Subthalamus
- **B.** Thalamus
- **C.** Hypothalamus
- **D.** Epithalamus

_____ **6.** What is the reticular activating system (RAS) responsible for?
- **A.** Blood pressure
- **B.** Respiration
- **C.** Heart rate
- **D.** Consciousness

_____ **7.** You are treating a patient that appears to have a fracture that has affected the upper jaw and the hard palate. What is the name for this fracture?
- **A.** Le Fort I
- **B.** Le Fort II
- **C.** Nasal fracture
- **D.** Mandibular fracture

_____ **8.** Which of the following is NOT advisable when covering an injured eye?
- **A.** Aluminum eye shield
- **B.** Gauze
- **C.** Sterile dressing
- **D.** Cup

_____ **9.** When a patient has a basilar skull fracture, which of the following signs or symptoms would you least expect to see?
- **A.** Raccoon eyes
- **B.** Battle's signs
- **C.** Blowout fracture of the eye
- **D.** Draining of blood and CSF from the ear

_____ **10.** What is the minimum CPP in an adult that is required to adequately perfuse the brain?
- **A.** 15 mm Hg
- **B.** 30 mm Hg
- **C.** 45 mm Hg
- **D.** 60 mm Hg

_____ **11.** You are treating a patient who has starred the windshield in a car crash. The patient reports that he cannot remember what happened before the collision. This is called:

A. anterograde amnesia.

C. amnesia.

B. retrograde amnesia.

D. focal brain injury.

_____ **12.** After you drop off the patient that you treated for a fall down the stairs, the doctor tells you she had bleeding into the brain tissue. You remember the medical term for this is:

A. epidural hematoma.

C. subarachnoid hemorrhage.

B. intracerebral hematoma.

D. subdural hematoma.

_____ **13.** What is the most important sign or symptom in evaluating a patient with a brain injury?

A. Bleeding from the ears

C. Level of consciousness

B. Pupil size and how the pupils react to light

D. Mechanism of injury (MOI)

_____ **14.** When using the Glasgow Coma Scale (GCS), what is the lowest and highest score a patient can get?

A. 0, 15

C. 3, 14

B. 0, 14

D. 3, 15

_____ **15.** What is the most important step in managing any type of head injury?

A. Airway and breathing

C. Assessment of where the bleeding is in the brain

B. Spinal immobilization

D. Establishing an IV

Labeling

Label the following diagrams with the correct terms.

1. Label the following structures of the eye:

A. Iris

B. Cornea

C. Pupil

D. Lens

E. Retina

F. Optic nerve

G. Sclera

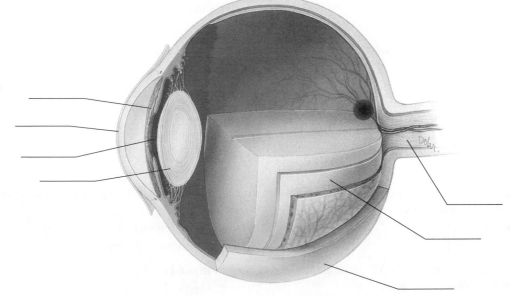

2. Label the following structures of the anterior part of the neck:

   A. Carotid arteries

   B. Thyroid cartilage

   C. Sternocleidomastoid muscle

   D. Cricoid cartilage

   E. Trachea

   F. Cricothyroid membrane

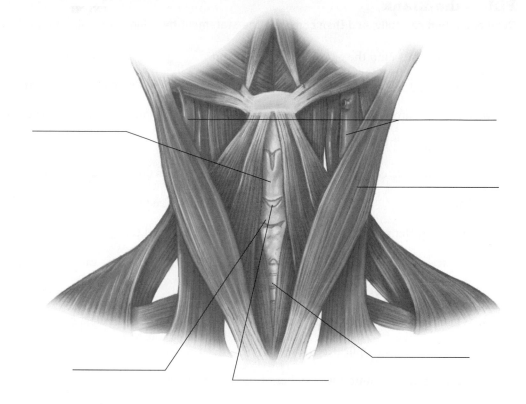

3. Label the following major regions of the brain:

   A. Diencephalon (hypothalamus, thalamus)

   B. Cerebrum

   C. Midbrain

   D. Pons

   E. Medulla

   F. Spinal cord

   G. Cerebellum

   H. Brain stem

   I. Skull

   J. Corpus callosum

   K. Meninges

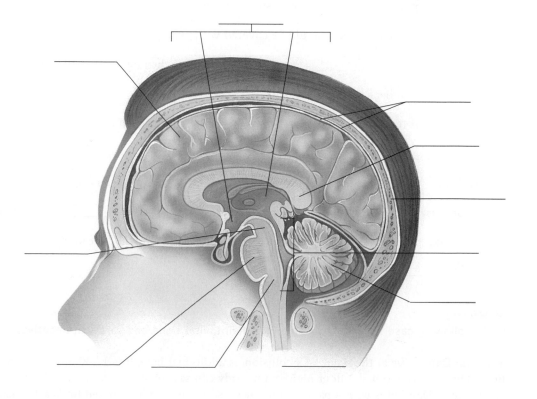

Fill-in-the-Blank

Read each item carefully, and then complete the statement by filling in the missing word(s).

1. The skull sits atop the _____ skeleton.

2. The _____ link the sutures in the skull and are soft when a child is born.

3. The bones around the eye are thin, and with significant trauma to the face the eye can be dislodged. This is called a/an

    _____ fracture.

4. The adjustable center of the iris that allows light to pass through the eye to the lens is called the _____.

5. The _____ is responsible for higher functions and is the largest portion of the brain.

6. The brain stem contains the midbrain, _____, and the _____.

7. The second layer of the meninges resembles a spider's web, so it is called the _____.

8. You should always assume _____ _____ precautions when the patient has facial trauma.

9. When dealing with an impaled object in the face, the only time you should remove the object is when you have

    _____ complications.

10. Bleeding into the anterior chamber of the eye is called _____.

11. _____, _____, and _____ rays can burn the eyes.

12. If you have a burn to the eyes caused by a strong alkali or acid, you should irrigate the eye for _____ minutes.

13. The only indication for removing a contact lens in the field is a/an _____ _____.

14. Reimplantation of a tooth may be successful for up to a/an _____ after it has been avulsed from the mouth.

15. Any open neck wounds should be covered with a/an _____ dressing.

16. A/an _____-_____ injury happens when the brain sloshes forward and hits the front skull and then recoils

    and hits the back part of the skull.

17. Increased ICP can produce signs of _____, bradycardia, and irregular respirations. This is known

    as _____ _____.

18. A/an _____ hematoma is the collection of blood between the dura mater and the skull.

19. Because of clenched teeth, the paramedic may have to perform _____ to safely intubate the head injury patient.

20. Unlike patients that are suffering from shock, the patient with a head injury can develop a very

    high _____ _____.

Identify

In the following case study, list the chief complaint, vital signs, and pertinent negatives.

Tom and Dan arrive at the scene of a collision as additional help. It is 12:30 at night and a carload of teenagers has rolled into a corn field. The corn is about shoulder high and nobody can say for sure how many kids were in the car. Tom begins a search around the crash site as Dan helps with a patient. Tom hears something to his left and finds a 17-year-old girl on the ground.

The girl is on her back with her arms drawn up to her chest and her feet seem to be rigid and slightly turned in. An initial assessment shows no life-threatening bleeding. The girl is "U" on the AVPU scale, and Tom determines she is an 8 on the GCS scale. Her respirations are 34 breaths/min and very deep, and oxygen saturation is 99%. Pupils are sluggish, blood pressure is 160/90 mm Hg, and her pulse is 72 beats/min. Skin is cool, but she has been lying on the ground for at least half an hour.

Help arrives and they apply a C-collar, secure her to a backboard, and get her in the unit.

The closest trauma center is half an hour away by helicopter, and so they call for the life flight crew to meet them on scene. Because she is unresponsive, Dan and Tom decide to insert an advanced airway and administer 100% supplemental oxygen to the patient. Two large-bore IVs are placed with normal saline. They are careful not to overload this patient with fluid because of the rising ICP. The ECG monitor shows a sinus bradycardia now at a rate of 56 breaths/min and the blood pressure is now 168/88 mm Hg. Life flight then takes over and flies her to the regional trauma center. They later find out that she does make it but has some neurologic defects that will take several months to years from which to recover.

1. Chief Complaint

2. Vital Signs

3. Pertinent Negatives

4. Why is it important to get this patient to the regional trauma center?

5. What does the patient's position on the ground tell you?

6. What are the patient's serial vital signs telling you?

Ambulance Calls

The following case scenarios provide an opportunity to explore the concerns associated with patient management and paramedic care. Read each scenario, then answer each question.

1. While enjoying a weekend off at a ski resort, you happen to see a young lady trip over the steps at the lodge and fall. As you rush to her assistance, you see blood coming from her mouth, and closer inspection reveals that she has knocked out one of her lower teeth entirely. What steps should you take?

   a. _____

   _____

   b. _____

   _____

   c. _____

   _____

   d. _____

   _____

   e. _____

   _____

2. You volunteer to accompany the young lady to the nearest hospital, some 2 hours away by road. Just as you are pulling away from the ski resort in a friend's car, the resort manager comes running after you, waving for you to stop. "I have someone else here who needs to go to the hospital," he says. Behind him, two ski instructors are leading a young man along. The patient had been involved in a fistfight and now has two black eyes. A thorough examination of an injured eye includes assessment what visible ocular structures and ocular functions?

   a. _____

   b. _____

   c. _____

   d. _____

   e. _____

   f. _____

   g. _____

   h. _____

3. A 12-year-old boy lost control of his bicycle as he was riding down a long, steep hill into town. At the base of the hill, his front wheel struck the curb, and he was catapulted from the bicycle straight through the show window of the local wedding dress shop. When you arrive, you find him bleeding from multiple lacerations. The most profuse bleeding seems to be coming from a large laceration on the left side of his neck.

   a. What are the principal dangers associated with the laceration of the neck?

_____

_____

_____

b. What should be done to the wound immediately?

_____

_____

_____

4. A 24-year-old driver is involved in a head-on collision. He was not wearing a seat belt. The windshield on the driver's side has a spiderweb crack. The patient is confused, and his breath smells of alcohol. The skin is warm. Breathing seems labored. The left pupil is larger than the right. His pulse is 56 beats/min and regular, respirations are 24 breaths/min and deep, and blood pressure is 190/110 mm Hg.

a. What three steps would you take at the scene?

(1) _____

(2) _____

(3) _____

b. What four steps would you take during transport?

(1) _____

(2) _____

(3) _____

(4) _____

5. A 34-year-old man has been injured in a road incident in which his head apparently struck the windshield with some force. When you first reach the scene, the patient is unconscious. He is breathing 8 breaths/min, inhaling approximately 500 mL of air with each breath.

a. What is his minute volume? per minute? _____

b. Is that volume greater or less than normal? _____

c. Therefore, you can conclude that the patient's arterial PCO_2 will tend to _____ (increase or decrease?), so his

pH will _____ (increase or decrease?). The net effect will be an acid–base disorder called a _____

(respiratory or metabolic?) _____ (acidosis or alkalosis?). The way you can help correct that abnormality is to

_____.

d. One reason to try to correct hypoventilation in a patient with a head injury is that hypoventilation may, through its effects on acid–base balance just mentioned, worsen cerebral edema and thereby accelerate the increase in intracranial pressure (ICP). How would you know if this patient is developing an increase in intracranial pressure? List five signs of increasing intracranial pressure.

(1) _____

(2) _____

(3) _____

(4) _____

(5) _____

    e. Here are the findings of your initial neurologic assessment of the patient:

- He opens his eyes only when pinched, not when spoken to.
- He pulls his whole arm and shoulder away when you pinch his hand.
- He makes garbled sounds that you cannot understand.

    (1) What is his AVPU? _____

    (2) What is his score on the Glasgow Coma Scale? _____

6. Score each of the patients described in the following scenarios according to the AVPU scale and the Glasgow Coma Scale (GCS).

    a. The patient is found unconscious. He opens his eyes in response to a loud voice. He does not follow commands, but he pulls his hand away when pinched and makes a few garbled noises that you cannot understand.

    AVPU scale _____   GCS score _____

    b. The patient is found apparently unconscious, but he opens his eyes at the sound of your voice. He can follow simple commands, but he is a bit confused and cannot tell you what month it is or what day of the week it is.

    AVPU scale _____   GCS score _____

    c. The patient is found unconscious. He does not open his eyes when pinched or try to pull away from the painful stimulus, but instead his arms flex spasmodically across his chest while his legs go into hyperextension. He makes no sound.

    AVPU scale _____   GCS score _____

    d. The patient is found conscious. He gives you a coherent account of what happened to him, his name, and the day of the week, and he can follow simple commands.

    AVPU scale _____   GCS score _____

7. You are called to attend to a patient injured in an altercation that took place in a downtown drinking establishment. In the course of the dispute, someone broke a whiskey bottle over the patient's head. You find the patient conscious, bleeding profusely from his scalp, and in a distinctly unfriendly frame of mind, which he manifests by hurling tables and chairs in all directions while screaming uncomplimentary names at his assailants. List the steps you would take in treating this patient.

    a. _____

    b. _____

    c. _____

    d. _____

True/False

If you believe the statement to be more true than false, write the letter "T" in the space provided. If you believe the statement to be more false than true, write the letter "F."

_____ 1. The cranial vault consists of 10 bones.

_____ 2. The cribriform plate allows for passage of the olfactory nerve filaments.

_____ 3. The hyoid bone is attached to the skull.

_____ 4. Hair movement at the organ of Corti forms nerve impulses that travel to the brain allowing us to "hear."

_____ 5. The glossopharyngeal nerve provides motor function to the tongue.

_____ 6. The brain uses 25% of the body's glucose.

_____ 7. The frontal lobe of the brain is responsible for personality traits.

_____ 8. The vagus nerve originates from the pons.

_____ 9. CSF is manufactured in the ventricles of the brain.

_____ 10. Bruising and swelling are your first clues to a maxillofacial fracture.

_____ 11. To maintain an airway it is okay to use a nasal airway when there are signs of facial fractures.

_____ 12. Blunt eye trauma can lead to a retinal detachment, and this is common in sports injuries.

_____ 13. It is not necessary to cover both eyes to prevent sympathetic eye movement.

_____ 14. When using a chemical ice pack for an avulsed part, place the part right on top of the ice pack.

_____ 15. It may be hard to determine the extent of bleeding in the mouth as a result of the patient swallowing the blood.

_____ 16. You should always use an occlusive dressing on an open neck wound to prevent air embolisms.

_____ 17. Motor vehicle crashes are the most common cause of head injury.

_____ 18. The body's response to a decrease of CPP is to increase MAP.

_____ 19. Decerebrate posturing is seen as the patient pulls the arms into the core of the body.

_____ 20. Subarachnoid hematoma will usually present with a sudden and severe headache.

Short Answer

Complete this section with short written answers using the space provided.

1. Injuries to the face may be quite frightening to look at, but facial injuries do not by themselves ordinarily pose an immediate threat to life. However, facial injuries may be associated with *other* conditions or injuries that *can* threaten life or limb. List two potentially serious or life-threatening conditions that may be associated with maxillofacial trauma.

   a. _____

   b. _____

2. In examining a trauma patient, what findings would lead you to suspect maxillofacial fracture? List five signs of maxillofacial fracture.

   a. _____

   b. _____

   c. _____

   d. _____

   e. _____

Crossword Puzzle

Use the clues in the column to complete the puzzle.

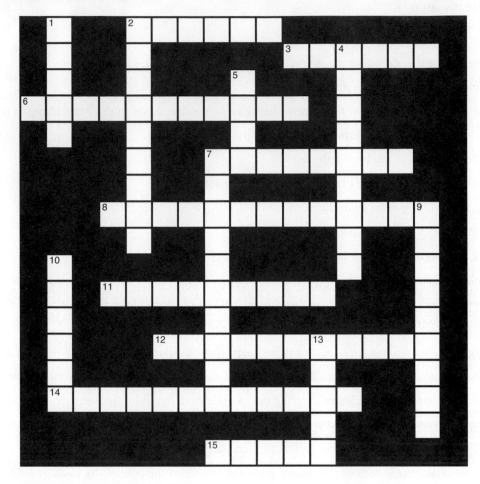

Across

2. A cone-shaped fossae that encloses and protects the eyes.

3. The "white" of the eye.

6. Medical term for chewing your food.

7. The speech center in the brain is located in the _____ __ lobe.

8. Where tears are produced.

11. The cheek bone is the _____ bone.

12. A mucous membrane that covers the sclera.

14. Blunt trauma can cause a misalignment of the teeth which is known as _____.

15. Most important organ in the body.

Down

1. The most common facial fracture is the _____ fracture.

2. The _____ lobe is where the optical nerves originate.

4. The vertebral arteries run _____ to the cervical vertebrae in the posterior part of the neck.

5. When treating an unconscious patient with no spinal injuries and suffering from epistaxis, you should position them on their _____.

7. The nerve that branches into the ophthalmic, maxillary, and mandibular nerves.

9. The top meninge of the brain that is referred to as the "tough mother."

10. The _____ separates the two nostrils.

13. The top portion of a tooth.

Fill-in-the-Table

Fill in the missing parts of the table.

1. Signs and Symptoms of Head Injury

Signs and Symptoms of Head Injury
■ Lacerations, _____, or _____ to the scalp
■ _____ or _____ noted on palpation of the scalp
■ Visible _____ or _____ of the skull
■ _____ sign or _____ eyes
■ CSF _____ or otorrhea
■ Pupillary abnormalities
– _____
– _____
■ A period of _____
■ _____ or disorientation
■ Repeatedly asking the same question(s) (_____)
■ Amnesia (_____ and/or _____)
■ _____ or other abnormal behavior
■ Numbness or _____ in the _____
■ Loss of _____ and/or _____
■ Focal _____-_____
■ Seizures
■ _____ triad: _____, _____, and irregular or erratic respirations
■ Dizziness
■ Visual disturbances, _____ vision, or _____ vision (diplopia)
■ Seeing "stars"
■ Nausea or _____
■ Posturing (_____ and/or _____)

2. Glasgow Coma Scale

GLASGOW COMA SCALE		
Eye Opening		
Spontaneous	4	
_____	3	
To Pain	2	
None	1	
Verbal Response		
Oriented	5	
_____	4	
Inappropriate Words	3	
_____	2	
None	1	
Motor Response		
Obeys Command	6	
_____	5	
Withdraws (pain)	4	
_____	3	
Extension (pain)	2	
None	1	
Glasgow Coma Score Total	**15**	

3. Brain Injury Classification Based on the GCS

Brain Injury Classification Based on the GCS
■ **13 to 15.** Mild traumatic brain injury
■ _____ Moderate traumatic brain injury
■ _____ Severe traumatic brain injury

C H A P T E R

22 Spine Injuries

Chapter Review

The following exercises provide an opportunity to test your knowledge of this chapter.

Matching

Match each of the following items to the appropriate type of shock.

A. Neurogenic shock

B. Hypovolemic shock

C. Spinal shock

_____ **1.** Skin cool and sweaty. Pulse 110 beats/min, regular, and somewhat weak; respirations 24 breaths/min, shallow, and regular; blood pressure 80 mm Hg systolic.

_____ **2.** Patient initially had feeling in the legs. Thirty minutes after incident, patient begins to lose feeling in the legs and the legs become flaccid.

_____ **3.** Skin warm and dry. Pulse 72 beats/min, full, and regular; respirations 20 breaths/min, regular; blood pressure 80 mm Hg systolic.

_____ **4.** Patient has been lying in a field for approximately 15 minutes. He shows signs of mottling on the back of his legs, but the legs are warm to the touch. He is hypotensive and bradycardic.

Match the correct term with the sentence.

A. Vertical compression

B. Primary spinal cord injury

C. Brown-Sequard syndrome

D. Central cord syndrome

E. Posterior cord syndrome

F. Incomplete spinal cord injury

_____ **1.** A hyperextension injury that rarely has fractures. The injury takes place in the cervical area. The patient will have more loss of function in the upper body than the lower body.

_____ **2.** This injury happens when the person either falls on the head or lands on the feet from a high fall. It causes a shattering effect or a burst fracture.

_____ **3.** After the initial injury the patient will retain some cord-mediated function below the insult. There may be some hope for recovery from the injury.

_____ **4.** This injury affects one side of the cord and complete damage to the cord-mediated side.

_____ **5.** This injury occurs at the moment of impact. Ischemia and hypoperfusion can lead to tissue necrosis, which then leads to permanent damage or loss of function.

_____ **6.** This is a rare syndrome and associated with an extension injury. It produces a decreased sensation to light touch and proprioception.

Multiple Choice

Read each item carefully, and then select the best response.

_____ **1.** What portion of the spine contains the largest bones in the vertebral column?

      A. Cervical   **C.** Lumbar

      B. Thoracic   **D.** Sacral

_____ **2.** How many pairs of spinal nerves are there?

      A. 12   **C.** 31

      B. 33   **D.** 5

_____ **3.** The _____ plexus innervates the diaphragm.

      A. Cervical   **C.** Lumbar

      B. Sacral   **D.** Brachial

_____ **4.** Which of the following is NOT associated with high-risk mechanisms of injury (MOI) for spinal injuries?

      A. Penetrating trauma near the spine   **C.** Unrestrained in a rollover crash

      B. Fall from two times the patient's height   **D.** Diving injury

_____ **5.** What is the initial step of assessment in a suspected spinal injury?

      A. Scene safety   **C.** Checking for a pulse

      B. Clearing the airway   **D.** Activating the trauma system

_____ **6.** What is the primary goal when immobilizing a patient with a spinal injury?

      A. Determining if the patient will be paralyzed   **C.** Preventing further injuries to the patient

      B. Determining where the exact injury is   **D.** Securing the airway of the patient

_____ **7.** Which of the following is NOT done prior to applying a cervical collar to a patient?

      A. Determine the need for the collar.   **C.** Assess extremities for distal PMS.

      B. Take manual stabilization of the head.   **D.** Check the patient's ability to move the neck.

_____ **8.** When should you NOT perform a rapid extrication?

      A. The patient's legs are tingling.

      B. The patient's condition needs immediate transport.

      C. The vehicle or scene is unsafe.

      D. You are unable to manage the airway.

_____ **9.** How many rescuers does it take to remove a helmet from a patient?

      A. One   **C.** Three

      B. Two   **D.** Never remove the helmet

_____ **10.** The nerve root located at T4 is responsible for what area dermatome?

      A. Umbilicus   **C.** Apex of axilla

      B. Back of the leg   **D.** Nipple line

Labeling

Label the following diagrams with the correct terms.

1. Label the cervical, thoracic, and lumbar spine areas.

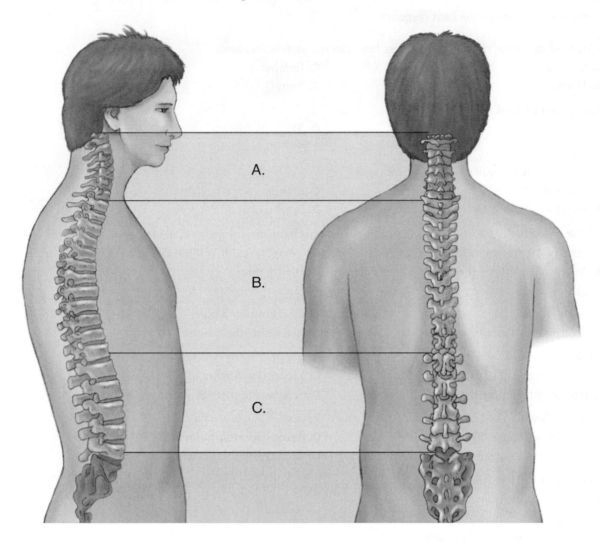

A. _____

B. _____

C. _____

2. Label the spinal cord and its layers.

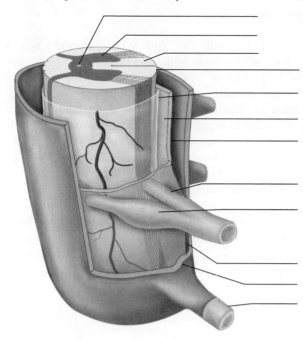

Fill-in-the-Blank

Read each item carefully, and then complete the statement by filling in the missing word(s).

1. Components of the vertebral body are the spinous process, _____, and the _____.

2. The two vertebrae in the cervical area that allow for the rotational movement of the skull are _____ and

_____.

3. The central nervous system consists of the _____ and the _____ _____.

4. The brain stem consists of the _____, _____, and _____.

5. The spinal cord attaches to the brain through the _____ _____, which is a hole in the base of the skull.

6. The sympathetic nervous system is controlled by the _____.

7. _____ spinal cord injury is total disruption of all tracts of the spinal cord, with all cord-mediated functions below

the level of transaction lost permanently.

8. The signs and symptoms of _____ _____ are hypotension and bradycardia, accompanied by warm, dry,

flushed skin.

9. The paramedic should always use the _____-_____ method for opening the airway of the patient with a

suspected spinal injury.

10. During an assessment of the feet of a patient when you stimulate the bottom of the feet, normally the feet move

_____; with a positive Babinski reflex the feet move _____.

Identify

In the following case study, list the chief complaint, vital signs, and pertinent negatives.

Your unit is called to a two-vehicle collision. It is a dark morning, and it is misting outside. Your patient is trapped in a vehicle that has landed on its wheels after rolling two or three times. Your patient is a young woman with long hair. Her hair is trapped between the roof of the car and the head rest, and you are unable to get inside because of the damage of the collision. You find that she responds to a few of your questions, but the only thing she can remember is her first name. You need the Jaws of Life to get her out. After the car is cut apart, you can finally get in the car to perform manual stabilization. A C-collar is applied, and you and your partners with some help from a firefighter do a rapid extrication, being very careful to move her in straight lines onto the backboard. En route you perform a rapid trauma assessment, which reveals no bleeding from anywhere. You patient is very cold, and you learn that the crash happened about an hour before anyone found the two cars. She has a blood pressure of 100/62 mm Hg and a pulse of 124 beats/min. Her oxygen saturation is 96% before applying supplemental oxygen via nonrebreathing at 15 L/min. Her rate of breathing is 26 breaths/min and somewhat shallow. Lungs are clear. You are unable to find a pulse in either of the feet. She is unable to move her legs and she doesn't respond to you when you touch or pinch her feet, knees, or her hips. The monitor shows sinus tachycardia with no ectopy. You start two large-bore IVs with warm normal saline and use active rewarming and turn the heat on high in the squad to help bring her body temperature back up. Her serial vital signs remain largely unchanged except for the oxygen saturation, which has come up to 98%. After a 500-mL bolus of fluid, her blood pressure has come up slightly to 108/64 mm Hg. The next day you learn she had a broken L2 vertebra and is paralyzed from there down.

1. Chief Complaint

_____

_____

_____

_____

2. Vital Signs

_____

_____

_____

_____

3. Pertinent Negatives

_____

_____

_____

_____

Ambulance Calls

The following case scenarios provide an opportunity to explore the concerns associated with patient management and paramedic care. Read each scenario, and then answer each question.

1. In the old cowboy movies, one of the standard ways of preventing the bad guys from making their getaway was to tie a rope securely between two trees on either side of the road, at a height about 8 or 9 feet off the ground. When the bad guys came galloping down the road, the rope would catch them across the chest or neck and throw them from their horses.

Imagine, then, that you are the Dodge City paramedic, called to attend a bad guy who has just been thrown from his horse after riding precipitously into a rope stretched across the road. You find the bad guy lying on the road moaning. His voice is quite hoarse as he replies to your questions about what happened, and he seems very short of breath. On examination, you find a prominent bruise over the anterior neck. The patient's face and neck appear bloated, and the skin there has a crinkly feel to it.

a. What serious injury or injuries do you have to consider in this patient, given the mechanisms of injury (MOI) and the findings on examination?

_____

_____

b. List the steps you would take in treating this patient.

(1) _____

(2) _____

(3) _____

2. A 15-year-old boy was shot in the abdomen during a gang dispute. You find him lying supine on the sidewalk. He is conscious, alert, and crying out, "I can't move my legs! I can't move my legs!" You find an entrance wound just to the left of the umbilicus. You cannot find an exit wound. On examination, sensation is absent from the toes up to the bottom of the ribs. The patient cannot move either leg, but he has normal strength in both hands.

a. At approximately what level of the spinal cord has this boy probably been injured?

_____

_____

b. Suppose that your examination also revealed a blood pressure of 80 mm Hg systolic. What could you conclude from that finding?

_____

_____

_____

_____

True/False

If you believe the statement to be more true than false, write the letter "T" in the space provided. If you believe the statement to be more false than true, write the letter "F."

_____ **1.** The outermost meninge is the dura mater.

_____ **2.** There are 32 pairs of spinal nerves that emerge from the spinal cord.

_____ **3.** The vagus nerve is part of the parasympathetic nervous system.

_____ **4.** A flexion injury is usually caused by a rapid deceleration or a direct blow to the occipital region.

_____ **5.** Most fractures sustained in a vertical compression are classified as unstable.

_____ **6.** In central cord syndrome, the patient will demonstrate a greater loss of function in the lower extremities than in the upper extremities.

_____ **7.** The diaphragm is innervated by the phrenic nerve between C3 and C5.

_____ **8.** When there is an absent pulse in a patient with a spinal cord injury, it is okay not to start CPR because of the region of the injury.

_____ **9.** A normal neurologic exam can immediately rule out a spinal cord injury.

_____ **10.** A drooping of the upper eyelid and a small pupil (Horner's syndrome) can indicate an injury to C3.

_____ **11.** The preferred method of immobilizing a person to a long spineboard is the two-person log roll method.

_____ **12.** You should assess the PMS functions in each extremity before and after placing the patient on a long backboard.

_____ **13.** A rapid extrication technique should be used for every patient that is in a seated position in a car crash.

_____ **14.** It is okay to release manual stabilization of the neck while you are measuring for a cervical collar. Make sure, however, to let your patient know not to move the head.

_____ **15.** If the patient is standing up and walking, it is okay to have the patient lay down on the backboard for transport.

_____ **16.** Autonomic dysreflexia is typically a late complication of SCI but can occur acutely.

Short Answer
Complete this section with short written answers using the space provided.

1. In a patient who has sustained potential injury to his spinal cord, it doesn't pay to wait until there are symptoms and signs of spinal cord damage—by then it may be too late to prevent permanent disability. The only sure way to prevent such disability is to anticipate spinal injury under the appropriate circumstances and to handle the patient in a way that will protect his spinal cord from damage. List eight high-risk mechanisms of injury (MOI) that strongly suggest spine injury:

a. _____

b. _____

c. _____

d. _____

e. _____

f. _____

g. _____

h. _____

2. When assessing a patient for traumatic injuries, you use the mnemonic DCAP-BTLS and PMS. Write the word for each letter as follows.

D _____

C _____

A _____

P _____

B _____

T _____

L _____

S _____

P _____

M _____

S _____

Word Find

Hidden in the following grid are 23 words or phrases related to what you have studied in this chapter. Find the hidden words in the grid below. Then use the words from the grid to answer the following questions (some words may be used to answer more than one of the questions).

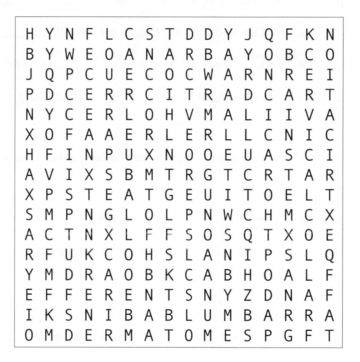

```
H Y N F L C S T D D Y J Q F K N
B Y W E O A N A R B A Y O B C O
J Q P C U E C O C W A R N R E I
P D C E R R C I T R A D C A R T
N Y C E R L O H V M A L I I V A
X O F A A E R L E R L L C N I C
H F I N P U X N O O E U A S C I
A V I X S B M T R G T C R T A R
X P S T E A T G E U I T O E L T
S M P N G L O L P N W C H M C X
A C T N X L F F S O S Q T X O E
R F U K C O H S L A N I P S L Q
Y M D R A O B K C A B H O A L F
E F F E R E N T S N Y Z D N A F
I K S N I B A B L U M B A R R A
O M D E R M A T O M E S P G F T
```

1. The _____ spine includes the largest bones in the vertebrae.

2. The pons, midbrain, and the medulla make up the _____ _____.

3. The _____ _____ acts as a transmitter between the body and the brain.

4. A person who hangs himself will sustain a/an _____ injury.

5. The paramedic should use a/an _____ _____ technique to place a patient on a long backboard.

6. Toes will move upward when the bottom of the feet is stimulated. This is called a positive _____ reflex.

7. Any deficits in a/an _____ examination must be noted and monitored.

8. A rigid device that holds the neck in place when there is a suspected spinal injury is known as a/an _____

_____.

9. When doing a rapid trauma assessment, you should look for _____ _____.

10. The sensory nerves are the _____, and the motor nerves are the _____. They are responsible for somatic functions of the spinal cord.

11. List in order from the head down the regions of the spine, _____, _____, lumbar, _____, and _____.

12. When a patient has a suspected spinal injury, you should open the airway with the _____-_____ maneuver.

13. You should always check the posterior side before placing a patient on a/an _____.

14. Spinal nerves innervate very specific areas of the body surface; these areas are called _____.

15. Never spend more than 10 minutes on a scene unless you have a long _____ time.

16. _____ _____ is a temporary loss of function as a result of an injury immediately following spinal trauma.

17. The opening at the base of the skull through which the spinal cord attaches to the brain is called the _____ _____.

18. Rapid deceleration such as a car crash can cause a _____ injury.

19. Hypovolemic _____ is associated with pale, cold, clammy skin and tachycardia.

Secret Message

Identify the following terms from the clues provided, and then use the letters to decode the secret message!

a. The _ _ _ _ _ _ _ _   _ _ _ _ _ _ _ system is made up of the brain and the spinal cord.
    17 20 41 36 30 1 43   8 26 11   3 46 38

b. The hypothalamus controls the _ _ _ _ _ _ _ _ _ _ _ _ nervous system.
    27 48 23 39 18 29   9   16

c. A temporary condition caused by swelling and edema: _ _ _ _ _ _   _ _ _ _ _ _
    40 44 22 19   12

d. Always use a _ _ _ _ - _ _ _ _ _ _ _ _ _ _ _ _ _ _ to open an airway on a suspected spinal injury patient.
    45 37   4 35   5 42 2   10   33 47

e. Sensor components of spinal innervate discrete areas of the body surface called _ _ _ _ _ _ _ _ _ _.
    24   6   25

f. To move a patient from the ground to a backboard you should use the _ _ _ _ _ -person _ _ _ _ _ _ _ _ _ _.
    14 31   7 34 15   13 32

Secret Message

_ _ _ _ _ _ _ _   _ _ _ _ _ _ _ _ _ _ _ _ _ _ _ _ _   _ X _ _ _ _ _ _ _ _ N ' _ _ _ _ _ _
1 2 3 4 5 6 7   8 9 10 11 12 13 14 15 16 17 18 19 20   22 23 24 25 26 27   29 30 31 32 33

_ _ _ _   _ _ _ _ _ _ _   I _ _ _ _ _ _.
34 35 36 37 38 39 40 41 42 43   44 45 46 47 48

Fill-in-the-Table

Fill in the missing parts of the table.

1. Landmark dermatomes

Landmark Dermatomes			
Nerve Root	**Anatomic Location**	**Nerve Root**	**Anatomic Location**
C2		T10	
C3		L1	Inguinal line
C5	Lateral side of antecubital fossa	L2	
C6		L3	Medial aspect of the knee
C7		L5	
C8	Little finger	S1-S3	
T2		S4-S5	Perianal area
T4			

C H A P T E R

23 Thoracic Injuries

Chapter Review

The following exercises provide an opportunity to test your knowledge of this chapter.

Matching

Certain signs identify specific lung injuries. Match the types of lung injuries to the signs.

_____ **1.** Hemoptysis, lack of tracheal deviation, dullness noted on the side affected during percussion.

_____ **2.** Jugular vein distention, and tracheal deviation and absence of breath sounds on affected side.

_____ **3.** Diminished breath sounds heard on auscultation, a find best heard anteriorly if the patient is in the supine position or in the apices if the patient is upright.

_____ **4.** A sucking chest wound may be noted and a bubbling wound may be noted.

_____ **5.** Evidence of underlying injury may include contusions, tenderness, crepitus, or paradoxical motion. Auscultation may reveal wheezes, crackles, or rales.

A. Simple pneumothorax
B. Open pneumothorax
C. Tension pneumothorax
D. Massive hemothorax
E. Pulmonary contusion

Match the physiology terms with the definitions and descriptions.

_____ **6.** The volume of blood delivered to the body in 1 minute.

_____ **7.** The process by which CO_2 is removed from the body.

_____ **8.** The process includes the delivery of oxygen from the air to the blood.

_____ **9.** This process includes both the delivery of oxygen to the body and the elimination of carbon dioxide from the body.

_____ **10.** The amount of blood per each beat of the heart.

A. Oxygenation
B. Ventilation
C. Cardiac output
D. Stroke volume
E. Breathing

Multiple Choice

Read each item carefully, and then select the best response.

_____ **1.** While riding his bicycle fast down a hill, a 16-year-old boy falls and sustains an injury to the chest. While palpating the chest during the rapid assessment of the chest, you feel what you believe to be fracture of a number of adjacent ribs and observe the patient is having paradoxical respirations. What you are feeling and observing is likely what type of injury?

    A. Flail chest

    B. Subcutaneous emphysema

    C. Commotio cordis

    D. Pulmonary contusion

_____ **2.** What is it called when a knife wound to the chest wall allows air to enter the thoracic space?

    A. Pulmonary contusion   **C.** Open pneumothorax

    B. Tension pneumothorax   **D.** Myocardial contusion

_____ **3.** While standing by with an ambulance at a college baseball game, you see a player get hit with a line drive to the chest and suddenly fall to the ground. You immediately go to the player's side and find he is in cardiac arrest. You attach the AED, and after the first defibrillation the patient gets a pulse and his eyes open. Which of the following is the condition you most likely observed?

    A. Myocardial rupture   **C.** Pulmonary contusion

    B. Commotio cordis   **D.** Diaphragmatic rupture

_____ **4.** Jugular vein distention (JVD) is measured when the patient is in what position?

    A. Sitting upright (Fowler's position)   **C.** Sitting at a 45° angle (semi-Fowler's position)

    B. Lying supine   **D.** Prone position

_____ **5.** On arrival at the scene of a motor vehicle crash, you find a man who owns up to not wearing a seat belt. During your assessment, you observe significant bruising. You suspect the patient has a pericardial tamponade. Which of the following is *not* a sign of Beck's triad?

    A. Hypotension   **C.** Muffled heart tones

    B. Jugular vein distention (JVD)   **D.** Hyperresonant chest sounds

_____ **6.** When are the ribs most pliable?

    A. In children   **C.** In young adults past puberty

    B. In elderly persons   **D.** In middle age

_____ **7.** Injuries to the great vessels are much more likely to occur with which of the following?

    A. Blunt trauma   **C.** Low-speed deceleration injury

    B. Penetrating injuries   **D.** Posterior blunt force

_____ **8.** Where are breath sounds most likely to diminish with an open pneumothorax?

    A. On both sides   **C.** Over the affected side

    B. Over the unaffected side   **D.** On neither side

_____ **9.** While performing an assessment on a patient involved in a high-speed motor vehicle crash, you observe decreased breath sounds and, upon palpation of the chest, you note hyperresonance. You immediately suspect which of the following conditions?

    A. Simple pneumothorax   **C.** Hemothorax

    B. Tension pneumothorax   **D.** Open pneumothorax

_____ **10.** You have a critical patient who has sustained a chest injury during a fall from about 15 to 20 feet. Your assessment reveals a tension pneumothorax, and you determine an immediate needle decompression must be performed. After preparing the site, where should you insert the needle?

    A. Below the third rib midclavicular   **C.** Above the third rib midaxillary

    B. Below the third rib midaxillary   **D.** Above the third rib midclavicular

Labeling

Label the following diagram with the correct terms.

Label the parts of the thorax

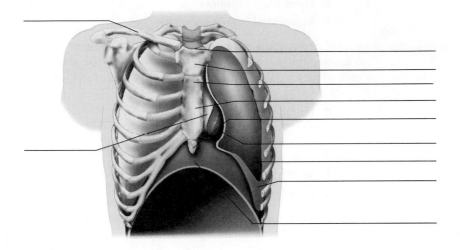

Fill-in-the-Blank

Fill in the possible injuries for each of the following situations.

Many if not most serious chest injuries cannot be specifically identified in the field. An understanding of the mechanism of injury (MOI), however, should enable you to anticipate the injuries that *might* be present in any given case and thereby to assess the potential urgency of the situation. For each of the following mechanisms of injury or associated injuries, indicate the serious chest injury or injuries that are likely to be present. The mechanism of injury (MOI), or easily detected injuries, may give clues to the presence of injuries that are harder to find.

If you find	The patient may have
1. Steering wheel imprint on anterior chest	
2. Caved-in door on driver's side	
3. Fall from a height	
4. Bullet entrance wound in fifth left intercostal space	
5. Fracture of ribs 5–7 in a young man	
6. Fracture of first and second ribs	

Identify

In the following case study, list the chief complaint, physical findings, and signs of Beck's triad.

1. A 35-year-old man was involved in a motor vehicle crash. The patient is quickly extricated from the vehicle. You are the first paramedic to evaluate the patient. He is verbal and when asked about pain and other symptoms, he states, "My chest hurts." During your assessment, you observe bruising on the lower chest, diaphoresis, cyanosis, dyspnea, and jugular vein distention.

While assessing the vital signs, you identify equal bilateral breath sounds, tachycardia, weak peripheral pulses, hypotension, and muffled heart tones. An ECG observes electrical alterans.

a. Chief Complaint

_____

_____

_____

b. Physical Findings

_____

_____

_____

c. Signs of Beck's Triad

_____

_____

_____

d. Do you suspect this patient has pericardial tamponade or a tension pneumothorax?

_____

2. In the following trauma scenario, list the physical findings that indicate pulmonary contusion. List the description of the Spaulding effect, inertial effects, and implosion.

You respond to an assault of a 16-year-old boy. Your patient has been struck in the chest with a baseball bat. Upon your arrival, he is conscious. You immediately perform an initial assessment. The airway is open and the patient is breathing with only mild distress. Crackles are heard upon auscultation. The pulse identifies a sinus tachycardia and other vital signs are within normal limits. An ECG shows ischemic changes. There are no other signs of hypovolemia. You apply supplemental oxygen and initiate an IV while en route to the hospital.

You suspect this patient has sustained a pulmonary contusion. You believe that the pressure waves generated by the blunt trauma disrupted the capillary-alveolar membrane. The pressure created by the trauma compresses the gases within the lung. The tissues accelerated and decelerated at different rates, causing a tear.

a. Physical Findings

_____

_____

_____

b. Spaulding Effect, Inertial Effects, and Implosion

_____

_____

_____

_____

_____

_____

c. Would you run the IV wide open for this patient?

_____

Ambulance Calls

The following case scenarios provide an opportunity to explore the concerns associated with patient management and paramedic care. Read each scenario, and then answer each question.

1. A 26-year-old woman was an unrestrained front-seat passenger in a car that was involved in a head-on collision. You find her lying unconscious on the front seat, her face covered with blood. The dashboard on her side is dented in, and the windshield in front of her is smashed.

   a. List four things that might jeopardize the _airway_ in this patient.

     (1) _____

     (2) _____

     (3) _____

     (4) _____

   b. Specify precisely what you would check in assessing her _breathing_ in the initial assessment.

     (1) Look for

       (a) _____

       (b) _____

       (c) _____

       (d) _____

     (2) Listen for

       (a) _____

       (b) _____

       (c) _____

     (3) Feel for

       (a) _____

       (b) _____

       (c) _____

   c. What steps would you take at this point to ensure adequate breathing?

     (1) _____

     (2) _____

d. Specify precisely what you would check in assessing her *circulation* in the initial assessment.

(1) _____

(2) _____

(3) _____

(4) _____

(5) _____

2. A 22-year-old man was shot at close range by a "friend" wielding a shotgun. You find the patient slumped in a chair in considerable respiratory distress. There is a ragged 2-inch hole in his left anterior chest, and the left chest does not seem to move with respirations.

a. This patient has a/an:

    (1) simple pneumothorax.   **(3)** open pneumothorax.

    (2) tension pneumothorax.   **(4)** spontaneous pneumothorax.

b. What steps would you take to manage this situation?

(1) _____

(2) _____

(3) _____

(4) _____

(5) _____

3. A 71-year-old woman was crossing the street when she was struck by a car and thrown to the ground. She is complaining of severe pain in her right chest (she points to the exact spot, over the fifth right rib in the anterior axillary line). She says the pain is much worse when she coughs or takes a deep breath. On examination, she is conscious and alert and leaning toward her right side. Her skin is warm and moist. There is no cyanosis. Her pulse is 88 beats/min and regular; respirations are 24 breaths/min and shallow. Blood pressure is 160/90 mm Hg. The neck veins are flat. There is no tracheal deviation. There is extreme tenderness over the right fifth rib in the anterior axillary line. Breath sounds are diminished over the right chest, which sounds somewhat hollow to percussion. The rest of the exam seems to be within normal limits.

a. This woman probably has _____.

b. What is the principal danger associated with the type of injury or injuries she has suffered?

_____

_____

c. What treatment is necessary in the field?

(1) _____

(2) _____

(3) _____

d. As you are transporting the woman to the hospital, a 20-minute drive from the collision scene, she suddenly becomes very restless and agitated and complains that she can't breathe. Her skin becomes cold and sweaty, and her pulse gets very weak. Her neck veins seem to bulge out.

(1) What do you think has happened?

_____

_____

_____

(2) What measures will you take?

_____

_____

_____

4. You are called to the scene of a two-car collision. A convertible going south on the interstate apparently jumped the median divider and plowed head-on into a station wagon traveling in the northbound lane. The driver of the convertible is lying unconscious in the road. Your initial assessment reveals gurgling respirations; broken teeth; flat neck veins; asymmetric chest movement; cold, sweaty skin; weak, rapid pulse; poor capillary refill; and brisk bleeding from wounds on the scalp and neck. You are 10 minutes from a regional trauma center. List in order the steps you would take in this case.

a. _____

b. _____

c. _____

d. _____

e. _____

f. _____

g. _____

5. A passenger was in a car that was struck from the right side by a truck running a red light. The right-hand front door of the car is rammed in, deforming the passenger compartment of the car. The patient, a middle-aged woman, is conscious and in considerable distress. Her skin is cold and moist. Her neck veins are distended. Her chest moves only minimally on respiration, and you have difficulty hearing breath sounds on the right. You can't really assess the percussion note because of all the noise at the scene. The woman's pulse is 120 beats/min and weak, and her respirations are 36 breaths/min and shallow.

a. What steps would you take at the scene?

(1) _____

(2) _____

(3) _____

(4) _____

b. What steps would you take during transport?

(1) _____

(2) _____

(3) _____

6. A passenger car has been involved in a head-on collision with a pickup truck. When you arrive at the scene, you find the driver of the passenger car propped up against a tree, where he had been placed by bystanders who pulled him from the wreckage. The patient has numerous cuts on his face and arms and is in severe respiratory distress. He seems confused. His skin is cold, cyanotic, and sweaty, and his pulse is rapid and very weak. He can barely talk, but he manages to gasp, "Can't breathe. . . ." You notice that the veins of his neck are bulging out. List in order the steps you would take in assessing and managing this patient.

Assessment

a. _____

b. _____

c. _____

d. _____

e. _____

f. _____

g. _____

Management

a. _____

b. _____

c. _____

d. _____

e. _____

f. _____

g. _____

h. _____

7. For each of the following patients, indicate what the most likely diagnosis is and list the steps of prehospital management.

A. Tension pneumothorax   **D.** Cardiac tamponade

B. Massive hemothorax   **E.** Traumatic asphyxia

C. Flail chest

a. _____ A 20-year-old driver of a car that rammed a utility pole at high speed. He is in severe distress. His pulse is rapid and feeble, and every so often you can hardly palpate a pulse at all. His neck veins are distended. There is a steering wheel imprint on his chest. The rib cage is stable. Breath sounds are equal bilaterally. It is too noisy to hear heart sounds. You are 30 minutes from the nearest hospital.

Steps of management:

(1) _____

(2) _____

(3) _____

(4) _____

b. _____ A 23-year-old driver of a car that rammed a utility pole at high speed. His face, neck, and chest are cyanotic and look very bloated. His eyes are bloodshot and bulging. He is vomiting blood. Breathing is labored. His pulse is rapid and very weak. The chest looks caved-in. You are 5 minutes from a regional trauma center.

Steps of management:

(1) _____

(2) _____

(3) _____

(4) _____

(5) _____

c. _____ A 70-year-old driver of a car that rammed a utility pole at high speed. He is conscious but in severe respiratory distress. The pulse is 92 beats/min, strong, and slightly irregular. Neck veins are flat. There are bruises on the anterior chest and point tenderness along the left sternal border and over the left fifth, sixth, seventh, and eighth ribs in the anterior axillary line. The chest seems to move asymmetrically on respiration. Breath sounds seem equal. It is too noisy to hear heart sounds. You are 10 minutes from the hospital.

Steps of management:

(1) _____

(2) _____

(3) _____

(4) _____

(5) _____

(6) _____

d. _____ A 42-year-old front-seat passenger in a car that was struck from the right side by an ambulance that ran a red light. The patient is in severe respiratory distress. Her pulse is rapid and very weak. Her skin is cold and sweaty. The neck veins are distended. Breath sounds are decreased on the right side of the chest, which is hyperresonant to palpation. It's too noisy to hear heart sounds. You are 15 minutes from the nearest hospital.

Steps of management:

(1) _____

(2) _____

(3) _____

(4) _____

e. _____ A 22-year-old man who was stabbed in the left chest. The patient is in severe distress. His pulse is rapid and very weak. His skin is cold and sweaty. His neck veins are flat. Breath sounds are decreased in the left chest, which is dull to percussion. It's too noisy to hear heart sounds. You are 15 minutes from the nearest hospital.

Steps of management:

(1) _____

(2) _____

(3) _____

True/False

If you believe the statement to be more true than false, write the letter "T" in the space provided. If you believe the statement to be more false than true, write the letter "F."

_____ **1.** Children's ribs are pliable, so underlying structures may be injured but the ribs won't be fractured.

_____ **2.** With a sucking chest wound, a large wound opening must occur to compromise ventilations.

_____ **3.** Pericardial tamponade is defined as fluid in the myocardium causing compression of the heart and decreasing cardiac output.

_____ **4.** Commotio cordis is when the thorax receives a direct blow during the critical portion of the heart's repolarization period, resulting in cardiac arrest.

_____ **5.** The aorta has only two layers (media and adventitia).

_____ **6.** Blunt disruptions of the diaphragm are usually associated with herniation of all or part of the liver into the right side of the chest.

_____ **7.** Esophageal injuries are not usually serious injuries.

_____ **8.** Jugular vein distention is usually an early sign of tension pneumothorax.

_____ **9.** Hypotension, as a late finding, should not be considered to either confirm or exclude the possibility of a tension pneumothorax.

_____ **10.** One physical finding of tension pneumothorax is distended neck veins.

Short Answer

Complete this section with short written answers using the space provided.

A 22-year-old man was shot in the right chest with a handgun at a range of 10 feet. There is an entrance wound in the right midclavicular line about 2 fingerbreadths below the right nipple. A slightly larger exit wound is visible 3 inches (7.5 cm) to the right of the vertebral column just below the lowest rib. What organs are most likely to have been in the path of the bullet?

_____

_____

Word Find

Hidden in the following grid are 22 words or phrases related to what you have studied in this chapter. Find the hidden words in the grid below. Then use the words from the grid to answer the following questions (some words may be used to answer more than one of the questions).

```
P B S E T R N M A Y X X A H E
B E U U I R U E N O A Z E O L
R N R B G N A E E R R M M A C
O I S I R A Z C O L O T S N I
N P I E C L H H H T P T A T V
C S T F H A T P H E O S V E A
H S F I X O R O O M A N A R L
I Y D T M S R D A S I N C I C
P E Z U G A H C I L E O K O L
O O E N X S H A R U E L P R I
N N U J Q F E O X Z M Q G L V
P L M E D I A S T I N U M Y E
M G A R H P A I D H E A R T R
A K Z D O P O O H O H N D F Y
A N E V X C E B S C A P U L A
```

1. The thoracic cavity lies within a bony, protective cylinder. The _____ encircle the whole thorax, articulating with the thoracic _____ posteriorly and the _____ _____. Also forming part of the bony protection on each side of the chest is the strong shoulder blade, or _____, posteriorly, and the collar bone, or _____, anteriorly. The inferior boundary of the thoracic cavity is formed by the _____.

2. The _____ nearly fill the thoracic cavity. Each of them is covered with a smooth, slippery membrane called the visceral _____; a similar membrane, the parietal pleura, lines the inner wall of the thoracic cavity. Ordinarily, there is no space between those two membranes. Injury to the chest, however, may permit air to enter between the two membranes, creating a _____; blood can also accumulate in the space between the two membranes, a situation called _____.

3. Some of the most important organs of the body are located in a region in the center of the thoracic cavity called the _____. The structures located there include the _____, _____, vena _____, _____, _____, and _____.

4. When two or more ribs are broken in two or more places, a condition called flail chest may develop. Tamponade occurs when the _____ becomes filled with blood, preventing the heart from contracting normally.

5. Because of the way the diaphragm is shaped, several abdominal organs actually lie partially or almost wholly within the chest, for example, the _____, the _____, and the _____. Those organs are thus liable to be injured whenever there is serious thoracic trauma.

Skill Drills

Test your knowledge of skill drills by placing the following photos in the correct order. Number the first step "1," the second step "2," etc.

Needle Decompression (Thoracentesis) of a Tension Pneumothorax

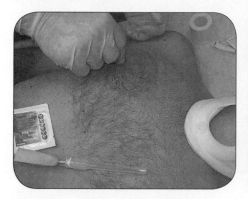

Cleanse the appropriate area using aseptic technique.

_____

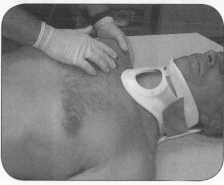

Assess the patient.

_____

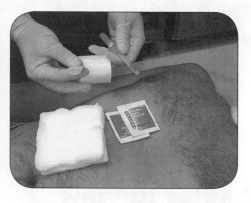

Prepare and assemble all necessary equipment. Obtain orders from medical control.

_____

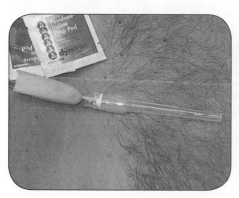

Make a one-way valve or flutter valve.

_____

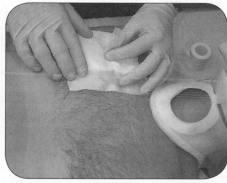

Secure the catheter in place. Monitor the patient closely for recurrence of the tension pneumothorax.

_____

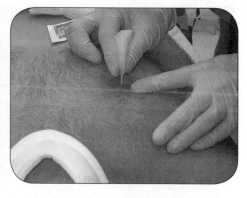

Remove the needle and listen for release of air. Properly dispose of the needle in the sharps container.

_____

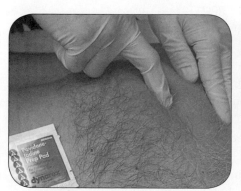

Locate the appropriate site between the second and third rib.

_____

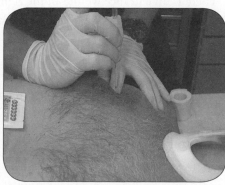

Insert the needle at a 90° angle.

_____

CHAPTER

24 Abdomen Injuries

Chapter Review

The following exercises provide an opportunity to test your knowledge of this chapter.

Matching

Match each of the items in the left column to the appropriate injury in the right column.

For each of the patients described here, given the mechanism of injury (MOI) and the clinical findings, indicate which injury from the righthand column he or she is *most* likely to have suffered. (*Note:* A patient may have sustained more than one of the injuries listed.)

_____ 1. A 15-year-old girl who was kicked in the left side by a horse. She is conscious and alert. Her pulse is rapid. She has a bruise over the left 10th rib in the anterior axillary line and has severe tenderness at that point.

_____ 2. A 50-year-old man was a passenger in a car that slammed into a wall. He was wearing a lap seat belt. He complains of shortness of breath and abdominal pain. He winces when he coughs. His vital signs are: pulse 92 beats/min and regular, respirations 36 breaths/min and shallow, and blood pressure 120/80 mm Hg.

_____ 3. An 18-year-old man shot in the right upper quadrant by his girlfriend wielding a .38 special at a distance of about 10 feet. The patient is conscious. He has cold, sweaty skin and a weak, rapid pulse. There is an entrance wound in the right upper quadrant, about 2 fingerbreadths below the costal margin in the midclavicular line. The exit wound is near the left buttock.

_____ 4. A 60-year-old man struck by a car as he was crossing the street. The patient presents with gross hematuria, suprapubic pain and tenderness, difficulty voiding, and abdominal distention, guarding, and rebound tenderness.

_____ 5. A 42-year-old construction worker is extricated from underneath a pile of concrete blocks that caved in on top of him. He is unconscious with cold and clammy skin. His pulse is very weak. There are no bruises on the chest, which moves symmetrically with respiration. The abdomen is not rigid, but there seems to be a fullness in the center of the lower quadrant. The pelvis is unstable.

_____ 6. Your team is assessing a conscious, alert 18-year-old man who was involved in a high-speed car crash versus bridge abutment. The patient was unrestrained. The patient has an odor of ethyl alcohol; he is currently complaint free. While you are evaluating the patient, you note ecchymosis of the flanks.

_____ 7. It's another weekend night and another stabbing. On arrival you have a conscious, alert male patient. He is lying on the ground with what appears to be exposed abdominal contents.

A. Diaphragm injury
B. Ruptured spleen
C. Liver laceration
D. Torn or ruptured bladder
E. Retroperitoneal injuries
F. Cullen's sign
G. Evisceration

_____ **8.** A patient is struck by falling debris. He was struck on the lower left quadrant and is found to be in profound shock. His lower left quadrant has point tenderness and is rigid.

_____ **9.** Your patient is a victim of blunt trauma; he is anxious and short of breath. He appears to have associated thoracic, abdominal, head, and extremity injuries.

_____ **10.** A woman fell from a height while hiking. You are assessing the patient and recognize that she has Kehr's sign. What injury should you anticipate?

Multiple Choice

Read each item carefully, and then select the best response.

_____ **1.** The focused history and physical exam of abdominal injuries includes all of the following, EXCEPT:

    A. inspect.   **C.** percussion.

    B. palpate.   **D.** vital signs.

_____ **2.** Patients who have suffered penetrating abdominal trauma should be treated by:

    A. removing the penetrating object to facilitate immobilization and transport.

    B. avoiding direct pressure in older patients with more flaccid abdominal walls.

    C. replacing protruding abdominal contents prior to transport.

    D. stabilizing and transporting in the position found.

_____ **3.** Patients with "open book" pelvic fractures are generally:

    A. categorized as stable to the pathophysiology of the injury.

    B. injured as the result of a side impact.

    C. injured as the result of an anteroposterior compression from a head-on collision.

    D. found with entrance and exit wounds.

_____ **4.** Hollow organs are less likely to be injured, *unless:*

    A. they are empty.

    B. the mechanism of injury (MOI) is a motor vehicle crash.

    C. they are full.

    D. the patient is a pregnant woman.

_____ **5.** There are numerous types of blast injuries. These include a/an:

    A. miscellaneous injury.   **C.** secondary blast injury.

    B. primary blast injury.   **D.** all of the above.

_____ **6.** Because of the nature of abdominal trauma in patients, which of the following is required?

    A. Ensuring an open airway   **C.** Administering analgesics

    B. Securing the cervical spine   **D.** Establishing IV access

_____ **7.** Injuries to the retroperitoneal space may include injuries to all of the following, EXCEPT the:

    A. rectum.   **C.** reproductive organs.

    B. ureters.   **D.** liver.

_____ **8.** Crushing injuries may be caused by:

    A. crushing of abdominal contents by the abdominal wall and the spinal column.

    B. the dashboard of a car.

    C. the hood of the car.

    D. all of the above.

_____ **9.** In penetrating trauma, it is helpful to:

      A. identify the type of weapon used.

      B. explore the wound to detect the path of destruction.

      C. cleanse the wound site to prevent life-threatening infection.

      D. remove all exposed foreign bodies.

_____ **10.** The initial assessment for abdominal injuries should include the following EXCEPT:

      A. road rash.   **C.** swelling.

      B. bruising.   **D.** epistaxis.

Labeling

Label the following diagrams with the correct terms.

1. Label the organs in the peritoneum.

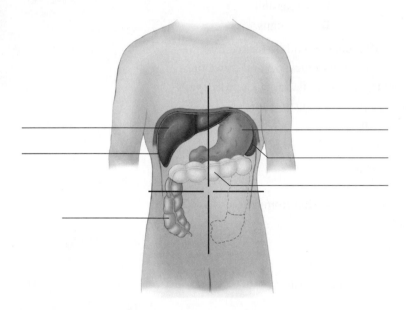

2. Label the organs in the retroperitoneal space.

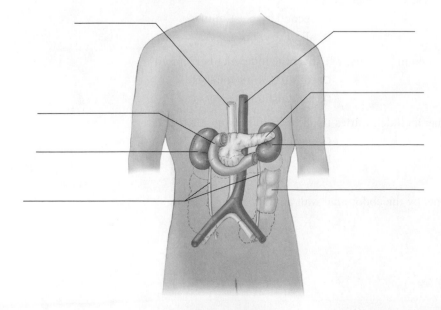

3. Label the organs in the pelvis.

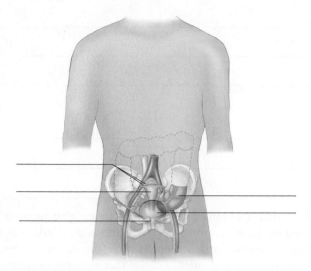

Fill-in-the-Blank

Read each item carefully, and then complete the statement by filling in the missing word(s).

1. _____ is a controversial treatment that can be used to stabilize the pelvis during rapid transports.

2. Retroperitoneal bleeding can lead to ecchymosis of the flanks, commonly referred to as _____ _____

_____.

3. Retroperitoneal bleeding can lead to ecchymosis around the umbilicus, commonly referred to as _____

_____.

4. Structures contained within the retroperitoneal cavity are the _____, _____, vascular structures,

and part of the small intestine.

5. The _____ detoxifies blood and produces bile.

6. The stomach is an intraperitoneal _____ organ that lies in the left upper quadrant and epigastric region.

Identify

In the following case studies, list the chief complaint, vital signs, and pertinent negatives.

1. You receive a priority one response for a conscious and alert 54-year-old man involved in domestic violence. When you arrive, you are advised that the scene is safe and secured by law enforcement. The patient is denying any complaint. You notice that the patient's shirt is blood soaked and the police have placed a kitchen knife in an evidence bag. The patient is not very cooperative, and he appears ashen, diaphoretic, and slightly short of breath. After several minutes of prodding, the patient agrees to remove his shirt. The patient denies any previous medical history. You observe a half inch laceration above his umbilicus. The wound is not actively bleeding. He denies chest pain or other injuries. His vital signs are: pulse 120 beats/min and regular; skin ashen, cool, and diaphoretic; oxygen saturation of 90%; blood pressure 86/60 mm Hg; and sinus tachycardia on the ECG.

a. Chief Complaint

_____

_____

_____

b. Vital Signs

_____

_____

_____

c. Pertinent Negatives

_____

_____

_____

2. Your unit is standing by at your local arena for indoor motocross. This is a high-speed motorcycle racing event, with numerous elevated jumps and turns. The riders are well protected by helmets and specialized outerwear. While watching, you observe a rider crash into a retaining wall. He initially appears unconscious. As you approach, the patient is alert and speaking clearly. He is attempting to stand and get back on his motorcycle. You quickly notice that bystanders are pointing to the patient's abdomen and you see what appears to be a small protrusion of abdominal contents from his left upper quadrant. It's obvious that the patient has an evisceration. You quickly assess ABCs and immobilize the patient. He has the following vital signs: pulse 100 beats/min and irregular; skin pale, warm, and dry; oxygen saturation of 97% on room air; blood pressure 160/90 mm Hg. After quickly treating the patient and initiating rapid transport you become suspicious because of the patient's vital signs. The patient states he has a history of atrial fibrillation and hypertension. He is currently denying chest pain.

a. Chief Complaint

_____

_____

_____

b. Vital Signs

_____

_____

_____

c. Pertinent Negatives

_____

_____

_____

Ambulance Calls

The following case scenarios provide an opportunity to explore the concerns associated with patient management and paramedic care. Read each scenario, and then answer each question.

1. You are called to the scene of a interstate collision in which an apparently intoxicated 25-year-old driver plowed his car into a bridge abutment at high speed. The front end of his vehicle is accordioned against the bridge. As you approach the disabled vehicle, your keen powers of observation enable you to perceive that the patient is conscious (he is screaming obscenities at a police officer). Describe the steps in evaluating this patient for possible abdominal injuries. In particular, what issues will you be looking for?

a. _____

_____

b. _____

_____

c. _____

_____

d. _____

_____

2. A 20-year-old man was the unrestrained driver of a car that was struck from the passenger side by another vehicle. The crash caused the empty bucket seat beside him to be jammed into his right side. On your arrival at the collision, you find the patient conscious, but anxious and restless. His skin color is ashen, cool, and diaphoretic. Patient has a delayed capillary refill greater than 2 seconds. His vital signs are a pulse of 140 beats/min and thready, respirations 40 breaths/min and shallow, and blood pressure 72/40 mm Hg. There is a bruise over the right lower ribs. A large portion of the small bowel is eviscerated through an avulsion in the right side of the abdomen. The right elbow appears to be fractured. List the injuries and your priorities in managing this case.

Injuries:

a. _____

b. _____

c. _____

d. _____

Priorities:

a. _____

b. _____

c. _____

d. _____

e. _____

f. _____

g. _____

3. During the usual Saturday night festivities at the local Knife & Gun Club, a 16-year-old boy is stabbed with a hunting knife in the left lower quadrant of the abdomen. When you arrive, you find him lying on the ground moaning. The knife is still embedded up to its hilt in the patient's abdomen. His skin is pale, warm, and moist. Vital signs are pulse of 100 beats/min, respirations 32 breaths/min, and blood pressure 100/80 mm Hg. List the steps you would take in managing this case.

a. _____

b. _____

c. _____

d. _____

True/False

If you believe the statement to be more true than false, write the letter "T" in the space provided. If you believe the statement to be more false than true, write the letter "F."

_____ **1.** Hollow organs are less likely to cause life-threatening injuries.

_____ **2.** Patients who suffer ruptured spleens in a traumatic event will likely have that organ removed during life-saving surgery.

_____ **3.** Cullen's sign is best described as ecchymosis around the umbilicus.

_____ **4.** Treatment of impaled abdominal objects includes removal of the object to allow for proper immobilization and transport.

_____ **5.** The leading cause of morbidity and mortality in all age groups is blunt abdominal trauma.

_____ **6.** The diaphragm plays a large role in the mechanical process of breathing.

_____ **7.** Penetrating trauma to the pelvis rarely causes life-threatening hemorrhage.

_____ **8.** PASG/MAST may cause an increase in bleeding by putting pressure on pelvic vessels.

Fill-in-the-Table

Fill in the missing parts of the table.

1. List the hollow and solid organs of the abdominal cavity.

Hollow Organs	Solid Organs
1.	1.
2.	2.
3.	3.
4.	4.
5.	
6.	
7.	

Short Answer

Complete this section with short written answers using the space provided.

1. Which of the abdominal organs is most likely to be injured in association with:

    a. Rapid deceleration in a motor vehicle crash or a fall from a height: Liver, _____, intestines, and spleen

    b. Right-sided chest trauma as well as abdominal trauma: _____

    c. Fracture of the pelvis: _____

    d. Stab wound to the right upper quadrant: _____

Crossword Puzzle

Use the clues in the column to complete the puzzle.

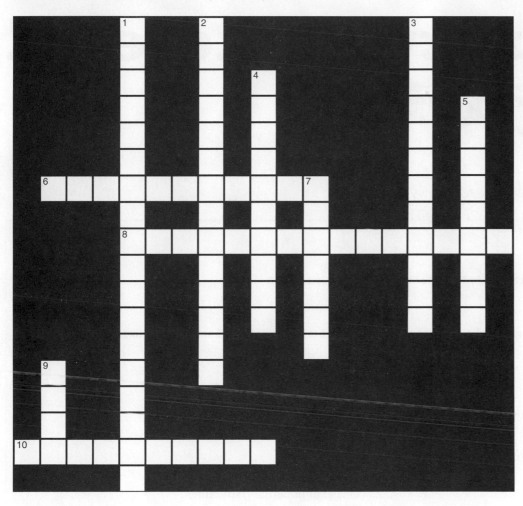

Across

6. Organs that are more resilient to blunt trauma

8. Preferred crystalloid solution used to replace fluid

10. Type of trauma that involves at least two thirds of all abdominal injuries

Down

1. RUQ, LUQ, RLQ, LLQ

2. The number of typical patterns of impacts in motor vehicle crashes

3. Divided into three sections

4. Listening to bowel sounds

5. Dome-shaped muscle separating the thoracic and abdominal cavity

7. The lining of the abdominal cavity

9. A collection of blood in the abdominal cavity

Secret Message

Identify the following terms from the clues provided, and then use the letters to decode the secret message!

a. Largest cavity in the body: _ _ _ _ _ _ _ _ _ _ _   _ _ _ _ _ _ _
　　　　　　　　　　　　　　1　　　　　　11　　　　　6

b. Largest solid organ in the body: _ _ _ _ _ _
　　　　　　　　　　　　　　　　2　　　7

c. Belly button: _ _ _ _ _ _ _ _ _ _
　　　　　　　　3

d. MOI: _ _ _ _ _ _ _ _ _ _ _ _   _ _   _ _ _ _ _ _ _
　　　　　10　　　　4　　　　　　　　9

e. Four different mechanisms: _ _ _ _ _   _ _ _ _ _ _ _ _
　　　　　　　　　　　　　　　8　5

Secret Message

_ _ _ _ _   _ _ _ _ _ _ _ .
1　2　3　4　5　　6　7　8　9　10 11

CHAPTER

25 Musculoskeletal Injuries

Chapter Review

The following exercises provide an opportunity to test your knowledge of this chapter.

Matching

Match the musculoskeletal injury in column A with the complication or other injury in column B that is most likely to be associated with it.

Column A

_____ **1.** Pelvic fracture

_____ **2.** Calcaneal fracture

_____ **3.** Humeral shaft fracture

_____ **4.** Posterior dislocation of the clavicle

_____ **5.** Elbow fracture

_____ **6.** Posterior dislocation of the hip

_____ **7.** Open fracture

_____ **8.** Patellar fracture

Column B

A. Fracture of L1/L2 of the spine

B. Volkmann's ischemic contracture

C. Fracture dislocation of the ipsilateral hip

D. Compartment syndrome

E. Deceleration injuries

F. Possible damage to underlying structures

G. Infection

H. Ruptured bladder

Multiple Choice

Read each item carefully, and then select the best response.

_____ **1.** Which of the following is considered one of the most common reasons that patients seek medical attention?

    A. Trauma

    B. Musculoskeletal injuries

    C. Dislocations

    D. Fractures

_____ **2.** Which of the following is considered one of the functions of the musculoskeletal system?

    A. Hematopoiesis

    B. Allowing the body to maintain an erect position

    C. Protecting internal organs

    D. All of the above.

_____ **3.** All of the following are types of joints EXCEPT:

    A. Fibrous

    B. Fused

    C. Synovial

    D. Cartilaginous

_____ **4.** Open fractures are often referred to as:

    A. compound.

    B. greenstick.

    C. comminuted.

    D. oblique.

_____ **5.** Crepitus is best described as a/an:

    A. loss of distal sensation.

    B. sure sign of a dislocation.

    C. sign that occurs with a sprain.

    D. grating sensation with fractures.

_____ **6.** Which of the following statements most accurately describes Achilles tendon rupture?

    A. It is rarely seen in adults.

    B. It often accompanies arthritis.

    C. It occurs with tendinitis.

    D. It can be identified with the Thompson test.

_____ **7.** Assessing extremity injuries should include all of the following EXCEPT:

    A. Scene size-up

    B. Auscultation

    C. Inspection

    D. Examination

_____ **8.** Splinting of fractured extremities most often results in:

    A. increased pain.

    B. delays in transport

    C. increased bleeding and nerve damage.

    D. reduced risk of further injury and less discomfort.

_____ **9.** Which of the following statements most accurately describes compartment syndrome?

    A. It can be one of the most devastating consequences of a musculoskeletal injury.

    B. It occurs as a result of loosely applied bandages.

    C. It does not occur with open fractures.

    D. It generally is not a painful injury.

_____ **10.** Pelvic fractures occur infrequently; however, they are:

    A. never fatal.

    B. responsible for a relatively high percentage of deaths.

    C. not to be splinted in the prehospital setting.

    D. rarely painful, and as a result they are often misdiagnosed.

Labeling

Label the following diagrams with the correct terms.

    1. Label the bones of the foot and ankle.

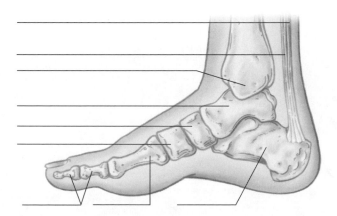

2. Label the types of fractures.

A   B   C   D   E

F

A. _____

B. _____

C. _____

D. _____

E. _____

F. _____

3. Label the three types of muscles.

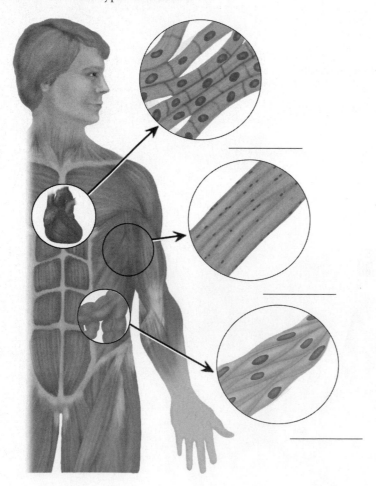

_____

_____

_____

Fill-in-the-Blank
Read each item carefully, and then complete the statement by filling in the missing word(s).

1. Vocabulary

   a. Wasting away of tissue is called _____.

   b. Inflammation of the joints is called _____.

   c. Location where two or more bones meet is the _____.

   d. The armpit is called the _____.

   e. The structure that acts as a strut is the _____.

   f. The shaft of a long bone is called the _____.

   g. The kneecap is also called the _____.

   h. When referring to the sole of the foot, you use the term _____.

   i. The shoulder girdle is also called the _____.

2. To detect a fracture, you have to know what a fractured extremity looks and feels like. Fill in the following signs and symptoms of fractures:

   a. Unnatural shape: _____ _____ F _____ _____ _____ _____ _____ _____

   b. Reduced length: _____ _____ _____ R _____ _____ _____ _____ _____ _____

   c. Fracture of the small finger: _____ _____ _____ E _____ _____ F _____ _____ _____ _____ _____ _____ _____

   d. Black-and-blue mark: _____ _____ C _____ _____ _____ _____ _____ _____ _____

   e. Grating: _____ _____ _____ _____ _____ T _____ _____

   f. Devastating consequence of musculoskeletal injuries: D _____ _____ _____ _____ _____ _____ _____ _____ _____

   g. Protecting from movement: _____ _____ _____ R _____ _____ _____ _____

   h. Hurts to touch it: _____ _____ _____ _____ _____ _____ _____ _____ _____ _____ E _____ _____

   i. Patient may report this: _____ _____ _____ _____ _____ _____ S _____ _____ _____

   j. Strange moves: _____ N _____ _____ _____ _____ _____ _____ _____ P _____ _____ _____ _____ _____ _____ _____

   k. Clavicle: _____ _____ _____ _____ _____ R _____ O _____ _____

   l. Seen in open fracture: _____ X _____ _____ _____ _____ _____ _____ _____ _____ _____ _____ N _____ _____

Identify
In the following case studies, list the chief complaint, vital signs, and pertinent negatives.

1. It is a snowy night in the Big Apple. Most people decided to stay indoors. You are dispatched to the scene where a 48-year-old man slipped on the ice and snow while working late on Wall Street. As you turn the corner to the scene, you notice that the NYPD is already on scene. You mentally note to yourself that the scene is safe.

Your patient states that he slipped and fell on the icy sidewalk. He complains of right ankle pain. The patient further states that he tried to catch himself and landed on his left wrist. He complains of severe wrist pain. You notice that the wrist is deformed and the patient appears to be supporting it against his chest with his right arm.

After questioning the patient, you realize that he has a previous medical history of angina, atrial fibrillation, and hypertension. He also takes one aspirin a day and an antihypertensive. He denies LOC and any head or neck pain. The patient denies any respiratory distress and denies any current chest discomfort. He denies any medical condition that may have caused him to fall. He adamantly states that he simply slipped on ice and fell. After quickly assessing the patient, you decide to move the patient into the warm ambulance for further treatment and evaluation.

His baseline vital signs reveal a pulse of 116 beats/min and irregular, respirations of 16 breaths/min and nonlabored, oxygen saturation on room air at 98%, and blood pressure of 150/90 mm Hg. His ECG is a rapid atrial fibrillation. Pupils Equal And Round, Regular in size, and react to Light (PEARRL). Normal capillary refill <2 seconds. Skin color is normal, warm, and dry.

a. Chief Complaint

_____

_____

_____

b. Vital Signs

_____

_____

_____

c. Pertinent Negatives

_____

_____

_____

2. Your patient is a 48-year-old woman who was injured while waiting in line for a popular clothing store to open during the annual President's Day sale. This is the one day of the year when all the designer handbags are on sale. Unfortunately, at "crunch" time, she tripped on the curb in the parking lot and fell to the ground. Luckily, she wasn't trampled by the hordes of bargain shoppers as the doors opened. She did catch herself with her two outstretched arms. Besides her injured pride, she complains of bilateral wrist injuries and is found in extreme pain. As you approach the patient she is sitting in a chair with ice packs already applied and mall security providing first aid. You notice that both her wrists appear bruised and deformed. Her initial mental status is conscious and alert. Her skin is slightly ashen and diaphoretic, and she has positive distal motor and neurologic sensations in both hands. She denies other injuries. Her capillary refill is > 2 seconds, and she has bilateral radial pulses that appear to be equal. Her blood pressure is obtainable only by palpation at 86 mm Hg. Her oxygen saturation is 96% on ambient air. She denies taking any medications or having allergies.

a. Chief Complaint

_____

_____

_____

b. Vital Signs

_____

_____

_____

c. Pertinent Negatives

_____

_____

_____

3. You believe that this is just another medical evacuation. As you take off from the hospital's rooftop pad and head toward the scene, you pay attention to the radio as the patient information, landing zone description, coordinates, and weather are relayed through your headset. You have a 25-minute ETA and request any vital signs and relevant patient information. After several minutes, you begin to realize that this call is anything but routine. The flight dispatcher describes a farm mishap where a tractor rolled on top of and is pinning a 64-year-old man. The flight dispatcher advises that the ground crew is requesting medicated facilitated intubation immediately on your arrival. Once again you request vital signs as you prepare the medications. Prior to arrival the patient is unresponsive with a GCS < 8, severe respiratory distress, and bilateral open femoral fractures and a possible dislocated or fractured hip or pelvis. Further transmissions indicate a delayed capillary refill, sinus tachycardia, a pulse of 128 beats/min, and a blood pressure of 64 by palpation. The ground medics were attempting IV access while rescue crews were attempting to extricate the patient.

a. Chief Complaint

_____

_____

_____

b. Vital Signs

_____

_____

_____

c. Pertinent Negatives

_____

_____

_____

Ambulance Calls

The following case scenarios provide an opportunity to explore the concerns associated with patient management and paramedic care. Read each scenario, and then answer each question.

1. There are injuries that frequently come in pairs because they share a common mechanism of injury (MOI). When you find one of such a pair, you should be alert for the presence of the other. For each of the following cases, indicate what _other_ injury or injuries you would look for in particular, given the injury already detected.

a. A young man jumped from a second-story window to escape a fire. He complains of severe pain in the left heel, which is quite black and blue and swollen. What other injury or injuries might you expect to find in this patient?

_____

_____

_____

_____

b. A 50-year-old woman was the front-seat passenger in a car that was hit head-on by an oncoming vehicle. Her right knee is bruised and swollen. What other injury or injuries might you expect to find in this patient?

_____

_____

_____

_____

c. A 60-year-old man fell sideways onto his outstretched hand. There is ecchymosis and tenderness at the base of his thumb. What other injury or injuries might you expect to find in this patient?

_____

_____

_____

_____

d. A construction worker has been extricated from under a pile of concrete blocks that fell on top of him, pinning him in a prone position, when part of a building collapsed. He has bruising over the left shoulder blade, and he cannot move the shoulder on that side. What other injury or injuries might you expect to find in this patient?

_____

_____

_____

_____

2. For each of the following patients, list the most likely diagnosis, answer any questions asked about the patient, and describe how you would manage the case.

a. A 14-year-old boy fell from his skateboard onto his extended right elbow. The elbow is massively swollen and ecchymotic. The right hand is cool and pale, and the patient cannot feel a pinprick over the dorsum of the hand in the web space between the thumb and index finger.

(1) What is the most likely field diagnosis? _____

_____

(2) Is there any particular danger in this case? _____ If so, what is the danger? _____

_____

(3) How would you manage this case? _____

_____

b. The mother of the boy just described fell over her son's skateboard as she was rushing to his assistance, and her outstretched left hand took the brunt of the impact as she hit the ground. As she walks toward the ambulance, she is gripping the dorsum of her left wrist with her right hand and holding the left wrist against her abdomen. When you inspect the left wrist from the side, it has a peculiar curve, rather like that of a dinner fork.

    (1) What is the most likely field diagnosis? _____

_____

    (2) Is there any particular danger in this case? _____ If so, what is the danger? _____

_____

    (3) How would you manage this case? _____

_____

c. A front-seat passenger in a car that hit a tree is found with his right hip flexed, adducted, and internally rotated. The right leg looks shorter than the left leg. There are no other obvious injuries, and baseline vital signs are normal.

    (1) What is the most likely field diagnosis? _____

_____

    (2) Is there any particular danger in this case? _____ If so, what is the danger? _____

_____

    (3) How would you manage this case? _____

_____

d. The driver of the vehicle in the same crash as above is unconscious behind the wheel. His skin is cold and sweaty. When you are extricating him from the vehicle, you notice that his hips are unstable.

    (1) What is the most likely field diagnosis? _____

_____

    (2) Is there any particular danger in this case? _____ If so, what is the danger? _____

_____

    (3) What would your initial assessment of this patient involve? How should this patient be managed? _____

_____

_____

_____

e. As your 250 lb partner leaps gracefully from the ambulance to attend to the patients of a car crash, his ankle buckles underneath him. "Ow," he says, "that is rather painful." He manages to complete his work at the scene by hopping around on one foot, but by the time he gets back to the station, his ankle is quite swollen and hurts a lot. Aside from the swelling, there is no obvious deformity and no ecchymosis.

    (1) What is the most likely field diagnosis? _____

_____

(2) Is there any particular danger in this case? _____ If so, what is the danger? _____

_____

(3) How would you manage this case? _____

_____

f. You are watching the championship football game pitting your local high school team against last year's regional champions. Your quarterback, who is about 5 feet 6 inches tall and weighs perhaps 150 pounds, is looking to pass when he gets sacked and buried under a horde of 225-lb defensive linemen from the other team. When they unpile the linemen, your quarterback is very slow in getting up. Of course, you race over to offer your assistance. After peeling off the boy's shirt, shoulder pads, and other gear, you notice that his chest is not symmetric. There seems to be a hollow area just to the left of the sternum, at the base of the neck, and that spot is very tender. The boy, meanwhile, is quite pale, and he gasps, "I'm choking."

(1) What is the most likely field diagnosis? _____

_____

(2) Is there any particular danger in this case? _____ If so, what is the danger? _____

_____

(3) How would you manage this case? _____

_____

g. A 25-year-old man was struck by a car while crossing the street. The bumper caught him in the middle of his shin. His lower leg is severely angulated and bleeding from an open wound. He complains of severe pain in his leg and of "pins-and-needles" in his foot.

(1) What is the most likely field diagnosis? _____

_____

(2) Is there any particular danger in this case? _____ If so, what is the danger? _____

_____

(3) How would you manage this case? _____

_____

h. Another 25-year-old man was shot in the thigh at close range. The left thigh is swollen compared to the right, and the left leg as a whole looks shorter than the right leg. The left dorsalis pedis pulse seems weaker than that on the right side.

(1) What is the most likely field diagnosis? _____

_____

(2) Is there any particular danger in this case? _____ If so, what is the danger? _____

_____

(3) How would you manage this case? _____

_____

_____

(4.) If your management of the case included a splint, why did you use a splint? List three reasons for splinting an injured extremity.

(A) _____

(B) _____

(C) _____

i. You are spending a weekend on the ski slopes. Sailing down a particularly challenging hill, you see a skier stopped in the middle of the slope, admiring the view. Seconds later, about five other skiers come careening down the slope and, one after another, pile into the stationary skier. When the pile is unraveled, the skier at the bottom is found to have a severely deformed right knee, which seems to be swelling before your eyes.

(1) What is the most likely field diagnosis? _____

_____

(2) Is there any particular danger in this case? _____ If so, what is the danger? _____

_____

(3) How would you manage this case? _____

_____

3. You are called to the scene of a hit-and-run collision. A 45-year-old man is lying unconscious in the street, surrounded by a crowd of highly agitated people. No one actually saw how the crash happened. At first glance, you can see that the man's right thigh is angulated, and the trouser leg on that side is soaked in blood.

a. Arrange the following steps in his management in the correct sequence. One step will be performed twice.

_____ Start an IV.

_____ Take the vital signs.

_____ Cut away the trouser leg.

_____ Determine whether he is breathing (he is).

_____ Secure the patient to a backboard.

_____ Apply the PASG/MAST (if your protocols allow), while holding the right leg in traction.

_____ Put manual pressure on the bleeding site.

_____ Open the airway (chin lift).

_____ Start transport.

_____ Move the patient to a backboard.

_____ Check for a carotid pulse (pulse is present).

_____ Check for a dorsalis pedis pulse on the right side.

_____ Do the AVPU "mental status" check.

_____ Check for an open or tension pneumothorax.

_____ Put a pressure dressing over the open wound on the leg.

b. Have any steps been omitted? _____ If so, which steps? _____

_____

_____

4. A 56-year-old woman was struck by a car as she was crossing the street. You find her lying in the street, near the curb, her left leg severely angulated and bleeding. She is conscious. There is no tenderness to palpation over the chest or spine (you don't want to take off her shirt there in the middle of the street to inspect the chest). Her skin is warm. Pulse is 108 beats/min and regular, respirations are 28 breaths/min, and blood pressure is 132/90 mm Hg. There is an open fracture of the left tibia. The dorsalis pedis pulses are equal, and sensation to pinprick is intact in both feet.

   a. What steps would you take at the scene?

   (1) _____

   (2) _____

   (3) _____

   (4) _____

   b. What steps would you take during transport?

   (1) _____

   (2) _____

   (3) _____

5. A backseat passenger, a 52-year-old woman, was wearing a lap seat belt when involved in a collision. She is shrieking, "My legs, my legs!" Her skin is warm. She has no tenderness over the chest, and the chest wall is stable. Pulse is 82 beats/min and regular, respirations are 30 breaths/min and slightly shallow, and blood pressure is 106/76 mm Hg. The patient cannot move her legs, and there is no sensation to pinprick from the toes up to around the iliac wings.

   a. What steps would you take at the scene?

   (1) _____

   (2) _____

   (3) _____

   b. What steps would you take during transport?

   (1) _____

   (2) _____

   (3) _____

True/False

If you believe the statement to be more true than false, write the letter "T" in the space provided. If you believe the statement to be more false than true, write the letter "F."

_____ **1.** Severely angulated fractures should be straightened before they are splinted.

_____ **2.** An air splint is also known as a pneumatic splint.

_____ **3.** There is no need to straighten or manipulate a fracture involving joints unless it has no distal pulse.

_____ **4.** A traction splint is contraindicated in an open femoral fracture because traction may drag broken bone ends back into the wound.

_____ **5.** Fingers or toes should be left out of the splint so that distal circulation can be monitored.

_____ **6.** A patient who sustained multi-trauma is in unstable condition. One should splint the whole axial skeleton as a unit, on a long backboard, rather than take time to splint individual fractures.

_____ **7.** Vacuum splints consist of a sealed mattress that is filled with air and small plastic beads.

Fill-in-the-Table

Fill in the missing parts of the table.

List the names of the bones that make up the following joints.

Joint	Bones That Make Up the Joint
Shoulder	
Elbow	
Wrist	
Hip	
Knee	
Ankle	

Short Answer

Complete this section with short written answers using the space provided.

1. Fractures of the forearm or lower leg may be complicated by a compartment syndrome when there is significant bleeding and swelling within one of the tight muscular compartments of the injured limb. A compartment syndrome, by cutting off the blood supply, can jeopardize the whole limb, so it is important to recognize the symptoms and signs that suggest that a compartment syndrome may be developing. List six symptoms and signs of compartment syndrome.

a. _____

b. _____

c. _____

d. _____

e. _____

f. _____

2. Review the case of the man injured on the ski slope, which is repeated here. List the steps you would take in examining him. Looking for the signs of compartment syndrome is, in fact, only part of the assessment of an injured extremity.

You are spending a weekend on the ski slopes. Sailing down a particularly challenging hill, you see a skier stopped in the middle of the slope, admiring the view. Seconds later, about five other skiers come careening down the slope and, one after another, pile into the stationary skier. When the pile is unraveled, the skier at the bottom is found to have a severely deformed right knee, which seems to be swelling before your eyes.

_____
_____
_____
_____
_____
_____
_____
_____
_____
_____
_____
_____
_____
_____

3. The equipment you should grab and take with you when you rush to the side of a severely injured patient should include the following items:

a. _____

b. _____

c. _____

d. _____

e. _____

f. _____

g. _____

Word Find

Hidden in the following grid are 26 words or phrases related to what you have studied in this chapter. Find the hidden words in the grid below. Then use the words from the grid to answer the following questions (some words may be used to answer more than one of the questions).

```
L A S R A T A T E M F P T D T
T L A L S R F N L M X X R T A
I L E C I U O I E A N B O B R
B E N B E I R T B A I H C S S
I T S O M T A E L U I X H U A
A A Q O N C A A M S L M A L L
T P R W A A H B C U S A N O I
M C K R Z P R H U K H B T E E
A P P E N D I C U L A R E L S
A A N L U U I L E M U T R L T
L Z U L M C L P D L G M L A E
A L U P A C S J Q P O U D M R
C L A V I C L E R A D I U S N
E N I P S P U B I S G L E J U
W I N W A L V G H M I I I S M
```

1. The part of the skeleton made up of the upper and lower extremities is called the _____ skeleton. The rest of the skeleton, the part made up of the _____, _____, _____, and _____, is called the _____ skeleton.

2. The highest point of the shoulder is called the _____.

3. The pelvis is made up of three bones, the _____, _____, and _____. The three come together laterally to form the depression called the _____ in which the head of the thigh bone fits.

4. "Translate" the following into technical terminology:

a. Shoulder blade: _____

b. Collarbone: _____

c. Funny bone: _____

d. The funny part of the funny bone: _____

e. The bone that articulates with the funny bone and whose name sounds funny: _____

   f. Kneecap: _____

   g. Shin bone: _____

   h. Finger bone: _____

   i. "Hip bone": greater _____

5. The bone that runs along the thumb side of the forearm is called the _____. It articulates at the wrist with the carpal

   bones, which in turn articulate with the _____ bones of the hand.

6. The _____, the smaller bone of the lower leg, forms the lateral _____ in its distal articulation with the

   _____ bones. Those in turn articulate with the _____ bones of the foot.

Fill-in-the-Table

Fill in the missing parts of the table.

   1. Indicate the potential blood loss from the following fracture sites.

Potential Blood Loss from Fracture Sites	
Fracture Site	**Potential Blood Loss (mL)**
Pelvis	
Femur	
Humerus	
Tibia or fibula	
Ankle	
Elbow	
Radius or ulna	

Problem Solving

Practice your calculation skills by solving the following math problems.

1. Your patient has a possible fractured humerus, radius, and ulna. What is the potential blood loss from these injuries?

   _____ mL

2. You are evaluating and treating the driver of a motorcycle involved in a high-speed crash. After assessing the patient, you believe that the patient may be suffering significant blood loss from a fractured pelvis and fractured femur. What is the potential blood loss?

   _____ mL

3. Your intoxicated patient jumped from a height of 20 feet off a roof while attending a party. He appears to have bilateral ankle fractures. How much blood loss would you estimate from this patient's injuries?

   _____ mL

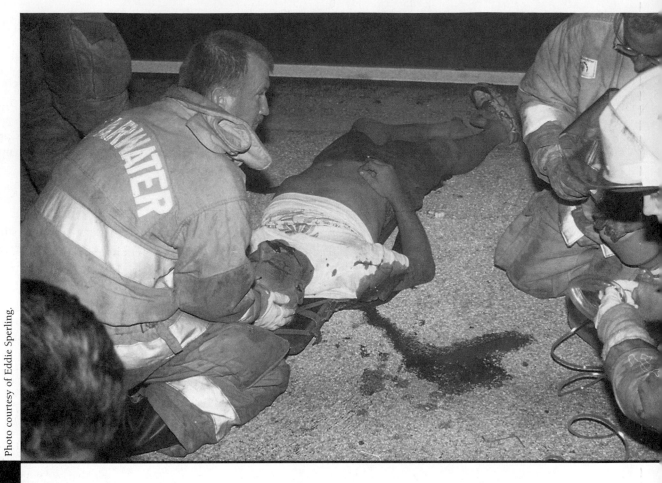

SECTION 4
CASE STUDY

50-Year-Old Male with Multiple Injuries

At 3:45 AM, your unit is dispatched to mile marker 540 on Interstate Highway 10 for a 50-year-old male who sustained injuries after being carjacked. While you are en route, an on-scene police officer radios you and advises you that the scene is secure.

You arrive at the scene. Fire personnel are maintaining manual stabilization of the patient's head. Apparently, the patient picked up a hitchhiker who stabbed him several times before pushing him from the slow-moving vehicle. You approach the patient, who is conscious and talking, and perform an initial assessment.

Initial Assessment

Mechanism of Injury	Stabbed and pushed from a slow-moving vehicle
Level of Consciousness	Conscious but restless
Chief Complaint	"My chest and hips are killing me!"
Airway and Breathing	Airway is patent; respirations, increased with adequate tidal volume.
Circulation	Radial pulse, weak and rapid; bleeding is noted from a large laceration to the upper left arm and from a stab wound to the left anterior chest; skin is pale, cool, and clammy.

1. What immediate care is required for this patient?

Fire personnel have retrieved a cervical collar, spine board, and straps from the ambulance. After completing the initial care of the patient, you perform a rapid trauma assessment. The patient remains conscious and is talking to your partner.

Rapid Trauma Assessment

Head	Several small scalp lacerations, no active bleeding, no deformities or depressions to the skull
Neck	Trachea is midline; jugular veins appear distended; no cervical spine deformities.
Chest	Single stab wound to the left anterior chest (sealed), multiple abrasions to the anterior chest, chest wall is stable to palpation, breath sounds are clear and equal bilaterally.
Abdomen/Pelvis	Abdomen is soft and nontender without bruising, rigidity, or distention; pain to the pelvis upon palpation.
Lower Extremities	Multiple abrasions, motor and sensory functions are grossly intact, pedal pulses are bilaterally absent.
Upper Extremities	Multiple abrasions, laceration to upper right arm (bleeding controlled), motor and sensory functions are grossly intact, radial pulses are bilaterally weak.
Posterior	The patient is not log rolled due to the pelvic pain; however, no obvious posterior bleeding is noted.

2. What does jugular venous distention in this patient suggest?

Upon completion of the rapid trauma assessment of the patient, a cervical collar is applied. Because he is experiencing pain to his pelvis, he is placed onto the long backboard with an orthopedic (scoop) stretcher. After fully immobilizing the patient's spine, you quickly load him into the ambulance. Your partner obtains baseline vital signs and a SAMPLE history while you prepare to initiate IV therapy.

Baseline Vital Signs and SAMPLE History	
Blood Pressure	90/60 mm Hg
Pulse	118 beats/min and regular, weak at the radial artery
Respirations	24 breaths/min, adequate tidal volume
Oxygen Saturation	96% (on 100% oxygen)
Signs and Symptoms	Laceration to the upper right arm, stab wound to the left anterior chest, pelvic pain, hypotension, tachycardia, jugular venous distention
Allergies	No known drug allergies
Medications	None
Pertinent Past History	Appendectomy 10 years ago
Last Oral Intake	Supper, approximately 8 hours ago
Events Leading to the Injury	"I picked up a hitchhiker. We were only traveling about 20 miles per hour when he stabbed me and then pushed me out of the car."

After establishing two large-bore IV lines of normal saline, transport is begun to a trauma center located 8 miles away. En route, you apply a cardiac monitor and assess the patient's cardiac rhythm **(Figure 4-1)**.

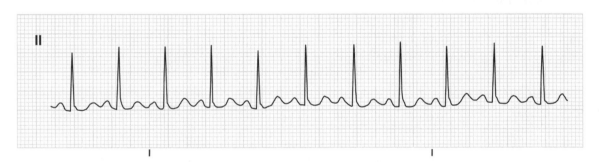

■ **Figure 4-1** Your patient's cardiac rhythm.

3. What additional signs may accompany jugular venous distention in a patient with penetrating chest trauma?

_____

_____

_____

_____

_____

4. What specific treatment is required to treat this patient's condition?

_____

_____

_____

Because the estimated time of arrival at the hospital is less than 5 minutes, you are unable to conduct a detailed physical exam, so you quickly perform an ongoing assessment and then call your radio report to the receiving facility.

Ongoing Assessment	
Level of Consciousness	Conscious, increasing restlessness
Airway and Breathing	Airway remains patent; respirations, 26 breaths/min with adequate tidal volume.
Oxygen Saturation	96% (on 100% oxygen)
Blood Pressure	80/66 mm Hg
Pulse	130 beats/min, weak and regular
ECG	Sinus tachycardia

You provide aggressive IV fluid resuscitation and continuous monitoring throughout transport. Upon arrival at the hospital, the physician assesses the patient and confirms a pericardial tamponade. An immediate pericardiocentesis is performed, after which the patient's blood pressure and clinical condition improve. He is taken to surgery, where his injury is repaired. A subsequent radiograph of the patient's pelvis reveals no fractures.

CHAPTER

26 Respiratory Emergencies

Chapter Review

The following exercises provide an opportunity to test your knowledge of this chapter.

Matching

Match each of the items in the left column to the appropriate term in the right column.

_____ **1.** A nose bleed	**A.** Emphysema
_____ **2.** Cells that produce mucus in the airway	**B.** Carpopedal spasm
_____ **3.** Substance that covers alveoli	**C.** Surfactant
_____ **4.** Peripheral pulse disappears upon inspiration	**D.** Carina
_____ **5.** Chronic destruction of terminal alveoli	**E.** Antitussives
_____ **6.** Used to suppress coughs	**F.** Epistaxis
_____ **7.** Hands and feet lock into claw-like position	**G.** Sellick maneuver
_____ **8.** May cause severe swelling of the tongue and lips	**H.** Pulsus paradoxus
_____ **9.** Pressure to the cricoid cartilage	**I.** Angioedema
_____ **10.** Point of bifurcation of the trachea	**J.** Goblet

Multiple Choice

Read each item carefully, and then select the best response.

_____ **1.** What is the opening at the top of the trachea called?

    A. Epiglottis   **C.** Larynx

    B. Glottis   **D.** Piriform fossa

_____ **2.** In a pneumothorax, where is air trapped?

    A. Inside the alveoli   **C.** Between visceral and parietal plura

    B. In the nasopharynx   **D.** Between the alveoli

_____ **3.** Which of the following substances are thin secretions in the airway so that the body can eliminate them by coughing?

    A. Antitussives   **C.** Diuretics

    B. Corticosteroids   **D.** Expectorants

_____ **4.** Right-side heart failure that has been caused by a chronic lung disease is known as which of the following?

    A. Guillian-Barre syndrome   **C.** Cor pulmonale

    B. Polycythemia   **D.** Atelectasis

5. Which of the following breathing patterns is characterized by breathing that becomes faster and deeper until there is a period of apnea before the pattern begins again?

    A. Cheyne-Stokes   **C.** Biots

    B. Kussmaul   **D.** Ataxic

6. What is another name for "rales"?

    A. Rhonchus   **C.** Crackles

    B. Wheezing   **D.** Death rattle

7. You respond to a patient that is having difficulty breathing. He is coughing up frothy sputum. What is the classic cause of frothy sputum?

    A. Bronchitis   **C.** Coronary heart failure

    B. Infection   **D.** Dehydration

8. What is the most common airway obstruction in an adult?

    A. Food   **C.** Vomit

    B. Tongue   **D.** Dentures

9. Which of the following is not used to treat asthma as defined in the asthma triad?

    A. Expectorants   **C.** Bronchodilator

    B. Corticosteroids   **D.** Hyperventilation

10. What is the correct name for a viral infection of the area around the glottis that strikes children between 6 months and 3 years of age usually in the middle of the night?

    A. Croup   **C.** Diphtheria

    B. Epiglottitis   **D.** Pneumonitis

Labeling

Label the following diagrams with the correct terms.

1. Label the missing parts of the upper airway.

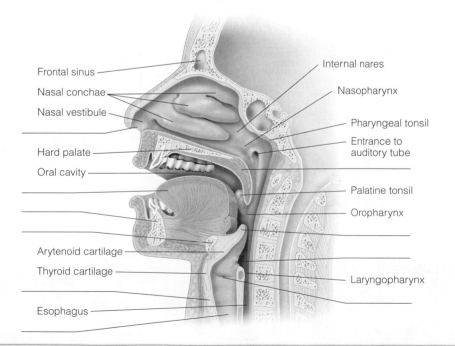

2. Label the parts of the larynx.

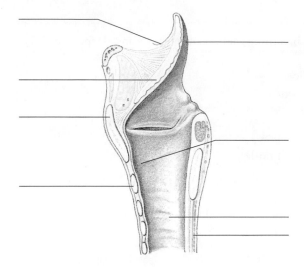

3. Label the respiratory patterns.

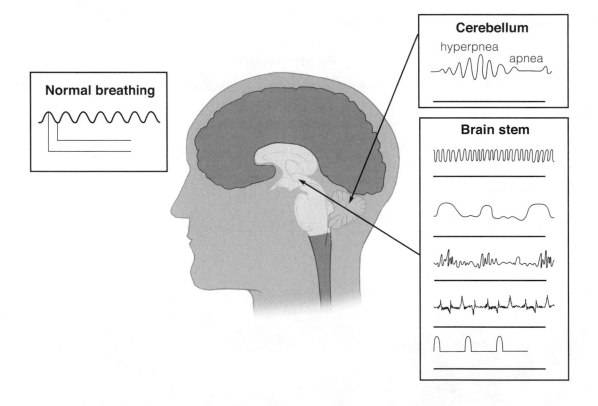

Fill-in-the-Blank

Read each item carefully, and then complete the statement by filling in the missing word(s).

1. Alveoli collapse is known as _____.

2. Hairlike structures (_____) move particulate matter up and out of the airway.

3. A surplus of red blood cells the body makes as a result of a chronic lung disease is called _____.

4. Your patient has two areas of broken ribs that are inhibiting her breathing. In your radio report, you report this as

a/an _____ _____.

5. The medical term for shortness of breath is _____, and the medical term for blue-tinged skin caused by lack of

oxygen is _____.

6. If your patient has been awakened with difficulty breathing during the night, this is known as _____

_____ _____.

7. _____ _____ are vibrations felt in the chest when a patient breathes.

8. There are _____ lobes in the right lung and _____ lobes in the left lung.

9. It is helpful during ventilation through an endotracheal (ET) tube that a/an _____ - _____ carbon

dioxide detector is used to confirm that gas exchange is happening.

10. You should reduce the risk of aspiration during ventilation by placing a/an _____ whenever possible.

Identify

In the following case study, list the chief complaint, vital signs, and pertinent negatives.

You respond to a call for a baby not breathing. As you approach the home, a mother comes running out holding a 1-year-old little boy. He is limp in her arms. You immediately jump out and take the child from her, get into the back of the unit, and lay him on the cot. The child is unconscious and blue, and he has no respirations. You begin the steps of CPR by opening the airway and trying to give two breaths. Your partner has crawled in the back along with the mother and is trying to calm her down and help you at the same time. Using a pediatric bag-mask device, you give a breath and notice no chest rise and fall. You reposition the head and try again, and once again there is no rise and fall of the chest. You check the brachial artery and find a faint pulse. Your partner has pulled out the intubation kit and is ready to try to insert an advanced airway. As he looks for the trachea, he hollers for the Magill forceps and suction. After suctioning and using the forceps, he removes a small plastic game piece from the boy. You immediately start to bag the child again with 100% supplemental oxygen. The child's chest rises now. His oxygen saturation is 54%, and the pulse is bradycardic at 46 beats/min. You are unable to get a blood pressure. Respirations are managed by you at one every 3 seconds. After a minute, the child is beginning to "pink" up, his "sats" come up to 85%, and his heart rate has been on a steady climb and at the moment is 92 beats/min. The child is regaining consciousness and begins to cry and fight you. He is breathing on his own. His mother wants the child transported to be checked out. Your partner has a pediatric nonrebreathing mask ready with 100% supplemental oxygen. Mom holds the nonrebreathing mask while you strap the child into a car seat and place mom in a seat belt. By the time you reach the emergency department (ED), little Tommy's heart rate is normal and his oxygen saturation is 99%; his mom, on the other hand, begins to cry with the realization of how close Tommy was to death.

1. Chief Complaint

_____

_____

_____

2. Vital Signs

_____

_____

_____

3. Pertinent Negatives

_____

_____

_____

Ambulance Calls

The following case scenarios provide an opportunity to explore the concerns associated with patient management and paramedic care. Read each scenario, and then answer each question.

1. You are called to an office building for a "possible heart attack." On arriving, you are somewhat surprised to find that the patient is a secretary who looks about 22 years old—not at all like your usual heart attack patient. The woman looks pale and anxious, however, and complains of stabbing pains in her chest that came on "out of the blue." She also complains of a "funny tingly feeling in my lips." On examination, her pulse is 110 beats/min and regular, respirations are 30 breaths/min and unlabored, and blood pressure is 140/84 mm Hg without significant variation during the respiratory cycle. There are no abnormal physical findings except that the patient's hands look a bit odd, almost like claws.

a. What is the most probable diagnosis in this case?

_____

_____

b. What steps will you take in managing this case?

(1) _____

(2) _____

_____

(3) _____

_____

c. This woman's arterial PCO_2 is probably _____ (higher or lower) than normal. Explain why.

_____

_____

_____

2. You are called late one night to the Koff family residence for a "man who can't breathe." The patient's wife answers the door, quite distraught, and hurries you into the bedroom, blurting, "This is the worst it's ever been. I kept telling him to leave those cigarettes alone—the doctor's been saying the same thing—but do you think he listens? Might as well be talking to a brick wall."

In the bedroom, you find a heavy-set man about 60 years old sitting up at the edge of the bed in obvious respiratory distress. In fact, his "obvious" respiratory distress is obvious only if you know the _signs_ of respiratory distress.

a. List five signs of respiratory distress.

(1) _____

(2) _____

(3) _____

(4) _____

(5) _____

b. What steps will you take at this point?

_____

_____

_____

_____

_____

_____

c. In due course, you learn that the patient called for an ambulance because he wakened from sleep unable to breathe. List seven questions you need to ask in taking his history.

(1) _____

(2) _____

(3) _____

(4) _____

(5) _____

(6) _____

(7) _____

3. As you proceed systematically through the physical assessment of this man, you will be looking for some specific abnormalities at each step. In the following table, indicate what in particular you will be looking for as you examine each part of the body indicated.

Part of the Body	What I Am Looking for in Particular
General appearance	
Vital signs	
Head	
Neck	
Chest	
Abdomen	
Extremities	

4. In the course of the focused history, you learn that the patient has been a three-pack-per-day cigarette smoker for about 45 years. He "keeps a cough," but lately it has been worse than usual, and he's been bringing up a lot more sputum. His feet have also begun swelling, to the point that he can hardly get his shoes on anymore. (Most of this you learn from the patient's wife; the patient is too short of breath to provide more than two or three words at a time.)

   a. This patient most likely has which of the following conditions?

       (1) Pulmonary embolism   **(4)** Pickwickian syndrome

       (2) Chronic obstructive pulmonary disease (COPD)   **(5)** Acute asthmatic attack

       (3) Pneumonia

   b. How will you manage this patient?

_____

_____

_____

_____

_____

5. A 56-year-old man calls for an ambulance because of severe dyspnea. His wife, who greets you at the door, tells you, "My husband, he's a heart patient. Please get him to the hospital quickly. I think he's having another heart attack."

    You find the patient in the living room, sitting in an armchair in obvious distress. "Hit me like a ton of bricks," he gasps. "Not like the heart attack"—gasp—"Can't get air"—gasp—"Hurts to breathe."

    On physical examination, his skin is cool and moist. Vital signs are pulse 120 beats/min and regular, respirations 32 breaths/min and shallow, and blood pressure 174/96 mm Hg. The neck veins look a bit distended, but otherwise there are no abnormal findings.

   a. This patient is most likely suffering from which of the following conditions?

       (1) Pulmonary embolism   **(4)** Pickwickian syndrome

       (2) Decompensated COPD   **(5)** Acute asthmatic attack

       (3) Pneumonia

   b. What steps will you take in managing this patient?

     (1) _____

     (2) _____

     (3) _____

     (4) _____

6. You are called to the scene of a three-alarm fire in a warehouse. The first casualty carried to your ambulance is a middle-aged fire fighter who was overcome by smoke. He seems very groggy.

   a. What is the first thing you should do for this fire fighter?

_____

_____

_____

   b. What are four questions about this patient and his exposure you would like to ask?

     (1) _____

     (2) _____

(3) _____

(4) _____

c. In examining the fire fighter, what would you be looking for in particular? That is, what signs would alert you to the possibility of respiratory injury? List five of them.

(1) _____

(2) _____

(3) _____

(4) _____

(5) _____

d. Among those signs, which one should alert you to the possibility that complete (severe) upper airway obstruction is imminent? If that sign is present, what action will you take?

_____

_____

_____

True/False

If you believe the statement to be more true than false, write the letter "T" in the space provided. If you believe the statement to be more false than true, write the letter "F."

_____ **1.** A tracheotomy allows inhaled air to skip the trip though the nose.

_____ **2.** Typically, anatomic dead space is equal to 5 mL per pound of body weight.

_____ **3.** Gas exchange only happens in the alveoli.

_____ **4.** A hiccup, yawn, or a sigh are all forms of breathing patterns.

_____ **5.** Laying a patient flat will help the patient breath better.

_____ **6.** Stridor is a result of a partial obstruction of the upper airway.

_____ **7.** A patient who is sitting in the Fowler's position and who can speak only in two- or three-word statements is a patient in distress.

_____ **8.** Patients that suffer from severe COPD often have jugular vein distension.

_____ **9.** The longer a stethoscope is, the less external sounds you will hear.

_____ **10.** Pulse oximetry is a tool that can give false readings because of low hemoglobin levels.

_____ **11.** A "blue bloater" is a person with chronic emphysema.

_____ **12.** Acute pulmonary embolism will sometimes present as a wheeze that sounds like an asthma attack.

_____ **13.** You should withhold high concentrations of oxygen for the patient who breathes with the hypoxic drive.

_____ **14.** A spacer device is used on a metered-dose inhaler for people that have difficulty in using these devices.

_____ **15.** A person with rib fractures should be encouraged to take deep breaths to prevent atelectasis.

_____ **16.** If you need to deliver medications via the ET tube, the dose should be 2 to 2½ times the normal dose.

_____ **17.** Immediate fast-acting medications used for bronchodilation are beta-1 agonists.

_____ **18.** When giving a corticosteroid as an IV bolus, you will see immediate results.

_____ **19.** Morphine can be used as a vasodilator and is helpful in the treatment of pulmonary edema.

_____ **20.** A continuous positive airway pressure (CPAP) machine cannot be used in the field.

Short Answer

Complete this section with short written answers using the space provided.

1. a. List four things that can cause a pulmonary embolism.

(1) _____

(2) _____

(3) _____

(4) _____

b. Discuss the clues to diagnosing a pulmonary embolism.

_____

_____

_____

_____

_____

_____

_____

_____

_____

2. What are the *contraindications* to supplemental oxygen therapy?

_____

_____

3. Not every patient who presents with dyspnea and wheezing has bronchial asthma. List four other conditions that can produce wheezing.

a. _____

b. _____

c. _____

d. _____

4. Asthma is common in children, so it's important to be able to distinguish a mild asthmatic attack from one that is potentially life-threatening. List at least five signs that an asthmatic attack is very severe and warrants urgent transport to the hospital.

a. _____

b. _____

c. _____

d. _____

e. _____

Crossword Puzzle

Use the clues in the column to complete the puzzle.

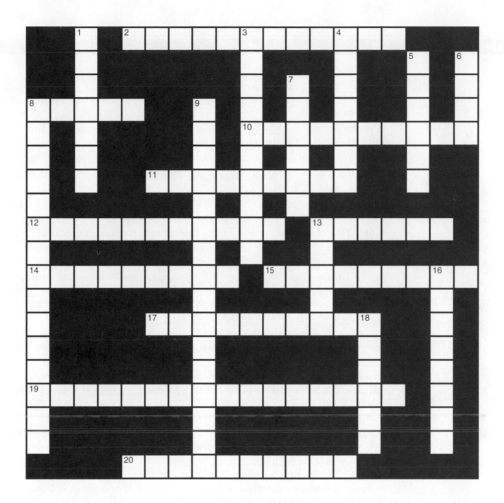

Across

2. Narrowing of the entire airway
8. Viral infection of the area around the glottis
10. Parts of the lung collectively together are known as the lung _____
11. Rapid breathing
12. In the elderly, chronic food aspiration causes _____
13. Muscle that surrounds the conducting airways
14. Wasted ventilation
15. Helps to reduce blood pressure and maintain fluid balance
17. The trap for particles as they are breathed in
19. A medication type that blocks the parasympathetic response
20. Patients with history of DVT have a/an _____ filter placed in the main vein

Down

1. A way to deliver liquid medications in the form of a fine mist
3. Blood in the sputum
4. A highly water-soluble toxic gas
5. Voice box
6. You should wear a/an _____ filter if you suspect your patient has TB
7. Point of bifurcation of the trachea
8. Hyperventilation will lead to the hands and feet in a claw-like position
9. Apply pressure on this to perform the Sellick maneuver
13. Some of the output of the right side of the heart doesn't reach the left side
16. Digital _____ is a sign of chronic hypoxia
18. A metered-dose inhaler should be equipped with this

Fill-in-the-Table

Provide signs and symptoms of various breathing patterns listed below.

Breathing Patterns

Breathing Patterns	
Pattern	**Signs and Symptoms**
Agonal	__(1)__ __(2)__ that are few and far between. Usually represent _(3)_ __(4)__ __(5)__ in the dying patient. It is not unusual for patients who are pulseless to have an occasional agonal gasp.
Apneustic	When the __(6)__ __(7)__ in the brain is damaged, the apneustic center causes a __(8)__ __(9)__ _(10)_ (_(11)_ __(12)__). This ominous sign indicates _(13)_ _(14)_ _(15)_ .
Ataxic	Completely __(16)__ respirations that indicate _(17)_ _(18)_ _(19)_ or _(20)_ _(21)_ __(22)__ .
Biot respirations	Respirations with an irregular __(23)__ , _(24)_ and __(25)__ with intermittent patterns of _(26)_ . Indicative of _(27)_ _(28)_ _(29)_ or _(30)_ _(31)_ __(32)__ .
Bradypnea	Unusually _(33)_ respirations.
Central neurogenic hyperventilation	Tachypneic __(34)__ . Rapid and deep respirations caused by __(35)__ __(36)__ __(37)__ or direct _(38)_ _(39)_ . Drives _(40)_ _(41)_ _(42)_ down and _(43)_ levels up, resulting in __(44)__ __(45)__ .
Cheyne-Stokes respirations	__(46)__ __(47)__ breathing with a period of _(48)_ between each cycle. It is not considered ominous unless grossly __(49)__ or in the context of a patient who has _(50)_ _(51)_ .
Cough	Forced exhalation against a closed _(52)_ ; an airway-clearing maneuver. Also seen when _(53)_ __(54)__ irritate the airways. Controlled by the cough center in the brain. __(55)__ medications work on the cough center to reduce this sometimes-annoying physiologic response.
Eupnea	_(56)_ __(57)__ .
Hiccup	Spasmodic contraction of the __(58)__ causing short __(59)__ with a characteristic sound. Sometimes seen in cases of diaphragmatic (or _(60)_ _(61)_) irritation from _(62)_ __(63)__ __(64)__ , ulcer disease, or __(65)__ __(66)__ .
Hyperpnea	Unusually deep __(67)__ . Seen in various __(68)__ or chemical disorders. Certain drugs may stimulate this type of breathing in patients who have __(69)__ . It does not reflect respiratory rate— only respiratory _(70)_ .
Hypopnea	_(71)_ __(72)__ __(73)__ .
Kussmaul respirations	The same pattern as _(74)_ __(75)__ __(76)__ , but caused by the body's response to metabolic __(77)__ ; the body is trying to rid itself of blood __(78)__ via the lungs. Kussmaul respirations are seen in patients who have _(79)_ __(80)__ , and are accompanied by a _(81)_ (acetone) breath odor. The mouth and lips are usually __(82)__ and _(83)_.
Sighing	Periodically taking a very deep breath (about _(84)_ the normal volume). Sighing forces open _(85)_ that close in the course of day-to-day events.
Tachypnea	__(86)__ _(87)_ __(88)__ . This term does not reflect _(89)_ of respiration, nor does it mean that the patient is __(90)__ (__(91)__ the carbon dioxide level by breathing too fast and too deep). In fact, patients who breathe very __(92)__ frequently move only small volumes of air and are __(93)__ (much like a panting dog).
Yawning	Yawning seems to be beneficial in the same manner that sighing is. It also appears to be __(94)__

1. _____   15. _____   29. _____   43. _____   57. _____   71. _____   85. _____
2. _____   16. _____   30. _____   44. _____   58. _____   72. _____   86. _____
3. _____   17. _____   31. _____   45. _____   59. _____   73. _____   87. _____
4. _____   18. _____   32. _____   46. _____   60. _____   74. _____   88. _____
5. _____   19. _____   33. _____   47. _____   61. _____   75. _____   89. _____
6. _____   20. _____   34. _____   48. _____   62. _____   76. _____   90. _____
7. _____   21. _____   35. _____   49. _____   63. _____   77. _____   91. _____
8. _____   22. _____   36. _____   50. _____   64. _____   78. _____   92. _____
9. _____   23. _____   37. _____   51. _____   65. _____   79. _____   93. _____
10. _____   24. _____   38. _____   52. _____   66. _____   80. _____   94. _____
11. _____   25. _____   39. _____   53. _____   67. _____   81. _____
12. _____   26. _____   40. _____   54. _____   68. _____   82. _____
13. _____   27. _____   41. _____   55. _____   69. _____   83. _____
14. _____   28. _____   42. _____   56. _____   70. _____   84. _____

Problem Solving

Practice your calculation skills by solving the following math problems.

1. Your patient weighs 200 lb. Typically, the dead space volume is 1 mL/lb. Also, a typical person loses 150 mL of air inside the bronchioles that are not used in the exchange of air.

   a. How much dead space volume does this patient have?

   _____

   _____

   b. If the patient's tidal volume is 700 mL, how many milliliters will reach the alveoli?

   _____

   _____

2. How about if your patient weighs 120 lb?

   a. How much dead space volume does this patient have?

   _____

   _____

   b. If the patient's tidal volume is 600 mL, how many milliliters will reach the alveoli?

   _____

   _____

CHAPTER

27 Cardiovascular Emergencies

Welcome to the cardiac chapter of the workbook. Because of the length and the amount of material covered in this chapter, we have divided the workbook chapter into three parts to facilitate your learning: Part 1: Cardiac Function, Part 2: Heart Rhythms and the ECG, and Part 3: Putting It All Together. Although you may not find all of the usual activities in each part, all of your favorites are represented in the three parts of this workbook chapter.

Part 1: Cardiac Function

Matching
Match each of the definitions in the left column to the appropriate term in the right column.

_____ **1.** High blood pressure

_____ **2.** Dilation or outpouching of a blood vessel

_____ **3.** Most common cause for right-sided heart failure

_____ **4.** Excessive fluid in the pericardium

_____ **5.** Another name for chronic heart failure

_____ **6.** The majority of acute myocardial infarctions (AMIs) occur because of this

_____ **7.** The first drug given by emergency medical services (EMS) providers during an AMI

_____ **8.** An excessive drop (more than 10 mm Hg) in the systolic blood pressure with each inspired breath

_____ **9.** An acute episode of shortness of breath that awakens the patient from sleep

_____ **10.** Sympathetic agent

A. Thrombus

B. Congestive heart failure

C. Epinephrine

D. Hypertension

E. Cardiac tamponade

F. Pulsus paradoxus

G. Left-sided heart failure

H. Paroxysmal nocturnal dyspnea

I. Oxygen

J. Aneurysm

Multiple Choice
Read each item carefully, and then select the best response.

_____ **1.** The innermost smooth layer of the heart is called the:

    A. myocardium.

    B. endocardium.

    C. epicardium.

    D. pericardium.

_____ **2.** The _____ separates the left atrium from the left ventricle.

     A. coronary sulcus   **C.** chordae tendineae

     B. mitral valve   **D.** tricuspid valve

_____ **3.** The normal dominant pacemaker for the heart is called:

     A. Purkinje fibers   **C.** bundle of His

     B. atrioventricular (AV) node   **D.** sinoatrial (SA) node

_____ **4.** The _____ component of the echocardiogram (ECG) represents the depolarization of the ventricles.

     A. P wave   **C.** R-R interval

     B. QRS complex   **D.** T wave

_____ **5.** The drug atropine is used to speed up the heart and is a:

     A. sympathetic (beta) agent   **C.** parasympathetic blocker

     B. sympathetic (alpha) agent   **D.** sympathetic blocker

_____ **6.** A statin is a drug that:

     A. lowers cholesterol   **C.** is a vasodilator

     B. is a beta blocker   **D.** is a calcium channel blocker

_____ **7.** An area of fat in the arteries that has calcified is known as a:

     A. bruit   **C.** thrombophlebitis

     B. phlebitis   **D.** plaque

_____ **8.** In a 65-year-old man, a systolic blood pressure of _____ would indicate hypertension.

     A. 120 mm Hg   **C.** 140 mm Hg

     B. 130 mm Hg   **D.** 150 mm Hg

_____ **9.** What symptom is NOT associated with an AMI or acute cardiac syndrome (ACS)?

     A. bulimia   **C.** palpitations

     B. dizziness   **D.** sweating

_____ **10.** The *M* in the mnemonic MONA stands for:

     A. myocardium   **C.** management

     B. morphine   **D.** monitor

Labeling

Label the following diagrams with the correct terms.

1. Label the coronary arteries.

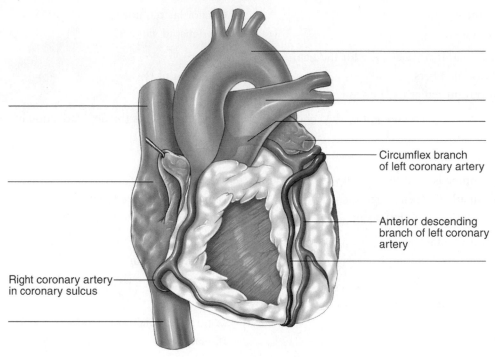

Circumflex branch
of left coronary artery

Anterior descending
branch of left coronary
artery

Right coronary artery
in coronary sulcus

2. Label the structures of a blood vessel.

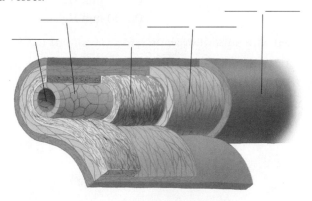

3. Label the major arteries and veins.

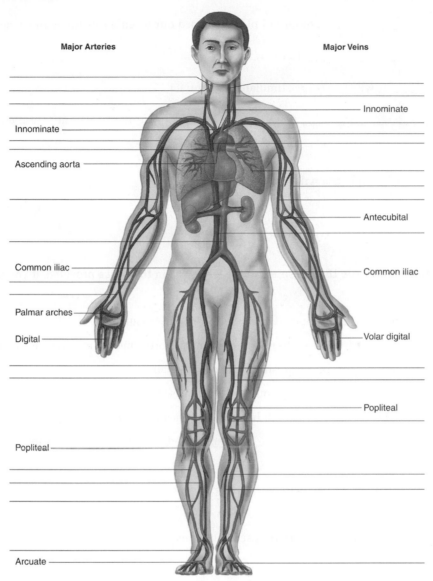

Major Arteries

Major Veins

Innominate

Innominate

Ascending aorta

Antecubital

Common iliac

Common iliac

Palmar arches

Volar digital

Digital

Popliteal

Popliteal

Arcuate

Fill-in-the-Blank

Read each item carefully, and then complete the statement by filling in the missing word(s).

1. Alternative routes of blood flow around the heart are known as _____ _____. These are used in case of a

blockage.

2. The _____ valve prevents blood from flowing back into the left ventricle.

3. The cardiac cycle comprises one complete phase of atrial and ventricular relaxation (_____), followed by one atrial

and ventricular contraction (_____).

4. The _____ _____ comprises the blood vessels between the right ventricle and left atrium, which receive

the output of the right side of the heart.

5. The smallest artery is known as a/an _____, and the largest artery in the body is the _____.

6. _____ _____ is the amount of blood pumped out by either ventricle in a single contraction.

7. The AV node serves as the _____ to the ventricles.

8. Muscle fibers _____ when they are stimulated to contract.

9. During the _____ _____ _____, the heart muscle will not contract because it is drained of all its energy.

10. Repolarization of the ventricles and atria will produce a/an _____ _____ marking on an ECG.

True/False

If you believe the statement to be more true than false, write the letter "T" in the space provided. If you believe the statement to be more false than true, write the letter "F."

_____ **1.** Labetalol and nitroglycerin are drugs that can lower blood pressure.

_____ **2.** The most characteristic physical finding in an abdominal aortic aneurysm (AAA) is decreased pedal pulse.

_____ **3.** An ECG will be very helpful in diagnosing cardiac tamponade.

_____ **4.** Management of left-side heart failure should be to decrease preload.

_____ **5.** Furosemide (Lasix) is a diuretic that will help with left heart failure.

_____ **6.** Percutaneous intervention can be used for a patient who does not qualify for fibrinolytic therapy.

_____ **7.** Fibrinolytic therapy should begin 2 hours after the AMI has occurred.

_____ **8.** Diabetic patients have incredible pain when suffering from an AMI.

_____ **9.** The most common symptom of AMI is chest pain.

_____ **10.** Stable angina follows a recurrent pattern, usually after exertion.

Crossword Puzzle

Use the clues in the column to complete the puzzle.

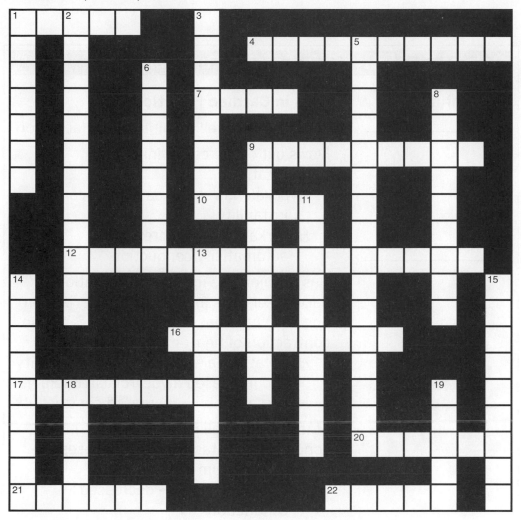

Across

1. Depolarization of the atria (on an ECG tracing)

4. The muscle layer of the heart

7. The left side of the heart is a _____-pressure pump.

9. The resistance against which the ventricle contracts

10. The upper chamber of the heart

12. The "wall" that separates the right and left side of the heart is the _____ septum.

16. These muscles are within the heart and keep the valves from inverting.

17. The _____ valve separates the right ventricle from the pulmonary artery.

20. Flows into a cell and causes depolarization

21. The normal dominant pacemaker

22. Primary nerve for the parasympathetic nervous system

Down

1. The pressure in which the ventricle fills is called the _____.

2. Generating electrical impulses without stimulation from a nerve

3. When muscle is deprived of oxygen

5. Calcium buildup that reduces the elasticity of the artery

6. Fibers that are throughout the ventricular muscle

8. The number of cardiac contractions in one minute

9. Another name for epinephrine

11. The amount of blood "kicked in" by the atrium

13. The right atrium collects blood from the _____.

14. Alpha or Beta (sites that cause a reaction)

15. The nervous system that controls involuntary actions

18. The opening within the blood vessel

19. _____ carry blood back to the heart.

Fill-in-the-Table

Fill in the missing parts of the table.

1. Role of Electrolytes in Cardiac Function

Role of Electrolytes in Cardiac Function	
Electrolyte	**Role in Cardiac Function**
_____	Flows into the cell to initiate depolarization

_____	Flows out of the cell to initiate repolarization
	    *Hypo*kalemia → increased myocardial irritability
	    *Hyper*kalemia → decreased automaticity/conduction

_____	Has a major role in the depolarization of pacemaker cells (maintains depolarization) and in myocardial contractility (involved in contraction of heart muscle tissue)
	    *Hypo*calcemia → decreased contractility and increased myocardial irritability
	    *Hyper*calcemia → increased contractility

_____	Stabilizes the cell membrane; acts in concert with potassium, and opposes the actions of calcium
	    *Hypo*magnesemia → decreased conduction
	    *Hyper*magnesemia → increased myocardial irritability

2. Components of the ECG

Components of the ECG	
ECG Representation	**Cardiac Event**
_____	Depolarization of the atria
P-R interval	_____
_____	Depolarization of the ventricles
	Period between ventricular depolarization and beginning of repolarization
_____	Repolarization of the ventricles
R-R interval	_____

Part 2: Heart Rhythms and the ECG

Matching
Match each of the items in the left column to the appropriate term in the right column.

_____ **1.** Where the RA lead is placed

_____ **2.** Where the LL lead is placed

_____ **3.** The point where the QRS complex ends and the ST segment begins

_____ **4.** Represents ventricular repolarization on an ECG

_____ **5.** A regular rhythm, 60 to 100 beats/min

_____ **6.** SA node pacemaker with a rate of 100 beats/min or more

_____ **7.** A rhythm in which the atria are contracting at a rate that is too fast for the ventricles to match

_____ **8.** When an impulse reaching the AV node is delayed and results in a PRI longer than 0.20 seconds

_____ **9.** Rhythm that occurs when the ventricles take over at a rate of 20 to 40 beats/min

_____ **10.** A delta wave is an indication of this

A. First-degree heart block

B. Heart rate

C. Left lower chest

D. T wave

E. Atrial flutter

F. Tachycardia

G. Right upper shoulder

H. Wolff-Parkinson-White (WPW) syndrome

I. J point

J. Idioventricular rhythm

Multiple Choice
Read each item carefully, and then select the best response.

_____ **1.** _____ is an electrolyte imbalance that causes very tall and pointed T waves.

    A. Hypokalemia

    B. Hyperkalemia

    C. Hyperglycemia

    D. Hypocalcemia

_____ **2.** The _____ is NOT a limb lead.

    A. I

    B. aVR

    C. aVF

    D. V_2

_____ **3.** During an AMI, the stage of injury appears as a/an _____ on the ECG.
    A. T wave inversion   **C.** ST-segment elevation
    B. ST-segment depression   **D.** spiked P wave

_____ **4.** Lead V$_5$ is placed on the patient on the _____.
    A. anterior axillary line   **C.** fourth intercostal space
    B. midaxillary line   **D.** left arm

_____ **5.** _____ is NOT a possible cause of pulseless electrical activity (PEA).
    A. Hypovolemia   **C.** Cardiac tamponade
    B. Hyperthermia   **D.** Pulmonary embolism

_____ **6.** The dosage of atropine used for sinus bradycardia is:
    A. 0.04 mg/kg   **C.** 0.5 mg
    B. 0.4 mg   **D.** 0.5 mg/kg

_____ **7.** When using paddles to shock a patient, you apply _____ lb of pressure to the chest with the paddles.
    A. 10   **C.** 20
    B. 15   **D.** 25

_____ **8.** The correct term for the use of a defibrillator to end an arrhythmia other than V-fib or pulseless V-tach is:
    A. cardioversion   **C.** defibrillation
    B. transcutaneous cardiac pacing   **D.** conversion

_____ **9.** A common treatment for chronic coronary heart failure or rapid atrial arrhythmias is:
    A. atropine   **C.** sodium bicarbonate
    B. digitalis   **D.** nitroglycerin

_____ **10.** One small box on the ECG strip represents _____ seconds.
    A. 0.04   **C.** 0.02
    B. 0.40   **D.** 0.20

Fill-in-the-Blank

Read each item carefully, and then complete the statement by filling in the missing word(s).

1. _____ _____ occurs when the SA node fails to fire and initiate an impulse, which in turns eliminates an entire cardiac cycle. After the missed set, a normal function returns.

2. A tachycardic rhythm that begins in the pacemaker above the ventricles is known as a/an _____ _____.

3. The SA node ceases to fire and the AV node takes over as the pacemaker; however, the rate is greater than 60 beats/min. This is called _____ _____ _____.

4. A/an _____-_____ _____ _____ occurs when there is no association between the AV node and the ventricles. Ventricular rate runs the heart.

5. _____ _____ occurs when the entire heart begins to quiver without any organized contractions.

6. The pattern _____ occurs when there is a normal complex followed by a premature ventricular complex. This pattern repeats itself. If every third beat is a premature ventricular complex, it is then called _____.

7. _____ occurs when the entire heart is at a standstill and there is no electrical activity.

8. A/an _____ _____ is an indication of Wolff-Parkinson-White syndrome.

9. When a premature ventricular complex comes from the same site, it is known as _____, but when the premature

   ventricular complexes come from different sites in the ventricles, the condition is known as _____.

10. The pacemaker is the SA node, but with a rate of less than 60 beats/min. This is called _____ _____.

True/False

If you believe the statement to be more true than false, write the letter "T" in the space provided. If you believe the statement to be more false than true, write the letter "F."

_____ 1. Lead II will give you the best view for monitoring a patient's rhythm.

_____ 2. P waves indicate the pacemaker for the heart is in the AV node.

_____ 3. The "6-second method" is the simplest, but not the most accurate, method for determining the heart rate when the rhythm is slow.

_____ 4. A heart rate of more than 100 beats/min is called tachycardia.

_____ 5. Wandering atrial pacemaker is most commonly seen in diabetic patients.

_____ 6. Prehospital treatment of atrial fibrillation is common.

_____ 7. Mobitz type I occurs when each successive impulse is delayed a little longer, until finally one impulse is not able to continue.

_____ 8. The ventricles will take over as the pacemaker if the SA node fails.

_____ 9. Polymorphic V-tach is more serious than monomorphic V-tach.

_____ 10. An agonal rhythm will produce a pulse.

Short Answer

Complete this section with short written answers using the space provided.

1. Discuss the basic principles in placing electrodes on a patient's chest.

   _____

   _____

   _____

2. Explain the cause for the P wave, P-R interval, QRS complex, and the T wave.

   _____

   _____

   _____

   _____

3. Describe how a 12-lead ECG helps to "look" at the heart.

   _____

   _____

   _____

4. What should you do if you find a patient in cardiac arrest?

_____

_____

_____

_____

5. If you are able to terminate cardiopulmonary resuscitation (CPR) in the field, what should you and your medical director do before you implement your protocols to terminate CPR in the field?

_____

_____

_____

_____

Word Find

Hidden in the following grid are 23 words or phrases related to what you have studied in this chapter. Find the hidden words in the grid. Then use the words from the grid to answer the following questions.

```
C C N P B Q N W V S L M X H Q P H I A
F O P O Q R W F C R H S Y D R T Y D T
K N M A I X A I H T Q P R E E N P I R
E L X P P S T D Y L O B C D B A O O I
Z J A R L E R H Y V M O O C U L K V A
E R O C R E R E O C R C P J L U A E L
E P Q U O L T L V D A C E Y H G L N L
K I I C A F E E I O S R R E U A E T A
I D W N P M I A H L I F D O Z O M R N
P N O W I S L T P E X D Q I B C I I O
S G U A A L O Q L O A N R V A I A C I
A V S N E V A W P U S R I A L T A U T
E J O A P O V Y M E M M T T C N V L C
S D D A I M H T Y H R R A B R A I A N
E S T A C H Y C A R D I A H L A W R U
N O I T A L L I R B I F E D C O T Q J
U N I F O C A L U U P F V P R N C E O
K G W B Y V R A Z A J N B R I G Y K S
K D N Z L P N X B T L N J O G Q P S N
```

1. Cardiac rhythm disturbance: _____

2. Impulse generated from the SA node: _____ _____

3. A button on a monitor used to cardiovert a patient: _____

4. A rate above 100 beats/min: _____

5. A rate below 60 beats/min: _____

6. An ectopic complex that is early and originates from the SA node: premature _____ complex

7. Occurs as a result of different SA node sites: _____ atrial tachycardia

8. The dominate pacemaker of the normal heart: _____ _____

9. Rhythm that occurs when the SA node fails and the AV node takes over: _____

10. Arising from a single site: _____

11. A rhythm originating in the ventricles: _____

12. When asystole presents with small sinusoidal complexes: _____ _____

13. A sharp pacer _____ is present with an artificial implanted pacemaker

14. Usually presents with a flat or apparently absent T wave and sometimes the development of a U wave: _____

15. Another name for third-degree AV block: _____ _____ _____

16. Another name for chest leads: _____ _____

17. Called when a patient goes into cardiac arrest: _____

18. A cause of pulseless electrical activity (PEA) as a result of low blood volume: _____

19. Electrical treatment for unstable tachycardia: _____

20. Electrical treatment for fibrillation of the heart: _____

21. The three major classes of drugs used to relieve angina: _____, beta blockers, calcium channel blockers

22. "Water pills": _____

23. Blood thinner drugs are known as: _____ drugs

Part 3: Putting It All Together

Matching

Match the generic name with the trade name for the following drugs.

_____ **1.** Amiodarone   **A.** Procardia
_____ **2.** Verapamil   **B.** Isoptin
_____ **3.** Furosemide   **C.** Lanoxin
_____ **4.** Procainamide   **D.** Trandate
_____ **5.** Nifedipine   **E.** Lasix
_____ **6.** Digoxin   **F.** Pronestyl
_____ **7.** Diltiazem   **G.** Inderal
_____ **8.** Labetalol   **H.** Cardizem
_____ **9.** Enalapril   **I.** Cordarone
_____ **10.** Propranolol   **J.** Vasotec

Labeling

1. Label the electrical conduction system of the heart.

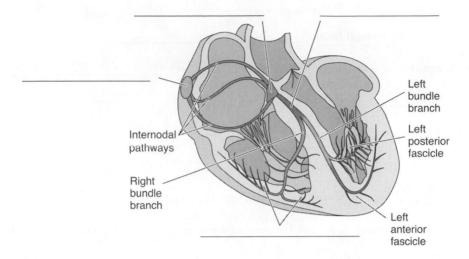

Internodal pathways

Right bundle branch

Left bundle branch

Left posterior fascicle

Left anterior fascicle

2. Label the missing schematic representations of a 12-lead ECG.

I	aVR	V₁	V₄
LCA		LCA	LCA
Lateral wall LV		Septum LV	Anterior wall LV
II	**aVL**	**V₂**	**V₅**
RCA	_____	_____	_____
Inferior wall LV	_____	_____	_____
III	**aVF**	**V₃**	**V₆**
_____	RCA	LCA	LCA
_____	Inferior wall LV	Anterior wall LV	Lateral wall LV

Ambulance Calls

Read each scenario, and then answer all the questions following the scenario.

1. You are called to see a 62-year-old man complaining of severe chest pain. He says that the pain came on an hour earlier and that it feels "like a thousand-pound weight on my chest." The patient is very restless and seems confused so it is hard to get much history. On physical examination, he is obviously in marked distress. His skin is pale and cold. His pulse is 82 beats/min and thready, respirations are 32 breaths/min and shallow, and blood pressure is 90/62 mm Hg. His oxygen saturation is 91% on room air.

    a. Identify the chief complaint and vital signs for this patient.

    Chief Complaint

_____

_____

    Vital Signs

_____

_____

b. What steps would you direct your partner to take at this time of the call?

(1) _____

(2) _____

(3) _____

(4) _____

c. After your partner hooks up the monitor, you run a 3-lead ECG strip and see this:

(1) Is the rhythm regular? _____

(2) What is the rate? _____

(3) Are the P waves present or absent? _____

(4) If present, is there a P wave before every QRS? _____

(5) P-R interval: _____ seconds

(6) QRS complex width: _____

(7) T waves present or absent? Upright? _____

(8) What is the name of this rhythm? _____

d. What field diagnosis will you give this patient and why?

_____

_____

_____

e. What treatment will you provide for this patient?

_____

_____

_____

2. You are called to see a patient whose chief complaint is dyspnea. He tells you in gasps that for several nights he's been waking up around 2:00 am unable to breathe. He has to get up and sit on the side of the bed to catch his breath. Tonight sitting up hasn't helped. "Must be those cigarettes," he wheezes. He tells you that he "keeps a cough," but lately he's been bringing up much more sputum than usual. On physical examination, he is in obvious respiratory distress, coughing periodically. His lips look rather blue. His pulse is 102 beats/min and irregular. His respirations are 60 breaths/min and labored, and his blood pressure is 170/94 mm Hg in both arms. His neck veins are distended to the angle of the jaw. His chest is a veritable symphony of crackles and wheezes, and his oxygen saturation is 86% on room air. There is a tender fullness in the right upper quadrant of his abdomen. Both feet are swollen well above the ankles.

a. Identify the chief complaint and vitals signs for this patient.

Chief Complaint

_____

_____

Vital Signs

_____

_____

b. What steps would you take at this point in the call?

(1) _____

(2) _____

(3) _____

(4) _____

c. What do you think the patient is experiencing?

_____

d. What can you do to help your patient?

_____

_____

3. The family of a 76-year-old woman calls for an ambulance after the woman fainted while preparing Sunday dinner. She is lying on the sofa when you arrive. She is conscious but somewhat confused. She was unharmed in the fall. Your partner begins with vital signs as you try to get a history. Her pulse is 44 beats/min and regular, respirations are 22 breaths/min and full, and oxygen saturation is 94%. She says that she is having some pain in her chest, but can't seem to rate the pain because of her confusion. Her blood pressure is 82/40 mm Hg, and her skin is cool. Her lungs are clear and she seems to be in good health otherwise. She takes a vitamin a day.

a. Identify the chief complaint and vital signs for this patient.

Chief Complaint

_____

_____

Vital Signs

_____

_____

b. List at least four reasons for a syncopal episode.

(1) _____

(2) _____

(3) _____

(4) _____

c. You hook up the monitor and see sinus bradycardia. What is your treatment for this patient now?

(1) _____

(2) _____

d. If pharmacologic therapies don't help, what else can you do to raise the heart rate in this patient?

_____

4. A 64-year-old man calls for an ambulance because he's been "feeling poorly." It's nothing he can really pin down. He's just been feeling very weak and washed out for the last few days, and so he thought maybe he ought to go to the hospital and have a doctor take a look at him. There are no striking findings on physical exam except for an irregular heartbeat. His pulse is about 76 beats/min but very irregular so that it is hard to count. His blood pressure is 110/74 mm Hg on both arms. He has no significant history and really hasn't been to a doctor except for a yearly checkup. His lungs are clear, and his oxygen saturation is 97%. His skin is a little cool. You hook up the heart monitor to take a quick peek and this is what you see.

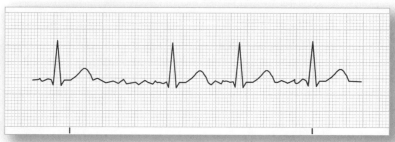

a. Identify the chief complaint and vital signs of this patient.
Chief Complaint

_____

_____

Vital Signs

_____

_____

b.

(1) Is the rhythm regular? _____

(2) What is the rate? _____

(3) Are the P waves present or absent? _____

(4) If present, is there a P before every QRS? _____

(5) Is there a QRS after every P? _____

(6) P-R interval: _____

(7) QRS complexes: _____ normal _____ abnormal

(8) Name of rhythm: _____

(9) Treatment: _____

5. You are taking a quick break at the emergency department (ED) after several hectic calls. You have made friends with the nurses, and they let you sit at the desk, where you can see the following heart monitors for different patients. Write the correct name of the rhythm on the line below the strip.

a.

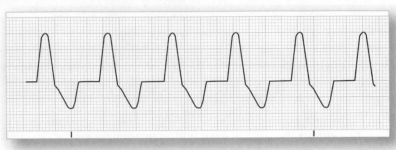

_____

b.

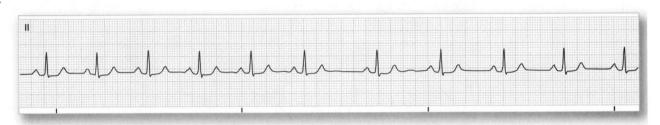

_____

c.

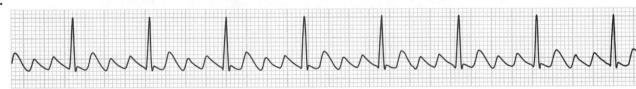

_____

d.

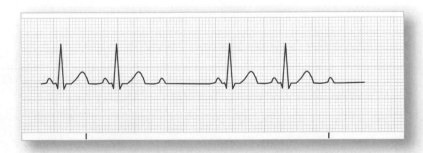

_____

e.

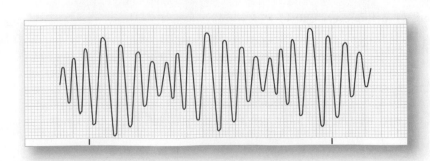

_____

f.

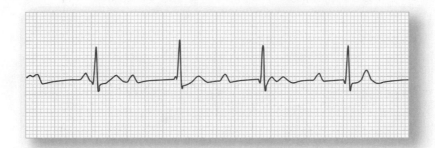

_____

g.

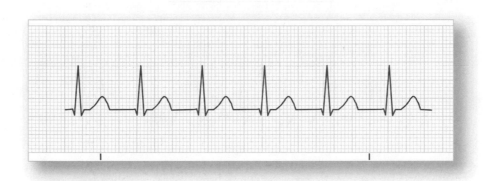

_____

h.

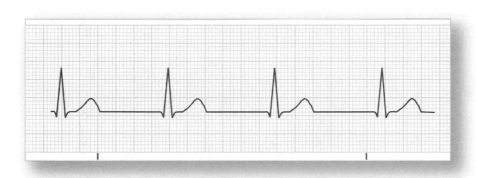

_____

i.

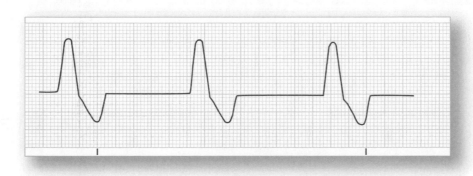

_____

j.

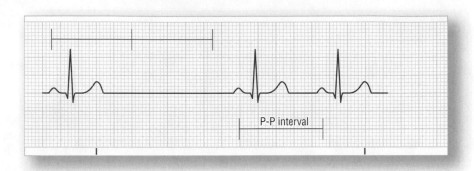

P-P interval

_____

k.

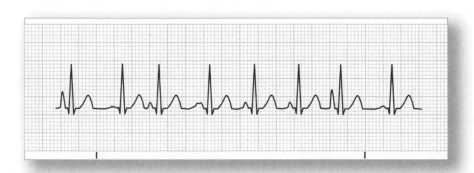

_____

l.

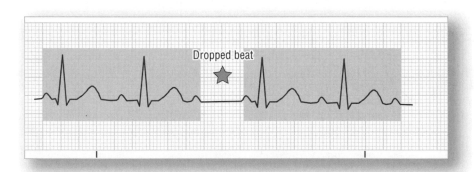

Dropped beat

_____

m.

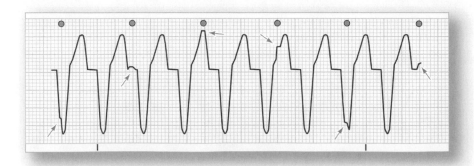

_____

n.

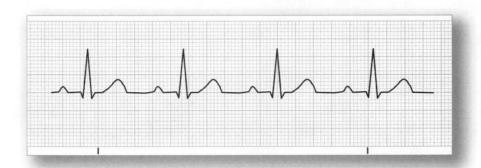

_____

o.

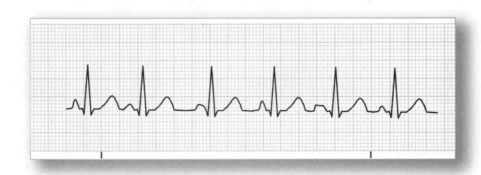

_____

p.

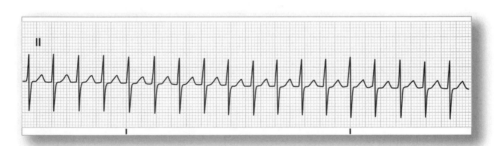

_____

q.

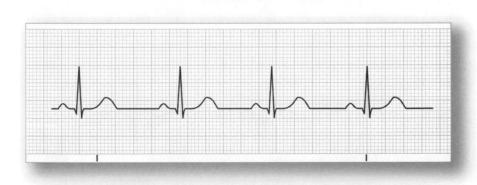

_____

r.

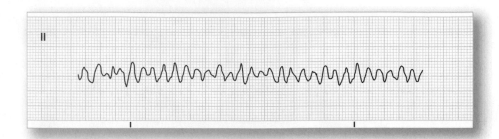

_____

6. The nurse hands you the following three strips and asks you if you can figure out what type of ectopic beat is present in each strip.

a.

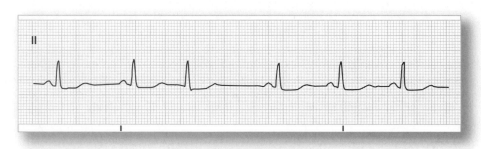

_____

b.

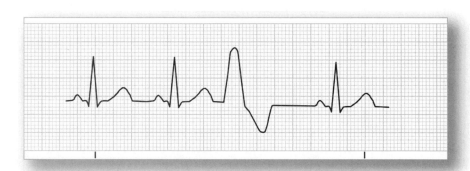

_____

c.

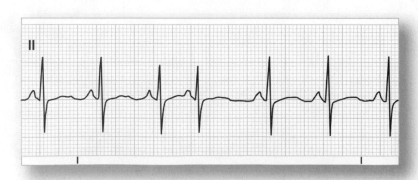

_____

Crossword Puzzle

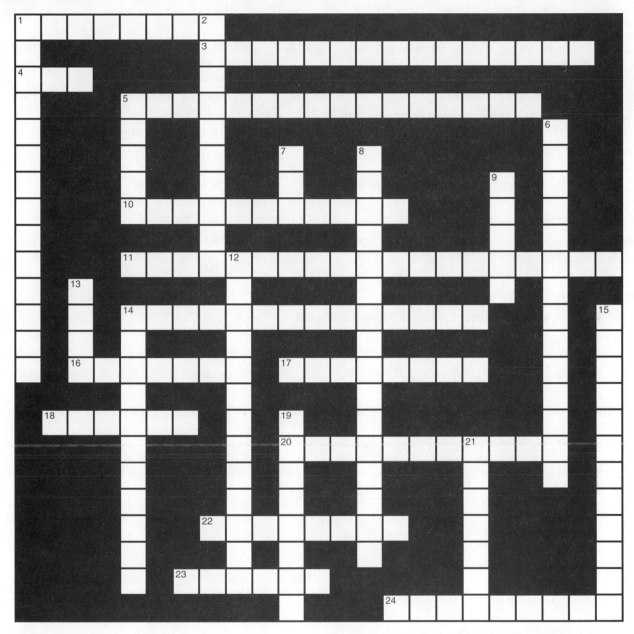

Across

1. The letter "P" in the mnemonic OPQRST stands for _____.

3. Another name for baseline on the ECG is _____ _____.

4. The right atrium and the right ventricle are _____ pressure pumps.

5. Straining against a closed glottis is also known as _____ _____.

10. The appropriate position in which to transport a patient suffering from an AMI is the _____-_____ position.

11. Alpha agents don't have much effect on the lungs; at most, they cause minor _____.

Down

1. Dyspnea, bubbling crackles and frothy sputum are signs and symptoms of _____ _____.

2. Another name for the separation of the arterial wall during an aneurysm is _____.

5. The main nerve for transmitting impulses from the parasympathetic nervous system is the _____ nerve.

6. The sympathetic nervous system uses _____ to convey its commands.

7. A delta wave is an indication for _____ (initials) syndrome.

8. Oxygenated blood reaches the heart through the _____ _____.

Across *(continued)*

14. The most common form of heart disease is _____ _____ disease.

16. A _____ will occupy the receptor site and will not allow a reaction to occur.

17. A sympathetic agent used at a low dose that increases the force of the cardiac contractions is called _____.

18. If a patient clenches a fist when describing chest pain, this is known as _____ sign.

20. The resumption of blood flow due to a reopening in the artery is called _____.

22. _____ were the first drugs to be used for the relief of angina.

23. The letter "O" in the mnemonic MONA stands for _____.

24. Swelling and pain along the veins that can lead to blood clots is called _____.

Down *(continued)*

9. In remembering cable placement, the color used for smoke is _____.

12. The ability of the heart to change the strength of the contraction without changing the stretch of the muscle is a property called _____.

13. Six of the leads—I, II, III, aVR, aVL, and aVF—are called _____ leads.

14. The other name for the parasympathetic nervous system is the _____ nervous system.

15. The sensations of a fast heart rate that the patient feels in his/her chest are known as _____.

19. Thick-walled muscular vessels that operate under a high pressure system are called _____.

21. The heart sound S2 is heard during _____.

Problem Solving

Practice your calculation skills by solving the following math problems.

1. Suppose a person at rest has a heart rate of 72 beats/min and a stroke volume of 75 mL/beat. What is his cardiac output (CO)? _____ mL/min.

2. Now that same person is running to catch a bus. His heart speeds up to 100 beats/min, and his stroke volume increases to 90 mL/beat. What is his cardiac output now? _____ mL/min

3. You must be able to decide quickly by the signs or symptoms if the patient could have left- or right-sided heart failure. Place an *L* for left and an *R* for right-sided heart failure before the following signs and symptoms.

a. _____ Dyspnea

b. _____ Jugular vein distention

c. _____ Swelling of the feet

d. _____ Crackles on auscultation

e. _____ Hepatomegaly

f. _____ Sacral edema

g. _____ Pink, frothy sputum

4. Find the mean arterial pressure (MAP) for the following blood pressures.

a. 160/94 mm Hg _____

b. 200/126 mm Hg _____

c. 148/86 mm Hg _____

5. How many seconds, or portions of a second, does a small box on an ECG graph paper represent? _____

6. How many small boxes does it take to make a large box on the ECG graph paper? _____

7. List the signs and symptoms that are present during a tachycardia that would make the patient "symptomatic" and a candidate for electric cardioversion.

a. _____

b. _____

c. _____

d. _____

e. _____

8. What is the initial drug of choice when dealing with a stable tachycardia with a regular rhythm that is not breaking with a

trial of vagal maneuvers? _____

9. What drug would be used on a stable tachycardia with a wide QRS? _____

10. You are faced with a third-degree heart block and a rate of 48 beats/min. Your patient is showing signs of poor perfusion. After starting an IV, what would you do next?

_____

_____

11. List the initial correct dosage of medication for the following.

a. Epinephrine in the care of cardiac arrest: _____

b. Vasopressin in the care of cardiac arrest: _____

c. Atropine in the care of cardiac arrest: _____

d. Atropine for a perfusing bradycardia: _____

e. Epinephrine for a conscious patient with a bradycardia and poor perfusion: _____

f. Adenosine for a stable, narrow, regular QRS tachycardia with pulses: _____

g. Amiodarone for an stable, wide, regular QRS tachycardia: _____

12. List the Hs and Ts that you might think of when dealing with a cardiac patient in asystole.

H _____   T _____

H _____   T _____

H _____   T _____

H _____   T _____

H _____   T _____

H _____

CHAPTER

28 Neurologic Emergencies

Chapter Review

The following exercises provide an opportunity to test your knowledge of this chapter.

Matching

For each of the following items, indicate whether the statement is an indication for or a contraindication against use of a fibrinolytic drug in a suspected stroke. Use the American Heart Association Fibrinolytic Checklist for Stroke.

A. Indication

B. Contraindication

_____ **1.** The patient has a history of intracranial bleeding.

_____ **2.** The patient had a witnessed seizure before calling 9-1-1.

_____ **3.** The patient is 55 years of age.

_____ **4.** The patient's symptoms began 45 minutes ago.

_____ **5.** Patient's blood pressure is 210/146 mm Hg.

_____ **6.** Patient has a broken arm.

_____ **7.** The patient takes warfarin (Coumadin).

_____ **8.** The patient's blood glucose level is 54 mg/dL.

_____ **9.** The patient had an acute myocardial infarction (AMI) 2 years ago.

_____ **10.** The patient has a measured neurologic deficit, with a positive clinical diagnosis of an ischemic stroke.

Multiple Choice

Read each item carefully, and then select the best response.

_____ **1.** The nervous system is responsible for all of the following functions EXCEPT:

    A. Heart rate   **C.** Breathing

    B. Blood pressure   **D.** Heart rhythm

_____ **2.** What area of the brain filters the information that you need for conscious thought?

    A. Pons   **C.** Diencephalon

    B. Medulla oblongata   **D.** Brain stem

_____ **3.** Which of the following acts as an "insulation" around the axon?

    A. Myelin

    B. Neuron

    C. Synapse

    D. Neurotransmitter

_____ **4.** When the brain receives too much oxygen, it can cause increased intracranial pressure (ICP). What happens to the cerebral arteries during this time?

    A. They vasodilate.

    B. They vasoconstrict.

    C. They will leak blood.

    D. They remain normal.

_____ **5.** You respond to a collision in which a woman has been thrown from a vehicle. She is unconscious and has her arms curled to her chest and her toes are pointed. How would you describe her position?

    A. Trismus posture

    B. Decerebrate posture

    C. Decorticate posture

    D. Pronation posture

_____ **6.** Pupils may be changed by many different things. Which of the following doesn't change the shape of a patient's pupils?

    A. Drugs

    B. Trauma

    C. Seizure

    D. Increased ICP

_____ **7.** You are treating a 17-year-old boy who is having a seizure. At this time, he is still except for his left arm, which is rocking back and forth in a rhythmic motion. What is the correct term for this activity?

    A. Clonic activity

    B. Tonic activity

    C. Intension tremors

    D. Parenthesis

_____ **8.** After using naloxone (Narcan) on a patient with a suspected narcotic overdose, which of the following patient reactions would you not expect?

    A. The patient would wake up quickly.

    B. The patient could become aggressive.

    C. The patient could act very fearful.

    D. The patient will be sleepy but easily awakened.

_____ **9.** Your patient suffers from an autoimmune disorder in which the body attacks the myelin sheath. What is this called?

    A. Dystonia

    B. Parkinson's disease

    C. Trigeminal neuralgia

    D. Multiple sclerosis

_____ **10.** What is the correct term for a patient that has a temporary paralysis of the seventh cranial nerve?

    A. Guillain-Barre syndrome

    B. Bell's palsy

    C. Poliomyelitis

    D. Myasthenia gravis

Labeling

Label the following diagrams with the correct terms.

1. Label the parts of the brain.

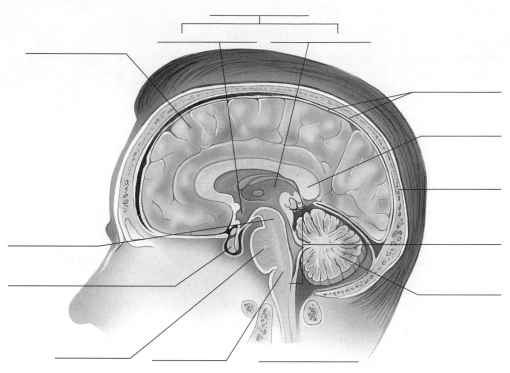

2. Label the parts of a neuron.

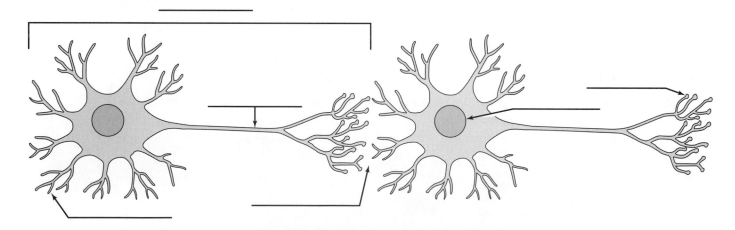

3. Indicate whether the following pupils are:

      A. Normal   **C.** Dilated

      B. Constricted (pinpoint)   **D.** Unequal

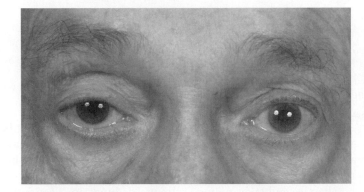

_____

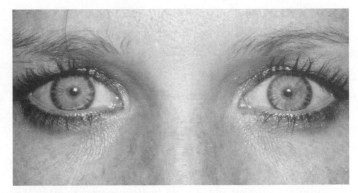

_____

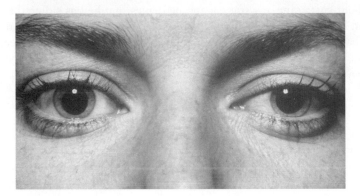

_____

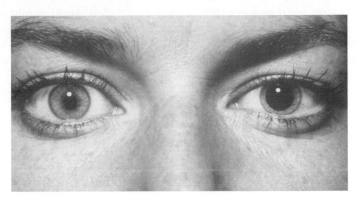

_____

Fill-in-the-Blank

Read each item carefully, and then complete the statement by filling in the missing word(s).

1. The _____ regulate how deeply you breathe and your respiratory rate.

2. Dopamine and epinephrine are two types of _____.

3. When gram-negative bacteria die inside our body, they release a protein that is called a/an _____.

4. The skull is filled with three substances; they are the _____, _____, and _____

    _____.

5. When a patient has increased ICP, the heart rate and respiratory rate will _____, and the blood pressure

    will _____.

6. The highest score on the Glasgow Coma Scale is _____, and the lowest score is _____.

7. You think your 80-year-old patient may be having a stroke. The patient can understand you, but is unable to speak clearly.

    This is called _____ _____.

8. _____ is the fuel for our brain. A normal reading is _____ mg/dL.

9. There are two types of strokes: _____ and _____.

10. An infant is more likely to suffer from a/an _____ seizure. There are two types of generalized seizures:

_____ and _____.

Identify

In the following case study, list the chief complaint, vital signs, and pertinent negatives.

You are called to a middle-class home for a 32-year-old man. He is alert and can answer all your questions. His main complaint is general weakness because he is unable to stand or squeeze your hands. His symptoms started this morning around 9 am and have intensified over the last 6 hours. He is having visual disturbances and doesn't want to open his eyes because the double vision he is experiencing is making him nauseous. You begin your assessment with vitals signs and a SAMPLE history. Blood pressure is 128/76 mm Hg, and his pulse is 84 beats/min and regular. He has no allergies and takes no medications. His lungs are clear and his oxygen saturation is 98% on room air. Because you still have no clue what is going on you place him on a nasal cannula at 4 L/min. Blood glucose check is 112 mg/dL, and he had a light lunch of a sandwich and soup around noon. He has no history of any illness and appears to be a very healthy individual. You question him about sustaining any trauma and he denies that he has suffered any in the last year. He doesn't have a headache or any pain anywhere in his body. He has no signs of any infections. You and your partner have spent a lot of time on scene looking for clues as to what is happening to him. One thing you are both sure of is that he needs to be seen at the emergency department. You provide supportive care and start an IV as a medication line in case the patient happens to get worse. Later you check in on the patient and find out that they are leaning toward a diagnosis of multiple sclerosis (MS).

1. Chief Complaint

_____

_____

_____

2. Vital Signs

_____

_____

_____

3. Pertinent Negatives

_____

_____

_____

Ambulance Calls

The following case scenarios provide an opportunity to explore the concerns associated with patient management and paramedic care. Read each scenario, and then answer each question.

1. The very next call is for a patient having seizures. This time it is one of the city's homeless whom the police found lying in an alley. He is having a generalized motor seizure when you arrive. It lasts about 3 minutes, and then subsides. You quickly open the airway by jaw lift, start supplemental oxygen, and prepare to start an IV, but before you can do so, the patient has another generalized motor seizure that lasts about 3 minutes.

   a. Urgent treatment measures will take priority over the rapid medical assessment. But when you do get around to examining this patient, what will you look for in particular?

      (1) _____

      (2) _____

      (3) _____

      (4) _____

      (5) _____

      (6) _____

      (7) _____

      (8) _____

      (9) _____

     (10) _____

   b. List the steps in the prehospital management of this patient.

      (1) _____

      (2) _____

      (3) _____

      (4) _____

   c. What medication is given in the field for repeated seizures? (You may need to refer to the pharmacology chapter.)

     _____

      (1) What are the _contraindications to this medication_?

        _____

        _____

      (2) What is the correct _dosage_ in the present situation, and how is it administered?

        _____

        _____

      (3) What possible adverse _side effects_ might occur when administering this medicine?

        _____

        _____

 2. You are called to the home of a 68-year-old woman for a "possible stroke." Arriving at the scene, you are greeted at the door by the woman's daughter. "I phoned and phoned all morning," she says, "and when no one answered, I figured I'd better come and check. I found Mother lying in the bathroom." You proceed to the bathroom, where you find the patient lying on the floor. She is conscious but does not seem to be able to answer your questions—she just makes garbled noises. Her skin is warm and dry. Her vital signs are a pulse of 70 beats/min and slightly irregular, respirations of 20 breaths/min and unlabored, and a blood pressure of 190/120 mm Hg. During the physical exam, you find no evidence of head injury, but the woman's face looks a bit lopsided, and tears are streaming down. The pupils are 4 mm, equal, and reactive. The gag reflex is absent. The right arm and right leg are flaccid. There is no evidence of injury.

a. Do you think the patient is right-handed or left-handed? _____ How did you reach that conclusion?

_____

_____

b. List the steps in treating this patient.

(1) _____

(2) _____

(3) _____

(4) _____

(5) _____

(6) _____

3. You are called to a department store where a woman who appears to be about 60 years old has been found unconscious in the ladies' restroom.

a. List nine possible causes of coma.

(1) _____

(2) _____

(3) _____

(4) _____

(5) _____

(6) _____

(7) _____

(8) _____

(9) _____

b. Now list eight things you would do to manage this comatose woman.

(1) _____

(2) _____

(3) _____

(4) _____

(5) _____

(6) _____

(7) _____

(8) _____

True/False

If you believe the statement to be more true than false, write the letter "T" in the space provided. If you believe the statement to be more false than true, write the letter "F."

_____ 1. The peripheral nervous system is responsible for conducting nerve impulses between the brain and the body.

_____ 2. The function of the midbrain is to regulate heart and respiratory functions.

_____ 3. The adrenal gland sends an impulse to the pituitary gland to release epinephrine and norepinephrine.

_____ 4. The medical term for cancer is *neoplasms*.

_____ 5. Emboli in the bloodstream may be caused by fat, air bubbles, and small blood clots.

_____ 6. The average pressure (MAP) is 100 to 120 mm Hg.

_____ 7. Trismus may result from head trauma, cerebral hypoxia, and seizures.

_____ 8. When you assess a stroke patient, you can ask the person to smile. This will show if the patient has ptosis.

_____ 9. Patients with apraxia will be unable to name a common object.

_____ 10. By stimulating the cough or gag reflex in a patient, you can decrease ICP.

_____ 11. At times you may need to give thiamine before D_{50} in chronic alcoholics or people that are malnourished.

_____ 12. Hyperglycemic patients do not need any fluid, so you must make sure to give less than 100 mL of fluid.

_____ 13. The Cincinnati Prehospital Stroke Scale uses a six-part criteria scale to assess for a stroke.

_____ 14. A little over one third of the patients who have a transient ischemic attack (TIA) will have a stroke soon after the initial event.

_____ 15. Usually an aura will precede a generalized (grand mal) seizure.

Short Answer

Complete this section with short written answers using the space provided.

1. Define the following vocabulary words:
   a. Hemiparesis

   _____

   _____

   b. Neuropathy

   _____

   _____

2. Over the course of a week of ambulance runs, you have found three patients in a coma. You don't have any information about any of them except for the medications found at the scene or on the patient's person. Nonetheless, based on those medications and assessment, you can make an educated guess at least as to each patient's underlying illnesses. For each of the comatose patients whose medications are listed here, indicate the most probable underlying illness(es).

a. Patient 1 is carrying phenobarbital (Luminal) and phenytoin sodium (Dilantin) in her purse.
Probable underlying illness(es):

_____

_____

b. Patient 2 is carrying human insulin (Humlin).
Probable underlying illness:

_____

_____

c. Patient 3 is carrying warfarin (Coumadin).
Probable underlying illness:

_____

_____

Word Find

Hidden in the following grid are 30 words or phrases related to what you have studied in this chapter. Find the hidden words in the grid below. Then use the words from the grid to answer the following questions (some words may be used to answer more than one question).

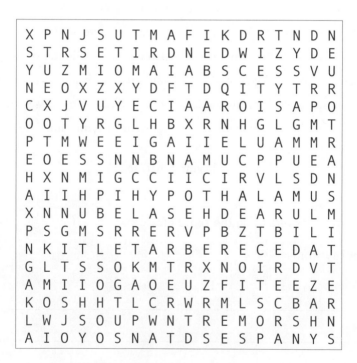

1. The _____ system has two branches, central and peripheral.

2. The _____ oblongata controls heart rate and blood pressure.

3. You wake up and fall asleep about the same time every day because of your _____ activating system.

4. Pleasure, hunger, and thirst are generated in the _____.

5. The _____ manages the complex movements of your body.

6. The slight gap between the nerve cells is called the _____.

7. Rage and anger are generated in the _____ system.

8. Acetylcholine is a/an _____.

9. _____ detect neurotransmitters and also release them in making connections with other nerve cells.

10. _____ increases the speed in which an impulse moves down an axon.

11. When a child is born with a portion of its nervous system outside its body, the condition is known

    as _____ _____.

12. _____ are proteins given off by bacteria or fungi to aid in the death and digestion of the surrounding cells.

13. An infection of the membranes surrounding the spinal cord and brain is called _____.

14. A trauma patient is found with his arms outstretched, palms down and toes pointed; the man is said to be in _____

    posturing.

15. When a patient does not respond to verbal or painful stimuli, she is in a/an _____.

16. The involuntary, rhythmic movement of the eyes of a stroke patient is called _____.

17. When you assess a patient that is suffering from a seizure, you find that the person's eyes are twitching. This is known as

    _____.

18. _____ is weakness of one side of the body.

19. The term _____ is used when a person is unable to perform coordinated motions such as clapping or

    walking.

20. Small alterations in smooth movements are _____.

21. The three major elements needed for the brain to function normally are _____, _____, and normal

    _____.

22. _____ can either be ischemic or hemorrhagic.

23. Partial or generalized, _____ can be life threatening.

24. After a seizure the patient will be _____. He or she will be very tired and very hard to wake up.

25. The temporary loss of consciousness that occurs suddenly is known as _____. The older patient will almost always

    be standing when it happens.

26. The body's response to an infection that it is unable to kill is to encase it, and that is known as a/an _____.

27. _____ is an abnormal muscle spasm that tends to be severe. It can cause the muscle group to distort, or cause a repetitive motion.

28. _____ _____ often affects the frontal lobe.

Fill-in-the-Table

Fill in the missing parts of the table.

1. Fill in the table with the basis for determining an adult's LOC.

Glasgow Coma Scale		
	Adult	**Pediatric Patient (< 5 y)**
Eye opening	4. Spontaneous	4. Spontaneous
	3.	3.
	2. Pain stimulation	2. Pain stimulation
	1.	1.
Verbal	5.	5.
	4. Disoriented	4. Cries, inappropriate words for age
	3.	3.
	2. Incomprehensible	2.
	1. None	1. None
Motor	6.	6.
	5. Localizes pain	5. Localizes pain
	4.	4.
	3.	3. Decorticate
	2.	2.
	1. None	1. None

2. List below all the words associated with each letter when dealing with the causes of seizures.

A: _____

B: _____

D: _____

F: _____

I: _____

O: _____

R: _____

S: _____

T: _____

U: _____

Problem Solving

Read the following scenario, and then list the portions of the scenario under the correct stroke scale or stroke screen.

You respond to a 69-year-old woman. Her daughter is waiting at the door for you when you arrive. Dispatch information said that the woman might be having a stroke. You enter the room to find "Betty" sitting in her recliner with her feet up. She acknowledges your entrance. "Hi, Mrs. Smith, my name is Jake Johnson and my partner is Julie Barnes. We are paramedics, and I am here at the request of your daughter. Can you tell me what is wrong today?" Mrs. Smith responds by telling you that her name is Betty, and she doesn't think anything is wrong with her. Her daughter is always fussing over her. You tell Betty that is because her daughter loves her and says that if Betty loves her daughter, she should be smiling about all the attention. Betty does respond with a smile, but the right side of her face doesn't respond as well as the left. Julie asks permission to do a set of vital signs, and Betty says to go right ahead. Julie gets a blood pressure of 136/82 mm Hg, and a pulse of 86 beats/min and regular, oxygen saturation of 97% on room air, respirations of 18 breaths/min, and lungs sounds are clear. She checks Betty's blood glucose, which is 110 mg/dL. During this time, you ask Betty to say "You can't teach an old dog new tricks." However, Betty can't seem to get the sentence out very clearly. You proceed by having Betty squeeze both your hands at the same time. Her grip strength is about half strength in the right arm. You then ask her to close her eyes and hold both arms up straight. When she does this, her right arm drifts downward. You then ask Betty and her daughter how long she has been having these symptoms. Betty's daughter says that she had no problems this morning when she was up fixing breakfast at 8:00 am, but she says she began to notice a few minor things around 11:00 am and that is when she decided to call 9-1-1. You take a SAMPLE history and find that Betty has never had any medical problems at all, she only takes a vitamin every morning. Both you and Julie feel she should be seen in the ED, and Betty agrees to go with you. You prepare to take Betty in.

You and Julie did a great job using both the Cincinnati Prehospital Stroke Scale and the Los Angles Prehospital Stroke Screen Assessments. Place portions of the preceding scenario under the correct screens. Remember, they might be on both assessments.

Cincinnati Prehospital Stroke Scale

1. _____

2. _____

3. _____

Los Angles Prehospital Stroke Screen

1. _____

2. _____

3. _____

4. _____

5. _____

6. _____

7. _____

8. _____

CHAPTER

29 Endocrine Emergencies

Chapter Review

The following exercises provide an opportunity to test your knowledge of this chapter.

Matching

Match each of the definitions in the left column to the appropriate terms in the right column.

_____ 1. A toxic condition caused by excessive levels of circulating thyroid hormone

_____ 2. Hormone that targets the adrenal cortex to secrete cortisol

_____ 3. The hormone secreted by the thyroid gland that helps maintain normal calcium levels in the blood

_____ 4. A form of acidosis in uncontrolled diabetes in which certain acids accumulate when insulin is not available

_____ 5. A hormone secreted by the posterior pituitary lobe of the pituitary gland that constricts blood vessels

_____ 6. A small region of the brain that contains several control centers for the body functions and emotions. It is the primary link between the endocrine system and the nervous system

_____ 7. Also known as hyperosmolar hyperglycemic nonketotic coma

_____ 8. Hormones produced by the adrenal medulla that assist the body in coping with physical and emotional stress by increasing the heart and respiratory rates and the blood pressure

_____ 9. Female gonads; they release eggs and secrete the female hormones

_____ 10. A hormone secreted by the parathyroids that acts as an antagonist to calcitonin; it is secreted when calcium blood levels are low

_____ 11. An essential element in the diet and an important component of thyroxine; without the proper level of intake, thyroxine can't be produced, and physical and mental growth are diminished

_____ 12. An extreme manifestation of untreated hyperthyroidism that is accompanied by physiologic decompensation

_____ 13. The hormone secreted by the thyroid gland that helps maintain normal calcium levels in the blood

_____ 14. One of the three major female hormones

A. Hypothalamus

B. Adrenocorticotropic hormone

C. Hyperosmolar nonketotic coma

D. Aldosterone

E. Thyrotoxicosis

F. Antidiuretic hormone

G. Diabetic ketoacidosis

H. Myxedema coma

I. Iodine

J. Progesterone

K. Ovaries

L. Calcitonin

M. Parathyroid hormone

N. Catecholamines

Multiple Choice

Read each item carefully, and then select the best response.

_____ 1. The endocrine system is made up of a network of glands that produce:
  A. homeostasis.
  B. glucose.
  C. calcium.
  D. hormones.

_____ 2. Agonists are molecules that bind to a cell's receptor and trigger a response by that cell; they produce some kind of action or:
  A. analgesic effect.
  B. fight-or-flight response.
  C. biologic effect.
  D. drug effect.

_____ 3. What part of the endocrine system has a role in hormone production as well as in digestion?
  A. Hypothalamus
  B. Pancreas
  C. Thyroid
  D. Parathyroid

_____ 4. The pituitary gland is often referred to as the:
  A. master gland.
  B. hypothalamus.
  C. guardian gland.
  D. none of the above.

_____ 5. The thyroid secretes:
  A. iodine.
  B. calcitonin.
  C. cardiac enzymes.
  D. norepinephrine.

_____ 6. The adrenal glands consist of two parts: an outer part, called the adrenal cortex, and an inner part, called the:
  A. adrenal cortex.
  B. adrenal medulla.
  C. posterior adrenal cortex.
  D. inferior medulla.

_____ 7. Epinephrine stimulates _____ nervous system receptors throughout the body.
  A. parasympathetic
  B. sympathetic
  C. dopamine
  D. neuron

_____ 8. Diabetes mellitus is referred to as:
  A. juvenile diabetes.
  B. adult-onset diabetes.
  C. diabetic hypoglycemia.
  D. sweet diabetes.

_____ 9. The most common form of diabetes is type 2 diabetes, also known as:
  A. insulin intolerance.
  B. insulin tolerance.
  C. insulin resistance.
  D. insulin opposition.

_____ 10. Patients in diabetic ketoacidosis (DKA) are seldom:
  A. comatose.
  B. asymptomatic.
  C. hyperglycemic.
  D. hypoglycemic.

_____ 11. What condition is characterized by hyperglycemia, hyperosmolarity, and the absence of ketosis?
  A. Hyperosmolar nonketotic coma (HONK)
  B. Hyperosmolar hyperglycemic nonketotic coma (HHNC)
  C. Cardiometabolic syndrome
  D. Both answers A and B

_____ 12. Signs and symptoms of acute adrenal insufficiency may appear suddenly and are commonly referred to as:
  A. addisonian crisis.
  B. adrenal insufficiency.
  C. severe infection.
  D. none of the above.

_____ **13.** Cushing's syndrome is caused by:
  A. an excess of cortisol production.
  B. an excess of glucocorticoid hormones.
  C. tumors of the pituitary gland or adrenal cortex.
  D. all of the above.

_____ **14.** An extreme manifestation of untreated hypothyroidism that is accompanied by physiologic decompensation is called:
  A. myxedema coma.   **C.** Cushing's syndrome.
  B. thyroid storm.   **D.** diabetic ketoacidosis.

_____ **15.** Thyrotoxicosis may also be called by all of the following names EXCEPT:
  A. goiters.   **C.** thyroid cancer.
  B. Grave's disease.   **D.** ketoacidosis.

Labeling

Label the following diagrams with the correct terms.

1. List the six-step process of the body's fight-or-flight response to stress.

Stress

Stress stops

2. Label the adrenal cortex and the adrenal medulla on the following kidney.

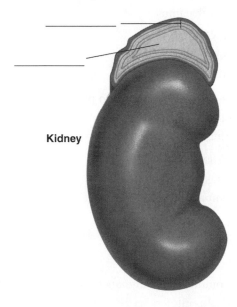

Adrenal gland

Kidney

Fill-in-the-Blank

Read each item carefully, and then complete the statement by filling in the missing word(s).

1. _____ _____ is a metabolic and cardiovascular emergency. If not diagnosed and treated immediately, the mortality rates are approximately 50%.

2. The anterior pituitary gland secretes _____-_____ _____ in response to secretion of thyrotropin-releasing hormone by the hypothalamus.

3. Aldosterone regulates and maintains the _____ and _____ balance in the blood.

4. The goals of prehospital treatment for diabetic ketoacidosis are to begin _____ and to correct the patient's _____ and acid–base abnormalities.

5. Diabetics are not immune to _____ _____, stroke, _____, meningitis, and other _____ injuries or conditions.

6. Symptoms of type 2 diabetes may include _____, nausea, frequent urination, and _____.

7. Two forms of diabetes exist: _____ _____ and _____ _____. Both types are serious conditions that affect many tissues and functions other than the glucose-regulating mechanism, and both require lifelong _____ _____.

8. The endocrine component is made up of the _____ _____ _____. These cell groups in the pancreas act like "an organ within an organ." The main hormones they secrete—_____ and _____—are responsible for the regulation of blood glucose levels.

9. The pituitary gland is often referred to as the _____ _____ because its secretions control, or regulate, the secretions of other _____ glands.

10. Hormones operate in _____ _____ to maintain an optimal internal operating environment in the body. Endocrine regulation, through _____ _____, is the most important method by which hormonal secretion is maintained within a physiologic range.

Identify

In the following case studies, list the chief complaint, vital signs, and pertinent negatives. Also identify the possible nature of the endocrine disorder.

1. It's a sunny but very cold mid-February day. You and your partner would be content to remain inside the station practicing your advanced life support (ALS) skills. The silence is broken with a dispatch to a priority 1 call for an unconscious, unresponsive patient waiting for a prescription at the neighborhood pharmacy. On arrival, you find the 29-year-old woman being attended by the pharmacist, who states the patient was waiting for an insulin prescription. The patient is unresponsive. You note respirations are shallow and the patient is diaphoretic. Her radial pulse is 118 beats/min. Her blood pressure is 104/88 mm Hg. Her blood glucose is 48 mg/dL. As you prepare the cardiac monitor and intravenous (IV) equipment, the pharmacist pulls her history.

a. Chief Complaint

_____

b. Vital Signs

_____

c. Pertinent Negatives

_____

d. Nature of the Endocrine Disorder

_____

2. It's cold and flu season, and today is no exception. It seems these ailments are what everyone is calling in for. On arrival at the scene, you locate an elderly man sitting in his rocker apparently short of breath. He states that he's had the flu for a number of days and can't stop vomiting. He speaks in full, complete sentences, but has an unusual breathing pattern and fruity breath odor. You quickly place the pulse oximeter probe on his finger. Surprisingly, his oxygen saturation is 95% on room air. You immediately follow up with high-flow supplemental oxygen as you begin your assessment. The patient states a long history of diabetes. He further states that he hasn't been able to keep food down for several days, but has been taking all of his medications. His blood glucose is 405 mg/dL. He is tachycardic with a blood pressure of 108/82 mm Hg. He has poor skin turgor, and skin tenting is present. The monitor is showing a sinus tachycardia. The patient complains of thirst.

a. Chief Complaint

_____

b. Vital Signs

_____

c. Pertinent Negatives

_____

d. Nature of the Endocrine Disorder

_____

3. Once again today, you are requested to respond to a call to the local nursing home for a "routine" transport to the emergency department. You are met by family members who are concerned that Grandma's mental status has been rapidly deteriorating, and she appears to be cold. The family states that the patient has suddenly become confused and psychotic. The nursing home chart indicates a history of hypothyroidism. Her pulse rate is slightly bradycardic. She is also hypotensive. You can't get an accurate pulse oximeter reading because of poor peripheral perfusion.

a. Chief Complaint

_____

b. Vital Signs

_____

c. Pertinent Negatives

_____

d. Nature of the Endocrine Disorder

_____

Ambulance Calls

The following case scenarios provide an opportunity to explore the concerns associated with patient management and paramedic care. Read each scenario, and then answer each question.

1. A 22-year-old woman is found unconscious in her apartment. Her roommate, who is nearly hysterical, tells you between sobs, "I went away for the weekend, and when I got back tonight, I found her like this. She won't die, will she?" A neighbor arrives and helps calm the roommate while you and your partner carry out the initial assessment. That accomplished, you proceed to the secondary survey. You find that the patient wakens to a painful stimulus but rapidly returns to sleep. Her skin is warm and flushed and tents when you pinch it. Her vital signs are as follows: a pulse of 110 beats/min and regular, respirations are 30 breaths/min and deep, and blood pressure is 90/60 mm Hg. Her eyes look sunken. Pupils are 5 mm, Equal And Round, Regular in size, and are reactive to Light (PEARRL). The breath smells like fruit-flavored gum. The neck is not rigid. The chest is clear. The abdomen is soft. There are multiple needle marks and skin changes over the anterior thighs. Completing your examination, you ask the patient's roommate, "Ma'am, is your friend by chance a diabetic?"

   "Oh, didn't I mention that?" sniffles the roommate.

   List the steps in treating this patient.

   a. _____

   b. _____

   c. _____

   d. _____

2. You are called to an office building where a young salesman apparently had a seizure while waiting for a meeting with his boss.

   a. List six possible causes of seizures.

      (1) _____

      (2) _____

      (3) _____

      (4) _____

      (5) _____

      (6) _____

   b. The secretary in whose office the patient had been waiting when the seizure occurred tells you that he had been "acting sort of strange" before the seizure. He complained of a headache and was very restless and irritable, which was entirely out of character for him ("Usually he's such a sweetheart!"). Then, he just fell to the ground and "started jerking all over."

      On examining the patient, you find him still unconscious, although he does respond to being pinched by pulling his arm away and mumbling some incomprehensible words. He is no longer seizing. His skin is cold, pale, and clammy. His vital signs are a pulse of 120 beats/min and weak, respirations are 16 breaths/min and unlabored, and his blood pressure is 130/44 mm Hg. His pupils are about 6 mm, equal and round, regular in size, and reactive to light (PEARRL). There are no unusual odors on the breath. The neck is not rigid. The only finding on head-to-toe exam is hyperactivity of the deep tendon reflexes.

      List the steps in treating this patient.

      (1) _____

      (2) _____

      (3) _____

(4) _____

(5) _____

(6) _____

(7) _____

(8) _____

(9) _____

(10) _____

(11) _____

c. As you finish carrying out the steps you just listed, you are very gratified to see that the patient rapidly becomes fully alert. "Gee, I sure am sorry to have caused you people all this trouble," he says. "I knew I shouldn't have skipped breakfast." What do you think caused his seizure? _____

d. What advice will you give this patient?

(1) _____

(2) _____

(3) _____

3. Over the course of a week of ambulance runs, four patients are found in a coma. You don't have any information about any of them except for the medications found at the scene or on the patient's person. Nonetheless, based on those medications, you can make an educated guess at least as to each patient's underlying illness(es). For each of the comatose patients whose medications are listed as follows, indicate the most probable underlying illness(es).

a. Patient 3 has glyburide (Micronase) on his bedside table.

Probable underlying illness(es):

_____

b. A vial of insulin is found in patient 4's refrigerator.

Probable underlying illness(es):

_____

c. This unconscious patient has what appears to be an insulin pump. The patient's Medical Identification Bracelet confirms your suspicion.

Probable underlying illness(es):

_____

d. This 35-year-old insulin-dependent woman had a sudden onset of a severe headache and blurred vision before she became unconscious and fell to the floor, striking her head on a concrete surface.

Probable underlying illness(es):

_____

True/False

If you believe the statement to be more true than false, write the letter "T" in the space provided. If you believe the statement to be more false than true, write the letter "F."

_____ 1. Cold, clammy skin is classically a sign of shock but may also signal severe hypoglycemia, as from an insulin reaction.

_____ 2. Supplemental oxygen is recommended in all cases of suspected respiratory involvement.

_____ 3. Adult hypothyroidism is sometimes called myxedema.

_____ 4. The anterior pituitary gland secretes thyroid-stimulating hormone (TSH) in response to the hypothalamus' secretion of thyrotropin-releasing hormone (TRH).

_____ 5. The primary clinical manifestation of adrenal crisis is atrial fibrillation.

_____ 6. The signs and symptoms of hypoglycemia and hyperglycemia can be quite similar.

_____ 7. Normal blood glucose is approximately 70 to 120 mg/dL; hypoglycemia occurs when blood glucose drops to 35 mg/dL.

_____ 8. Type 2 diabetes may be related to metabolic syndrome.

_____ 9. Symptoms of type 2 diabetes may include fatigue; nausea; frequent urination; thirst; unexplained weight loss; blurred vision; frequent infections and slow healing of wounds; crankiness, confusion, or shakiness; unresponsiveness; and seizure.

_____ 10. Most diabetic patients do not live a normal lifespan, even if they adjust their lives to the demands of the disease, especially their eating habits and activities.

_____ 11. Endocrine disorders can be caused by either hypersecretion or insufficient secretion of a gland.

_____ 12. The islets of Langerhans secrete glucagon and insulin, which are responsible for the regulation of blood glucose levels.

_____ 13. When sodium is reabsorbed into the blood, water is secreted; this action decreases both blood volume and blood pressure.

_____ 14. Iodine is an important component of thyroxine. Without the proper level of dietary iodine intake, thyroxine can't be produced.

_____ 15. Exocrine glands excrete chemicals for absorption.

Short Answer

Complete this section with short written answers using the space provided.

1. Define the following vocabulary words:

   a. Hypoglycemia:

   _____

   b. Diabetic ketoacidosis (DKA):

   _____

   c. Thyrotoxicosis:

   _____

   d. Insulin:

   _____

   e. Cushing's syndrome:

   _____

2. Explain the treatment for the following conditions:

　a. Myxedema coma:

　_____

　_____

　b. Adrenal insufficiency:

　_____

　_____

　c. Hyperosmolar nonketotic coma:

　_____

　_____

Fill-in-the-Table

Fill in the missing parts of the tables.

1. Hormones of the Adrenal Glands

Hormones of the Adrenal Glands	
Cortisol	Increases _____ rate, using fat and _____ for energy
Aldosterone	Reabsorbs _____ and water from the _____, and _____ excess potassium
Epinephrine/norepinephrine	Stimulates _____ nervous system _____

2. Hormones of the Gonads

Hormones of the Gonads	
Male	
Testosterone	Main sex hormone in males Responsible for _____ sex characteristics: _____ deepening, growth of facial_____, muscle development,_____hair, growth spurts
Female	
Estrogen	Responsible for secondary sex characteristics: _____ growth, fat accumulation at _____ and _____, pubic hair, growth spurts Involved in _____ Regulation of _____ cycle
Progesterone	Involved in pregnancy Regulation of _____ cycle Prevents _____ of additional egg during _____

3. Diabetic Emergencies

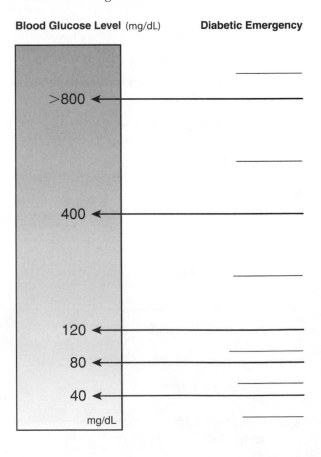

Blood Glucose Level (mg/dL)   Diabetic Emergency

Crossword Puzzle

Use the clues in the column to complete the puzzle.

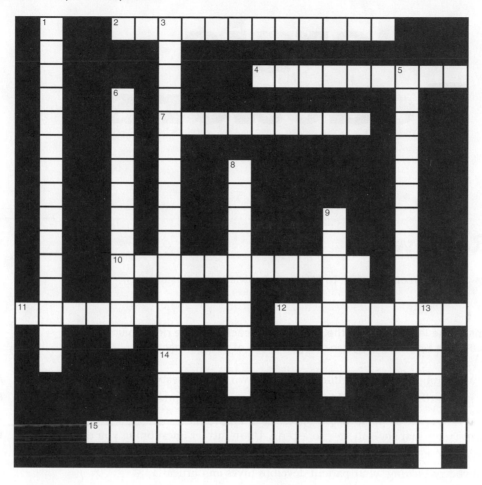

Across

2. The _____ is a small region of the brain (not a gland) that contains several control centers for body functions and emotions. It is the primary link between the endocrine system and the nervous system.

4. The hypothalamic–_____ system controls the function of multiple peripheral endocrine organs.

7. _____, the body's major metabolic hormone, stimulates energy production in cells, which increases the rate at which cells consume oxygen and use carbohydrates, fats, and proteins.

10. _____ stimulates the kidneys to reabsorb sodium from the urine and excrete potassium by altering the osmotic gradient in the blood.

11. The thyroid gland also secretes _____, which helps maintain normal calcium levels in the blood.

12. _____ affects almost every organ and tissue in the body. Its primary role is to assist with the body's response to stress.

14. _____ _____ is an extreme manifestation of untreated hypothyroidism that is accompanied by physiologic decompensation.

15. Type 1 diabetes generally strikes children as opposed to adults; it has been referred to as _____ _____.

Down

1. _____ _____ is caused by atrophy or destruction of both adrenal glands, leading to deficiency of all the steroid hormones produced by these glands.

3. The parathyroid gland assists in the regulation of calcium. However, the _____ _____, when secreted by the parathyroid, acts as an antagonist to calcitonin.

5. _____ are molecules that bind to a cell's receptor and block the action of agonists. Hormone antagonists are widely used as drugs.

6. Maintaining _____ requires a response to any change in the body, such as low glucose or calcium levels in the blood.

8. The most common form of diabetes is called _____-_____ diabetes, in which blood glucose levels are elevated.

9. The _____ is a digestive gland that is considered both an endocrine gland and an exocrine gland. It secretes digestive enzymes into the duodenum through the pancreatic duct.

13. In women, the gonads are the _____, which release the eggs and secrete the hormones estrogen and progesterone.

CHAPTER

30 Allergic Reactions

Chapter Review

The following exercises provide an opportunity to test your knowledge of this chapter.

Matching

Match each of the items in the left column to the appropriate reaction in the right column.
Each of the following patients would be experiencing what type of allergic reaction?

_____ **1.** A patient was stung by hornets while raking his lawn. He is sweaty, weak, nauseous, vomiting, pale, and diaphoretic. He is suffering from severe respiratory distress and is hypotensive.

_____ **2.** Your patient states that she's allergic to aspirin. Upon further questioning you discover that it may cause mild nausea.

_____ **3.** While strawberry picking, your patient develops hives and urticaria.

_____ **4.** One of your partners suffers a tick bite while searching the woods for a missing person. The area is swollen and red. It is painful and itchy to touch.

_____ **5.** It is hay fever season again. With the mild winter conditions, your runny nose and swollen eyes indicate it's going to be severe.

_____ **6.** Thank goodness for credit cards. At least this bee sting wasn't as severe as the last patient you treated. Scraping away the stinger certainly minimized the pain, swelling, and redness.

_____ **7.** You are preparing the IV site. Prior to using any antiseptics you repeatedly ask the patient if he's allergic to any medications. He explains that he's allergic to iodine. Upon further questioning he states that he gets extremely short of breath, has chest pain, and can't swallow.

_____ **8.** After administering nitroglycerine spray to your cardiac patient, he is still complaining of 9 on 10 chest discomfort (1 to 10 scale, 10 being the worst pain). You choose to administer morphine sulphate. The patient states that he's allergic to pain killers such as codeine. You ask him what type of reaction he typically has to those drugs. Your patient states "nausea."

_____ **9.** You have a new partner today. She is helping you complete your rig check. She notices that you are carrying latex gloves. She complains because she is allergic to latex. When you ask her what type of reaction she gets, she states that her skin cracks and itches, not to mention that messy powder.

A. Local reaction
B. Systemic reaction
C. Hypersensitivity
D. Anaphylaxis

_____ **10.** While standing by at a minor league professional baseball game you are notified of a young child having severe respiratory distress, and he appears to be choking. As you rush toward the patient, you notice that his face is red, swollen, and he has hives all over. Nearby on a seat is a popular baseball game snack. The upset grandfather states that he didn't realize that it had peanuts.

Multiple Choice
Read each item carefully, and then select the best response.

It's been a slow shift, so you decide to grab a quick dinner at Joe's Steak 'n Lobster. You park your rig outside and find a table near the door, in case you have to leave in a hurry on a call. You've just had your medium-rare sirloin placed in front of you when you notice a woman at the next table who does not look well. You ask her if there is anything the matter. "I don't know," she says in a very squeaky voice. "I have this lump in my throat, and I feel like I'm going to die," whereupon she collapses to the floor.

_____ **1.** This woman is most likely suffering from:
   A. food poisoning.   **C.** strep throat.
   B. choking.   **D.** anaphylaxis.

_____ **2.** The treatment you need to give most urgently is to:
   A. pump out her stomach.   **C.** have her gargle with salt water.
   B. administer 6 to 10 manual abdominal thrusts.   **D.** administer epinephrine 1:1,000, 0.5 mL SQ.

_____ **3.** Assuming the patient is suffering from an acute anaphylactic reaction, what other medications might be helpful?
   A. Nitroglycerin sublingual   **C.** Morphine sulfate
   B. Solu medrol   **D.** Narcan

_____ **4.** You finally decide to administer diphenhydramine (Benadryl). You determine that Benadryl is most helpful at this time because it blocks:
   A. beta receptor site.   **C.** neurotransmitters that cause respiratory distress.
   B. alpha receptor sites.   **D.** histamine receptors.

_____ **5.** While assessing and treating your patient, you discover a used EpiPen next to her collapsed body. The EpiPen auto injector (if used properly) would have administered:
   A. 1 mg of 1:10,000 solution IM.   **C.** 0.3 mg of 1:1,000 solution SQ.
   B. 1 mg of 1:10,000 solution IV.   **D.** 0.3 mg of 1:1,000 solution IM.

_____ **6.** The patient is responding slowly to the epinephrine. The following medication(s) may also be helpful:
   A. Glucagon   **C.** Decadron (dexamethasone)
   B. Albuterol   **D.** All of the above

The patient's mother explains that the baby had been up all night tugging at her ear and crying inconsolably. She has been running a low-grade fever that appears to respond well to pediatric Tylenol (acetaminophen). Today the baby went to the pediatrician who prescribed liquid amoxycillin for an ear infection. After the first dose of the stawberry-flavored antibiotic, the baby began to vomit and appeared to stop breathing. EMS was called. On your arrival, the child appeared conscious and alert and acting appropriately for her age. Based on the preceding scenario, please answer the following questions:

_____ **7.** The baby was most probably suffering from an:
   A. anaphylactic reaction.
   B. localized reaction.
   C. no reaction; sometimes sick children vomit and appear to hold their breath.
   D. a systemic reaction.

8. If the small child were having a reaction to the antibiotic, what would be the correct course of treatment?

    A. Check level of consciousness, open her airway, place an oral or nasal airway, ventilate with 100% supplemental oxygen, initiate IV access and pharmacologic treatment and initiate rapid but safe transport to an appropriate facility.

    B. Intitiate rapid transport and perform all assessment and treatment modalities en route.

    C. After securing the patient's ABCs, administer IM Benadryl (diphenhydramine) immediately.

    D. Contact medical control for further instructions.

9. Because of the small size of the patient, what assessment skills/tools may be helpful in determining proper medication dosages and equipment sizes?

    A. Paramedics should be able to rely on their memory exclusively. Time shouldn't be wasted using fancy adjuncts.

    B. Put the "rubber on the road." This child doesn't need a paramedic. She needs a doctor and quickly.

    C. A calm professional demeanor and approach to this possible anaphylactic reaction can make all the difference. It's okay to use charts, tapes, and calculators. You may get only one chance to get this right.

    D. Children don't have medication reactions. It's her first time getting this antibiotic. It must be something else.

10. What was the "route" of exposure?

    A. Exposure   **C.** Ingestion

    B. Inhalation   **D.** Injection

Labeling

Use the following figure to complete the following questions regarding anaphylaxis.

1. What is the first form of attack on the human body?

_____

_____

_____

2. What types of cells are released?

_____

3. What signs and symptoms may be present in the respiratory system?

_____

_____

_____

4. What are the negative cardiovascular signs/symptoms that may be present?

_____

_____

_____

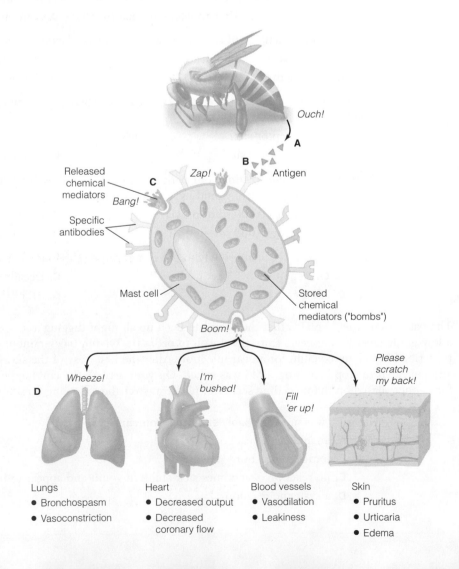

5. Are there any effects to the circulatory system? If so, describe them.

_____

_____

_____

6. The skin is often the first place to show signs/symptoms; what are they?

_____

_____

_____

Fill-in-the-Blank

Read each item carefully, and then complete the statement by filling in the missing word(s).

1. The immunity the body develops as part of exposure to an antigen is _____ _____.

2. The immunity the body develops as part of being exposed to an antigen and developing antibodies is _____

   _____.

3. A protein the body produces in response to an antibody is a/an _____.

4. _____ cells meet and greet invaders.

5. _____ is a chemical found in mast cells.

6. A _____ _____ _____ is an early sign of impending airway occlusion due to swelling.

7. An anaphylactic reaction is a _____-_____ reaction and must be treated as such.

8. Patients who receive _____ must be monitored closely for adverse effects.

9. If a patient does not respond to epinephrine, _____ may be indicated.

10. High-flow _____ should be given to each anaphylactic patient.

Identify

In the following case studies, list the chief complaint, vital signs, and pertinent negatives.

1. You are treating a 16-year-old girl who was stung by a bee at her pool. She complains of hives and itching at the sting site. She denies respiratory distress or trouble swallowing. She states that she has never been stung before and doesn't carry an EpiPen. She is conscious and alert. Her skin color is normal, warm, and dry. Capillary refill is normal. Her oxygen saturation is 99% and her blood pressure is 112/68 mm Hg, PEARRL (Pupils Equal And Round, Regular in size, react to Light).

   a. Chief Complaint

   _____

   _____

   _____

b. Vital Signs

_____

_____

_____

c. Pertinent Negatives

_____

_____

_____

2. You are called to a rural location for a 23-year-old man who states that he was bitten by a tick. He appears scared but other than being "grossed-out" has no complaint. The tick is still attached to his leg. After removing the tick, you assess his vital signs. He is conscious and alert. His pulse is 110 beats/min and regular. Blood pressure is 142/84 mm Hg, PEARRL (Pupils Equal And Round, Regular in size, react to Light), skin is warm and moist. Our patient has no previous medical history, no allergies, and no known drug allergies.

   a. Chief Complaint

_____

_____

_____

   b. Vital Signs

_____

_____

_____

   c. Pertinent Negatives

_____

_____

_____

3. A priority one response directs you to Uptown Elementary School for an eighth grader complaining of trouble breathing and swallowing after ingesting doughnuts brought by a classmate. The student is in a class that has signs posted designating it as a "peanut-free" environment. The student has a MedicAlert bracelet indicating a severe allergy to peanuts and any byproducts. The school nurse believes that the student accidentally ingested peanuts that were ingredients in the doughnuts. The student is conscious and alert, anxious, and speaking in a raspy voice. He has redness around his face and neck. Vital signs are a pulse of 124 beats/min, oxygen saturation of 90%, and a blood pressure of 90/62 mm Hg.

   a. Chief Complaint

_____

_____

_____

b. Vital Signs

_____

_____

_____

c. Pertinent Negatives

_____

_____

_____

4. It's about 10:00 pm. You respond to a call for an allergic reaction to seafood. On arrival, you are met by a 32-year-old woman who states that she's allergic to shellfish and iodine. She speaks in complete full sentences and complains of nausea and vomiting. While giving her medical history, she indicates that she has never had a reaction previously to eating fish. While assessing your patient you note the following vital signs: She has a pulse of 124 beats/min and regular, oxygen saturation of 90% on ambient air, and her blood pressure is easily auscultated at 112/62 mm Hg.

a. Chief Complaint

_____

_____

_____

b. Vital Signs

_____

_____

_____

c. Pertinent Negatives

_____

_____

_____

5. It's late in the morning, and you are responding to a reported allergic reaction in a 10-month-old boy. Dispatch advises that the child was at the pediatrician today for a well baby check. While there, the child received several immunizations. The child is now lethargic and gasping for breath. The child presents with urticaria all over. The baby has no other reported medical history or reported allergies. Vital signs are an apical pulse of 190 beats/min. The infant has delayed capillary refill and mottled skin.

a. Chief Complaint

_____

_____

_____

b. Vital Signs

_____

_____

_____

c. Pertinent Negatives

_____

_____

_____

Ambulance Calls

The following case scenarios provide an opportunity to explore the concerns associated with patient management and paramedic care. Read each scenario, and then answer each question.

1. You are called to the suburban home of a 52-year-old man with "shortness of breath." You learn that while gardening, the patient was stung by a bee; several minutes later he noticed a tight feeling in his chest. Now, 15 minutes after the sting, he looks flushed and very apprehensive. His vital signs are a pulse of 124 beats/min and slightly irregular, respirations 36 breaths/min and shallow, and blood pressure 90/60 mm Hg.

   a. List the steps in managing this patient.

   (1) _____

   (2) _____

   (3) _____

   (4) _____

   (5) _____

   (6) _____

   (7) _____

   (8) _____

   b. One of the drugs that you will be giving is epinephrine. List the possible adverse effects of epinephrine if given in an excessive dosage.

   (1) _____

   (2) _____

   (3) _____

2. You are dining out on your night off at Fish Fare, a local restaurant. As you are just about to dig into your red snapper, you notice a woman at a nearby table looking distressed. "Aunt Gertrude, what's the matter?" asks another woman at the table.

   "I don't know," squeaks the distressed woman. "I feel so peculiar. Like there's a lump in my throat. And my chest feels so tight."

   Without waiting to hear another word, you bolt over to the telephone, dial 9-1-1, and ask for an ambulance posthaste. Then you go over to the woman in distress and introduce yourself as a paramedic. You notice that the woman's face is very flushed, and her eyes look puffy. Her pulse is weak and rapid.

   "Oh, dear, I think I'm going to be sick," she says.

Just then the ambulance pulls up. List the steps in treating this patient.

a. _____

b. _____

c. _____

d. _____

e. _____

f. _____

3. Which of the following patients is most likely to be experiencing an anaphylactic reaction? (For those who are *not*, indicate what you think they *are* suffering from.)

a. A 25-year-old man is dining at a fast-food joint. Suddenly he grows very pale, lurches back from the table clutching his throat, with his eyes popping. He staggers to his feet, and then collapses to the floor—all in complete silence. His problem is most likely _____.

b. You are summoned for a 60-year-old man having a "bad reaction" to a medicine. Earlier in the day, the patient was prescribed erythromycin for a respiratory infection. Now he complains of severe abdominal distress and nausea. On physical examination, his skin is slightly pale and cool. His pulse is 72 beats/min and regular, his respirations are 22 breaths/min and unlabored; his blood pressure is 160/94 mm Hg. His problem is most likely _____.

c. A 22-year-old man is found sitting on the sidewalk in marked distress. He tells you hoarsely that he just got "a shot" at the VD clinic down the street, and right after he was given the shot and sent home, he started to feel "real strange." He says he got hot and itchy all over, and now he feels like he's going to die. On physical examination, his face looks quite flushed and puffy. His pulse is 140 beats/min and thready, his respirations are 32 breaths/min and shallow, and his blood pressure is 110/60 mm Hg. His problem is most likely _____.

4. Describe how you would manage the patient who is having an anaphylactic reaction.

a. _____

b. _____

c. _____

d. _____

e. _____

5. After you report in to medical command, the physician instructs you, in addition, to give diphenhydramine (Benadryl). What are the *contraindications* to giving diphenhydramine?

a. _____

b. _____

c. _____

d. _____

e. _____

6. What are the correct *dosage* and *route of administration* in this case?

_____

7. What *side effects* of diphenhydramine (Benadryl) should you anticipate?

a. _____

b. _____

c. _____

d. _____

e. _____

True/False

If you believe the statement to be more true than false, write the letter "T" in the space provided. If you believe the statement to be more false than true, write the letter "F."

_____ **1.** All patients who exhibit signs and symptoms of allergic reaction should receive epinephrine.

_____ **2.** Patients should be educated to wear MedicAlert tags and carry their prescribed anaphylaxis kit.

_____ **3.** IM epinephrine is more effective than IV.

_____ **4.** Epinephrine has beta-1 properties that cause the blood vessels to constrict, reducing vasodilation.

_____ **5.** Bee stings are best removed with sharp, pointy tweezers.

_____ **6.** More than 40 million Americans are at risk for anaphylaxis.

_____ **7.** Allergens can invade the body through the skin, respiratory tract, or GI tract.

_____ **8.** The respiratory system usually protects the human body from substances and organisms that are considered foreign to the body.

_____ **9.** Use of the polio vaccine has resulted in "herd immunity."

_____ **10.** Epinephrine is generally not a first-line drug as a result of its delayed response.

Short Answer

Complete this section with short written answers using the space provided.

1. When an antigen combines with a specific antibody on the surface of a mast cell, the mast cell loses its chemical bombs ("degranulates," to use the technical term), releasing a variety of powerful mediators, such as histamine and serotonin. List seven effects produced by those mediators.

a. _____

b. _____

c. _____

d. _____

e. _____

f. _____

g. _____

2. Besides bees, what other agents are commonly responsible for anaphylactic reactions? List at least four.

a. _____

b. _____

c. _____

d. _____

Word Find

Hidden in the following grid are 19 words or phrases related to what you have studied in this chapter. Find the hidden words in the grid below. Then use the words from the grid to answer the following questions (some words may be used to answer more than one question).

```
P M M D B U K N N E E U U J G
B D P W E C R I H H D Y P H W
L Z M A O Y K T C L I E L T F
O G B H P O A A I C F Y M W Q
A N S C A I D R A C Y H C A T
T I W F I A C S Z Q A D S R W
I H M K E T O S E Y R R K M H
N S Z H P S D E T T G I I J E
G U P Y T Y A N I G N A V A E
A L E M S Y A E H R R A I D Z
E F F P A M H S T R I D O R E
S I N Q I R A R I C O U G H S
U E H X U P C A R Y Q P G T F
A F T N F Q N O K A E B N W Y
N T I G H T C H E S T W F Q D
```

1. Find the signs and symptoms.

2. Sort out the signs and symptoms according to the organ system they affect.

SIGNS AND SYMPTOMS
Cardiovascular

a. _____   c. _____

b. _____   d. _____

Respiratory

e. _____   h. _____

f. _____   i. _____

g. _____   j. _____ chest

Gastrointestinal

k. _____   m. _____

l. _____   n. _____

Skin

o. _____   q. _____

p. _____   r. _____

Central Nervous

s. _____

Secret Message

Identify the following terms from the clues provided, and then use the letters to decode the secret message!

Our thought for today comes to us in a somewhat squeaky voice. Decode it in the usual fashion.

a. Protective protein: _ _ _ _ _ B _ _ _ _
               59 40 8 16   51 32 56

b. Substance that evokes item a above: _ _ _ _ _ G _ _
                      24 7 50 30   27 34

c. Form of definition of item b that produces hypersensitivity: _ _ L _ _ _ _ _ _
                                          3 44   61 19 35 6 28

d. Overwhelming allergic reaction: _ _ _ _ _ Y _ _ _ _ _ _
                    1 31 42 23 47   43 33 57 10 21

e. Chemical mediator of item "d": _ _ _ _ _ _ _ N _
                   55 20 13 41 52 49 26   36

f. Possible cause of item "d": _ _ _ _ _
                 9 22 53 2

g. Pruritus: _ _ C _
         48 4   12

h. What capillaries do in item "d": _ _ _ _ _
                   38 37 5 54

i. Wife of a person who suffers from item "d": _ _ _ _ _ W
                         46 58 17 45

j. Wrongful conduct that gives rise to a suit: _ _ _ _ _
                          60 18 15 11

k. What the prefix *ad-* means: _ _
                  29 39

l. Abbreviation for "drop": G _ _
                 25 14

Secret Message

_ _ _ _ _ _ _ _ _ _ _ _ _ _ _ _ _ _ _ _ _ _ _ _ _ _ _ _ _ _ _ _ _ _ _ _ _ _ _ _ . _ _ _ _
1 2 3 4 5 6 7 8   9 10 11 12   13 14 15 16 17 18 19   20 21   22   23 24 25 26 27 28 29   30 31   32 33 34 35 36 37   38 39 40 41

_ _ _ _ _ _ _ _ _ _ _ _ _ _ _ _ _ _ _ _ .
42 43 44 45 46   47 48 49   50 51   52 53 54 55 56 57 58 59 60 61

Fill-in-the-Table

Fill in the missing parts of the table with examples of the common substances associated with anaphylaxis.

Antigen	Examples
Drugs	
Insect stings	
Foods	
Latex	
Animals	

Problem Solving

Practice your calculation skills by solving the following math problems.

1. Medical control orders you to administer 0.3 to 0.5 mg epinephrine 1:1,000 SQ to your patient. How many milliliters of fluid will you draw up?

_____

_____

2. Your partner was able to rapidly obtain IV access. What would be the correct dose and concentration of epinephrine?

_____

_____

3. Your patient is improving but still symptomatic. Medical control orders an epi drip at 2 mcg/min. You are using a 250-mL bag of normal saline and a 60-gtt infusion set. You have on hand 1 mg of 1:10,000 epi (10 mL). How many drops per minute would you run the IV?

_____

_____

4. Along with epinephrine, what other drug orders might you anticipate and at what dose?

_____

_____

CHAPTER

31 Gastrointestinal Emergencies

Chapter Review

The following exercises provide an opportunity to test your knowledge of this chapter.

Matching

Match each of the items in the left column to the appropriate definition in the right column.

Term

_____ **1.** Feculent
_____ **2.** Diarrhea
_____ **3.** Melena
_____ **4.** Urticaria
_____ **5.** Hematochezia
_____ **6.** Borborygmi
_____ **7.** Ascites
_____ **8.** Suprapubic
_____ **9.** Epigastric
_____ **10.** Peristalsis
_____ **11.** Portal vein
_____ **12.** Striae
_____ **13.** Murphy's sign
_____ **14.** Endoscopy
_____ **15.** Peptic ulcer disease

Definition

A. Stretch marks on the abdomen caused by size changes

B. A large vessel created by the intersection of blood vessels from the gastrointestinal (GI) system that empties into the liver

C. Blood with the stool that is separate; caused by lower GI bleeds

D. Abrasion of the stomach or small intestine

E. Pain when pressure is applied to the right upper quadrant of the abdomen in a specific manner; helps detect gallbladder problems

F. Smelling of feces

G. Liquid stool

H. Abdominal edema typically caused by liver failure

I. The insertion of a flexible tube into the esophagus with the intent of visualizing and repairing damage or disease

J. Dark, tarry, very odorous stools caused by an upper GI bleed

K. An itching rash

L. A bowel sound characterized by increased activity in the bowel

M. The right upper region of the abdomen directly inferior to the xyphoid process and superior to the umbilicus

N. The region of the abdomen superior to the pubic bone and inferior to the umbilicus

O. The rhythmic contractions of the intestines and esophagus that help material to move

Multiple Choice

Read each item carefully, and then select the best response.

_____ **1.** A 42-year-old man calls for an ambulance because of "burning" epigastric pain of several hours' duration. He says that yesterday he noticed his bowel movement was "black as pitch," and about an hour ago he vomited some "stuff that looked like coffee grounds." He also feels quite dizzy. He takes no medications except Mylanta (alumina/

magnesia/simeth) "for my heartburn." On physical examination, he looks pale and anxious, and he sits leaning forward. His skin is cold and sweaty. His pulse is 140 beats/min and regular; his respirations are 20 breaths/min and slightly labored; his blood pressure is 90/60 mm Hg. His abdomen is diffusely tender, especially over the epigastrium. There is guarding but no real rigidity. Peripheral pulses are intact. This patient's findings are most consistent with which of the following conditions?

A. Peptic ulcer disease

B. Diverticulitis

C. Mesenteric ischemia

D. A leaking abdominal aortic aneurysm

_____ **2.** A 70-year-old woman calls for an ambulance because of abdominal pain of 4 hours' duration. "I just knew I shouldn't have eaten all that rich, fatty food," she says. "It never agrees with me. Oh, I hate to cause everyone so much bother." And she starts to cry. On questioning, she says she had some diarrhea, but it didn't relieve the pain. Her past medical history is notable for two previous acute myocardial infarctions. On physical examination, the woman appears to be in considerable distress. Pulse is 108 beats/min and slightly irregular; respirations are 20 breaths/min and shallow; blood pressure is 160/100 mm Hg in both arms. The chest is clear. The patient has a positive Murphy's sign. This patient most likely has which of the following conditions?

A. Peptic ulcer disease

B. Diverticulitis

C. Gallbladder attack

D. Leaking abdominal aortic aneurysm

_____ **3.** A 52-year-old woman called for an ambulance because of severe abdominal pain. She says the pain started a couple of days ago as a kind of steady ache (she points to the left lower quadrant), and it just kept getting worse and worse. Now her whole abdomen hurts. It's been 2 days since she had a bowel movement. On physical examination, the patient is in obvious distress. She lies very still on the stretcher and cries out with pain when your partner accidentally bumps the stretcher. Her pulse is 128 beats/min and regular; respirations are 28 breaths/min and shallow; blood pressure is 150/80 mm Hg. The abdomen is slightly distended, and it does not move with respiration. On palpation, it feels like a slab of concrete. The pedal pulses are equal. This patient's findings are most consistent with which of the following conditions?

A. Peptic ulcer disease

B. Diverticulitis

C. Mesenteric ischemia

D. A leaking abdominal aortic aneurysm

_____ **4.** A 30-year-old man contacts the emergency medical dispatcher by calling 9-1-1. He states he has severe abdominal pain in the lower right quadrant. He states a history of rectal bleeding, diarrhea, arthritis, and fever. He further states episodic periods of similar symptoms. This patient's findings are most consistent with which of the following conditions?

A. Peptic ulcer disease

B. Diverticulitis

C. Crohn's disease

D. A leaking abdominal aortic aneurysm

_____ **5.** Pain that originates in the abdomen and that causes pain in a distant location as a result of similar paths for the peripheral nerves of the abdomen and the distant location is considered _____ pain.

A. referred

B. parietal

C. somatic

D. rebound

_____ **6.** On arrival, you discover that your patient is a 28-year-old woman complaining of severe vomiting. You arrive to find that the patient is in the first trimester of pregnancy. She explains that she has been suffering from morning sickness. Her vomiting is so severe that she is now vomiting blood. She most likely has which of the following conditions?

A. Peptic ulcer disease

B. Hemorrhoids

C. Pancreatitis

D. Mallory Weiss syndrome

_____ **7.** The proper treatment for esophageal varices includes:

A. narcotic pain relief.

B. treatment with 5% dextrose and water.

C. fluid resuscitation.

D. placement of a laryngeal mask airway (LMA) to prevent aspiration.

_____ **8.** Acute hepatitis is not generally a concern for paramedics because:

      A. paramedics should be immunized against hepatitis.

      B. Body substance isolation (BSI) precautions should prevent infections.

      C. transmission occurs only from IV drug abusers and prostitutes.

      D. hepatitis is bacterial and not viral.

_____ **9.** You receive an emergency call for a conscious, alert 26-year-old man with a sudden onset of severe abdominal pain. He is complaining of an associated fever, nausea, and vomiting. The pain appears isolated to the right lower quadrant (RLQ). Your patient most likely has which of the following conditions?

      A. Hypovolemia   **C.** Esophageal varices

      B. Inflammation of the interstitial lining   **D.** Appendicitis

_____ **10.** The following may cause a bowel obstruction EXCEPT:

      A. paralysis of the intestines.   **C.** infection.

      B. an immune attack against the GI tract.   **D.** kidney disease.

Labeling

Label the following diagrams with the correct terms.

   1. Label the abdominal organs.   **2.** Label the parts of the stomach.

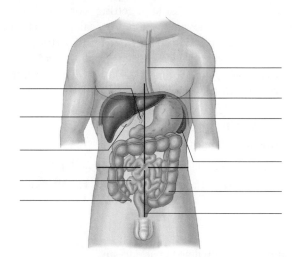
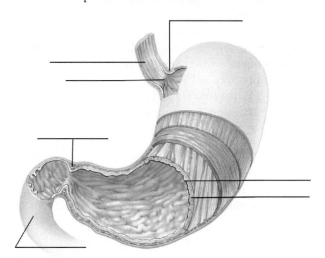

Fill-in-the-Blank

Read each item carefully, and then complete the statement by filling in the missing word(s).

   1. When patients have _____, any drug that is given may remain active within the body for _____ than anticipated.

   2. Chronic consumption of _____ or _____ may increase the acidity in the stomach beyond the limits of the protective _____ layer.

   3. The _____ vein transports _____ blood from the GI tract directly to the liver for processing of the nutrients that have been _____.

   4. The small intestine is divided into three sections: the _____, the _____ , and the _____.

5. People who are _____ are more likely to have a poor outcome from _____ - _____ illness.

6. Most peptic ulcers are the result of infection of the stomach with _____ _____. Another major cause is chronic use of _____ inflammatory drugs.

7. _____ is caused by obstruction of the cystic duct leading from the _____ to the _____,

8. The typical patient with _____ is older than 40 years old.

9. _____ _____ is a disease of the young; most patients are between 15 and 30 years of age. It occurs with equal incidence in men and women. There is a strong _____ component to this disease.

10. Many GI diseases involve pain and/or _____. As blood volume begins to drop, the body tries to compensate for this change by releasing _____ in the form of _____ and norepinephrine.

Identify

In the following case studies, list the chief complaint, vital signs, and pertinent negatives.

1. "Medic 640, respond Priority One, for a 63-year-old male patient, near syncope. Patient is now conscious and alert." As you enter the apartment, you recognize the odor. It smells as though the patient has melena stools. Your paramedic instructor was right; it's an unforgettable smell even for a brand-new, inexperienced paramedic. The patient is found to be sitting on the commode in the bathroom. He appears ashen, diaphoretic, and barely able to sit up. You and your partner lift him off the commode and lay him on the floor, which you've covered with towels. His skin color slightly improves and his level of consciousness (LOC) improves as well. You immediately place the patient on high-flow supplemental oxygen and begin your initial assessment. You already have formed your general impression and realize that the patient is suffering from a GI bleed. His vital signs are a pulse oximetry of 89%, a pulse rate (laying flat) of 118 beats/min, blood pressure of 88/P mm Hg. His abdomen is slightly distended. The patient tells you that he has an extensive history of rectal bleeding.

   a. Chief Complaint

   _____

   _____

   _____

   b. Vital Signs

   _____

   _____

   _____

   c. Pertinent Negatives

   _____

   _____

   _____

2. You are dispatched to a reported "man down." On arrival, you find law enforcement standing next to a man who presents as very unkempt. He has an empty bottle of Wild Irish something in his hands. You assume that this is a street person. Regardless

of your feelings, you understand the importance of remaining professional. Law enforcement explains that the patient is highly intoxicated and is a danger to himself and needs to be transported to a detox unit. You begin to assess the patient and decide that he looks much older than his real age of 42. Assessment reveals a male patient with an odor of ethyl alcohol (ETOH) and urine. He is conscious and alert, but slurring his words. He is mostly cooperative. The patient has icteric sclera, and right upper quadrant (RUQ) pain on palpation. His blood glucose is 110 mg/dL. His oxygen saturation level is 94%, pulse rate is 104 beats/min and regular, and his blood pressure is 142/86 mm Hg. His skin is jaundiced, but cool and dry. He has equal bilateral motor neurologic function to all extremities. His lungs are essentially clear and equal bilaterally. Patient has slightly delayed capillary refill. He has sinus tachycardia on the monitor and appears to have had several bowel movements that appear to have been alcoholic in nature. The patient denies any recent injury or falls. He's not a very good historian.

a. Chief Complaint

_____

_____

_____

b. Vital Signs

_____

_____

_____

c. Pertinent Negatives

_____

_____

_____

3. It's New Year's Eve and your patient is a 45-year-old slightly overweight woman. She is complaining of severe right upper quadrant (RUQ) pain. She states that she knows better than to eat fatty foods, but after all it's New Year's Eve. She is in pain that she describes as "worse than childbirth." She is slightly nauseated and complains of gas pains. She denies any recent injury or trauma. She states a history of gallbladder disease that is usually controlled by diet. But tonight the pain is "unbearable." She further states that tonight's episode is consistent with other bouts of gallbladder attack. She says that after tonight she's going to "finally have it taken out." Her vital signs are a pulse of 92 beats/min, strong and regular. She has equal bilateral radial pulses. The abdomen is tender in the right upper quadrant (RUQ). Her oygen saturation is 99%. ECG: Sinus rhythm, normal capillary refill, skin color is normal, skin is warm and slightly diaphoretic. Your patient is crying for pain relief.

a. Chief Complaint

_____

_____

_____

b. Vital Signs

_____

_____

_____

c. Pertinent Negatives

_____

_____

_____

Ambulance Calls

The following case scenarios provide an opportunity to explore the concerns associated with patient management and paramedic care. Read each scenario, and then answer each question.

1. You are assessing and treating a conscious, alert 23-year-old man with a sudden severe onset of periumbilical pain that migrates to the right lower quadrant. He states that he can't find a position of comfort and also feels slightly nauseated and febrile.

   a. What is your initial impression of this patient's presentation?

_____

_____

   b. Your patient denies any other previous medical history, he isn't on any medications, and he denies allergies to medications. His vital signs would be considered within normal limits. How would you treat this patient?

     (1) _____

     (2) _____

     (3) _____

     (4) _____

     (5) _____

     (6) _____

   c. Your patient is very nauseated and is vomiting frequently. You have a choice of the following standing order medications in your drug box: Diphenhydramine, Hydroxyzine, Promethazine. Describe the contraindications of each.

_____

_____

_____

_____

_____

2. Your patient presents with a history of esophageal varices. He is vomiting copious amounts of undigested blood. What would your prehospital treatment for this patient include?

   a. _____

   b. _____

c. _____

d. _____

3. You respond to a call for a 76-year-old woman with a possible bowel obstruction. In the prehospital setting, there might not be much you can do to treat this particular patient. List the general treatment guidelines for patients with gastrointestinal disease.

a. _____

b. _____

c. _____

d. _____

e. _____

f. _____

g. _____

True/False

If you believe the statement to be more true than false, write the letter "T" in the space provided. If you believe the statement to be more false than true, write the letter "F."

_____ **1.** Promethazine is a drug for managing patients with nausea and vomiting.

_____ **2.** Ulcerative colitis presents with a chronic complaint of abdominal pain, often in the lower right area. This pain corresponds to the location of the ileum. Rectal bleeding, weight loss, and diarrhea are some symptoms of this condition.

_____ **3.** All types of acute hepatitis, regardless of their etiology, are associated with the same signs and symptoms.

_____ **4.** Patients with peptic ulcers experience a classic sequence of burning or gnawing pain in the stomach that subsides or diminishes immediately after eating, and then reemerges 2 to 3 hours later.

_____ **5.** Deep palpation can help you discern some of the organs and structures in the cavity and requires a level of technique usually employed in the prehospital setting.

_____ **6.** Pain is often an unimportant finding with GI patients. The patient's complaint of pain is something that a paramedic must learn to expect.

_____ **7.** The major effects from GI disease typically relate to the nervous, cardiovascular, and respiratory systems and result from pain, hypovolemia, and infection.

_____ **8.** True absent bowel sounds, which are characterized by no sounds heard for 2 minutes, are typically not practical to discover in the prehospital setting.

_____ **9.** The foul-smelling stools that accompany GI emergencies are to be expected.

_____ **10.** Orthostatic vital signs are only relevant when dealing with abdominal trauma.

Short Answer

Complete this section with short written answers using the space provided.

1. Define the following vocabulary words:

a. Borborygmi

_____

_____

b. Cholecystitis

_____

_____

c. Scaphoid

_____

_____

d. Mallory Weiss syndrome

_____

_____

2. A 15-year-old girl complains of sharp pain in the right lower quadrant. The pain is made worse by coughing or moving around. The spot she points to is the spot that is most tender to palpation. She lies very still, with her right leg flexed at the hip and knee.

a. What *type* of abdominal pain is this?

_____

b. What *mechanism* is most likely to produce this type of pain?

_____

c. Describe the *causes* of this type of pain.

_____

_____

3. Your patient is complaining of pain localized to the right upper abdomen. The patient describes the pain as sharp and as the worse pain he's ever felt. He also states that he is nauseous and has vomited several times. Physical exam reveals fever, tachycardia, hypotension, and muscle spasms in the extremities.

a. What type of abdominal pain is this?

_____

b. When does this type of pain usually occur?

_____

_____

Word Find

Hidden in the following grid are 10 words or phrases related to what you have studied in this chapter. Find the hidden words in the grid below. Then list the words from the grid, which include the structures of the gastrointestinal system.

```
G G N G Z L V H I D T S D B U
A E M V I Y C E L G N B I O I
L V O V Y A R O E K P L M I C
L Q E M M E G H U O E C U B M
B R M O C B X H M D V T N J N
L S T L R E C T U M G U U N P
A S A I G F P C O L Q Z J S E
D E K E O M T X M U P D E D F
D M E B R F H P P L J J J Q U
E C K L X C M U U O V H F V N
R W O W E X N V T J B J N F F
Z Q E L O N R A L B H U E V J
S B K U O Z P F P E D I K O I
Y H Z I P N S U T Y A C D C D
M U N E D O U D J Z X V C N I
```

GASTROINTESTINAL SYSTEM

1. _____

2. _____

3. _____

4. _____

5. _____

6. _____

7. _____

8. _____

9. _____

10. _____

Fill-in-the-Table

Fill in the missing parts of the table.

1. In the course of a busy week (is there any other kind?), you have several calls for patients with abdominal pain. Each time you have to evaluate a different story and a different set of physical findings. Among the findings in the patients you cared for were those listed here. For each finding, explain its clinical significance.

Finding	What the Finding Tells Me
Coffee-ground vomitus	
Severe bradycardia	
Melena	
Tenting of the skin	
Patient very still	
Pulsatile abdominal mass	
Rigid abdomen	

CHAPTER

32 Renal and Urologic Emergencies

Chapter Review

The following exercises provide an opportunity to test your knowledge of this chapter.

Matching

Match each of the items in the left column to the appropriate term in the right column.

_____ 1. Progressive and irreversible inadequate kidney function.

_____ 2. Peaked T waves are a classic sign of this problem.

_____ 3. Normal flora bacteria enters the urethra and begins to grow.

_____ 4. Insoluble salt or uric acid crystallizes in the urine and produces this.

_____ 5. A sudden decrease in filtration through the glomeruli.

_____ 6. Hypoperfusion of the kidneys caused by hypovolemia.

_____ 7. This is caused by an obstruction of urine flow from the kidneys.

_____ 8. Increased waste products and urea in the blood.

_____ 9. Chronic inflammation of the interstitial cells around the nephrons.

_____ 10. When the urine output drops below 500 mL/day.

A. Hyperkalemia

B. Acute renal failure (ARF)

C. Urinary tract infection

D. Chronic renal failure

E. Kidney stones

F. Uremia

G. Interstitial nephritis

H. Prerenal ARF

I. Oliguria

J. Postrenal ARF

Multiple Choice

Read each item carefully, and then select the best response.

_____ 1. Which of the following is not considered part of the urinary system?

    A. Ureters

    B. Kidney

    C. Liver

    D. Bladder

_____ 2. How much blood does the kidney filter per day in the normal adult?

    A. 200 mL

    B. 200 L

    C. 2,000 L

    D. 200 quarts

_____ 3. Each minute _____ of the body's systemic cardiac output of blood flows through the kidneys.

    A. One tenth

    B. One quarter

    C. One half

    D. Two thirds

_____ 4. What structure inside the kidney is the main filter for the blood entering the kidney?

    A. Peritubular capillaries

    B. Renal pyramids

    C. Calyces

    D. Glomerulus

_____ **5.** What is the most common composition of kidney stones?

        A. Calcium   **C.** Glucose

        B. Salt   **D.** Fat

_____ **6.** When a patient is suffering pain from a kidney stone, it is important to remember that the greater the pain,

        A. the lower the blood pressure and pulse will be.

        B. the higher the blood pressure and pulse will be.

        C. the higher the blood pressure will be and the lower the pulse will be.

        D. the lower the blood pressure will be and the higher the pulse will be.

_____ **7.** What is the name of the condition when urine output stops completely?

        A. Oliguria   **C.** Anuria

        B. Uremia   **D.** Hematuria

_____ **8.** When reading an ECG, what is a classic finding of hyperkalemia?

        A. Peaked T waves   **C.** Atrial flutter

        B. Inverted T waves   **D.** No T waves at all

_____ **9.** Which of the following is _not_ a sign of air embolism caused by a loose dialysis system?

        A. Cyanosis   **C.** Hypotension

        B. Hypertension   **D.** Dyspnea

_____ **10.** How much normal saline would you give to a dialysis patient who is suffering from hypotension as a result of dialysis?

        A. 50 mL   **C.** 5 mL/kg

        B. 100 mL   **D.** 50 mL/kg

Labeling

Label the following diagrams with the correct terms.

1. Label the urinary system.

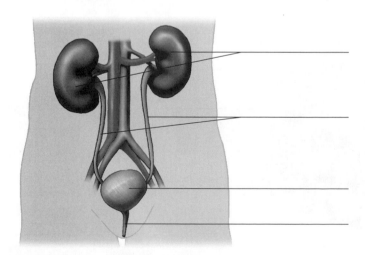

2. The glomerulus of the kidneys. The nephron carries out three blood-filtering processes. Label them below.

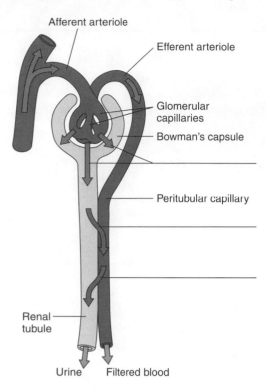

Afferent arteriole

Efferent arteriole

Glomerular capillaries

Bowman's capsule

Peritubular capillary

Renal tubule

Urine   Filtered blood

3. Label the parts of the male reproductive system.

SIDE VIEW

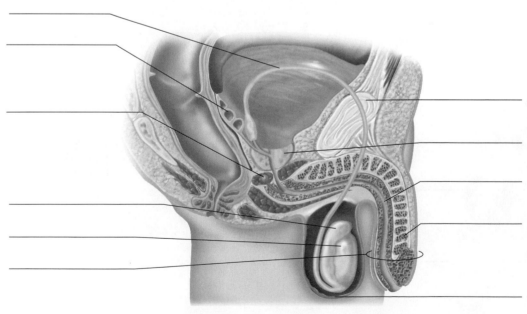

4. Label the parts of the female reproductive system.

SIDE VIEW

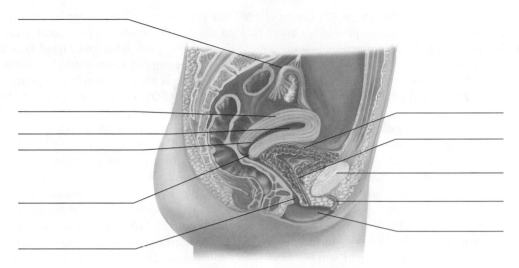

Fill-in-the-Blank

Read each item carefully, and then complete the statement by filling in the missing word(s).

1. When managing a patient whose chief complaint is renal calculi, your focus should be on _____ and

_____.

2. The kidneys' internal anatomy is divided into three regions: the _____, the _____, and the

_____.

3. _____ _____ is produced by the hypothalamus and is secreted when the solute concentration of the

blood increases.

4. During _____, the patient's blood circulates through a dialysis machine that works the same way the patient's

kidneys function.

5. _____ _____ occurs during dialysis and happens because of the water shifting from the bloodstream into

the cerebrospinal fluid (CSF).

6. Sickle cell disease can cause _____ in the male. Usually, this condition is caused by trauma.

7. _____ pain is usually associated with hollow organs and presents with a crampy, aching pain deep within the body.

8. You should always monitor the patient's _____ functions when dealing with a renal patient.

9. Treatment of kidney stones in the prehospital setting should revolve around _____ _____ for the patient.

10. Urinary tract infections usually occur in the _____ urinary tract.

Identify

In the following case study, list the chief complaint, vital signs, and pertinent negatives.

You're just about to hit the hay after a long day at the fire station. Unfortunately, Bill, the paramedic on duty, is not feeling very well, and so you have to fill in for him. He has had a crampy pain in his lower back all day, and he is worried he is coming down with the flu. At about 1 am, Bill wakes you and tells you something is really wrong. He is having pain in his lower quadrants, and he can't take it any more. You give him a little ribbing about all the potato chips he has been eating and the gallons of sports drink he drinks each day. You tell him to go back to sleep. It is just an upset stomach. He tells you he is about to jump through his skin because it hurts so badly and asks you to get up and haul him in to the emergency department (ED). You decide that maybe Bill is having some problems, and so you wake up the other EMT-B and start an assessment on Bill. He is 47 years old, he is alert, his oxygen saturation is 98%. You put him on a nasal cannula at 4 L/min just for good measure. Your partner takes his pulse, which is 104 beats/min, and the heart monitor shows a sinus tachycardia. Blood pressure is 148/94 mm Hg, respirations are 18 breaths/min, and all lung fields are clear. His skin is warm and dry, and he has a normal temperature. Not wanting to miss anything on Bill, you measure his blood glucose, which is 96 mg/dL. His pain is a 10 on a 10 scale, and he is really hurting. Bill doesn't smoke and, other than a fast-food diet, he keeps in good shape. Both you and Bill right now are suspecting a kidney stone. You start an IV and give him a 500-mL bolus of normal saline on the way to the hospital. Medical direction agrees with you about the possibility of a stone and orders 5 mg morphine for the pain. Bill is feeling a lot better when you reach the ED. His pain is down to a 4 on a 10 scale. You check back with him in the morning when you get off shift. He says that he passed a stone about 4 hours after you brought him in. They will run a few more tests, but he thinks he will be out of the hospital around noon. He is now swearing off sports drinks and promises water is his new buddy.

1. Chief Complaint

_____

_____

_____

2. Vital Signs

_____

_____

_____

3. Pertinent Negatives

_____

_____

_____

Ambulance Calls

The following case scenarios provide an opportunity to explore the concerns associated with patient management and paramedic care. Read each scenario, and then answer each question.

1. A 42-year-old man complains of crampy abdominal pain that builds up to a peak, subsides, and then builds again. When you ask where the pain is, he points to the general area of the umbilicus, but when you palpate his abdomen, the part that is tender is in the left lower quadrant. He tells you that he has been vomiting nearly since the pain started, about 6 hours ago.

   a. What *type* of abdominal pain is this?

   _____

   _____

b. What *mechanism* is most likely to produce this type of pain?

_____

_____

_____

c. Describe the *causes* of this type of pain.

_____

_____

_____

2. On the first hot day of the summer, a 35-year-old construction worker calls for an ambulance because of "excruciating" abdominal pain. He was hit in the back lower right quadrant by a steel beam that was being moved into place by a crane. It knocked him down, but he didn't want to appear hurt to his coworkers. So, after catching his breath, he went back to work. He has come home for lunch and now is hurting badly. His wife admits you to the house, where you find the patient in the bedroom, writhing about on the bed, tears rolling down his face. "I can't take it, I can't take it," he says. "Please give me something for the pain." His wife says that he came home from work complaining of back pain and then pain in his groin, and it just got worse and worse. He has been vomiting for the past hour or so. On physical examination, he is clearly in severe distress. His pulse is 124 beats/min and regular, respirations are 30 breaths/min, and blood pressure is 160/80 mm Hg. There is some guarding in the abdomen and tenderness on the left side, but no rigidity. This patient's findings are most consistent with which of the following conditions?

    A. Peptic ulcer disease   **D.** Leaking abdominal aortic aneurysm

    B. Diverticulitis   **E.** Trauma to the kidneys

    C. Mesenteric ischemia   **F.** None of the above

3. The following ambulance calls involve dialysis patients. For each situation described, indicate what you think is the problem and what you would do about it.

    a. A patient is due for dialysis today but says he feels "too weak and dizzy even to get out of bed." His ECG shows a rate of 40 beats/min, flattened P waves, wide QRS complexes, and tall, pointy T waves. You are 30 minutes from the hospital ED.

        (1) What do you think is the problem?

_____

_____

_____

        (2) What steps will you take to manage the problem?

           (a) _____

           (b) _____

           (c) _____

           (d) _____

           (e) _____

b. The patient calls for an ambulance because of dyspnea that wakened him from sleep. You find him sitting bolt upright, struggling for breath, and coughing up foamy, pink sputum. The lungs are full of crackles. The ECG shows sinus tachycardia (120 beats/min). His blood pressure is 190/120 mm Hg.

(1) What do you think is the problem?

_____

_____

_____

(2) What steps will you take to manage the problem?

(a) _____

(b) _____

(c) _____

(d) _____

c. The patient just got home from a dialysis session at the local kidney center. He complains of a severe headache and nausea. He has vomited twice since getting home. On physical examination, he seems a little confused. His pulse is 56 beats/min and regular, respirations are 16 breaths/min, and blood pressure is 180/102 mm Hg.

(1) What do you think is the problem?

_____

_____

_____

(2) What steps will you take to manage the problem?

(a) _____

(b) _____

(c) _____

(d) _____

True/False

If you believe the statement to be more true than false, write the letter "T" in the space provided. If you believe the statement to be more false than true, write the letter "F."

_____ **1.** When you suspect a patient to be in acute renal failure, you should put the patient in the shock position.

_____ **2.** Hyperkalemia presents with an inverted T wave on the ECG.

_____ **3.** The "cleft" of the kidney is called the renal medulla.

_____ **4.** Nephrons are the functioning units inside the kidney that form urine.

_____ **5.** The only absorption of water and electrolytes occurs in the loop of Henle.

_____ **6.** Aldosterone is produced in the hypothalamus.

_____ **7.** When the body becomes low on water, the pituitary gland releases ADH, which causes reabsorption of water into the bloodstream.

_____ **8.** The female urethra is much shorter than the male urethra.

_____ **9.** Men are more prone to urinary tract infections (UTIs) than women are because of the length of their urethra.

_____ **10.** Prerenal acute renal failure (ARF) is caused by a lack of blood flow to the kidneys.

Short Answer

Complete this section with short written answers using the space provided.

1. Use a medical dictionary to look up the following words, and then write the dictionary definition beside each word:
   a. Oliguria

   _____

   _____

   b. Perinephric

   _____

   _____

   c. Hepatomegaly

   _____

   _____

   d. Anasarca

   _____

   _____

   e. Polyuria

   _____

   _____

   f. Hepatoma

   _____

   _____

   g. Cytoscopy

   _____

   _____

   h. Uremia

   _____

   _____

2. Many patients with chronic renal failure are kept alive by periodic hemodialysis. Although dialysis does remove toxic wastes from the blood and helps restore fluid and electrolyte balance, it does not by any means solve all the patient's problems. Patients maintained on long-term dialysis for chronic renal failure are much more vulnerable than patients with normal kidneys. List eight medical problems to which patients with chronic renal failure are particularly susceptible.

   a. _____

b. _____

c. _____

d. _____

e. _____

f. _____

g. _____

h. _____

Crossword Puzzle

Use the clues below to complete the puzzle.

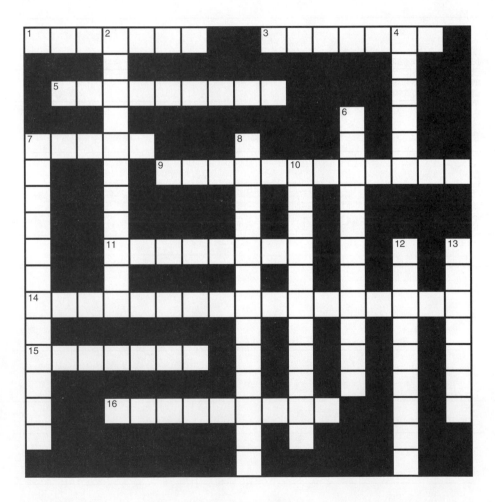

Across

1. Middle layer of the kidney

3. Common kidney stone is made up of

5. A muscle that can retract the testicle

7. An enzyme that initiates reactions in the body to produce angiotensin I

9. An infection of the urethras

11. A condition of urine output that is less than 500 mL/day

14. A sudden decrease in filtration through the glomeruli

15. Irreversible inadequate kidney function because of permanent nephron loss is _____ renal failure

16. Blood in the urine

Down

2. A powdery accumulation of uric acid
4. Fluid and waste product build up in the blood is known as _____
6. A/an _____ unit is where kidney stones are disintegrated

7. The most common acute renal disease
8. An arteriovenous fistula
10. Connective tissue that anchors the kidney to the abdominal wall
12. Chemicals that increase urinary output
13. Transports urine from the kidneys to the bladder

Fill-in-the-Table

Fill in the missing parts of the table.

Signs and Symptoms of Acute Renal Failure

Signs and Symptoms of Acute Renal Failure	
Prerenal acute renal failure	Hypotension
	_____
	Dizziness
	_____
Intrarenal acute renal failure	_____
	Joint pain
	_____
	Hypertension
	_____
	_____
	Seizure
Postrenal acute renal failure	_____
	Oliguria
	_____
	Peripheral edema

CHAPTER

33 Toxicology: Substance Abuse and Poisoning

Chapter Review

The following exercises provide an opportunity to test your knowledge of this chapter.

Matching

Match the definitions in the left column to the appropriate terms in the right column.

_____ **1.** A synthetic narcotic not derived from opium

_____ **2.** A common houseplant; ingestion leads to burns of the mouth and tongue and, possibly, paralysis of the vocal cords

_____ **3.** Chemicals that are acids or alkalis; cause direct chemical injury to the tissues they contact

_____ **4.** A naturally occurring alkaloid found in a variety of plants (such as tea leaves)

_____ **5.** The total effects are greater than the sum of the independent effects of the two substances

_____ **6.** Withdrawal syndrome seen in people with alcoholism who are deprived of ethyl alcohol

_____ **7.** Psychiatric medication used primarily to treat atypical depression by increasing norepinephrine

_____ **8.** A plant that contains cardiac glycosides used in making digitalis

_____ **9.** A seed that contains the poison ricin

_____ **10.** The emotional state of craving a drug to maintain a feeling of well-being

_____ **11.** Compounds made up principally of hydrogen and carbon atoms mostly obtained from the distillation of petroleum

_____ **12.** The cornerstone drug for the treatment of bipolar disorder

_____ **13.** Class of drugs that increase alertness and excitation

_____ **14.** Drugs used to treat severe depression and manage pain; minimal dosing errors can cause toxic results

_____ **15.** Physiologic adaptation to the effects of a drug such that increasingly larger doses of the drug are required to achieve the same effect

A. Caustics

B. Monoamine oxidase inhibitors

C. Hydrocarbons

D. Castor bean

E. Tricyclic antidepressants

F. Amphetamines

G. Foxglove

H. Lithium

I. Theophylline

J. Opioid

K. Tolerance

L. Delirium tremens

M. Psychological dependence

N. Dieffenbachia

O. Synergism

Multiple Choice

Read each item carefully, and then select the best response.

_____ **1.** Poisoning in adults is usually a result of:

   A. improperly labeled over-the-counter medications.

   B. improperly dispensed prescribed medications.

   C. suicide attempts.

   D. workplace mishaps involving chemicals and toxic exposures.

_____ **2.** All of the following are common routes of poisoning EXCEPT:

   A. inhalation.   **C.** injection.

   B. ingestion.   **D.** excretion.

_____ **3.** Alcoholism usually consists of two distinct phases that include _____ drinking.

   A. problem   **C.** medicinal

   B. social   **D.** binge

_____ **4.** Alcohol abuse may cause a number of medical consequences, including:

   A. deterioration of memory and higher thinking.   **C.** a higher risk of mouth and esophageal cancers.

   B. acute gastric distress.   **D.** all of the above.

_____ **5.** Alcohol withdrawal may have life-threatening consequences, including delirium tremens. Delirium tremens, or the "DTs," are best characterized by:

   A. tremors.   **C.** restlessness.

   B. confusion.   **D.** all of the above.

_____ **6.** The general assessment approach for toxicologic emergencies includes the following tasks EXCEPT:

   A. There is no "general assessment"; these patients are neither medical nor trauma.

   B. initial assessment.

   C. scene size-up.

   D. physical exam.

_____ **7.** You are called to the scene of a 4-year-old who ingested a common house plant. The _best_ source of information regarding the accidental ingestion is:

   A. referring to the Department of Transportation (DOT) _Emergency Response Guidebook_ (_ERG_).

   B. contacting the poison center.

   C. contacting CHEMTREC.

   D. contacting medical control.

_____ **8.** A chronic disorder characterized by the compulsive use of a substance resulting in physical, psychological, or social harm to the user who continues to use the substance despite the harm, is considered:

   A. tolerance.   **C.** substance abuse.

   B. drug addiction.   **D.** antagonist.

_____ **9.** The treatment for patients abusing cocaine, amphetamine, or methamphetamine is fundamentally the same. This treatment includes the following tasks EXCEPT:

   A. establishing and maintain the airway. Consider an advanced airway as needed.

   B. establishing vascular access.

   C. applying the ECG monitor, pulse oximeter, and capnometer.

   D. contacting medical control for chemical restraint when behavior is violent.

_____ **10.** Signs and symptoms of overdose with cardiac drugs may include:

    A. hypotension.

    B. weakness or confusion.

    C. nausea and vomiting.

    D. all of the above.

_____ **11.** Salivation, lacrimation, urination, defecation, gastric upset, and emesis are symptoms associated with a toxic exposure to:

    A. psychedelics.

    B. narcotics.

    C. ketamine.

    D. organophosphates.

_____ **12.** Physical examination of a patient who has been poisoned with cyanide may reveal a/an:

    A. altered mental state.

    B. respirations that are rapid and labored and that become slow and gasping.

    C. rapid and thready pulse.

    D. all of the above.

_____ **13.** The most common symptom of a tricyclic antidepressant overdose is:

    A. an altered mental status.

    B. abdominal pain.

    C. internal bleeding.

    D. burning of the eyes, nose, and throat.

_____ **14.** All of the following may alter the presentation of salicylate overdose EXCEPT:

    A. patient's age.

    B. dose ingested.

    C. duration of respiratory distress syndrome.

    D. duration of exposure.

_____ **15.** Death from Hymenoptera stings usually occurs as a result of:

    A. acute respiratory distress.

    B. psychogenic shock.

    C. anaphylactic shock.

    D. infection.

Fill-in-the-Blank

Read each item carefully, and then complete the statement by filling in the missing word(s).

1. A/an _____ is a substance that is toxic by nature, no matter how it gets into the body or in what quantities it is taken. By contrast, a/an _____ is a substance that has some therapeutic effect.

2. _____ _____ usually fall under one of two general headings: _____ and _____. Poisoning in adults is commonly intentional.

3. Toxins cannot exert their effects until they enter the body. The four primary methods of entry are _____, _____, _____, and _____.

4. _____ are useful for remembering the assessment and management of different substances that fall under the same _____ _____.

5. People with alcoholism tend to have chronic _____ and fall frequently, increasing the likelihood of head _____ or other trauma.

6. The most immediate danger to an acutely intoxicated person is death of _____ _____ and/or aspiration of vomitus or stomach contents secondary to a suppressed _____ _____.

7. Shortly after injecting _____, a user will appear to pass out. However, the user is typically quite _____ and remains aware of what is being done or said.

8. Signs and symptoms of overdose with cardiac drugs may include _____, weakness or confusion, nausea and vomiting, _____ _____, headache, and difficulty _____.

9. Treatment of carbon monoxide (CO) _____ in the field is aimed at providing the highest concentration of _____ possible to attempt to displace CO molecules from the _____.

10. Acids tend to be more _____-_____ than _____, and so they are often diluted relatively quickly. With _____, it is more important to keep water continually flowing because it usually takes much longer to rinse away an alkali.

11. The most dangerous drugs that increase sexual gratification include erectile dysfunction medications such as _____, which are contraindicated for patients who take _____ for cardiac problems. Their use by people taking nitrites may result in severe _____ or total cardiovascular collapse.

12. Long-term _____ abuse can lead to permanent loss of mental function as evidenced by a variety of neuropathies, such as loss of _____, loss of fine motor _____, balance and _____ disorders, and occasionally _____.

13. Hydrocarbon products cause _____ _____, which results in severe abdominal _____, diarrhea, and belching. At the other end of the spectrum, just a single hydrocarbon substance exposure may cause life-threatening _____ and on occasion, sudden _____.

14. With a serious toxic exposure of _____ _____, be alert for ventricular _____, hypotension, respiratory _____, QT prolongation on the ECG, and _____.

15. When taken in toxic levels, _____ _____ inhibitors can be lethal because they can produce _____, metabolic _____, and rhabdomyolysis.

Identify

In the following case studies, identify the appropriate toxidrome and list two drugs associated with that particular toxidrome.

1. You arrive on scene to find a 22-year-old woman who appears confused, has a blood pressure of 88/60 mm Hg, is slurring her speech, and is somewhat sleepy.

   a. Identify the appropriate toxidrome: _____

   b. Name two drugs that may fit this toxidrome.

   (1) _____

   (2) _____

2. Your advanced life support (ALS) ambulance arrives on scene at the request of law enforcement for a very agitated 42-year-old man. He won't stop talking and is paranoid.

   a. Identify the appropriate toxidrome: _____

   b. Name two drugs that may fit this toxidrome.

   (1) _____

   (2) _____

In the following case studies, identify the possible causative agent based on the presenting symptoms.

3. On arrival, you discover a 16-year-old boy with severe nausea and vomiting. You begin assessing the patient and immediately notice an odor that appears to be alcohol.

   _____

   _____

   _____

   _____

4. You are dispatched to a "Delta" response (high priority) for a patient seizing. On arrival, you discover a 56-year-old man who is actively seizing and has snoring respirations. Family members state the patient has been recently depressed and withdrawn.

   _____

   _____

   _____

   _____

Ambulance Calls

The following case scenarios provide an opportunity to explore the concerns associated with patient management and paramedic care. Read each scenario, and then answer each question.

1. You are called to a somewhat rundown apartment building where the police have forcibly entered an apartment after neighbors reported that the occupant of the apartment has not been seen for a few days and has not answered his telephone. Inside, you find a man who looks to be about 30 years old lying unconscious on a sofa in the living room. Some neighbors are milling around, giving information to the police officers.

   a. List six questions you would ask the neighbors about the patient.

   (1) _____

   (2) _____

   (3) _____

   (4) _____

   (5) _____

   (6) _____

b. Besides the neighbors, what other sources of information might be present? What places in the apartment would you check? What would you be looking for?

(1) _____

(2) _____

(3) _____

c. When you examine the patient, you detect the following findings. For each finding listed, indicate its possible diagnostic significance.

Finding	Possible Diagnostic Significance
Cold, dry skin	
Pulse = 110 beats/min, thready	
Blood pressure = 90/60 mm Hg	
Respirations = 12 breaths/min and shallow	
Pupils dilated and do not react to light	
Breath smells of alcohol	
Left arm is cold and blue	

d. In assessing this patient's level of consciousness, you find the following:
- He does not open his eyes.
- His arms flex when you pinch his leg.
- He does not make any sound in response to your calling his name or pinching him.

In view of those findings, he is best described as:

      (1) drowsy.

      (2) lethargic.

      (3) comatose.

      (4) stuporous.

      (5) obtunded.

(Circle the best answer.)

e. List in order the steps in managing this patient.

(1) _____

(2) _____

(3) _____

(4) _____

(5) _____

(6) _____

(7) _____

(8) _____

(9) _____

2. You are called to the home of a frantic young couple who discovered their 3-year-old happily consuming the contents of a bottle from the cleaning cupboard. List five questions you would ask in taking the history of the incident.

a. _____

b. _____

c. _____

d. _____

e. _____

3. A middle-aged man is found unconscious in his garage. He has left a suicide note on the car windshield, but the hood of the car is cold, so you are reasonably sure the engine has not been run recently. List five things to which you would give particular attention in the physical examination of this patient.

a. _____

b. _____

c. _____

d. _____

e. _____

4. A 15-year-old boy swallowed about 35 of his father's antihypertensive pills in a suicide gesture after a family argument. You arrive at the scene, some 30 minutes distant from the nearest hospital, about 15 minutes after the ingestion. In a telephone consultation, Poison Control advises you to administer activated charcoal. The boy is alert, and vital signs are all within normal limits.

a. What is the purpose of giving activated charcoal? That is, what is the therapeutic effect?

_____

_____

_____

_____

b. List three poisonings in which activated charcoal is *contraindicated*.

(1) _____

(2) _____

(3) _____

c. What is the *dosage* of activated charcoal for this patient?

_____

d. List in order the steps in treating this patient.

(1) _____

(2) _____

(3) _____

(4) _____

(5) _____

5. A 35-year-old man ingested "about a tablespoon" of drain buildup remover (Drano) crystals 10 to 15 minutes before your arrival. He is fully alert and complaining of severe pain in his throat and chest. His lips and mouth are very red, and there are still crystals sticking to the mucous membranes in his mouth.

a. List the steps in treating this patient.

(1) _____

(2) _____

(3) _____

(4) _____

6. You are summoned to a location near the railway tracks where the local "down-and-outs" gather. A police officer at the scene gestures you toward two of the group members congregated there. "They looked in pretty bad shape," he says, "so I thought I'd better call EMS."

"Been drinking real bad stuff," one of the group chimes in. "Told 'em to stay away from that rotgut—you can go blind from drinkin' stuff like that."

The first patient is in severe respiratory distress. He says he hasn't had a drink since the previous day, when he drank "some stuff they left lying around the gas station—I don't know what it was—tasted pretty good." He says he threw up a few times about 6 hours after that. On physical examination, the patient is alert. There is no alcohol odor on his breath. His vital signs are a pulse of 120 beats/min and regular, respirations of 36 breaths/min and noisy, and blood pressure is 180/105 mm Hg. The pupils are midposition, equal, and reactive to light. The gag reflex is present. The chest is full of crackles.

a. What do you think is this patient's problem?

_____

_____

_____

_____

b. List the steps you would take in managing this patient.

(1) _____

(2) _____

(3) _____

(4) _____

(5) _____

The second patient appears intoxicated. His speech is slurred, and he can scarcely walk. "Why ish it shnowing in Sheptember?" he mumbles. His breath smells of alcohol. His pulse is 108 beats/min and regular, his respirations are 30 breaths/min and deep, and his blood pressure is 140/86 mm Hg. There is no evidence of head injury. The pupils are about 6 mm and equal and react sluggishly to light. The gag reflex is present. The chest is clear. The abdomen is very tender and nearly rigid to palpation.

c. What do you think is this patient's problem?

_____

_____

_____

_____

d. List the steps you would take in managing this patient.

(1) _____

(2) _____

(3) _____

(4) _____

(5) _____

(6) _____

7. You are called to the home of a 46-year-old woman who swallowed an unknown quantity of silver polish in a suicide attempt. A bevy of agitated family members is hovering around her, all talking at once. As far as you can determine, the ingestion took place sometime during the past hour. While your partner telephones Poison Control for a rundown on the exact composition of that brand of silver polish, you examine the patient. You find her very confused and sleepy. There is a funny smell on her breath that you can't quite place—a little like almonds? The skin is flushed. The pulse is 132 beats/min and thready, respirations are 32 breaths/min and labored, and blood pressure is 90/64 mm Hg.

a. What do you think is this patient's problem?

_____

_____

_____

_____

b. What *drug* is indicated to treat this problem to "buy time" until you reach the emergency department?

_____

c. How is it given?

_____

d. What *side effects* should you anticipate?

_____

_____

_____

_____

e. List the steps you would take in managing this patient.

(1) _____

(2) _____

(3) _____

(4) _____

(5) _____

(6) _____

(7) _____

8. You are staying with a bunch of friends at their cabin in the mountains for a nice ski weekend. Your host takes considerable pride in the cabin, which he built himself. "Snug as a bug in a rug," he says, "not a draft in the place." You have to admit that he did a good insulation job and that the place is nice and cozy with the Franklin stove in the corner.

　　When you get up the next morning, your friend's wife, asks, "Will you have a look at the baby? She's sick with something. She's been throwing up all morning." You don't know much about babies, and you don't feel so hot yourself, but you take a look at the baby. You find her pale and dehydrated, with a bounding pulse but no fever. As you are examining her, she has a grand mal seizure. "It must be the flu," says the baby's mother, "because I'm coming down with something, too. I feel real sick to my stomach." Meanwhile, your friend, just getting up, says, "Boy, do I have a headache; it's like Niagara Falls roaring through my skull."

a. What do you think is the baby's problem?

_____

_____

_____

b. What steps should you take in this situation?

(1) _____

(2) _____

(3) _____

(4) _____

(5) _____

(6) _____

(7) _____

9. One fine Sunday afternoon, you are called to a suburban home for a "possible heart attack." On arrival, you find a middle-aged man, clad in shorts and a T-shirt, sprawled out on the sofa in the living room. "I don't know what happened," he says. "I was just sitting outside on the lawn, and I started to feel real dizzy and sick to my stomach, and real weak. And there's this tight feeling in my chest. . . ."

"It's that stuff Mr. Dimbledirt was spraying," his wife chimes in. "I'm sure of it. Why he has to spray his precious roses precisely when *we're* sitting in the garden is beyond me."

While you begin your assessment of the patient, your partner goes next door to talk with Mr. Dimbledirt. You find the patient in considerable distress. His skin is pale and diaphoretic. His vital signs are a pulse of 42 beats/min and regular, respirations are 28 breaths/min and labored, and blood pressure is 140/80 mm Hg. The pupils are very constricted. The patient is salivating profusely, and his breath smells like garlic. The neck veins are flat. The chest is full of wheezes. As you are completing the examination, your partner returns carrying a bottle labeled "parathion."

a. What do you think is this patient's problem?

_____

_____

_____

_____

b. What *drug* is used to treat this problem?

_____

c. What is the correct *dosage* in this situation?

_____

d. List all the steps in treating this patient.

(1) _____

(2) _____

(3) _____

(4) _____

(5) _____

(6) _____

(7) _____

(8) _____

(9) _____

10. You are called to a local junior high school where a 12-year-old boy had a grand mal seizure. The school nurse, who is kneeling on the floor of the boys' restroom beside the boy, tells you that the boy has no known seizure history. The boy is unconscious but can be roused by painful stimuli. You cannot find any abnormalities on physical examination save for signs that he indeed just had a seizure (slight bleeding of the tongue, incontinence). A search of his pockets, however, reveals a few small bottles of typewriter correction fluid. What steps will you take in managing this patient?

a. _____

b. _____

c. _____

d. _____

e. _____

True/False

If you believe the statement to be more true than false, write the letter "T" in the space provided. If you believe the statement to be more false than true, write the letter "F."

_____ **1.** Your call to the Poison Control Center helps the center collect data on poisonings in your region. These data may be analyzed to help detect trends, spot developing public health problems, and evaluate current treatment protocols for different poisonings.

_____ **2.** Oxygen has a greater affinity than carbon monoxide (CO) to bind to hemoglobin on the red blood cells.

_____ **3.** Intact skin provides an adequate barrier against the body absorbing poisons. As a result, the seriousness of absorbed poisons is often minimal.

_____ **4.** The major toxidromes are produced by stimulants, narcotics, cholinergics, anticholinergics, sympathomimetics, sedatives, and hypnotics.

_____ **5.** The more frequently consumption of alcohol takes place, the greater the irritation of the digestive system.

_____ **6.** The severity of alcohol withdrawal can vary according to the length and intensity of the alcoholic habit. Minor withdrawal is characterized by restlessness, anxiousness, sleeping problems, agitation, and tremors.

_____ **7.** Prolonged heavy use of alcohol may cause ulcers, hiatal hernias, and cancers throughout the digestive tract.

_____ **8.** In a poisoning, the container and the remaining contents should never be taken with the patient to the hospital for fear of contaminating the emergency department.

_____ **9.** If the person decides to quit using stimulants, the likelihood that he or she will succeed over the long term is virtually nil. Sadly, the only way out of methamphetamine or cocaine addiction is often an early death.

_____ **10.** Patients who take lithium and nonsteroidal anti-inflammatory drugs (NSAIDs) have slowed renal clearance of the lithium, increasing the likelihood that they will inadvertently reach a toxic lithium level.

_____ **11.** Most patients who have swallowed caustic substances present with severe respiratory distress and pain in the mouth, throat, or chest.

_____ **12.** The primary goals when dealing with a patient who has inhaled hydrocarbons are to remove the patient from the noxious environment, give high-concentration supplemental oxygen, and promptly transport to the appropriate facility.

_____ **13.** When tricyclic antidepressants exert their toxic effects, the most common cause of death is cardiac arrhythmia.

_____ **14.** Field treatment of a salicylate overdose should include the "universal antidote."

_____ **15.** Ticks should only be removed with a scraping motion with an item such as a credit card to avoid squeezing the tick's body.

Short Answer

Complete this section with short written answers using the space provided.

1. List ten medical problems to which alcoholics are particularly susceptible.

a. _____

b. _____

c. _____

d. _____

e. _____

f. _____

g. _____

h. _____

i. _____

j. _____

Word Find

Hidden in the following grid are 13 words or phrases related to what you have studied in this chapter. Find the hidden words in the grid. Then, use the words from the grid to answer the following questions.

```
A A N J C I L S Z D C B T S C F H E
M N X O I Y K L A S A L C G B E S P
P A G Q I V A Z F R L I M A R O G B
H U S G D T E N B G T Y E O D L X S
E J Y E C A A I I O M R I R K I Q B
T I A D Y A T U C D P N E F I T J Q
A R Y C V U R R T Z E V R O T H M O
M A V F R L A B R I O Q P D J I R J
I M K A Y N W H O E B I L X W U Q S
N A T D P U V L T N J A M Y W M F C
E E D M C P I A D U M Y H M K T P Z
S X U K A L L L T L C O A S T W S S
K A B L G Y P K V J W X N I Z R S R
Y F G O C X S N O B R A C O R D Y H
V A S I L N H H W Y I N M Q X W H F
M P L N G I G H F B N L G S O I M Q
Y A C O C A I N E R R P V E F E D P
S E D A T I V E H Y P N O T I C S E
```

1. Speedball: _____ and _____

2. Weed, pot, dope, smoke: _____

3. Increases alertness and excitation: _____

4. Reds, yellows, yellow jackets, blues, blue heavens, rainbows: _____

5. Benzodiazepines: _____-_____

6. One of the most rapid-acting and deadly poisons: _____

7. Opiates, opioids: _____

8. Causes more poisoning deaths than any other substance: _____ _____

9. Found in a variety of products around the home, including cleaning and polishing products: _____

10. Cornerstone drug for the treatment of bipolar disorder: _____

11. Psychological dependence on a drug or drugs: _____

12. Ingestion of 150 mg/kg or less will usually make a person "mildly toxic": _____ _____

Fill-in-the-Table

Fill in the missing parts of the table.

1. Although it is advisable to consult Poison Control for definitive identification of any ingested substance, it is nonetheless worthwhile to have a general knowledge of the categories of poisons and some of the more commonly encountered examples of each category. Fill in the following table with examples of each type of poison mentioned.

Type of Poison	Examples
Strong acid	
Strong alkali	
Volatile hydrocarbon	
Toxic plant	

2. Fill in the amount of time it takes for the four stages of acetaminophen toxicity.

Signs and Symptoms of Acetaminophen Toxicity		
Stage	Timeframe	Signs and Symptoms
I		Nausea, vomiting, loss of appetite, pallor, malaise
II		Right upper quadrant abdominal pain; abdomen tender to palpation
III		Metabolic acidosis, renal failure, coagulopathies, recurring GI symptoms
IV		Recovery slowly begins, or liver failure progresses and the patient dies

CHAPTER

34 Hematologic Emergencies

Chapter Review

The following exercises provide an opportunity to test your knowledge of this chapter.

Matching

Match each of the items in the left column to the appropriate definition in the right column.

_____ **1.** Sickle cell disease	**A.** Red blood cells
_____ **2.** Leukopenia	**B.** Antigen classification given to blood
_____ **3.** Coagulation	**C.** Making an incision into a vein to take blood
_____ **4.** Erythrocytes	**D.** Bloody stool
_____ **5.** Neoplastic cells	**E.** Disease causing RBCs to be misshaped
_____ **6.** ABO system	**F.** Itching
_____ **7.** Hemoglobin	**G.** Iron-rich protein in blood that carries oxygen
_____ **8.** Phlebotomy	**H.** Clotting
_____ **9.** Melena	**I.** Term for cancer cells
_____ **10.** Pruritus	**J.** Reduction in the number of WBCs

Multiple Choice

Read each item carefully, and then select the best response.

_____ **1.** During the focused history and physical exam of hematologic patients, it is important to do all of the following EXCEPT:

    A. look for changes in LOC.

    B. obtain a SAMPLE history.

    C. obtain an ECG.

    D. interview the family; confidentiality rules dictate that the family not be present.

_____ **2.** Common findings with patients with blood disorders include which of the following?

    A. Bone fractures   **C.** "Clubbed" nails

    B. Mental health disorders   **D.** Epistaxis

_____ **3.** Assessment and management of patients with hemophilia include which of the following procedures?

    A. Controlling bleeding   **C.** Administering an analgesic

    B. Administering high-flow supplemental oxygen   **D.** All of the above

_____ **4.** The following organs assist in the production of red blood cells EXCEPT the:

    A. medulla.
    C. spleen.

    B. liver.
    D. bone marrow.

_____ **5.** The Rh antigen was first found in:

    A. pig cells.
    C. Rhesus monkeys.

    B. horse serum.
    D. cow liver.

_____ **6.** Which blood type is considered the universal donor?

    A. AB
    C. O

    B. A
    D. B

_____ **7.** Leukemia patients may have which of the following signs/symptoms?

    A. Frequent urinary tract infections
    C. Frequent bleeding

    B. No symptoms
    D. Spontaneous pneumothorax

_____ **8.** Disseminated intravascular coagulopathy (DIC):

    A. has a mortality rate of 75%.
    C. is rarely fatal.

    B. has a mortality rate of 10% to 15%.
    D. can be prevented with large fluid bolus.

_____ **9.** Assessment and management of patients with multiple myeloma include which of the following procedures?

    A. IV therapy using a BIG device
    C. Supplemental oxygen via CPAP

    B. Pain management
    D. Transport with PASG/MAST in place

_____ **10.** Blood performs which of the following functions?

    A. Transports oxygen from the lungs to the tissues
    C. Carries nutrients

    B. Ferries waste products
    D. All of the above

Labeling

Label the following diagrams with the correct terms.

    1. Label the main components of the body related to the blood system.

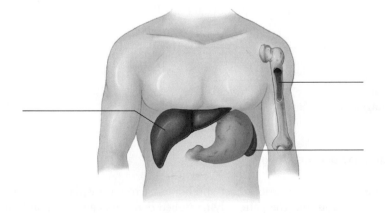

2. Label the red blood cells and sickle cells.

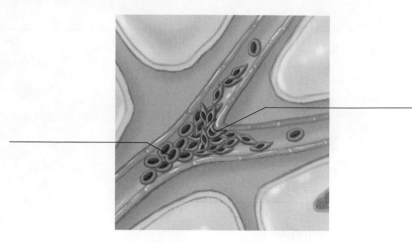

Fill-in-the-Blank

Read each item carefully, and then complete the statement by filling in the missing word(s).

1. Blood is the fluid of _____.

2. The _____ system includes blood components and the organs involved in their development and production.

3. The formed elements of blood include _____ _____ _____, _____

_____ _____, _____, and _____.

4. Red blood cell production occurs within _____ _____.

5. _____ _____, _____ _____, and _____ are three common blood tests

done on blood samples.

6. _____ are responsible for the clotting of blood.

7. _____ _____ disease is a bleeding disorder in which clotting occurs insufficiently.

8. The leading inherited blood disorder is called _____ _____ _____.

9. Leukemia patients frequently present with _____, _____, or _____.

10. Patients with lymphoma may require _____ management.

Identify

In the following case studies, list the chief complaint, vital signs, and pertinent negatives.

1. You are called to the home of a 42-year-old woman with a history of metastatic cancer and bone marrow transplant. Her chief complaint is extreme weakness, fatigue, and exertional dyspnea. You find the patient lying in bed conscious and alert, although she appears very "withdrawn" and weighs about 90 lb. She denies chest pain or shortness of breath. She tells you that she doesn't have any energy, and the doctor's office wants her back in the hospital. Her vital signs are as follows: pulse is 86 beats/min, slightly irregular, and difficult to palpate; blood pressure is also difficult to auscultate but appears to be 92/P mm Hg. Her skin is pale, warm, and dry. She has an oxygen saturation of 91% on ambient air. Her Pupils are Equal And Round, Regular in size, and are reactive to Light (PEARRL). She has a central IV port in place.

a. Chief Complaint

_____

_____

_____

b. Vital Signs

_____

_____

_____

c. Pertinent Negatives

_____

_____

_____

2. Your unit is dispatched to a priority one response to Middle of the Road Elementary School. The dispatch information indicates a 10-year-old boy with near syncope. Once inside the nurse's office, you recognize your patient. You've transported him several times in the past. For years, he's been treated for leukemia. His mom is on the scene, and she appears comforted to see a familiar face. She explains that he was just able to return to school full time after his latest round of treatments. As you speak to the patient, it's apparent that his mental status is slightly altered. However, when you ask him about his most favored topic, baseball, he becomes quite talkative. En route to the hospital his vital signs indicate that he is now conscious and fully alert. He doesn't remember the near syncope. His radial pulses are equal bilaterally and regular at 86 beats/min. He currently denies any complaints as the baseball conversation continues. Blood pressure is 98/64 mm Hg. His skin is jaundiced, but cool and dry. Pupils are Equal and Round, Regular in size, reactive to Light (PEARRL). His oxygen saturation is 98% on a nonrebreathing mask. The patient has central IV access. You contact medical control for direction and are told to continue transport while monitoring his ABCs. His IV will be activated in the ED.

a. Chief Complaint

_____

_____

_____

b. Vital Signs

_____

_____

_____

c. Pertinent Negatives

_____

_____

_____

3. It's been a rather busy day with mostly routine emergency calls. However, this call is a little different. A man with a history of sickle cell disease is having an acute crisis and is in extreme pain. He states that the pain is breaking through his oral morphine tablets and fentanyl transdermal patch. He states that his pain is a 9 on a 1 to 10 scale for pain. He states that it's the worst sickle cell pain that he's ever had. His vital signs are pulse of 112 beats/min and regular; skin pale, warm, and moist; and a blood pressure of 148/96 mm Hg. Pupils are Equal and Round, Regular in size and reactive to Light (PEARRL). His pulse oximetry is 91%. He is anxious and keeps telling you to "get the rubber on the road."

a. Chief Complaint

_____

_____

b. Vital Signs

_____

_____

_____

c. Pertinent Negatives

_____

_____

_____

Ambulance Calls

The following case scenarios provide an opportunity to explore the concerns associated with patient management and paramedic care. Read each scenario, and then answer each question.

1. You are transporting a patient from the local community hospital to a regional trauma center. The patient's vital signs are stable when you start the transport. He has a unit of blood running. Shortly after you set out, the patient begins complaining of severe back pain. Soon thereafter he breaks out in a cold sweat, his lips take on a bluish tinge, and his neck veins seem to bulge out. You check his pulse, and it is 60 beats/min. A few minutes later, when you check it again, it is 110 beats/min.

a. The patient is showing signs of a/an:

(1) allergic reaction to the transfusion.

(2) hemolytic reaction to the transfusion.

(3) air embolism.

(4) pyrogenic reaction to the transfusion.

(5) thrombophlebitis.

b. List the steps you will take to deal with the situation.

(1) _____

(2) _____

(3) _____

(4) _____

2. Your crew receives a call for a 16-year-old boy with a severe hemorrhage. On arrival you find the patient's 19-year-old sister hysterical on the front porch. She states that her brother is "bleeding to death." She is too excited and emotional to provide any additional information. You enter the house and are directed to the bathroom. You are met by a rather pleasant but obviously frustrated 16-year-old boy. There is a minimal amount of blood in the sink. He is holding a tissue to his carotid region and states that he cut himself shaving. He is very apologetic for and embarrassed about his sister's behavior. He states that he has a history of von Willebrand disease and he wears a MedicAlert® bracelet.

a. What is von Willebrand disease and what are some of the symptoms?

_____

_____

_____

_____

b. How would you treat a patient that exhibits signs and symptoms of von Willebrand disease? What broad class of diseases does this fall under?

_____

_____

_____

_____

_____

_____

_____

_____

_____

_____

_____

True/False

If you believe the statement to be more true than false, write the letter "T" in the space provided. If you believe the statement to be more false than true, write the letter "F."

_____ **1.** White blood cells are responsible for transporting oxygenated blood.

_____ **2.** Red blood cell production occurs in the pancreas.

_____ **3.** "Clot busters" activate the fibrinolytic system, resulting in clot decomposition.

_____ **4.** The "universal donor" is a person with AB blood type.

_____ **5.** Malignant diseases that occur within the lymphoid system are called lymphomas.

_____ **6.** Phlebotomy is the treatment of choice for patients with disseminated intravascular coagulopathy.

_____ **7.** In multiple myeloma, abnormal plasma cells infiltrate the bone marrow.

_____ **8.** Patients with hematologic diseases might have symptoms that include vertigo, fatigue, or syncopal episodes.

_____ **9.** Oxygen is generally contraindicated for patients with red blood cell abnormalities.

_____ **10.** Paramedics should be compassionate providers, especially to patients with blood disorders.

Short Answer

Complete this section with short written answers using the space provided.

1. Blood disorders present differently from other typical injuries and diseases encountered by paramedics. Please provide some of the common findings as they relate to the following organs and systems:

   a. Skin

   _____

   _____

   _____

   _____

   b. Gastrointestinal tract

   _____

   _____

   _____

   _____

   c. Cardiovascular system

   _____

   _____

   _____

   _____

2. Assessment and treatment of patients with blood disorders may differ slightly from assessment and treatment of patients with more typical diseases encountered by paramedics. Please describe how the treatment and assessment of the following diseases differ.

   a. Leukemia

   _____

   _____

   _____

   _____

b. Hemophilia

_____

_____

_____

_____

_____

c. Polycythemia

_____

_____

_____

_____

_____

3. Provide definitions for the following terms:

a. Leukopenia

_____

b. Polycythemia

_____

c. ABO system

_____

d. Reticuloendothelial system

_____

e. Pruritus

_____

f. Hematocrit

_____

g. Melena

_____

Word Find

Hidden in the following grid are 18 words or phrases related to what you have studied in this chapter. Find the hidden words in the grid below. Then use the words from the grid to answer the following questions (some words may be used to answer more than one of the questions).

```
R O B Y S O Q Y E B X T E R W S A S H
L E L O I N H F A Z H H S Y L I I T E
E X D M N T E S T R C T A L I S M E M
G H Z R M E O G O L I Z E E K A E M A
R O T Q O P M M I R D C S Y N T K C T
A C A X H S B A C T D K I X C S U E O
J G U I E O I O R O N A D D A O E L P
K T L C C F T D O R M A L A U E L L O
V S B Y Q A S L C S O B L L N M E S I
I U T D M O B W A I O W E Y X O R T E
L E U E H E Z L T K T C C W I H D V T
S I H E T S P L E E N Y E C Z A P A I
W M V I U N I V E R S A L D O N O R C
C H H E M O G L O B I N K O E R O G M
L W Q Z R N P O F Q J W C V M J M L J
A I M E H T Y C Y L O P I C R E D Z P
S A M O H P M Y L N T S S B P R H X R
E R Z R W T G G C R I C U D I Z S X U
R O N M D T T T S A A V A S G P S Y T
```

1. Blood is made up of two main components, _____ and formed elements (cells).

2. The _____ system is the blood components and the organs involved in their development and production.

3. RBC production occurs within _____ _____.

4. The three laboratory tests commonly performed on blood are RBC count, hemoglobin level, and _____.

5. The patient's blood is considered balanced if the _____ level is one third of the hematocrit and the RBC count is one third of the hemoglobin level.

6. Leukocytes are _____ _____ _____.

7. Platelets are _____.

8. _____ are also known as MAST cells.

9. The bone marrow, liver, and _____ are the major players of the hematologic system.

10. The _____ _____ is the primary site for cell production.

11. As old RBCs enter the _____, they are broken down into bile.

12. If a patient has blood type O, that person is considered to be a/an _____ _____.

13. Substances identified as foreign to the body are _____.

14. The body works within a close balance, referred to as _____.

15. A disorder related to the breakdown of RBCs is _____ _____.

16. The leading inherited blood disorder is _____ _____ _____.

17. _____ is a disease that develops in the lymphoid system.

18. An overabundance or overproduction of RBCs is _____.

Fill-in-the-Table

Fill in the missing parts of the table.

Complete the table with the proper blood donor types.

Blood Types			
Blood Type	ABO Antigens	ABO Antibodies	Acceptable Blood Donor Types
A	A	Anti-B	
B	B	Anti-A	
AB	A, B	None	
O	None	Anti-A Anti-B	

CHAPTER

35 Environmental Emergencies

Chapter Review

The following exercises provide an opportunity to test your knowledge of this chapter.

Matching

Place the letters **HP** next to the factors that increase heat production and the letters **HL** next to factors that predispose heat loss.

_____ **1.** Wind chill

_____ **2.** Physical exertion

_____ **3.** Impaired judgment from drugs or alcohol

_____ **4.** Diabetic peripheral neuropathies

_____ **5.** Hyperthyroidism

_____ **6.** Response to infection

_____ **7.** Wet clothes

_____ **8.** Drug overdoses such as cocaine, caffeine, Ecstasy

_____ **9.** Cold water drowning

_____ **10.** Vasodilatation from acute spinal injury

_____ **11.** Agitated and tremulous state (such as from Parkinson's disease or drug withdrawal)

Multiple Choice

Read each item carefully, and then select the best response.

_____ **1.** Heat syncope is seen in nonacclimated people who may be under heat stress and typically occurs in all the following situations EXCEPT:

    A. standing suddenly.   **C.** prolonged standing.

    B. mass outdoor gatherings.   **D.** after swimming on a very hot day.

_____ **2.** The major contributors to the basal metabolism rate (BMR), the heat energy produced at rest from normal body metabolic reactions, are:

    A. spleen and lungs.   **C.** liver and skeletal muscles.

    B. kidneys and heart.   **D.** kidneys and gall bladder.

_____ **3.** The loss of heat that takes place when moving air picks up heat and carries it away is:

    A. evaporation.   **C.** radiation.

    B. convection.   **D.** conduction.

_____ **4.** A call to the scene of an outdoor high school track meet is for a 15-year-old student who was running the mile race. It is a humid day with the temperature in the 90s. The patient presents with muscle pain in the lower extremities and abdomen. Based on these symptoms, what is the most likely problem?

    A. Heat cramps   **C.** Heat stroke
    B. Heat exhaustion   **D.** Heat syncope

_____ **5.** You are called to an apartment building on a hot July afternoon for a bedridden 78-year-old woman. Upon entering the apartment, you notice that it is extremely hot, and the patient is very warm with dry skin. The SAMPLE history identifies that the patient has congestive heart failure (CHF) and is taking beta-blockers and diuretics. Her blood glucose is normal. You should suspect:

    A. exertional heat stroke.   **C.** neuroleptic malignant syndrome.
    B. malignant hyperthermia.   **D.** classic heat stroke.

_____ **6.** Each of the following factors increase heat loss EXCEPT:

    A. vasoconstriction.   **C.** alcohol.
    B. wet clothes.   **D.** diabetic neuropathies.

_____ **7.** What unique finding might be observed on an ECG of a patient with a low core body temperature?

    A. Alterans   **C.** Spiked waves
    B. Osborn waves   **D.** Inverted T waves

_____ **8.** You are called to a local boat dock for a patient returning from a scuba dive. His dive computer shows the maximum depth was 120 feet. The patient is reported by his buddy to have had inappropriate behavior while getting ready to ascend. The ascent was controlled with a safety stop for a few minutes at around 20 feet. Back in the dive boat, the patient complained of tingling in his lips and legs. He has no other reported symptoms. You most likely suspect that the patient may have a mild case of:

    A. arterial gas embolism.   **C.** pulmonary overpressurization syndrome.
    B. nitrogen narcosis.   **D.** barotitis externa.

_____ **9.** You are dispatched to the pool at a private residence for an unconscious teenager. Upon arrival you are told that he was competing with a friend to see who could hold his breath underwater the longest. He was swimming underwater, and while coming to the surface, went limp and was pulled from the water. You find the patient is breathing, and you administer supplemental oxygen and continue with an assessment. What do you expect is the patient's problem?

    A. Decompression sickness   **C.** Shallow water blackout
    B. Barotrauma   **D.** Bends

_____ **10.** Deep frostbite usually involves the hands or feet, and the extremity may initially exhibit all of the following colors EXCEPT:

    A. white.   **C.** mottled blue-white.
    B. yellow-white.   **D.** gangrene.

Labeling
Label the following diagrams with the correct terms.

1. Label the appropriate physiologic responses to the hot or cold environment when the hypothalamus is stimulated.

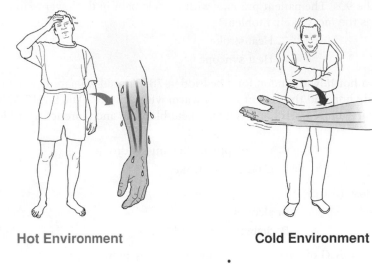

Hot Environment   **Cold Environment**

•   •

•   •

•   •

Body temperature *decreases*   Body temperature *increases*

Fill-in-the-Blank
Read each item carefully, and then complete the statement by filling in the missing word(s).

1. The core temperature of the human body at any given moment represents a balance between the heat produced by the body and the heat shed by the body.

   a. List the potential sources of body heat and the mechanisms by which body heat can be dissipated.

   Sources of Body Heat   **Ways of Shedding Heat**

   (1) _____   (1) _____

   (2) _____   (2) _____

   (3) _____   (3) _____

   (4) _____

   b. The body's mechanisms for dissipating excess heat have certain limitations. First, all of the mechanisms depend on

   _____ _____ to shunt blood from the core to the body surface. Furthermore, to be effective, three

   of the body's cooling mechanisms require a temperature gradient between the body and the outside. None of these three

   mechanisms—_____, _____, or _____—can work if the outside temperature is not at

   least a few degrees cooler than the body core. Finally, one of the body's cooling mechanisms is dependent on the ambient humidity. When the humidity is high, that mechanism—namely, _____ _____ _____—is

ineffective in lowering the core temperature.

c. A hatless hiker standing still on a mountaintop on a windless day loses heat from his head by _____.

A breeze picks up. Now the hiker loses heat by _____ as well.

d. A white-water enthusiast who capsizes his canoe in a swift-running river loses body heat by _____.

e. A soldier on maneuvers in the desert in ambient temperatures of more than 37.7°C (100°F) can shed heat only by

_____ _____ _____.

Identify

In the following case studies, list the chief complaint, vital signs, and pertinent negatives.

1. You are riding on Squad 5 and are dispatched to a person who fell through the ice at a local pond. Upon arrival, you find an 18-year-old man who is shivering with a blanket wrapped around him. It is reported that a Good Samaritan threw a rope and helped the patient get to shore. When you question the patient, he says that he was trying to walk home and didn't realize he had gotten lost. There is a smell of alcohol on the patient's breath. You immediately place the patient in your squad and turn the heat on high. The wet clothes are removed and the patient is wrapped in a number of blankets. He is placed on supplemental oxygen and a cardiac monitor. The ECG rhythm is regular, and you observe Osborne waves. You establish an IV using warm crystalloid solution. The patient is transferred to the regional trauma center that is 15 minutes away. You continue to monitor the patient and perform an ongoing assessment. You take vital signs every 5 minutes.

a. Chief Complaint

_____

_____

_____

b. Vital Signs

_____

_____

_____

c. Pertinent Negatives

_____

_____

_____

d. What three pieces of information that are not included in this scenario would be helpful to know?

(1) _____

(2) _____

(3) _____

e. Based on this scenario, which of the following four methods of heat loss is most responsible for the greatest amount of heat lost by this patient?

A. Radiation	**C.**	Convection	
B. Conduction	**D.**	Evaporation	

f. You determine the patient is moderately hypothermic. How much IV fluid should you infuse initially?

_____

_____

Ambulance Calls

The following case scenarios provide an opportunity to explore the concerns associated with patient management and paramedic care. Read each scenario, and then answer each question.

1. At morning briefing, you are told that you will be doing a stand-by at an outdoor festival at a local college campus. These assignments are usually boring, but you will make the best of it. It is a very hot and humid day in late spring, and except for a few scrapes and blisters you have little request for service. The concert has been going for about an hour when you are called to a person who has passed out. When you arrive, you find an unresponsive man about 20 years old. His friends tell you that he had been standing listening to the concert and suddenly fell. As you are assessing the patient, he starts to regain consciousness. You can tell he has been drinking. You ask how many beers he had, and he tells you he drank two. In your mind, you at least double that number. You load the patient into the ambulance and turn up the air conditioner. The assessment indicates dehydration.

   a. What is the probable cause of the syncopal episode, and what may be some contributing underlying causes?

   _____

   _____

   _____

   _____

   b. How would you mange this patient?

   _____

   _____

   _____

   _____

   c. If the patient does not recover and stabilize quickly, what may be another presenting problem to consider?

   _____

   _____

   _____

   _____

2. You are called to the local high school playing field on a hot, sticky August afternoon to deal with a "casualty" of preseason training—a 16-year-old fullback who "became crazy" during practice. You see him over near the goalposts, where several of his teammates are trying to restrain him. "None of my boys ever messed around with drugs before," the coach tells you, "and I sure never would have pegged Chuck as a junkie. But I don't know how else to explain his behavior. He's been touchy all afternoon, and he just started acting crazy."

   You find the fullback agitated and combative. He seems completely disoriented. His skin is warm and sweaty. His vital signs are as follows: a pulse of 120 beats/min and bounding, respirations are 30 breaths/min and shallow, and blood pressure is 150/90 mm Hg, and oral temperature is 41.7°C (107°F). The pupils are widely dilated and react only sluggishly to light.

   a. This boy is most likely suffering from _____.

b. List the steps in managing this case.

(1) _____

(2) _____

(3) _____

(4) _____

(5) _____

(6) _____

(7) _____

3. The following day, it is even hotter, but mercifully the humidity has dropped considerably. You are called to the very same playing field for another casualty of preseason training, this time a 14-year-old running back. You find him lying at midfield writhing in pain. "I swear I didn't clip him," one of the other players is insisting. "I didn't even get near him. He just fell down by himself."

"Sure, sure," says the coach, who is trying to massage the cramps out of the boy's legs. When you ask the boy what his problem is, he just moans and says, "My legs, my legs."

On examination, his skin is cool and sweaty. His pulse is 100 beats/min and regular, respirations are 30 breaths/min and shallow, blood pressure is 110/70 mm Hg, and oral temperature is 37°C (98.6°F). There are no signs of injury to the extremities.

a. This boy is most likely suffering from _____ .

b. List the steps in managing this case.

(1) _____

(2) _____

(3) _____

(4) _____

4. "As long as you folks are already here," says the coach, "maybe you could take a look at our quarterback. I think he's coming down with something, and I have to decide whether to send him home."

You find the quarterback sitting on the bench looking quite miserable. He says that his girlfriend has mononucleosis, and he thinks he may be coming down with it too because he feels very tired and achy. On examination, he is sweating profusely, and his skin feels clammy. His pulse is 110 beats/min and somewhat weak, respirations are 28 breaths/min and shallow, blood pressure is 100/60 mm Hg, and oral temperature is 39.4°C (103°F).

a. This boy is most likely suffering from _____ .

b. List the steps in managing this case.

(1) _____

(2) _____

(3) _____

(4) _____

(5) _____

c. What advice should you give the football coach?

_____

_____

_____

_____

5. On the very same day, you are called to a local supermarket for a "sick baby." You arrive to find a nearly hysterical woman who looks scarcely out of her teens holding a comatose baby. "I just left her in the car for a minute while I ran in to buy a couple of things," she says, although you note three full shopping bags in the woman's cart. The baby, a 6-month-old, is unconscious (AVPU = U). The pulse is 180 beats/min, respirations are 60 breaths/min, and blood pressure is 100/80 mm Hg. The rectal temperature is 43.3°C (110°F).

a. This baby is most likely suffering from _____.

b. List the steps in managing this case.

(1) _____

(2) _____

(3) _____

(4) _____

(5) _____

(6) _____

(7) _____

6. You are enjoying a week off at a mountain ski resort. On your first morning there, the manager of the resort asks for volunteers to join a search-and-rescue party that is going out to look for three skiers who failed to return to the lodge the previous night. You, of course, volunteer, and you set off with a team on skis to comb the slopes. You are all carrying two-way radios so that you can summon a snowmobile to help transport the lost skiers if you find them. Eventually, you locate two of the skiers, about 15 miles from the ski lodge, dug into a makeshift shelter in the snow (and unaware that only about 50 meters away, beyond a stand of trees, is an empty cabin). Both skiers are alert.

a. The first skier tells you that he lost all sensation in his left leg sometime during the night. On examination the leg is white, cold, and very hard. He is most likely suffering from _____.

b. Describe how you would manage this patient.

(1) _____

(2) _____

(3) _____

(4) _____

(5) _____

c. The second skier says, "I think I've got the same problem in my left foot." On examination, the foot has a waxy, white appearance. The skin feels very stiff, but there is "give" underneath when you press down hard on the skin. He is most likely suffering from _____.

d. How would you manage *this* patient?

(1) _____

(2) _____

(3) _____

(4) _____

(5) _____

e. Not long after those two skiers have been evacuated on stretchers by snowmobile, you find the third skier. He is sitting up against a tree, unconscious. Apparently, he did not realize that he had come within a 100 meters of the main road. His skin is very cold. You cannot detect any pulse. His pupils are dilated and unreactive. He does seem to be breathing, although only about once or twice a minute. You radio for a paramedic-staffed ambulance to meet you at the road. What is this patient suffering from? _____

f. Describe the management of this patient until the ambulance comes and en route to the hospital.

(1) _____

(2) _____

(3) _____

(4) _____

(5) _____

(6) _____

(7) _____

(8) _____

7. You and your crew are at the local lake on a chilly November afternoon, covering an annual speedboat race that invariably produces a few minor casualties (mostly from indigestion among the picnicking spectators). Making a hairpin turn at high speed, one of the speedboats capsizes. After what seems like a very long time, you see the boat's driver bob to the surface of the water (he is wearing a life jacket) and begins swimming for shore. Describe the actions you should take in this situation.

a. _____

b. _____

c. _____

d. _____

e. _____

f. _____

g. _____

h. _____

8. During the first spell of bitter cold weather of the season, you are called to the downtown bus terminal for a "man down." When you reach the scene, a police officer waves you over. "Sorry to bother you folks with this," he says. "Just a vagrant who's been sleeping in the place for a few days, and probably all he needs is a night in the lockup to sober up." You find the patient, being restrained by another police officer, over in a corner. His speech is slurred, and he staggers when he tries to walk. His breath smells of wine. His skin is pale and cold.

a. List at least three diagnoses you must consider in this case.

(1) _____

(2) _____

(3) _____

b. In view of the diagnostic possibilities, describe how you would manage this case.

(1) _____

(2) _____

(3) _____

(4) _____

(5) _____

(6) _____

(7) _____

9. You decide to take a week's vacation to do some climbing in the Canadian Rockies. Of course, you are carrying a medical kit because it's hard for you to accept the idea that you are *really* on vacation. On your first day out, one of your buddies starts complaining of a headache—"probably because I didn't sleep really well last night," he says. You're a little concerned that he might be suffering from the altitude, but he shrugs it off and insists that you all keep going.

a. At that point, how could you check if your friend is suffering from a serious case of acute altitude sickness?

_____

_____

_____

_____

b. As things turn out, you decide to continue climbing. About an hour later, you feel a tug on the rope and look back to see your friend really dragging. He seems out of breath. Now you're really concerned. List four signs or symptoms that would suggest your friend may be suffering from high-altitude pulmonary edema.

(1) _____

(2) _____

(3) _____

(4) _____

c. Assuming that you do find signs of high-altitude pulmonary edema, what steps should you take to treat your friend?

(1) _____

(2) _____

(3) _____

10. When your next vacation comes up, you decide you won't make the same mistake twice: no more mountains where emergencies will spoil your relaxation. Instead, you sign up for a cruise to the West Indies—a week of sun and sand and steel drum bands. On the ship with you are a group of scuba enthusiasts, who don't miss any opportunity to explore the local coral reefs each time you anchor.

One fine afternoon, as you are sunning yourself on deck with a rum swizzle in hand, you hear a commotion off to the starboard side of the ship. You leap from your chair and peer over the rail to see some of the diving crowd in a state of agitation in the rubber raft from which they've been diving. One of their number is lying motionless in the raft, and another two are just emerging from the water and climbing into the raft to join them. The captain, meanwhile, having spotted the situation, has already lowered a winch to bring up the raft and everyone in it.

As soon as the divers are back aboard the ship, you race to the side of the diver who is unconscious. His friends tell you that he was the least experienced of their group. He had surfaced first, and a minute or so after being pulled onto the raft, he complained of chest pain and his voice had sounded funny. Then, he just blacked out.

a. What do you think has happened to this diver?

_____

_____

_____

_____

b. What steps should you take to manage this situation?

(1) _____

(2) _____

(3) _____

(4) _____

(5) _____

(6) _____

c. About an hour later, while you are monitoring the condition of the diver pending more definitive treatment, you hear one of his friends who was in the water with him saying to another member of the group, "Gee, my back is sure killing me. I must have pulled a muscle when I did my back flip off the raft. The hell of it is that I can't pee either." You perk up your ears when you hear that because that bit of information makes you suspect that the speaker has suffered:

_____.

True/False

If you believe the statement to be more true than false, write the letter "T" in the space provided. If you believe the statement to be more false than true, write the letter "F."

_____ **1.** A superficial frostbitten extremity is best warmed in front of a campfire or heater.

_____ **2.** In deep frostbite, the extremity feels cold and rock hard.

_____ **3.** If rescue circumstances require it, a patient with deep frostbite may walk on a frostbitten leg without causing major additional damage to the limb.

_____ **4.** Antibiotic ointment should be applied gently over frostbitten areas to prevent infection.

_____ **5.** A frostbitten extremity will be excruciatingly painful until it is rewarmed.

_____ **6.** Frost nip most often affects the tips of the ears, nose, fingers, and toes.

_____ **7.** Heat exhaustion is a clinical syndrome thought to represent a milder form of heat illness on a continuum leading to heat stroke.

_____ **8.** Classic heat stroke is less apt to affect older patients with chronic illnesses.

_____ **9.** Patients with heat stroke usually have dilated pupils.

_____ **10.** Radiation accounts for more than 65% of heat loss in a cooler setting.

Short Answer

Complete this section with short written answers using the space provided.

1. The body's normal response to entering a hot environment can place considerable stress on a person who has a limited cardiovascular reserve. Explain why.

_____

_____

_____

_____

2. Anyone can succumb to a heat wave, but some people are more vulnerable than others. List five factors that increase a person's risk of suffering significant heat illness in response to heat stress.

   a. _____

   b. _____

   c. _____

   d. _____

   e. _____

3. Paramedics, like other public safety personnel, do not have the luxury of postponing heavy exertion until weather conditions are favorable; they must do their job whatever the weather, which means they may be exposed to a significant risk of heat illness during periods of high temperature.

   a. List five measures you can take to reduce your risk of becoming ill from the heat.

   (1) _____

   (2) _____

   (3) _____

   (4) _____

   (5) _____

   b. If you do start to experience early symptoms of heat illness, you must stop your activities immediately. But to do so, you need to be able to recognize the warning symptoms of heat illness when they occur. List four warning symptoms of heat illness.

   (1) _____

   (2) _____

   (3) _____

   (4) _____

4. No one would ever suffer cold injury if they simply heeded the advice of their mother. Mothers always know, even without taking a paramedic course, how to keep warm on cold days. Following are several statements you have heard at least once from Mother. Each statement reflects an intuitive knowledge of the ways in which the body generates and loses heat. For each statement, explain why Mother was right.

   a. "Don't go out without a hat and scarf; it's freezing out there."

   Mother was right because:

   _____

b. "Stop rolling around in the snow. You'll get a death of a chill."
Mother was right because:

_____

c. "Get out of those wet clothes this minute."
Mother was right because:

_____

d. "Those skates are much too tight. Your toes will fall off."
Mother was right because:

_____

e. "Make sure you wear your windbreaker. It's blowing a gale out there."
Mother was right because:

_____

f. "Eat. Eat. You have to have something to keep going in this weather."
Mother was right because:

_____

5. In addition to Mother's advice, the body has only a limited repertoire of defenses against the cold. List three ways the body can defend itself against a drop in core temperature.

a. _____

b. _____

c. _____

6. Although anyone can suffer cold injury, certain factors *predispose* a person to suffer ill effects from the cold.
a. List four factors that predispose a person to suffer frostbite when exposed to freezing conditions.

(1) _____

(2) _____

(3) _____

(4) _____

b. List four factors that predispose a person to suffer hypothermia.

(1) _____

(2) _____

(3) _____

(4) _____

7. The stories that many of us learned as children contain many cautionary tales about cold exposure.

a. When the three little kittens lost their mittens, they became most vulnerable to _____.

b. Sitting on an ice-cold tuffet on a winter day, Little Miss Muffet was losing heat from her body by _____.

c. Who is at greater risk of suffering hypothermia—Jack Sprat or his wife? _____

d. Before venturing outside to try out his new ice skates, little Jack Horner retreated to a corner and ate his Christmas pie. Was that a good idea? Why or why not?

_____

_____

e. Swinging about in the treetop is baby in his cradle. When the wind blows, the cradle will rock. Furthermore, when the wind blows, baby will lose heat from his body by the process called _____.

Word Find

Hidden in the following grid are 25 words or phrases related to what you have studied in this chapter. Find the hidden words in the grid. Then, use the words from the grid to answer the following questions.

```
W Z U T G A C E W C X F E A P L V
Q I M A T N N L I M H Z A L I A L
N K N A X E I L A Y E I P T N T O
N O X D R P O N B S M C H I T N R
I I I G C B O L W R S E R T S E T
A V N S A H A R E O R I P U O M H
H A Q T S C I H D M R R C D R N O
G O E T K E T L O R K D R E F O S
E M M O Q R R L L W E L S W Z R T
D R U E E H Y P O N A T R E M I A
U T O P O S G M M N R N F S G V T
T C Y B I S C O A O R D J A K N I
I H S S K S T N A R C O S I S E C
S Y M E J L Z A V E Z E B Q L R Y
S N O I T A R U T A S C D S H O T
A O X R A D I A T I O N F F O C R
L H L A R B E R E C S P M A R C H
```

1. _____ is caused at least in part by the return of cold blood from the body surface to the body core.

2. _____ illness is caused by the effects of hypobaric hypoxia on the central nervous system (CNS) and pulmonary system as a result of unacclimatized people ascending to altitude.

3. Inability to coordinate the muscles properly; the word often used to describe a staggering gait is _____.

4. Shallow water _____ occurs when a person hyperventilates just before submerging underwater and loses consciousness before resurfacing.

5. High-altitude _____ edema is altitude illness in which there is a change in mental status and/or ataxia.

6. _____ heat stroke usually occurs during heat waves and is most likely to strike the very old, very young, or bedridden persons.

7. The temperature in the part of the body that includes the heart, lungs, and brain is called _____ body temperature.

8. Heat _____ are acute and involuntary muscle pains, usually in the lower extremities and abdomen, and occur as a result of profuse sweating and sodium loss.

9. _____ sickness refers to a broad range of signs and symptoms caused by nitrogen bubbles in blood and tissues coming out of solution during ascent.

10. _____ is the process of experiencing respiratory impairment from immersion in liquid.

11. _____ emergencies are medical conditions caused or worsened by weather, terrain, or unique atmospheric conditions.

12. Early frostbite, characterized by numbness and pallor without significant tissue damage, is called _____.

13. _____ is permanent cell death.

14. _____ refers to body processes that balance the supply and demand of the body's needs.

15. Malignant _____ can occur as a result of common anesthesia medications, notably succinylcholine.

16. A concept closely related to sodium-depleted heat exhaustion is exertional _____.

17. Condition of listlessness and fatigue is called _____.

18. The liver and skeletal muscles are major contributors to the basal _____ rate.

19. Nitrogen _____ is the state of altered mental status caused by breathing compressed air (including nitrogen) at depth.

20. Blood pressure drop when the patient tries to sit or stand from the recumbent position is called _____ hypotension.

21. A unique wave seen on an ECG with hypothermic patients is called a J wave or _____ wave.

22. _____ is the transfer of heat by electromagnetic waves, accounting for more than 65% of body heat lost in a cooler setting.

23. _____ diving is when the diver remains at depth for prolonged periods.

24. The release of stored heat and energy from the body is called _____.

25. The _____ factor measures the chilling effect of a given temperature at a given wind speed.

Fill-in-the-Table

Fill in the missing parts of the table.

Hypothermia affects every system in the body. In the following table, list some of the effects of a drop in core temperature on each body system mentioned.

Body System	Effects of Hypothermia
Central nervous system	
Cardiovascular system	
Respiratory system	
Muscular system	
Metabolic system	

CHAPTER

36 Infectious and Communicable Diseases

Chapter Review

The following exercises provide an opportunity to test your knowledge of this chapter.

Matching

Match each of the items in the left column to the appropriate term in the right column.

_____ **1.** Time during which a person is capable of transmitting a disease to someone else	**A.** Reservoir
_____ **2.** Local or systemic disease process caused by a microorganism	**B.** Carrier
_____ **3.** Inanimate object that can transmit disease microorganisms from one person to another	**C.** Fomite
	D. Incubation period
_____ **4.** Place where microorganisms live and multiply	**E.** Communicable period
_____ **5.** Time between exposure to a microorganism and the development of symptoms	**F.** Nosocomial
_____ **6.** Relating to a hospital or other health care setting	**G.** Contamination
_____ **7.** Presence of harmful microorganisms on or in a person, animal, or object	**H.** Infection
_____ **8.** One who harbors an infectious agent and can transmit it to others, although the person is not ill	**I.** Skin
	J. Bloodborne diseases
_____ **9.** Primary barrier that prevents infections	
_____ **10.** Hepatitis, HIV	

Multiple Choice

Read each item carefully, and then select the best response.

_____ **1.** Agencies responsible for protecting public health include the following EXCEPT:

    A. OSHA.
    B. CDC.
    C. state health departments.
    D. National Sanitary Foundation.

_____ **2.** Communicable diseases may be transmitted by:

    A. indirect contact.
    B. inhalation.
    C. vectors.
    D. all of the above.

_____ **3.** Host resistance refers to:

    A. drug-resistant antibiotics.
    B. bloodborne pathogens infecting a weak immune system.
    C. virulence of the invading microorganism.
    D. period of contagiousness.

_____ **4.** Which of the following best defines the Ryan White law?

    A. Federally mandated Designated Infection Control Officer

    B. Part of the postexposure reporting network

    C. Notified within 48 hours after a workplace exposure

    D. Federal law

_____ **5.** Personal protective equipment (PPE) needs to be worn when a paramedic is working in the following situations EXCEPT:

    A. at a collision scene.   **C.** while treating contaminated patients.

    B. at a multiple-casualty incident (MCI).   **D.** only while working in the "clinical setting."

_____ **6.** Most exposures to health care workers in the prehospital setting occur:

    A. by needlestick injuries.   **C.** because exposure to infected droplets.

    B. because of broken glass at crash scenes.   **D.** when using pocket masks without other barriers.

_____ **7.** A comprehensive exposure plan for employees includes:

    A. mandatory drug and alcohol testing.

    B. anonymous blood tests.

    C. CDC-recommended vaccinations.

    D. identifying "at-risk populations" in your response area.

_____ **8.** Most droplets and airborne disease exposures can be prevented by:

    A. placing a mask on patients with fevers and rashes.

    B. doing nothing; confining the patient's face may exacerbate secretions.

    C. the crew wearing level III biohazard suits.

    D. notifying the hospital in advance and having the patient decontaminated prior to admission.

_____ **9.** All of the following are highly communicable viral diseases EXCEPT:

    A. measles.   **C.** pertussis.

    B. mumps.   **D.** meningitis.

_____ **10.** Lice and scabies infections may affect:

    A. patients.   **C.** crews.

    B. families.   **D.** All of the above.

Fill-in-the-Blank

Read each item carefully, and then complete the statement by filling in the missing word(s).

1. _____ _____ is the term used to describe infection control practices that reduce the opportunity of an exposure to occur in the daily care of patients.

2. A paramedic's major protective measure is _____.

3. Unfortunately, paramedics get exposed to communicable diseases. The third line of defense is considered _____

    _____-_____.

4. Paramedics treating patients with suspected infectious diseases should first focus on _____-_____ _____.

5. Mononucleosis is caused by the _____-_____ virus. Transmission occurs via direct contact with _____

    secretions.

6. Paramedics who work while infected with the cold or flu could endanger patients who are _____.

7. Gonorrhea, syphilis, herpes, and HIV are all considered _____ _____ _____.

8. An inflammation of the liver that may be produced by five distinct forms of virus is called _____ _____.

9. MRSA is believed to be transmitted from _____ to _____ via _____ hands.

10. Severe Acute Respiratory Syndrome (SARS) arose from the merger of viruses from _____and _____.

Identify

In the following case studies, list the chief complaint, vital signs, and pertinent negatives.

1. Your unit is called to the airport to meet an inbound flight. There is a patient reported to have flulike symptoms that include fever, chills, and dry cough. The patient is conscious and alert but very weak. He is assisted from the aircraft when it arrives at the terminal gate. You note that the flight appears to be domestic in origin. While you are taking the patient's history, he denies any type of international travel but has been traveling extensively this past week. He denies other previous medical history. He denies medications and allergies to medications or prescription drugs. His skin is warm and dry. He feels febrile. After further discussion, you discover that his school-aged children were recently sick with a viral infection. His vital signs are respiratory rate of 20 breaths/min and oxygen saturation on ambient air is 95%, pulse is 106 beats/min and regular, and blood pressure is 128/68 mm Hg.

a. Chief Complaint

_____

_____

_____

b. Vital Signs

_____

_____

_____

c. Pertinent Negatives

_____

_____

_____

2. It's a hot, humid day in the mid 90s and your advanced life support unit is dispatched to assist the police department. You arrive on-scene to discover several patrol vehicles located outside an unkempt house. You are met by one of the officers who explains that the police department received a call from an out-of-town relative to check on the welfare of the elderly resident. Once inside the house, the police officers noticed a severe lice infestation. Many of the officers are exposed to the nasty critters. Although the exposure is not life-threatening, the officers appear annoyed. They describe the conditions as squalid. You request that the exposed officers assist the elderly patient out to his front yard so that you can properly decontaminate him and minimize the lice exposure to any additional providers and equipment. Once outside, the patient appears emaciated, wearing soiled clothing, yet states he just put on the clean clothes this morning. He has a bag of prescription medications that seem to indicate a mental health and cardiac history but says he rarely needs to take any pills. His vital signs are a pulse of 88 beats/min and irregular, blood pressure of 98/72 mm Hg, and an oxygen saturation of 88%. He is tachypneic, and there is obvious skin tenting and delayed capillary refill.

a. Chief Complaint

_____

b. Vital Signs

c. Pertinent Negatives

3. While preparing for an ALS interfacility transport, you are told by the nurse's station that the patient has Methicillin-resistant *Staphylococcus aureus* (MRSA). The patient has a number of drip medications along with strict respiratory precautions. You are told that the patient is "stable" for transport. He is also on a nonrebreathing face mask and is conscious and alert. The patient is on a cardiac monitor and is in a sinus rhythm. His blood pressure as noted on the noninvasive monitor is 98/54 mm Hg with a heart rate of 62 beats/min. He has a lengthy medical history, including kidney transplant. He is on several immunosuppressants.

a. Chief Complaint

b. Vital Signs

c. Pertinent Negatives

Ambulance Calls

The following case scenarios provide an opportunity to explore the concerns associated with patient management and paramedic care. Read each scenario, and then answer each question.

1. You are called to transport a 22-year-old college student from the college infirmary to the hospital. The nurse tells you that the student has a high fever. He complains of a severe headache and stiff neck, and he seems rather confused. He vomits twice en route to the hospital.

   a. What is the patient experiencing?

   _____

   _____

   b. How can the paramedic minimize the risk of catching the illness?

   _____

   _____

2. A 54-year-old man calls for an ambulance after he coughed up some blood. He says that over the past several weeks he's been waking up in the middle of the night with his pajamas and bedclothes soaked through with sweat. He's lost about 25 pounds in the last 2 or 3 months, and today he started noticing some blood in his sputum.

   a. What is the patient experiencing?

   _____

   _____

   b. How can the paramedic minimize the risk of catching the illness?

   _____

   _____

3. A 28-year-old man calls for an ambulance because he "feels lousy." He says that for a week or so, he hasn't had any energy at all. He doesn't feel like eating or doing anything; he just feels "done in." Even cigarettes "taste like cow dung." This morning, he noticed that his urine was very dark, and he got panicky. On examination, you observe that his eyes have a yellow tinge and there are needle tracks on his arms.

   a. What is the patient experiencing?

   _____

   _____

   b. How can the paramedic minimize the risk of catching the illness?

   _____

   _____

4. You are called to transport an 8-year-old boy who fell and sustained a laceration to his forehead. "I told him to stay in bed," his mother says, "but no, he has to go horsing around with his brother." According to the mother, both children have been sick for a week with a fever and sore throat. On examining the 8-year-old, you find a 2-inch laceration on the left side of the forehead, and you control the bleeding with pressure. He does seem a little warm, and the angles of his jaw are indistinct, as if there is something swollen there.

   a. What is the patient experiencing?

   _____

   _____

b. How can the paramedic minimize the risk of catching the illness?

_____

_____

5. It's back to the college infirmary for another patient with a fever—this time a 19-year-old woman. She complains of headache and says the light bothers her a lot. Her eyes are reddened, and she is coughing. She has a blotchy, red rash over her face and neck, and when you examine her throat you notice some little white spots on the mucous membranes in her mouth.

a. What is the patient experiencing?

_____

_____

b. How can the paramedic minimize the risk of catching the illness?

_____

_____

6. You are called late one night to the scene of a two-car collision on the interstate. One of the vehicles involved in the crash skidded into a ditch and flipped upside down. The driver is unconscious inside. There is blood and broken glass everywhere. At the least, you are going to have to deal with this patient's bleeding, stabilize his spine, extricate him, and start an IV.

a. List at least four precautions you will take to protect yourself from possible infection during the care and extrication of this patient.

(1) _____

(2) _____

(3) _____

(4) _____

b. List the routine measures you will employ for cleaning the ambulance and its equipment after this call.

_____

_____

c. While you are putting fresh linens on the stretcher, your partner emerges from the "crash room" where the patient has been taken. "You oughta see that guy's eyes," he says, "they're yellow as a canary. I didn't notice it in the vehicle, but with these fluorescent lights, you can't miss it." Given that information, what further measures should you take?

_____

_____

True/False

If you believe the statement to be more true than false, write the letter "T" in the space provided. If you believe the statement to be more false than true, write the letter "F."

_____ **1.** AIDS is a highly contagious disease.

_____ **2.** Approximately 60 million people worldwide are infected with the HIV virus.

_____ **3.** Patients with AIDS are abnormally susceptible to many infectious diseases.

_____ **4.** AIDS can be acquired through casual contact, such as shaking hands with an HIV-positive patient.

_____ **5.** AIDS is a highly communicable disease.

_____ **6.** HIV type 1 was first identified in the late 1970s.

_____ **7.** Many health care workers have acquired HIV through contact with the blood or body fluids of patients.

_____ **8.** The majority of AIDS cases that have occurred in health workers as a result of occupational exposure have been among EMS personnel.

_____ **9.** Complications of syphilis can include cardiac, ophthalmic, auditory, and central nervous system complications.

_____ **10.** STDs require special standard precautions.

Short Answer

Complete this section with short written answers using the space provided.

1. Carry out the following research project before you begin employment as a paramedic.

   a. Check off the illnesses you had as a child or up to this point:

   ___ Measles

   ___ Mumps

   ___ Chickenpox

   ___ German measles (rubella)

   ___ Polio

   ___ Hepatitis B

   b. Check off the immunizations you have had up to this point, and fill in the dates (obtain the records from your family doctor or the clinic where you received your immunizations):

   ___ Measles   Date immunized: _____

   ___ Mumps   Date immunized: _____

   ___ Rubella   Date immunized: _____

   ___ DPT (diphtheria/pertussis/tetanus)

       #1 Date immunized: _____

       #2 Date immunized: _____

       #3 Date immunized: _____

   ___ Most recent   Date immunized: _____
   tetanus booster

   ___ Oral polio #1   Date immunized: _____

   ___ Oral polio #2   Date immunized: _____

   ___ Oral polio #3   Date immunized: _____

   ___ Hepatitis B   Date immunized: _____

   c. Based on the preceding data you have compiled, what immunizations do you need to get before you start work?

   _____

   _____

2. With all the hysteria over AIDS, it is crucial that health professionals be as knowledgeable as possible on the subject.

   a. List three ways that AIDS can be transmitted from one person to another.

   (1) _____

   (2) _____

   (3) _____

b. List three things you can do to minimize the risk of acquiring HIV from a patient.

(1) _____

(2) _____

(3) _____

Crossword Puzzle
Use the clues below to complete the puzzle.

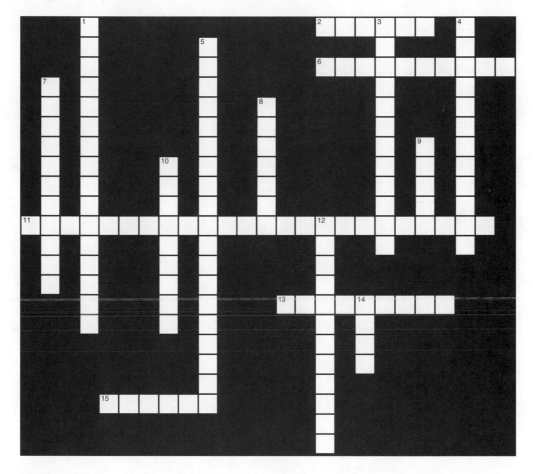

Across

2. Kills HBV

6. Inflammation of the membranes that cover the brain or spinal cord

11. Leading cause of lower respiratory tract infections in infants, older people, and immunocompromised persons

13. Live in or on another living creature

15. Should be nonlatex, vinyl, nitrile, or rubber

Down

1. Period between exposure and symptom onset

3. Caused by a virus that occurs naturally in the bird population

4. A common normal organism of the GI tract

5. Formally called universal precautions

7. Tick-borne disease first discovered in Connecticut

8. Type of injury prevention that begins at home

9. Acquired from contact with decaying organic matter

10. Bacterial infection characterized by an irritating cough

12. Once widespread in the United States

14. Gonorrhea, syphilis, genital herpes, chlamydia

Secret Message

Identify the following terms from the clues provided, and then use the letters to decode the secret message!

a. Object that transmits a disease agent: _ _ _ _ _ _
82 73 39 20 26 60

b. Type of microbe that causes hepatitis: _ _ _ _ _
87 64 33 74 56

c. Skin test to detect TB: _ _ _ _ _ _ U _ _ _
50 13 4 88 85 91   93 43 21

d. Sign of hepatitis: _ _ _ _ _ U _
29 24 41 63 15   70

e. Painful complication of mumps: _ _ _ _ _ _ I _
32 75 47 76 40 1   80

f. Symptom of gonorrhea: _ _ _ U _ _ _
57 72 65   35 53 17

g. Sign of measles: _ _ _ _
89 9 38 2

h. Sign of TB: _ I _ _ _ _ _ _ _ _ _
78   52 28 66 6 68 86 77 42 59

i. Another sign of TB: _ _ U _ _
27 67   31 71

j. Symptom of hepatitis: _ _ _ I _ _ _
10 46 7   45 55 84

k. Another symptom of hepatitis: _ _ U _ _ _
49 19   8 5 81

l. Bluish skin in hypoxemia: C _ _ _ _ _ _ _
90 69 30 54 62 58 22

m. Protective reflex: _ _ _
18 92 12

n. What arteries do in neurogenic shock: _ I _ _ _ _
79   94 14 34 3

o. Good source of K⁺: B _ _ _ _ _
61 37 25 44 51

p. Nickname for U.S. transportation agency: _ _ _
16 48 83

q. Caffeine-containing drink: _ _ _
23 11 36

Secret Message

_ _ _ _ _ _ _ _ _ _ _ _ _ _ _ _ _ _ _ _ _ _ _ _ _ _ _ _ _ _ _ _
1 2 3   4 5 6 7   8 9 10 11 12 13 14 15 16   17 18 19 20 21 22 23   24 25 26 27 28 29 30 31   32 33

_ _ _ _ _ _ _ _ _ _ _ _ _ _ _ _ _ _ _ _ _ _ _ _ _ _ _ _ _ _ _ _ _ _ _ _
34 35 36 37 38 39 40 41 42 43 44 45   46   47 48 49 50 51 52 53 54 55 56   57 58 59 60 61 62 63   64 65   66 67

_ _ _ _ _ _ _ _ _ _ _ _ _ _ _ _ _ _ _ _ _ _ _ _ _ _ _ _ _.
68 69 70 71   72 73 74 75   76 77 78 79 80   81 82 83 84 85   86 87 88 89 90   91 92 93 94

Fill-in-the-Table

Fill in the missing parts of the table.

1. Complete the following table for the PPE necessary for the prevention of transmission of HIV and Hepatitis B. Indicate "yes" or "no" for each task or activity.

Recommended Personal Protective Equipment for Prevention of Transmission of HIV and Hepatitis B Virus in the Prehospital Setting				
Task or Activity	**Disposable Gloves**	**Gown**	**Mask**	**Protective Eyewear**
Bleeding control with spurting blood	Yes			Yes
Bleeding control with minimal bleeding	Yes	No		
Emergency childbirth		Yes		Yes, if splashing is likely
Blood drawing		No	No	
Starting an intravenous line			No	
Endotracheal intubation, laryngeal mask airway, Combitube use	Yes		No, unless splashing is likely*	
Oral/nasal suctioning, manually cleaning airway		No		
Handling and cleaning instruments with microbial contamination	Yes			No
Measuring blood pressure		No		No
Measuring temperature	No		No	
Giving an injection		No		No

*Splashing is often likely, so use PPE accordingly.
Adapted from: Centers for Disease Control and Prevention.

2. For each of the illnesses in the following box, list its usual mode(s) of transmission and the measures a paramedic can take to minimize the risk of contracting the illness from a patient.

Disease	Mode(s) of Transmission	Protective Measures
AIDS		
Hepatitis type A		
Hepatitis type B		
Meningitis		
Mumps		
Syphilis		
Tuberculosis		

CHAPTER

37 Behavioral Emergencies

Chapter Review

The following exercises provide an opportunity to test your knowledge of this chapter.

Matching

Match each of the items in the left column to the appropriate description in the right column.

1. For each of the following signs and symptoms, indicate whether it is:

_____ **1.** Obsessional thinking

_____ **2.** Flat affect

_____ **3.** Delirium

_____ **4.** Distractibility

_____ **5.** Compulsions

_____ **6.** Visual hallucinations

_____ **7.** Confabulation

_____ **8.** Anxiety

_____ **9.** Coma

_____ **10.** Circumstantial thinking

O More typical of *organic* brain syndrome

P More typical of *psychiatric* illness

B Apt to be seen in *both* organic and psychiatric illnesses

2. For each of the psychiatric signs and symptoms listed, indicate whether it is a disturbance of:

_____ **1.** The patient cannot name three objects that you listed out loud 5 minutes earlier.

_____ **2.** The patient is pacing back and forth.

_____ **3.** The patient smiles pleasantly as he tells you that his daughter was run over by a truck.

_____ **4.** The patient keeps shifting his attention from you to the television or to the window.

_____ **5.** The patient seems to be having a conversation with an invisible friend.

_____ **6.** The patient thinks it's 1931.

_____ **7.** The patient also thinks that he is Albert Einstein.

_____ **8.** He tells you, "All the world is my kingdumbell and I'm the pellmellery scullop."

_____ **9.** The patient is terrified of spiders.

_____ **10.** He puts two fingers to his forehead in a salute every time he finishes speaking.

_____ **11.** He complains of palpitations, nausea, tightness in his chest, and numbness around his lips.

_____ **12.** He thinks that the sound of the wind is someone calling his name.

A. Consciousness

B. Motor activity

C. Speech

D. Thinking

E. Affect or mood

F. Memory

G. Orientation

H. Perception

Multiple Choice

Read each item carefully, and then select the best response.

_____ **1.** In an acute behavioral emergency, paramedics are best able to treat:

    A. hypoglycemia.   **C.** drug and alcohol intoxications.

    B. severe infections.   **D.** dementia.

_____ **2.** Pressured speech, neologisms, echolalia, and mutism are examples of:

    A. disorders of thinking.   **C.** disorders of motor activity.

    B. disorders of mood and affect.   **D.** disorders of speech.

_____ **3.** During the initial assessment of patients with behavioral disorders it is important for a paramedic to:

    A. hurry the call; you can't really assist the patient. **C.** convey that you have the time and concern.

    B. assess the patient only en route to the hospital. **D.** not gain consent because consent is never required.

_____ **4.** The mental status exam includes:

    A. perception.   **C.** memory.

    B. affect and mood.   **D.** All of the above.

_____ **5.** Guilt, depressed appetite, sleep disturbances, lack of interest, low energy, and suicide are diagnostic features of:

    A. depression.   **C.** mood disorders.

    B. anxiety.   **D.** manic-depressive illness.

_____ **6.** Paramedics need to always take scene safety seriously. The following are risk factors for violence EXCEPT:

    A. posture.   **C.** motor activity.

    B. speech.   **D.** prescription medication.

_____ **7.** Restraining a violent patient should involve:

    A. a police presence.   **C.** lots of duct tape.

    B. a Reeves stretcher.   **D.** no more than two paramedics.

_____ **8.** A psychiatric emergency exists when a patient:

    A. threatens to harm him- or herself.   **C.** is delusional.

    B. threatens to harm other people.   **D.** All of the above.

_____ **9.** All of the following drugs may sometimes cause a psychotic state EXCEPT:

    A. steroids.   **C.** digitalis.

    B. Wellbutrin (bupropion).   **D.** LSD and PCP.

_____ **10.** Which of the following are considered disturbances of behavior?

    A. Anxiety disorder   **C.** Head injury

    B. Organic brain syndrome   **D.** CVA

Fill-in-the-Blank

Read each item carefully, and then complete the statement by filling in the missing word(s).

1. The three categories that may cause abnormal behavior include _____ or organic causes, _____ causes, and

    _____ causes.

2. Identify yourself _____. Tell the patient who you are and what you are trying to do. If the patient is _____or _____

    _____, you may have to explain yourself at _____ intervals.

3. Overwhelming feelings of _____ and _____ characterize panic disorder.

4. Posttraumatic stress disorder is characterized by the patient reliving the _____ and _____ of the original situation.

5. _____ and _____ are common trade names for tricyclic antidepressants.

6. MOA inhibitors' most notable side effect is a _____ _____.

7. _____ is the third leading cause of death among 15- to 24-year-olds and the fourth leading cause of death among the 25- to 44-year age group.

Identify

List the behavioral medications in the following scenarios.

1. You respond to a domestic dispute. When you arrive on-scene, you are told by law enforcement that the scene is secure and safe. You and your partner proceed inside. The patient's wife is holding a bag of the patient's medications. The patient denies any complaint and simply states that he has a cardiac history and takes furosemide (Lasix) and digoxin. While you calm the patient, your partner reviews the bag of medications. He finds the furosemide and digoxin along with glyburide, fluoxetine (Prozac), and diazepam (Valium).

_____

_____

2. You are called to an outpatient mental health clinic for a patient requiring voluntary in-patient hospitalization. The patient has a history of hypercholesterolemia and depression. The patient is taking over-the-counter omega-3 and garlic. The patient is on the following prescription medications: phenelzine (Nardil), buproprion (Wellbutrin), simvastatin (Zocor), and atorvastatin (Lipitor).

_____

_____

3. You receive an emergency call for a "psychotic" patient. As you evaluate your patient, you review her medication list and discover the following prescriptions: tamaxofin, niacin (Niaspan), fluticasone/salmeterol inhaled (Advair), aripiprazole (Abilify), and famotidine (Pepcid).

_____

_____

Ambulance Calls

The following case scenarios provide an opportunity to explore the concerns associated with patient management and paramedic care. Read each scenario, and then answer each question.

1. The following is the transcript of an interview between an inexperienced paramedic and a disturbed patient. The interview illustrates several errors in approach. Read through the interview. Then, list the points in the interview that you think could have been handled or phrased in a better way.

PARAMEDIC (entering an apartment in which there is a lot of noise and confusion): Okay, which one of you is the patient?

(Someone points to a young woman crouching in a corner, crying.)

PARAMEDIC (approaching the woman and standing in front of her): Now, dearie, what's the trouble?

(Patient continues crying.)

PARAMEDIC: Now come on, get hold of yourself. Big girls don't cry.

PATIENT (sobbing): Everything's just so hopeless.

PARAMEDIC: Things are never hopeless. You're probably just making a mountain out of a molehill, and by tomorrow you'll wonder what you were making such a big fuss about.

(Patient sits crying to herself.)

PARAMEDIC: Well, if you don't want to tell me what's wrong, maybe one of your friends here can tell me. Is there anyone here who can tell me what's going on?

(Immediately the noise and confusion resume, as everyone starts talking at once. The patient huddles farther into the corner.)

List the things you think were done incorrectly in this interview (include errors of omission and errors of commission).

a. _____

_____

b. _____

_____

c. _____

_____

d. _____

_____

e. _____

_____

f. _____

_____

g. _____

_____

h. _____

2. You are called to a downtown apartment building for a "sick man." Reaching the corridor outside the man's apartment, you are intercepted by a neighbor who had called for the ambulance. "I feel a little silly troubling you folks," she says, "but Mr. Crosby next door—he's just not himself lately—doesn't even poke his head out of that apartment, doesn't want to see no one—he just says, 'Go away,' when I knock. So I got to worrying. I mean I don't even think he's got himself anything to eat in there."

You knock on Mr. Crosby's door. There isn't any response. You knock several more times.

"Who's there?" someone finally says.

"We're paramedics, from the city ambulance service."

"Well, what do you want with me?"

"We just want to talk with you a bit," you say. "There are folks worried about you."

It takes some persuading, but finally Mr. Crosby opens the door and admits you to his apartment. The place is in complete disarray, and it appears as if no one has washed a dish or tidied up in months. Here and there you note an empty liquor bottle lying around on the floor.

"So what do you want?" Mr. Crosby asks listlessly.

a. Where would you go from here? List some of the questions you would ask Mr. Crosby at this point.

_____

_____

_____

b. In the course of your interview with Mr. Crosby, which seems to go very slowly, you learn that he is a 62-year-old widower. He has one son ("I never hear from him"). He used to be a watchmaker, "but I haven't been worth anything since I got this arthritis 10 years ago." In response to your query about why he has stopped going out of the apartment, he says, "What's there to go out for? Anyway, I don't have the energy to go rambling around the city."

"Don't you have to shop for food?" you ask.

"What for? I don't feel much like eating these days anyway."

This patient is showing clear symptoms of depression. List the symptoms of depression present in this case.

(1) _____

(2) _____

(3) _____

(4) _____

c. List four other symptoms or signs of depression.

(1) _____

(2) _____

(3) _____

(4) _____

d. List the risk factors for suicide present in this patient's history.

(1) _____

(2) _____

(3) _____

(4) _____

(5) _____

e. List four other risk factors for suicide.

(1) _____

(2) _____

(3) _____

(4) _____

f. List three questions you would ask to try to evaluate the patient's risk of suicide.

(1) _____

(2) _____

(3) _____

3. You are called to a downtown office building for a "possible heart attack." When you reach the building, you are escorted into an office by a harried-looking businessman. "It's my secretary," he says. "She's having some kind of cardiac attack." In the midst of a buzzing group of people, you see a woman who looks to be about 24 years old sitting wide-eyed and pale. People are fanning her with file folders and trying to get her to drink some water. You make your way through the crowd and ask the woman what her problem is.

"Can't breathe," she gasps. "Chest all tight (gasp). Feel like I'm going to pass out (gasp). Everything is unreal (gasp), like I'm dying (gasp)."

"Quick! Quick!" squeaks one of the bystanders. "Get her to the hospital!"

Ignoring the chorus demanding that you leave immediately for the hospital, you begin taking the woman's vital signs. Her pulse is 112 beats/min and regular, her respirations are 30 breaths/min and deep, and her blood pressure is 160/88 mm Hg. You notice that her skin is cold and sweaty and her hands are shaking.

a. What do you think is this patient's problem?

_____

_____

b. What signs and symptoms led you to that conclusion?

(1) _____

(2) _____

(3) _____

(4) _____

(5) _____

(6) _____

(7) _____

c. Are there any other diagnoses you need to take into consideration? If so, what diagnoses?

(1) _____

(2) _____

(3) _____

(4) _____

(5) _____

d. How will you manage this patient?

(1) _____

(2) _____

(3) _____

(4) _____

(5) _____

4. You and your partner are called to a downtown bar to see a man who has apparently become disruptive there. A police officer meets you at the entrance to the bar. "Listen," he says, "the barkeeper called *us* to deal with an unruly customer, but personally I think the guy's a psycho case—so I thought maybe you folks ought to take a look at him."

You enter the bar and find a well-dressed but disheveled man pacing rapidly up and down. "One week from today," he is announcing, "one week from today, I'll be one of the richest men in America. I'm putting together a business empire now that will rule Wall Street." He is talking a mile a minute, cracking jokes, and gesturing extravagantly. He catches sight of you and your partner and says, "Well, hello, fellas. Bartender, give these fine young people a drink, on me. They do a great public service. This country was built on public service, yes indeed it was. So give them a public service drink."

"You haven't paid for the drinks you already ordered," says the bartender.

"Listen, fathead, I said give these nice people a drink."

"Uh, sir," you break in, "we're not allowed to drink while on duty. And we thought maybe you'd like to take a little ride with us to the hospital."

"Hospital? What do I need to go to the hospital for? Never felt better in my life. By next week, I'll be able to buy the hospital, buy this bar too, buy the whole damned town."

The police officers says, "Maybe you *ought* to go with them, sir, just to get a checkup."

"Any of you puts a hand on me," replies the man, "I'll sue the whole lot of you. Assault. Battery. False imprisonment. I'll sue you for the whole lot, and let me tell you, you don't want to tangle with *my* team of lawyers. Best legal talent in the country. You wouldn't stand a chance."

a. What do you think is this man's problem?

_____

_____

b. What symptoms and signs led you to that conclusion?

(1) _____

(2) _____

(3) _____

(4) _____

c. How will you manage this patient?

_____

_____

5. You are called to a downtown street corner where several police officers are standing around apparently trying to talk to a somewhat wild-eyed man who could be anywhere from 55 to 75 years old. He is dressed in about six layers of tattered clothes and wearing a naval officer's cap. He clearly hasn't had a bath, shave, or haircut in weeks. "He was just walking down the middle of Main Street," says one of the police officers, "as if he didn't even notice the traffic—and all those horns blowing, people screeching on their brakes."

You introduce yourself to the man and ask whether you can be of help. He mumbles something that sounds like, "Dogs and cats."

"Sorry," you say, "I didn't quite catch what you said."

"Salt and pepper," he says. "Black and blue, I didn't, dontcha know, I didn't."
The police officer gives you a meaningful look.
How will you manage this case?

_____

_____

_____

_____

_____

6. A middle-aged woman calls for an ambulance because "my son is acting real strange." When you arrive at the designated address, the woman greets you at the door. She tells you that her 20-year-old son won't come out of his room. He's been in there for 2 days now. Sometimes she hears him talking to someone, but there isn't anyone else there. "I'm sure it's all that karate stuff," she says. "It just went to his head, made him crazy, all that black belt business."

You go up to the son's room and knock on the door.

"You're not going to get me," says a voice from the other side of the door. "You won't take me alive."

"Sir, we're paramedics. We've just come to talk with you."

"You can't fool me. I know you're from the FBI. Well, you'll have to shoot me to take me."

You try the door and find it's unlocked. Inside, a young man clothed in karate garb is sitting in an armchair, gripping the armrests.

You introduce yourselves again. The patient looks away.

"You won't take me alive," he says again in a monotone. He looks suddenly toward the wall. "I know, I know," he says to the wall.

"Who are you talking to?" you ask.

He looks startled. "The voices said you would come. They killed John Lennon, and the FBI is after me. The voices said not to let you take me alive."

a. This patient is showing signs of _____

  (1) a panic attack.

  (2) psychosis.

  (3) depression.

  (4) mania.

  (5) disorganization.

b. Are there any indications that he might become violent?

_____

c. If so, what are the indications?

  (1) _____

  (2) _____

  (3) _____

  (4) _____

d. How will you manage this case?

_____

_____

_____

_____

True/False

If you believe the statement to be more true than false, write the letter "T" in the space provided. If you believe the statement to be more false than true, write the letter "F."

_____ **1.** The most important thing a paramedic can do to help a disturbed patient is to remain calm and steady.

_____ **2.** There should be a maximum sense of urgency in evacuating a disturbed patient to the hospital because there is nothing that can be done to help the patient in the field.

_____ **3.** It is essential to correct a patient's misinterpretations of reality.

_____ **4.** The disturbed patient should be reassured that everything will turn out all right.

_____ **5.** The paramedic should remain with the disturbed patient at all times until the emergency department staff takes over the patient's care.

_____ **6.** Police intervention is usually required to transport a disturbed patient against his or her will.

Short Answer

Complete this section with short written answers using the space provided.

1. Certain situations have a higher potential for violence than others do. List three scenarios that should activate the paramedic's "nose for danger."

a. _____

b. _____

c. _____

2. List four diagnostic groups that would activate the paramedic's "nose for danger."

a. _____

b. _____

c. _____

d. _____

Secret Message

Identify the following terms from the clues provided, and then use the letters to decode the secret message!

Your thought for the day can be decoded in the usual fashion.

a. Seeing or hearing things that aren't there: __ __ __ __ __ __ __ __ __ __ __ __ __
  62 106 87 7 31 68 11 51 22 93 56 14 103

b. A fixed, false idea: __ __ __ U __ __ __ __
  39 80 112   76 34 53 92

c. Repetitive expression of a single idea: __ __ __ __ E __ __ __ __ __ I __ __
  98 83 81 71   17 97 107 73 90   65 35

d. Intense, irrational fear: __ __ __ __ __ __ __
  58 2 94 78 24 84

e. Having two opposite feelings at once: __ __ B __ __ __ __ __ __ __ __
  6 49   88 5 99 111 46 85 61 108

f. Describing repetitive, purposeless behavior: __ __ E __ __ __ __ __ __ __ __
47 95   19 91 30 1 113 21 50 33

g. Disorientation and impaired understanding: __ __ N __ __ __ __ __ __
105 77   54 75 89 67 63 26

h. Type of memory loss: __ __ __ __ E   __ __ A __ __
109 38 66 110   45 104   52 4

i. Speech disorder with compulsive repetition of sounds heard: __ __ __ O __ __ __ I __
16 36 29   64 43 32   69

j. Feeling of uneasiness: __ __ X __ __ __ __
9 42   101 40 72 60

k. Inability to sit still: R __ __ __ __ __ __ __ __ __ __
102 48 10 37 25 59 28 13 18 57 79

l. Affect that shows little or no feeling is called: __ __ __ __
15 70 41 100

m. Flight of ideas is a disorder of: __ __ __ __ G __ __
74 96 12 8   55 27

n. Syphilis is one: __ __ __
44 23 86

o. Jealousy: __ N __ __
3   82 20

Secret Message

___ ___ _____ __ _____ _____ _____
1 2 3   4 5 6 7 8 9 10 11 12 13   14 15   16 17 18 19 20   21 22 23 24 25 26 27   28 29 30 31 32 33

_____ __ _____ __ ___ _____
34 35 36 37 38 39 40   41 42   43 44 45 46 47 48 49 50 51 52   53 54   55 56 57   58 59 60 61 62 63 64 65 66 67 68 69 70

_____ _____ ____ _____ __ ___ _____
71 72 73 74 75 76   77 78 79 80 81 82 83   84 85 86   87 88 89 90 91 92   93 94   95 96 97   98 99 100 101 102 103 104

_____.
105 106 107 108 109 110 111 112 113

Fill-in-the-Table

Fill in the missing parts of the table with the conditions and substances that can produce psychotic symptoms.

Selected Disease States That May Produce Psychotic Symptoms	
Disease State	**Psychotic Symptoms**

Toxic and deficiency states	■ Drug-induced psychoses, especially from:
	  • _____
	  • _____
	  • Disulfiram
	  • _____
	  • LSD, PCP, and other psychedelics
	■ Nutrition disorders:
	  • Alcohol abuse
	  • _____
	■ Poisoning with bromide or other heavy metals
	■ _____
	■ _____

Infections	■ Syphilis ■ Parasites ■ _____ ■ _____
Neurologic disease	■ _____ ■ Primary and metastatic tumors of the brain ■ _____ ■ Cerebrovascular accident ■ _____
Cardiovascular disorders	■ _____
Endocrine disorders	■ Thyroid hyperfunction (thyrotoxicosis) ■ _____ _____
Metabolic disorders	■ _____ _____ ■ Hypoglycemia ■ _____

Skill Drills

Test your knowledge of skill drills by placing the following photos in the correct order. Number the first step "1," the second step "2," etc.

1. *Restraining a Patient*

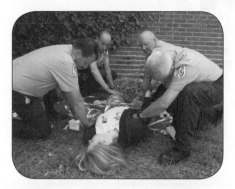

Each team member should grasp the assigned body part and carefully, with the least amount of force, bring the patient to the ground.

_____

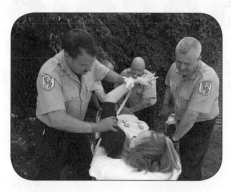

Carefully place the patient on the stretcher or carrying device in a face-up position.

_____

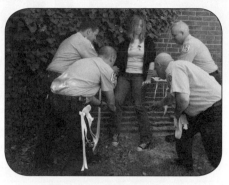

On the direction of the team leader, move together toward the patient.

_____

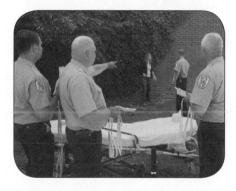

Assign positions to each team member: four extremities and the head.

_____

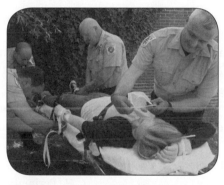

Tie the patient with soft restraints at each wrist and ankle as well as the chest and pelvis sheets. If the patient is spitting, place an oxygen mask or surgical mask on his or her face.

_____

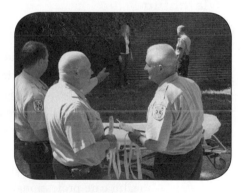

Assemble 4 or 5 rescuers and have the stretcher or carrying device and soft restraints nearby. Designate a leader.

_____

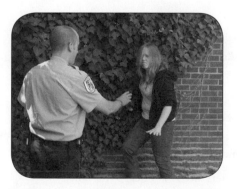

If possible, corner the patient in a safe area.

_____

CHAPTER

38 Gynecologic Emergencies

Chapter Review

The following exercises provide an opportunity to test your knowledge of this chapter.

Matching

Match each of the items in the left column to the appropriate term in the right column.

_____ **1.** Area between the vaginal opening and anus

_____ **2.** Glands that secrete lubrication for intercourse

_____ **3.** A cyclic and periodic vaginal discharge

_____ **4.** The onset of the first menses

_____ **5.** Vaginal bleeding lasting several days longer than normal for the patient

_____ **6.** A t-shaped device inserted into the uterus by a health care professional

_____ **7.** Dome-shaped rubber disk that covers the cervix

_____ **8.** The medical term for pregnancy

_____ **9.** Blood in the abdominal cavity

_____ **10.** Term for live delivery

A. Hypermenorrhea

B. Parity

C. Bartholin

D. Diaphragm

E. Menstruation

F. Gravid

G. IUD

H. Perineum

I. Hemoperitoneum

J. Menarche

Multiple Choice

Read each item carefully, and then select the best response.

_____ **1.** How many days is the average "cycle" of a woman?

    A. 5 days

    B. 10 days

    C. 28 days

    D. 30 days

_____ **2.** What is the onset of the first menses is called?

    A. Menopause

    B. Premenstrual syndrome

    C. Menstruation

    D. Menarche

_____ **3.** During an ectopic pregnancy, where do 97% of eggs implant?

    A. In the uterus

    B. In the fallopian tube

    C. In the ovary

    D. In the cervical opening

_____ **4.** Which of the following is a symptom associated with gonorrhea?

    A. A growth in the genital area

    B. Painful urination with a foul, yellowish vaginal discharge

    C. Prolonged high fever, headache, and malaise

    D. Lower abdominal pain, and pain during intercourse

_____ **5.** When you estimate blood loss, what kind of vitals signs do you expect to find in a second-stage hemorrhage?

    A. Elevated heart rate, respiration no change, blood pressure no change

    B. Anxiety, tachycardia, decreased pulse pressure, tachypnea

    C. Hypotension, decreased heart rate, coma

    D. Hypertension, increased heart rate, alert

_____ **6.** Which of the following is not considered a life-threatening gynecologic condition?

    A. Child birth   **C.** Tubo-ovarian abscess

    B. Ectopic pregnancy   **D.** Ruptured ovarian cyst

_____ **7.** Referred pain caused by gallbladder problems tends to radiate where?

    A. Lower left quadrant   **C.** Right shoulder

    B. Left shoulder   **D.** Lower right quadrant

_____ **8.** Besides constant pain on one side, what other symptom might occur in the patient suffering from an ectopic pregnancy?

    A. Blurred vision   **C.** Soft abdomen

    B. Hypertension   **D.** Vaginal bleeding

_____ **9.** When dealing with a victim of sexual assault, which of the following statements is true?

    A. You should try to gain as much information as possible about the assault.

    B. You should place the patient's articles in a paper bag.

    C. You should place the patient's articles in a plastic bag to preserve DNA.

    D. You should allow the patient time to wash him- or herself.

_____ **10.** Which one of the date rape drugs is a stimulant?

    A. GHB   **C.** Ecstasy

    B. Ketalar   **D.** Rohypnol

Labeling

Label the following diagrams with the correct terms.

1. Label the parts of the female reproductive system.

FRONT VIEW   SIDE VIEW

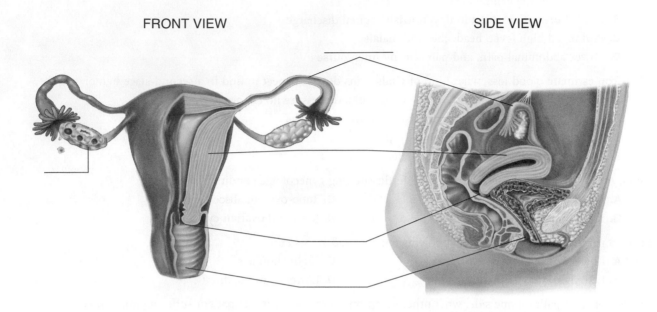

2. Label the parts of the female reproductive system with an ectopic pregnancy.

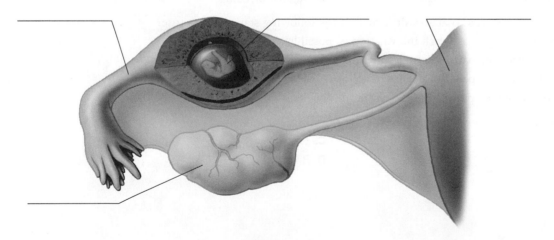

Fill-in-the-Blank

Read each item carefully, and then complete the statement by filling in the missing word(s).

1. The lower portion of the birth canal is also called the _____.

2. In some cases, a/an _____ _____ will completely cover the vaginal orifice.

3. The cessation of menses is known as _____.

4. _____ is when a woman is no longer able to bear children.

5. Endometrial tissue grows outside the uterus and causes _____.

6. _____ _____ _____ is a form of septic shock.

7. _____ _____ is the first thing to ensure when called to a gynecologic emergency.

8. At all times, you should try to protect a patient's _____ when treating a gynecologic emergency.

9. _____ sign or _____ - _____ sign may indicate internal bleeding.

10. _____ _____ is mainly used as a veterinary anesthetic.

Identify

In the following case study, list the chief complaint, vital signs, and pertinent negatives.

Your unit has been called to the local high school for a young woman with severe abdominal pain. When you arrive, the 16-year-old girl is doubled up in pain. She is crying. You begin your assessment with the MS-ABCs and apply supplemental oxygen via a nonrebreathing mask. Lucy rates her pain as 10 on 10. Your partner Abe begins with her baseline vital signs as you gather a personal history. Lucy's heart rate is 120 beats/min, and her ECG rhythm is sinus tachycardia, blood pressure is 140/92 mm Hg. Her oxygen saturation is 99%, and respirations are 20 breaths/min. Skin is very warm and her temperature is 102°F. Pupils are Equal And Round, Regular in size, and reactive to Light (PEARRL). Lung sounds are clear. She has no history of illness or trauma. She denies being sexually active yet. A physical exam reveals guarding of the abdomen. She has rebound tenderness, and her abdomen is distended. She says she is going to be sick and throws up. You feel that this is a load-and-go priority patient, and so your partner gets an IV started and you load the patient quickly and get to the local hospital as quickly as possible.

1. Chief Complaint

_____

_____

_____

2. Vital Signs

_____

_____

_____

3. Pertinent Negatives

_____

_____

_____

Ambulance Calls

The following case scenarios provide an opportunity to explore the concerns associated with patient management and paramedic care. Read each scenario, and then answer each question.

1. A 25-year-old woman calls for an ambulance because of abdominal pain. She says the pain started yesterday and has just gotten worse and worse. It is a "heavy," aching pain in the lower abdomen. This afternoon, she started having chills as well, and she threw up once. Her last menstrual period (LMP) was 5 days ago and was normal. She uses an intrauterine device (IUD) for contraception. On physical examination, the patient looks ill. Her skin feels hot and dry. Her pulse is 110 beats/min and regular while sitting, 116 beats/min while standing; respirations are 24 breaths/min and unlabored; and the blood pressure is 122/74 mm Hg. The abdomen is *very* tender to palpation in all quadrants.

a. This woman is most likely to be experiencing which of the following conditions?

    A. A threatened abortion   **D.** An ectopic pregnancy

    B. An inevitable abortion   **E.** Pelvic inflammatory disease (PID)

    C. A septic abortion

b. List the steps you would take in managing this patient.

    (1) _____

    _____

    (2) _____

    _____

2. A 24-year-old woman calls for an ambulance because she says, "I think I have appendicitis." She says she's been having some crampy pain in the right lower quadrant for a couple of days, but today it got much worse. She can't remember exactly when her last menstrual period was, "But I think I'm getting my period now, because I had some spotting this morning." She is certain, in any case, that she couldn't possibly be pregnant. On physical examination, she appears anxious and in moderate distress. Her skin is cool and moist. Her pulse is 100 beats/min and regular while sitting, 124 beats/min while standing; her respirations are 24 breaths/min and regular; her blood pressure is 110/70 mm Hg. Her abdomen is very tender to palpation.

a. What is your field diagnosis of this patient?

    A. A threatened abortion   **D.** An ectopic pregnancy

    B. An inevitable abortion   **E.** Pelvic inflammatory disease (PID)

    C. A septic abortion

b. List the steps you would take in managing this patient.

    (1) _____

    (2) _____

    (3) _____

    (4) _____

    (5) _____

    (6) _____

    (7) _____

    (8) _____

True/False

If you believe the statement to be more true than false, write the letter "T" in the space provided. If you believe the statement to be more false than true, write the letter "F."

_____ **1.** The paramedic should take a detailed history of the rape incident to enable the victim to ventilate her feelings about what happened.

_____ **2.** All superficial wounds and abrasions suffered by a rape victim should be carefully cleaned and covered with sterile dressings before transport to prevent infection.

_____ **3.** The patient should be discouraged from cleaning up before being examined in the emergency department.

_____ **4.** The rape victim's external genitalia should be routinely inspected for injury.

_____ **5.** The diagnosis on your trip sheet for a victim of sexual assault should read "Alleged rape" rather than "Rape."

_____ **6.** Gonorrhea can cause the Bartholin glands to become cystic and abscessed.

_____ **7.** Dysmenorrhea means the patient has excessive blood flow during menses.

_____ **8.** Endometritis is hereditary and runs in families.

_____ **9.** When using the mnemonic ACHES-S, the *E* stands for ectopic pregnancy.

_____ **10.** If a woman has had three pregnancies and two live births, she is classified as a gravid 3, para 2.

Short Answer

Complete this section with short written answers using the space provided.

1. You are summoned to a downtown apartment for a "sick woman." On arrival, you find a 24-year-old woman complaining of severe abdominal pain.

    a. List 10 questions you would ask in taking this woman's history.

      (1) _____

      (2) _____

      (3) _____

      (4) _____

      (5) _____

      (6) _____

      (7) _____

      (8) _____

      (9) _____

     (10) _____

    b. List two things you would look for in particular in performing the physical examination.

      (1) _____

      (2) _____

2. Ectopic pregnancy is more likely in some women than in others. List two factors that predispose a woman to ectopic pregnancy.

    a. _____

    b. _____

3. Three findings in the history make up the classic diagnostic triad for ectopic pregnancy, and a woman who has those three findings must be considered to be experiencing an ectopic pregnancy until proven otherwise. What three findings make up the classic triad for ectopic pregnancy?

    a. _____

    b. _____

    c. _____

Crossword Puzzle

Use the clues in the column to complete the puzzle.

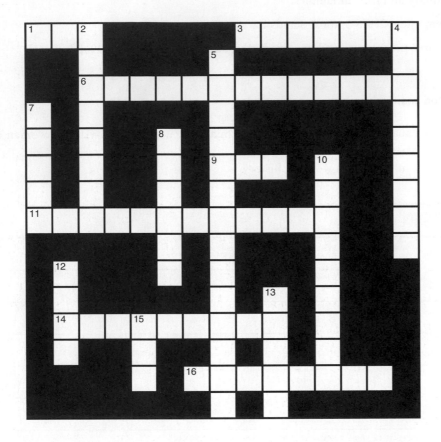

Across

1. Menstruation disorder occurring 7 to 14 days prior to the menstrual cycle (initials)
3. Located away from a normal position
6. A menstrual cycle that occurs more often than a 24-day interval
9. An infection of the female upper reproductive organs (initials)
11. Painful menses
14. The most common cause of amenorrhea
16. The female external genitalia is known as the _____

Down

2. STD caused by the bacterium *Treponema pallidum*, it has three stages
4. "C" in the mnemonic LORDS TRACHEA
5. Blood in the abdominal cavity
7. 30% to 40% blood volume loss is known as a/an _____ grade hemorrhage
8. A disk-shaped polyurethane device containing the spermicide nonoxynol-9
10. An infection that causes ulcers of the genitals
12. The most common sexual assault
13. The vaginal orifice is protected by the _____
15. Date rape drug which is a colorless liquid with a salty taste that is mixed in drinks (initials)

Fill-in-the-Table

Fill in the missing parts of the table.

1. Estimating Blood Volume Loss

Estimating Blood Volume Loss				
Grade of Hemorrhage/ Blood Loss	Heart Rate	Respiratory Rate	Blood Pressure	Central Nervous System
First/< 15%	Minor tachycardia		No change	
Second/15%–30%		Tachypnea		Anxiety or combativeness
Third/30%–40%	Marked tachycardia		Systolic hypotension	
Fourth/> 40%		Marked tachypnea		Comatose/unresponsive

Source: Adapted from United States Department of Defense. *Emergency War Surgery Nato Handbook.* 2004:Table 7-1. Available at: http://www.bordeninstitute .army.mil/emrgncywarsurg/Chp7Shock&Resuscitation.pdf. Accessed May 18, 2006.

CHAPTER

39 Obstetrics

Chapter Review

The following exercises provide an opportunity to test your knowledge of this chapter.

Matching

Match each of the items in the left column to the appropriate term in the right column.

_____ **1.** A woman who has had two or more pregnancies	**A.** Primigravida
_____ **2.** A woman who is pregnant for the first time	**B.** Primipara
_____ **3.** A woman who has had two or more deliveries	**C.** Multigravida
_____ **4.** A woman who has never delivered	**D.** Multipara
_____ **5.** A woman who has had only one delivery	**E.** Nullipara
_____ **6.** Arises when a malfunction of the egg or sperm creates a problem at the fertilization stage, resulting in an abnormal placenta	**F.** Antepartum
	G. Abruptio placenta
_____ **7.** Before delivery	**H.** Placenta previa
_____ **8.** A severe disorder of pregnancy with potentially life-threatening consequences	**I.** Molar pregnancy
_____ **9.** The placenta is implanted low in the uterus and, as it grows, it partially or fully obscures the cervical canal	**J.** Pseudocyesis
	K. Ectopic pregnancy
_____ **10.** A false pregnancy that develops all the typical signs and symptoms of pregnancy	
_____ **11.** Premature separation of a normally implanted placenta from the wall of the uterus	

Multiple Choice

Read each item carefully, and then select the best response.

_____ **1.** An abortion that is spontaneous and cannot be prevented is called:

    A. missed abortion.   **C.** threatened abortion.

    B. inevitable abortion.   **D.** incomplete abortion.

_____ **2.** What is the condition in which the placenta is implanted low in the uterus and, as it grows, it partially obscures the cervical canal?

    A. Abruptio placenta   **C.** Pseudocyesis

    B. Molar pregnancy   **D.** Placenta previa

3. Which of the following words describes a woman who has had two or more pregnancies?

   A. Multigravida   **C.** Multipara

   B. Primipara   **D.** Parity

4. When the baby's head enters the birth canal, the _____ stage of labor begins.

   A. fourth   **C.** second

   B. third   **D.** first

5. The Apgar scoring system is an evaluation tool for the newborn's vital functions and is recommended to be taken at what intervals after birth?

   A. 2 minutes and 10 minutes   **C.** 5 minutes and 10 minutes

   B. 1 minute and 5 minutes   **D.** 1 minute and 2 minutes

6. _____ of blood loss after delivery is considered postpartum hemorrhage.

   A. 1,000 mL   **C.** 750 mL

   B. 150 mL   **D.** 500 mL

7. What medication can be used to control postpartum hemorrhage in the prehospital setting?

   A. Oxytocin   **C.** Magnesium sulfate

   B. Terbutaline   **D.** Diphenhydramine

8. The fallopian tube is composed of three layers of tissues. _____ is NOT one of these layers.

   A. Mucosa   **C.** Serosa

   B. Muscularis   **D.** Fundus

9. The normal gestational period for an infant to develop in the uterus is how many weeks?

   A. 30   **C.** 38

   B. 32   **D.** 42

10. A pregnant woman's heart rate gradually increases during pregnancy by an average of how many beats/min by term?

   A. 15 to 20 beats/min   **C.** 20 to 25 beats/min

   B. 5 to 10 beats/min   **D.** 15 to 30 beats/min

Labeling

Label the following diagrams with the correct terms.

1. Label the structures of the pregnant uterus.

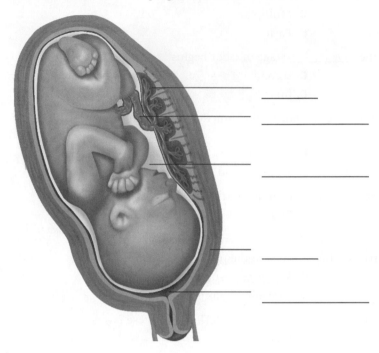

_____

_____

_____

_____

_____

2. Label the following figures with the correct cause of hemorrhage listed as follows.

    A. Abruptio placenta

    B. Placenta previa

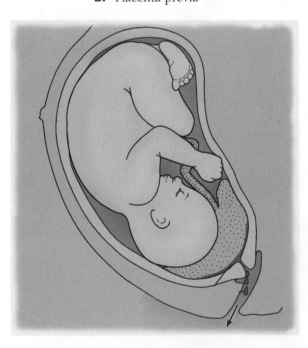 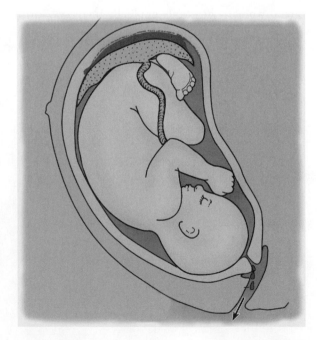

_____   _____

Fill-in-the-Blank

Read each item carefully, and then complete the statement by filling in the missing word(s).

1. The inner lining of the uterus is called the _____.

2. The _____ _____ connects the placenta to the fetus.

3. A pregnant woman's heart rate gradually _____ during pregnancy.

4. _____ is the most serious of the hypertension disorders that occurs during pregnancy.

5. A _____ _____ occurs naturally, affecting about 1 in every 5 pregnancies.

6. _____ _____ _____ is when the placenta is implanted low in the uterus and, as it grows, it partially or fully obscures the cervical canal.

7. _____ is a term used to describe a woman who has had two or more pregnancies.

8. The _____ _____ of labor begins as the baby's head enters the birth canal.

9. In a/an _____ presentation, the fetus lies crosswise in the uterus and may wave at the paramedic with one hand protruding from the vagina.

10. _____ _____ is a drug used in pregnancy as the principal management for eclampsia.

Identify

In the following case study, list the chief complaint, vital signs, and pertinent findings.

You are called to a private residence for a report of a pregnant patient who has vaginal bleeding. The patient is lying in bed, and when you ask what is wrong she tells you, "I am bleeding from my vagina." You see blood on the sheets. You and your partner start a quick assessment. You take the vital signs and your partner obtains a SAMPLE history. The patient is 35 years old and states she started to bleed about half an hour ago. Upon questioning, she tells you there is no pain, the blood was bright red, this is her third pregnancy, and she is in her eighth month. Both the previous pregnancies were full term and delivered by cesarean section. She states that she had strong contractions, but they have decreased. She feels weak and asks if she can have a drink of water. She has no allergies, is taking vitamin supplements per doctor's orders, has no significant past medical history, and had a light breakfast of toast and juice about 2 hours ago. Your partner reports the pulse to be 110 beats/min and thready, respirations are 24 breaths/min, blood pressure is 100/70 mm Hg, and she is pale and diaphoretic. The patient tells you that the blood pressure reading you just measured is lower than the pressure the doctor measured last week at her checkup appointment. You put the patient on 100% supplemental oxygen using a nonrebreathing mask, place a loose trauma pad over the vagina, prepare for immediate transport, start a large-bore IV in the ambulance, contact medical control to get an order for magnesium sulfate, and notify the hospital so they can be properly prepared upon your arrival. You arrive at the receiving facility in 15 minutes and are told to go immediately to the delivery room. Later that evening while delivering another patient to the same hospital, you are informed that the mother delivered, and although the baby's birth weight is low, both the mother and the baby are expected to be fine.

1. Chief Complaint

_____

_____

_____

2. Vital Signs

_____

_____

_____

3. Pertinent Findings

_____

_____

_____

Ambulance Calls

The following case scenarios provide an opportunity to explore the concerns associated with patient management and paramedic care. Read each scenario, and then answer each question.

1. A 22-year-old woman calls for an ambulance because of vaginal bleeding. She states that she is "about 3 months pregnant" and that the bleeding started yesterday, when she thinks she passed some tissue. She has used about 10 sanitary napkins since then. On examination, her skin feels cool and wet. Her pulse is 120 beats/min and weak, and her blood pressure is 90/60 mm Hg.

   a. This woman is likely to be experiencing a/an:

        A. threatened abortion.

        B. inevitable abortion.

        C. incomplete abortion.

        D. missed abortion.

        E. septic abortion.

   b. List the steps in the prehospital management of this patient.

        (1) _____

        (2) _____

        (3) _____

        (4) _____

        (5) _____

2. A 32-year-old woman calls for an ambulance because she is "feeling poorly." She states that she is "about 6 months along" in a pregnancy. She has not had any prenatal care. She had some vaginal bleeding "early on," but it lasted only a few days, and then stopped. Now for several days, the patient has felt vaguely unwell. She has had a brownish vaginal discharge that smells rank, and "things are very quiet in there." On physical examination, the patient does not appear to be in any distress. Her pulse is 74 beats/min and regular, respirations are 18 breaths/min and unlabored, and blood pressure is 120/80 mm Hg. On abdominal examination, you can feel the uterine fundus just above the pelvic brim; it feels quite hard. You are not able to hear fetal heart tones, but the room is noisy, and so you are not sure what to make of that finding.

   a. This woman is likely to be experiencing a/an:

        A. threatened abortion.

        B. inevitable abortion.

        C. incomplete abortion.

        D. missed abortion.

        E. septic abortion.

b. List the steps in the prehospital management of this patient.

(1) _____

(2) _____

3. A 20-year-old primigravida calls for an ambulance because of vaginal bleeding. She states that she is in her fourth month of pregnancy and has been fine up to now, but this morning she noticed some bleeding. She denies abdominal pain or cramping. On physical examination, there are no abnormal findings.

a. This woman is likely to be experiencing a/an:

    A. threatened abortion.

    B. inevitable abortion.

    C. incomplete abortion.

    D. missed abortion.

    E. septic abortion.

b. List the steps in the prehospital management of this patient.

(1) _____

(2) _____

4. You are called to a suburban home for a "sick girl." The patient is a 16-year-old girl with a high fever. She insists on giving you her history privately, without her parents in the room. After her parents exit, the girl tells you that she had gone that morning to "some hole in the wall" to have an abortion. A few hours after she got home, she started to feel sick, and she has been having a bad-smelling, bloody vaginal discharge ever since. On examination, she looks very ill. Her pulse is 120 beats/min and weak, respirations are 28 breaths/min and shallow, blood pressure is 80/60 mm Hg, and oral temperature is 40°C (104°F).

a. This woman is likely to be experiencing a/an:

    A. threatened abortion.

    B. inevitable abortion.

    C. incomplete abortion.

    D. missed abortion.

    E. septic abortion.

b. List the steps in the prehospital management of this patient.

(1) _____

(2) _____

(3) _____

(4) _____

(5) _____

5. You are called to the home of a weeping 26-year-old woman in the 15th week of pregnancy. "It's happening again," she sobs, "I just know it's happening again." She tells you that she has had three miscarriages in the past and that this morning she started having severe abdominal cramps and bleeding, "just like all the other times." She has used six sanitary napkins since the bleeding started about 3 hours ago. On physical examination, she is very distraught. Her pulse is 110 beats/min and regular, respirations are 24 breaths/min and unlabored, blood pressure is 110/70 mm Hg, and she is febrile. On palpating the abdomen, you can feel the uterine contractions.

a. This woman is likely to be experiencing a/an:

    A. threatened abortion.

    B. inevitable abortion.

    C. incomplete abortion.

    D. missed abortion.

    E. septic abortion.

b. List the steps in the prehospital management of this patient.

(1) _____

(2) _____

(3) _____

(4) _____

(5) _____

6. You are called to the home of a 36-year-old grand multipara whose chief complaint is bleeding. She is in her 11th pregnancy and "due any day now." She states that the bleeding, a bright red blood, started a few hours ago, without any warning. She has not had any cramps or other symptoms, and "the baby is still kicking like a football player." On physical examination, the woman looks a little pale and apprehensive. Her pulse is 124 beats/min and regular, respirations are 28 breaths/min and unlabored, and blood pressure is 100/68 mm Hg; she is afebrile. On gentle palpation, you find the abdomen soft. The fundus is at the level of the xiphoid, and fetal heart tones are audible. The fetal heart rate is 140 beats/min.

a. List three possible causes of this woman's bleeding.

(1) _____

(2) _____

(3) _____

b. Of those three causes, which do you think is the most likely cause in her case?

_____

c. What signs led you to this diagnosis?

(1) _____

(2) _____

(3) _____

(4) _____

d. List the steps you will take in managing this patient.

(1) _____

(2) _____

(3) _____

(4) _____

7. You are called to see a 28-year-old woman in her 35th week of pregnancy after she had a "fainting spell." The patient's husband greets you at the door and tells you, "We were just sitting there talking—Agnes was lying in bed and I was sitting in the chair—and suddenly I look over and I see that she's out cold. Not sleeping, just out." The patient has meanwhile regained consciousness. She says she feels rather dizzy and has a slight headache, but otherwise feels all right. She denies vaginal bleeding. On physical examination, her pulse is 104 beats/min and regular, her respirations are 24 breaths/min and unlabored, and her blood pressure is 90/60 mm Hg. When you have her roll onto her side, and then recheck her vitals a couple of minutes later, her pulse is 88 beats/min and her blood pressure is 120/72 mm Hg. Her fundus is nearly at the level of the xiphoid, and fetal heart tones are present at a rate of 160 beats/min.

   a. This woman is most probably suffering from which of the following?

       A. Inevitable abortion

       B. Preeclampsia

       C. Eclampsia

       D. Abruptio placenta

       E. Supine hypotensive syndrome

   b. List the steps in the prehospital care of this patient.

     (1) _____

     (2) _____

     (3) _____

     (4) _____

8. You are called to a downtown department store, where an obviously pregnant woman has fallen and twisted her ankle. You find her surrounded by a knot of agitated people, none of them more agitated than the store manager. As you are checking the woman's pedal pulses, you notice that *both* ankles are swollen, not just the one she injured. You decide you had better get a set of vital signs because you vaguely remember learning that vital signs should be measured in *every* patient, especially every *pregnant* patient. In this woman, you find the pulse is 110 beats/min and regular, respirations are 20 breaths/min and unlabored, and blood pressure is 150/90 mm Hg. As you are taking the radial pulse, you notice that the patient's hands seem puffy. It is too noisy in the store to even bother trying to listen for fetal heart tones, but the woman tells you that the baby is "kicking away."

   a. This woman is most probably suffering from:

       A. inevitable abortion.

       B. preeclampsia.

       C. eclampsia.

       D. abruptio placenta.

       E. supine hypotensive syndrome.

   b. List the steps in the prehospital care of this patient.

     (1) _____

     (2) _____

     (3) _____

   c. En route to the hospital, you find yourself locked in a traffic jam on the freeway. Meanwhile, your patient starts complaining of cramping abdominal pains. "I've never had a baby before," she says, "but I think these are labor pains." While you look helplessly at the line of cars stretching endlessly in front of and behind the ambulance, the woman's eyes suddenly roll back, and she has a grand mal seizure. What steps will you take *now*?

     (1) _____

     (2) _____

     (3) _____

     (4) _____

     (5) _____

9. A 26-year-old woman in her 30th week of pregnancy was the driver of a car that skidded off the road and plowed head-on into a tree. The woman was wearing a shoulder/lap seat belt. Sitting in the passenger seat of the same car was a woman in her 28th week of pregnancy (they were returning together from a natural childbirth class), also wearing a seat belt. En route to the call, you try to review in your mind the injuries you will need to look for in particular because you remember that pregnancy makes a woman more vulnerable to trauma.

a. List five anatomic or physiologic changes of pregnancy that affect a woman's susceptibility or response to trauma.

(1) _____

(2) _____

(3) _____

(4) _____

(5) _____

b. On reaching the scene of the accident, you find the driver of the car conscious, still sitting behind the wheel of the car. She complains of thirst. On physical examination, her skin is cool and moist. Her pulse is 120 beats/min and regular, respirations are 24 breaths/min and shallow, and blood pressure is 110/68 mm Hg. There is a steering wheel bruise on the upper abdomen. The abdomen is not particularly tender, and it is not rigid. The conditions are too noisy to try to hear fetal heart tones. List the steps in managing this patient.

(1) _____

(2) _____

(3) _____

(4) _____

(5) _____

(6) _____

c. The front-seat passenger is also fully conscious. She complains of a "whiplash," but otherwise thinks she feels all right. "At least the baby's all right," she says. "I can feel him moving around." On physical examination, her skin is warm and moist. Her pulse is 100 beats/min and regular, respirations are 20 breaths/min and unlabored, and her blood pressure is 124/70 mm Hg. You do not find any evidence of injury. Can you conclude that there has been no injury to the fetus? _____ Explain the reason for your answer.

_____

_____

10. For each of the following cases, indicate one of the following:

T   There is time to transport the woman to the hospital for delivery.

D   You will have to assist in emergency delivery in the field.

For each case that you decide requires prehospital delivery, indicate what, if any, complications you must anticipate.

a. _____ A 20-year-old woman in her first pregnancy. She says her water broke about 6 hours ago. Now her contractions are about 2 minutes apart, and she feels a need to move her bowels. You are 20 minutes from the hospital.

What, if any, complications may occur?

_____

_____

b. _____ A 32-year-old multipara (gravida 10, para 8) who has been in labor about 5 hours. Her contractions are 3 minutes apart. She says she thinks the baby's coming. You are 10 minutes from the hospital.

What, if any, complications may occur?

_____

_____

c. _____ A 25-year-old nullipara (gravida 1, para 0) who has been in labor for 9 hours. Her contractions are 4 to 5 minutes apart. You are 20 minutes from the hospital.

What, if any, complications may occur?

_____

_____

d. _____ A 30-year-old gravida 4, para 3 who has been in labor for 6 hours. She had two of her three children by cesarean section. Her contractions are 2 minutes apart, and she is crowning. You are 5 minutes from the hospital.

What, if any, complications may occur?

_____

_____

e. _____ A 28-year-old gravida 1, para 0 whose contractions started 24 hours ago. They do not come at regular intervals, and they have not gotten much more intense since they started. You are 25 minutes from the hospital.

What, if any, complications may occur?

_____

_____

f. _____ A 24-year-old gravida 3, para 2 who announces, as you enter her apartment, "Hurry, the twins are coming any minute!" She says she has been in labor "quite a while," and you time her contractions as coming less than 2 minutes apart. You are 20 minutes from the hospital.

What, if any, complications may occur?

_____

_____

11. You are assisting in the delivery of a baby in the lingerie section of a downtown department store.

a. The baby's head delivers spontaneously, and you notice that it is covered with a membrane. What should you do?

_____

_____

b. You deal with that problem successfully. The next thing you notice is that the umbilical cord is wound tightly around the baby's neck. What should you do about that?

_____

_____

c. List the steps in carrying out the remainder of the delivery (second and third stages).

(1) _____

(2) _____

(3) _____

(4) _____

(5) _____

(6) _____

(7) _____

(8) _____

(9) _____

12. During another one of your weekends off at the ski lodge, when you are cheerfully snowed in, one of the other guests arrives in the lounge and asks, "Does anyone here know anything about delivering a baby? My wife seems to be in labor." You shrivel up into a corner of your chair, hoping someone else will come forward, but there doesn't seem to be any obstetricians among the skiers. So, with a sigh, you stand up and follow the distraught husband to his room. There you find a woman in active labor, already crowning. Inspecting the presenting part, you note that it looks awfully smooth, and it has a sort of crack running down the middle.

a. What are you dealing with?

_____

b. Describe how you will manage this case.

(1) _____

(2) _____

(3) _____

(4) _____

(5) _____

(6) _____

(7) _____

13. The day after you get back to work, your very first call is another "possible OB." The patient is a 24-year-old woman in her first pregnancy whose labor started about 10 hours earlier. "This wasn't supposed to happen for another month and a half," she tells you. The contractions are now about 2 minutes apart. When you inspect her to see whether she is crowning, you see a short length of umbilical cord protruding from her vagina. Describe how you will manage this case.

a. _____

b. _____

c. _____

d. _____

e. _____

f. _____

14. You are called to the home of a 30-year-old gravida 6, para 5 who has gone into labor. "It's twins," she announces as soon as you come in the door. "I'm carrying twins, and they're coming at any moment, I can feel it." And indeed, when you examine the woman, you find that she is crowning.

   a. Describe the special measures necessary in this case.

   (1) _____

   (2) _____

   b. After delivery of the placenta, the mother continues bleeding quite briskly from her vagina. Did this woman have any risk factors for postpartum hemorrhage? _____ If so, what risk factor(s)?

   _____

   _____

   c. List three other risk factors for postpartum hemorrhage.

   (1) _____

   (2) _____

   (3) _____

   d. Describe how you will manage this situation.

   (1) _____

   (2) _____

   (3) _____

   (4) _____

   (5) _____

   (6) _____

True/False

If you believe the statement to be more true than false, write the letter "T" in the space provided. If you believe the statement to be more false than true, write the letter "F."

_____ 1. If you are transporting a woman in labor, and she begins crowning when you are only a minute or two from the hospital, you should instruct her to cross her legs until you reach the emergency department.

_____ 2. If the fetal heart rate is less than 120 beats/min, the fetus is in danger.

_____ 3. A woman should be discouraged from sitting up or squatting for delivery of her baby because those positions are counter to natural physiology and increase the demand on the mother's energy.

_____ 4. If the baby is coming fast, it is more important to control the delivery than it is to drape the mother with sterile towels.

_____ 5. If the cut ends of the umbilical cord are oozing blood, you should unclamp them and reapply the clamps more tightly.

_____ **6.** If the placenta has not delivered within 20 minutes of the baby's delivery, you should exert gentle traction on the umbilical cord while you vigorously massage the uterus.

_____ **7.** With the exception of buttocks breech, all other abnormal presentations must be delivered in the hospital.

Short Answer

Complete this section with short written answers using the space provided.

By the second or third week of pregnancy, the placenta starts to develop inside the maternal uterus. The placenta is a specialized organ of pregnancy whose overall task is to nurture the developing fetus. List four specific functions that the placenta carries out for the fetus.

a. _____

b. _____

c. _____

d. _____

Fill-in-the-Table

Fill in the missing parts of the table.

1. Fill in the amount of time needed for the three stages of labor for a nullipara and for a multipara.

The Stages of Labor: Nullipara Versus Multipara		
Stage of Labor	**Nullipara**	**Multipara**
First stage	8 to 12 hours	
Second stage		
Third stage		5 to 60 minutes

Word Find

Hidden in the following grid are 19 words or phrases related to what you have studied in this chapter. Find the hidden words in the grid below. Then use the words from the grid to answer the following questions (some words may be used to answer more than one question).

```
O F G P U O N G L V Y U G D R
Y S B Y U G N P E A G Y V R W
S Y X H B I L R U M O U C O C
E B U T N A I P O L L A F C P
S F B W C U B Y N V S C X L R
S D O E Z C T Z A C A K I A E
L R N M U V O E I X J K V C P
C T Y L N O I T R O B A R I A
A E A P S B O P D U X L E L R
F M O V D I V A R G S E C I T
E B V I N V A G I N A D O B U
T R Z M P R I M I P A R A M M
U Y A O V U L A T E D Z R U R
S O D H W D O U N T X N K R E
K E D O S U T K K F F H B H T
```

On around the 14th day of the cycle, women _____, that is, a Graafian follicle located in the left or right ovary ruptures and releases an egg, or _____. If a sperm should happen along just about the time when the egg is released, fertilization may take place, usually in the _____ _____, where the fertilized egg remains for about 3 days before entering the _____ and implanting in the endometrium. Between the third and eighth week of development, the fertilized egg is called a/an _____. Thereafter, it is called a/an _____ until delivery. After delivery, it is officially a/an _____.

Specialized structures develop during pregnancy to support the developing baby. The baby is enclosed in a fluid-filled _____ _____. It is nourished by a large, vascular organ of pregnancy called the _____, which attaches to the baby via the _____ _____.

At about 40 weeks after conception, the baby reaches maturity, or _____, and is ready to make its debut in the world. (When a baby is expelled early, before the 20th to 28th week of gestation, the woman is said to have had a miscarriage, or _____.) At that point, the woman goes into labor, the process by which the baby is expelled from the womb, and the pregnant, or _____, womb begins contracting. As it does so, the _____ progressively effaces and dilates until the womb becomes continuous with the birth canal, or _____. The period of uterine contractions are of shorter duration in a/an _____, a woman who has already had a delivery in the past, than they are in a nullipara. Delivery is imminent when the presenting part becomes visible, that is, when _____ occurs. At that point, it is important to control the rate at which the baby emerges; otherwise, there may be injury to the mother's external genitalia (_____) or to the skin between the anus and the opening of the birth canal, an area called the perineum. All events occurring before delivery are called antepartum, or _____, while those occurring after delivery are called postpartum.

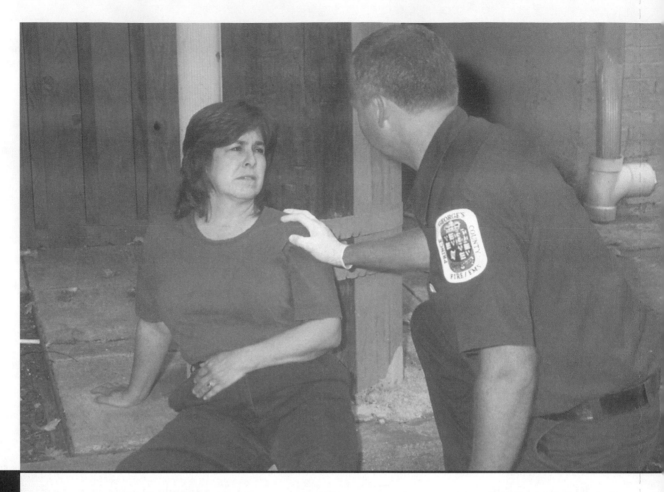

45-Year-Old Female with a Severe Headache

At 9:44 am, you are dispatched to a convenience store in the 1600 block of North Main St for a 45-year-old female with a severe headache. The patient's husband stopped at the convenience store and asked the clerk to call EMS. Your response time to the scene is approximately 5 minutes.

You arrive at the scene at 9:50 am, where you find the patient, who appears confused and disoriented, sitting on the sidewalk outside the convenience store. You introduce yourself to the patient, and begin an initial assessment.

Initial Assessment

Level of consciousness	Confused and disoriented
Chief complaint	"My head is killing me!"
Airway and breathing	Airway is patent; respirations are normal
Circulation	Pulse is regular and bounding, rate appears normal, skin is flushed and warm

1. What initial management is indicated for this patient?

As your partner is performing the required initial management, the patient's husband tells you that his wife has high blood pressure and depression, and takes medications for both conditions.

Your partner attaches the ECG leads to the patient, as you perform a focused history and physical examination. The patient's husband provides you with the information you need.

Focused History and Physical Examination	
Description of the episode	"She had a headache when she awoke this morning."
Onset	"I don't know exactly when the headache began."
Duration	"She has had this headache since she woke up."
Associated symptoms	"She complained of nausea and double vision."
Evidence of trauma	None
Interventions prior to EMS arrival	None
Seizures	"She has not had any seizures."
Fever	The patient is afebrile
Blood glucose	130 mg/dL

You ask the patient when she last took her blood pressure medication. Still confused and disoriented, she tells you that she cannot recall. Your partner hands you the patient's cardiac rhythm strip **(Figure 5-1)**.

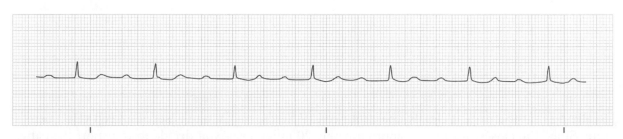

■ **Figure 5-1** Your patient's cardiac rhythm.

2. What is your interpretation of this cardiac rhythm?

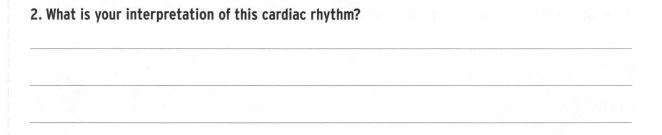

The patient complains that the sun is making her headache worse, so you move her into the ambulance and dim the lights. As your partner establishes an IV of normal saline, you obtain baseline vital signs and a SAMPLE history.

Baseline Vital Signs and SAMPLE History	
Blood pressure	210/170 mm Hg
Pulse	64 beats/min, regular and bounding
Respirations	16 breaths/min and unlabored
Oxygen saturation	98% (on 100% oxygen)
Signs and symptoms	Confusion, nausea, diplopia and photophobia, headache, and hypertension
Allergies	"I am allergic to Novocain."
Medications	"I take prazosin, Diuril, and Luvox."
Pertinent past history	"I have high blood pressure, and am always depressed."
Last oral intake	"I can't remember when I last ate."
Events leading to present illness	"I woke up this morning with this headache, which is the worst headache that I have ever had."

3. What is your field impression of this patient?

_____

_____

_____

_____

4. Are the patient's vital signs and SAMPLE history findings consistent with your field impression?

_____

_____

_____

Realizing that the patient clearly does not need IV fluids, the IV line is set at a keep vein open rate. Since the closest hospital is approximately 20 miles away, you decide to transport the patient at once, while performing further interventions en route.

5. What specific treatment is required for this patient's condition?

_____

_____

_____

_____

Following your next intervention, you reassess the patient's blood pressure, and note that it is 170/110 mm Hg. The patient, who is still complaining of a severe headache, appears less confused and disoriented. You complete your ongoing assessment and then notify the receiving hospital of your impending arrival.

Ongoing Assessment

Level of consciousness	Conscious, less confused and disoriented
Airway and breathing	16 breaths/min and unlabored
Oxygen saturation	98% (on 100% oxygen)
Blood pressure	168/106 mm Hg
Pulse	60 beats/min and regular, less bounding

6. Is further treatment required for this patient?

_____

_____

_____

_____

7. Are there any special considerations for this patient?

_____

_____

_____

_____

The patient's condition continues to improve with your treatment. She is delivered to the emergency department, where her blood pressure is treated definitively.

A CT scan of her head shows no abnormalities. She is admitted to the medical intensive care unit with a diagnosis of acute hypertensive encephalopathy, and is discharged home 1 week later without neurologic deficit.

CHAPTER

40 Neonatology

Chapter Review

The following exercises provide an opportunity to test your knowledge of this chapter.

Matching

Match each of the definitions in the left column to the appropriate term in the right column.

_____ **1.** A dark green fecal material that accumulates in the fetal intestines and is discharged around the time of birth

_____ **2.** First pregnancy

_____ **3.** Used to describe an infant delivered at less than 37 weeks gestation

_____ **4.** Respiratory pause greater than or equal to 20 seconds

_____ **5.** A fissure or hole in the palate (roof of the mouth) that forms a communicating pathway between the mouth and nasal cavities

_____ **6.** Infant during the first month after birth

_____ **7.** Oxygen administered via oxygen tube and a cupped hand on patient's face

_____ **8.** A narrowing or blockage of the nasal airway by membranous or bony tissue; a congenital condition, meaning it is present at birth

_____ **9.** Used to describe an infant delivered at 38 to 42 weeks of gestation

_____ **10.** Abnormal location of the placenta in the lower part of the uterus, near or over the cervix

_____ **11.** Scale used to assess newborn infant status (range 0 to 10)

_____ **12.** A substance formed in the lungs that helps keep the small air sacs, or alveoli, from collapsing and sticking together; a low level in a premature baby contributes to respiratory distress syndrome

_____ **13.** A pulse rate of less than 100 beats/min in the newborn

_____ **14.** Blood vessel in umbilical cord used to administer emergency medications

A. Apnea

B. Neonate

C. Term

D. Free-flow (blow-by) oxygen

E. Choanal atresia

F. Umbilical vein

G. Placenta previa

H. Meconium

I. Preterm

J. Surfactant

K. Cleft palate

L. Bradycardia

M. Apgar score

N. Primigravida

Multiple Choice

Read each item carefully, and then select the best response.

_____ 1. As the baby is delivered, a rapid series of events must occur to enable the baby to breathe; this process is called fetal:

      A. transportation.
      B. transposition.
      C. transmission.
      D. transition.

_____ 2. An infant delivered at less than 37 weeks of gestation is considered:

      A. preterm.
      B. term.
      C. postterm.
      D. none of the above.

_____ 3. The Apgar score, named after Dr. Virginia Apgar, who developed this measure in 1953, helps determine the need for and the effectiveness of resuscitation. The Apgar score is determined on the basis of the newborn's condition at _____ minutes after birth.

      A. 2 and 10
      B. 5 and 10
      C. 1 and 5
      D. 1 and 3

_____ 4. Fewer than 1% of deliveries involve bradycardia that requires treatment with chest compressions. The most common etiology for bradycardia in a neonate is:

      A. fetal alcohol syndrome.
      B. maternal drug abuse.
      C. hypoxia.
      D. prolapsed cord.

_____ 5. Infants do not normally pass stool before birth, but if they do and then inhale the meconium-stained amniotic fluid either in utero or at delivery, their airways may become plugged and hypoxia may ensue. This, in turn, can lead to:

      A. atelectasis.
      B. pneumonitis.
      C. pneumothorax.
      D. all of the above.

_____ 6. A fluid bolus in an infant consists of _____ mL/kg of normal saline IV given over 5 to 10 minutes.

      A. 10
      B. 15
      C. 5
      D. 20

_____ 7. After ensuring the patency of the airway by bulb suctioning of the newborn's mouth and nose, dry and stimulate the infant. Flick the soles of the baby's feet and:

      A. slap the baby's back.
      B. slap the baby's buttocks.
      C. aggressively rub the baby's back.
      D. gently rub the baby's back.

_____ 8. A diagnosis of diaphragmatic hernia is suspected clinically in a newborn with:

      A. apnea.
      B. heart sounds shifted to the left.
      C. scaphoid abdomen.
      D. all of the above.

_____ 9. Primary apnea is often characterized by:

      A. hypoxia, rapid breathing, apnea, and bradycardia.
      B. hypoxia, apnea, and bradycardia.
      C. apnea and bradycardia.
      D. none of the above.

_____ 10. The lungs of a premature infant are weak, so use:

      A. the maximum allowable ventilatory pressure to expand lung tissue.
      B. mechanical devices to administer positive-pressure ventilation.
      C. small puffs from your cheek with a pocket mask to ventilate.
      D. the minimum pressure necessary to move the chest when you are providing positive-pressure ventilation (PPV).

Labeling

The following is a portion of the algorithm used for the resuscitation of a distressed newborn. Fill in the appropriate time and heart rate that corresponds to the lines left blank in the following diagram.

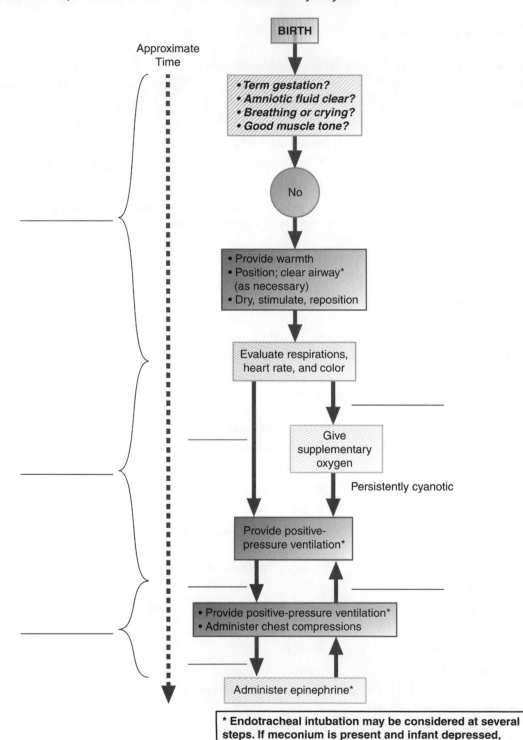

A. 30 seconds (approximate time)

B. 30 seconds (approximate time)

C. 30 seconds (approximate time)

D. Breathing, heart rate (HR) >100 beats/min but cyanotic

E. Apneic or HR < 100 beats/min

F. HR < 60 beats/min

G. HR > 60 beats/min

H. HR < 60 beats/min

BIRTH

Approximate Time

• Term gestation?
• Amniotic fluid clear?
• Breathing or crying?
• Good muscle tone?

No

• Provide warmth
• Position; clear airway*
 (as necessary)
• Dry, stimulate, reposition

Evaluate respirations, heart rate, and color

Give supplementary oxygen

Persistently cyanotic

Provide positive-pressure ventilation*

• Provide positive-pressure ventilation*
• Administer chest compressions

Administer epinephrine*

* Endotracheal intubation may be considered at several steps. If meconium is present and infant depressed, intubate and suction trachea before stimulating.

Fill-in-the-Blank

Read each item carefully, and then complete the statement by filling in the missing word(s).

1. During fetal _____, the newborn's lungs need to expand with air within seconds. As the baby's lungs become filled with air, the _____ pressure drops and blood begins to flow to the lungs, picking up _____.

2. An infant delivered at less than _____ completed weeks of gestation is considered preterm; an infant born at _____ to _____ weeks of gestation is described as term; and an infant born at more than _____ weeks of gestation is described as postterm.

3. If the _____ _____ comes out ahead of the baby, the _____ _____ through the umbilical cord may be cut off. In this case, relieving _____ on the cord can be lifesaving.

4. All newborns are _____ immediately after birth. If the newborn remains _____ and quickly becomes pink, ongoing observation and continued _____ with direct skin-to-skin contact with the mother should be maintained while on the way to a local hospital.

5. You should use caution when squeezing the ventilation bag to avoid inadvertently delivering too much volume, potentially resulting in a/an _____. After providing 30 seconds of adequate ventilation by PPV with 100% supplemental oxygen via a bag-mask device, check the infant's pulse. If the rate is less than 60 beats/min, begin chest _____. Effective chest compressions should result in _____ pulses.

6. Oral airways are _____ used for neonates, but they can be lifesaving if airway _____ leads to respiratory failure. Bilateral _____ _____ can be rapidly fatal, but usually responds to placement of an oral airway.

7. Gastric _____ using a/an _____ tube is indicated for prolonged bag-mask ventilation, if abdominal distention is impeding ventilation, or in the presence of a/an _____ hernia.

8. Jitteriness is often confused with a/an _____. Jitteriness is characteristically a disorder of the _____ and is rarely seen at a later age.

9. Many newborns with serious life-threatening _____ may actually see their core _____ drop; these infants are at a higher risk for _____ and _____ acidosis.

10. Symptoms of _____ may include cyanosis, _____, irritability, poor sucking or _____, and hypothermia. These symptoms may also be associated with _____, tremors, twitching or _____, and coma.

11. Vomiting _____, occasionally _____ streaked, in the first few hours of life is not _____.

12. _____ should not be administered in the field. The infant may be dehydrated, however, and may need fluid _____. Dry mucous membranes, tachycardia, or a sunken _____ are clues that the patient needs hydration.

13. The newborn's airway and ventilation may be compromised if he or she is severely _____ and is _____, so ensure that adequate oxygenation and ventilation is available. Perform chest _____ in addition to PPV in a newborn if the pulse rate is less than 60 beats/min.

14. Because the average _____ _____ cannot provide the specially trained doctors and nurses or the expensive _____ needed for such care, it sometimes becomes necessary to transfer the critically ill infant to a/an _____ _____, where the infant may benefit from highly skilled personnel and sophisticated equipment.

15. The most common cause of acute diarrhea in children is _____ _____.

Identify

In the following case studies, identify the appropriate resuscitation steps.

1. You are dispatched to the scene of a full-term pregnancy. Mom is in active labor and the baby is crowning. You've appropriately decided to move her to your Advanced Life Support unit with the heater turned on and have requested a second unit in the event of complications. To your surprise, you discover the presentation of a prolapsed cord.

    a. How do you treat this emergency?

    (1) _____

    (2) _____

    (3) _____

    (4) _____

    (5) _____

    (6) _____

    (7) _____

2. After assisting in the delivery of a full-term newborn boy, you bulb suction the infant's mouth and nose, and dry and stimulate the baby.

    a. After 30 seconds, the baby is centrally cyanotic of the trunk and mucous membranes. What treatment would you now initiate?

    (1) _____

    (2) _____

    b. After 30 seconds of adequate ventilation by PPV with 100% supplemental oxygen via a bag-mask device, the infant's pulse rate is now less than 60 beats/min. What treatment would you now initiate?

    (1) _____

    (2) _____

    (3) _____

Ambulance Calls

The following case scenarios provide an opportunity to explore the concerns associated with patient management and paramedic care. Read each scenario, and then answer each question.

1. You are called to attend a 38-year-old woman who is in active labor at home. She has not had any prenatal care. She tells you that "this baby is a month late according to my calendar and is sure a long time in coming." Her contractions started about 10 hours ago and are now 2 minutes apart. Her "bag of waters" broke 10 minutes before your arrival, and you notice greenish stains on the bedclothes. The woman says she feels as if she has to move her bowels.

   a. Are there any indications that this may be a complicated delivery or that you may have problems with the baby after delivery? _____. If so, list the risk factors in this delivery.

      (1) _____

      (2) _____

      (3) _____

      (4) _____

      (5) _____

   b. List four other risk factors, not present in this case, that indicate a high likelihood of complications during delivery or immediately thereafter.

      (1) _____

      (2) _____

      (3) _____

      (4) _____

   c. You immediately set up for delivery—and none too soon! You scarcely have your gloves on before the baby is crowning, and a moment later, the head is delivered. It is covered with a thick, greenish substance. List the steps you would take at this point.

      (1) _____

      (2) _____

   d. What further steps should you take when the baby is fully delivered?

      (1) _____

      (2) _____

      (3) _____

      (4) _____

      (5) _____

2. You are called to a movie theater where a 23-year-old woman who is gravida 4, para 3 went into active labor while watching *Return of the Spider Monster.* You find the patient in a cold, drafty ladies' room, sitting on the floor, panting. "I'm only in my seventh month," she says. "This can't be happening." As she makes that statement, the baby's head delivers spontaneously, and so you scramble to the floor to control the rest of the delivery. Within seconds, you find yourself holding a very red, wrinkled, little baby.

a. List the steps you would take at this point in the sequence in which you would perform them.

(1) _____

(2) _____

(3) _____

(4) _____

b. At what point would you clamp and cut the baby's umbilical cord? (Explain the reasoning behind your answer.)

_____

_____

_____

c. What steps can you take to prevent the baby from becoming hypothermic?

(1) _____

(2) _____

(3) _____

(4) _____

(5) _____

(6) _____

d. What other special measures should be taken in caring for this baby, besides ensuring that it stays warm?

(1) _____

(2) _____

(3) _____

3. You are called to a downtown apartment for a "sick woman." You arrive to find a teenage girl sitting on the toilet, having given birth only seconds before. The placenta has not yet delivered. You quickly remove the newborn from the toilet.

a. List the steps you would take at this point.

(1) _____

(2) _____

(3) _____

(4) _____

(5) _____

b. What would be the indications for starting artificial ventilation on this baby?

(1) _____

(2) _____

(3) _____

c. As it turns out, the baby has one of those indications, so you start artificial ventilation with a bag-mask device and 100% supplemental oxygen. After a minute, you reassess the baby and find that its heart rate is 84 beats/min. What should you do now?

_____

_____

d. After another minute or so, you reassess again. The baby's heart rate is now 56 beats/min. What should you do now?

_____

_____

e. Under what circumstances should you administer epinephrine to this baby?

(1) _____

(2) _____

f. If ordered to give epinephrine, what dosage will you give? (The baby weighs 3 kg.) _____

True/False

If you believe the statement to be more true than false, write the letter "T" in the space provided. If you believe the statement to be more false than true, write the letter "F."

_____ 1. Oropharyngeal suctioning may stimulate the vagus nerve in a newborn and cause severe bradycardia.

_____ 2. Even slight meconium staining of the amniotic fluid indicates a need to intubate the newborn immediately after delivery.

_____ 3. If the fetal heart rate is less than 120 beats/min at any point during labor, you should roll the mother onto her side and give her supplemental oxygen to breathe.

_____ 4. Clamping and cutting of the umbilical cord should ordinarily be carried out after the cord stops pulsating.

_____ 5. Infants may die of cold exposure at temperatures adults find comfortable.

_____ 6. Most newborns who require resuscitation will need cardiopulmonary resuscitation (CPR).

_____ 7. The umbilical vein is a large, thin-walled vessel usually found at the 4 o'clock position, as compared to the two thick-walled umbilical arteries usually found at 12 and 8 o'clock.

_____ 8. Birth injuries account for 20% to 30% of all infant deaths.

_____ 9. A normal number of stools per day for an infant is five to six, especially if the infant is breastfeeding, when infants often produce stool after every feeding.

_____ 10. Meconium-stained amniotic fluid, which is present in 10% to 15% of deliveries, carries a high risk of morbidity.

Short Answer

Complete this section with short written answers using the space provided.

1. Neonatal IV access under the best circumstances can be difficult and stressful. An important alternative is catheterization of the umbilical vein. Detail the steps necessary to perform this task.

   a. _____

   b. _____

   c. _____

   d. _____

   e. _____

2. One of the most important skills that a paramedic must acquire and maintain is the ability to intubate neonates. Describe the steps necessary to properly intubate a neonate.

   a. _____

   b. _____

   c. _____

Word Find

Hidden in the following grid are 18 words or phrases related to what you have studied in this chapter. Find the hidden words in the grid below. Then use the words from the grid to answer the following questions (some words may be used to answer more than one question).

```
Y Q F O J S N P I N I F F D N W S
T R E V E Q L L S I S O D I C A H
M I E T F O R A M E N O V A L E U
R U E T W J E C V V M B M X F E N
P J I R R T R E T L D C M L M A T
L R O N A A N N Y A R Y U Y D G X
A C E N O A L T L C U T E R U S C
Y E O M C C H A G I A Z N A U N E
M E N A A X E N C L D T I V Y R K
N I V P D T B M V I N K R O Y I R
F A A S A X U L V B L C E I O J M
B H H O H U X R C M I I P W A K I
L E R P U E W E E U K O B G L G C
O T G B P T Z N Q S C I X M W S F
A D V N G X D W K C V F K I U P R
V Q C J Z N K C O H S Z N M L Z G
S U S O I R E T R A S U T C U D B
```

1. Oxygenated blood from the _____ enters the fetus in the _____ _____. It flows through the liver into the inferior _____ _____. Leaving that vessel, a large proportion of the oxygenated blood flows directly across the _____ through a hole called the _____ _____, thereby bypassing the lungs. When blood goes from the right side of the heart to the left side of the heart without picking up oxygen in the lungs, it is called a/an _____. Another direct connection, the _____ _____, links the fetal pulmonary artery to the _____. Both of these connections close very soon after birth. After circulating through the fetus, blood enters a/an _____ _____ to return to the placenta.

2. The newborn, or _____, is very vulnerable to hypothermia. It is important to try to prevent hypothermia from occurring in the newborn because hypothermia may lead to _____, which in turn may lead to _____. A baby born before the 38th week of pregnancy or weighing less than 2.5 kg is considered to be _____ and is at higher risk of hypothermia.

3. When fetal stool, called _____, is expelled into the amniotic fluid, it may find its way into the fetal airway before birth and then be aspirated deep into the airway when the baby takes its first breath. The result may be a complete failure to breathe at all, called _____.

4. The womb: _____

5. The organ where eggs reside: _____

6. The region between the vagina and the anus: _____

Fill-in-the-Table

Complete the table by filling in the causes of neonatal seizures.

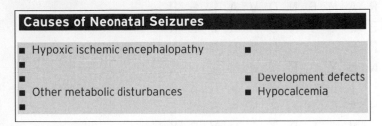

Causes of Neonatal Seizures	
■ Hypoxic ischemic encephalopathy	■
■	
■	■ Development defects
■ Other metabolic disturbances	■ Hypocalcemia
■	

Problem Solving

Practice your calculation skills by solving the following math problems using the Apgar score.

You have just assisted in the delivery of a full-term newborn.

1. At 1 minute, the baby is centrally blue, pale, and the pulse rate is 100 beats/min; the baby grimaces, has some extremity

flexion, and has a slow and irregular respiratory effort. The Apgar score is _____.

2. At 5 minutes, the baby is pink with blue extremities, has a pulse rate of 120 beats/min, is actively crying with a strong effort,

and has active motion. The Apgar score is _____.

Skill Drills

Test your knowledge of skill drills by placing the following photos in the correct order. Number the first step with a "1," the second step with a "2," and so forth.

Intubation of a Neonate

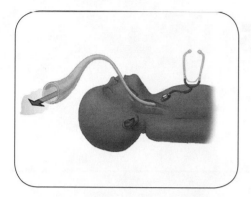

Confirm placement. Observe chest rise, auscultate laterally and high on the chest, note the absence of significant air sounds over the stomach, and note mist in the ET tube.

_____

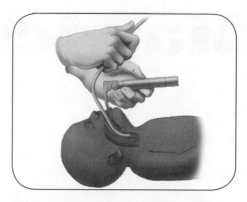

Place the laryngoscope blade in the oropharynx. Visualize the vocal cords. Place the endotracheal (ET) tube between the vocal cords until the black line on the ET tube is at the level of the cords.

_____

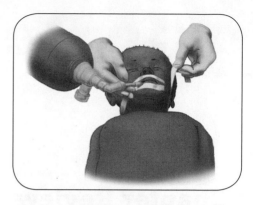

Tape the ET tube in place. Monitor the newborn closely for complications.

_____

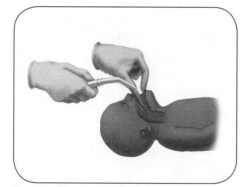

Suction the oropharynx. Provide bag-mask ventilation if bradycardia results.

_____

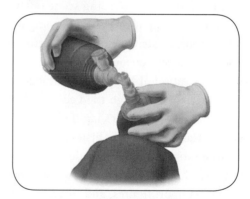

Preoxygenate the infant by bag-mask ventilation with 100% supplemental oxygen.

_____

CHAPTER

41 Pediatrics

Chapter Review

The following exercises provide an opportunity to test your knowledge of this chapter.

Matching

Match the following statements with the age group(s) most applicable to each. The statements may apply to more than one age group.

_____ **1.** Don't let your guard down regarding scene safety

_____ **2.** Can be distracted by jangling keys and cooing noises

_____ **3.** Give the child appropriate choices, and control whenever possible, and provide ongoing reassurance and encouragement

_____ **4.** Begins with observation of the child's interactions with the caregiver, vocalizations, and mobility, measured through the Pediatric Assessment Triangle

_____ **5.** Should be examined on mother's lap if stable

_____ **6.** Can provide at least some of the history

_____ **7.** During the first months of life, they do not do very much other than eat, sleep, and cry

_____ **8.** Tailor the physical exam to the child's age and developmental stage

_____ **9.** Friends are key support figures, and this is a time of experimentation and risk-taking behaviors

_____ **10.** Child abuse or maltreatment comes in many forms: physical abuse, sexual abuse, emotional abuse, and child neglect

_____ **11.** He or she becomes much more analytic and capable of abstract thought. At this age, the child can understand cause and effect

_____ **12.** Use play and distraction techniques whenever possible

_____ **13.** Make sure that your hands and stethoscope are warm

_____ **14.** Once secondary sexual characteristics have developed, the child should be treated as an adult

_____ **15.** Will be able to tell you what hurts and may have a story to share about the illness or injury

A. Neonate and infant

B. Toddler

C. Preschooler

D. School-age child

E. Adolescent

Multiple Choice

Read each item carefully, and then select the best response.

_____ **1.** Although child abuse can generate a big emotional response from the emergency medical services (EMS) crew, remember that your primary focus should be:

    A. documenting the suspected abuse for further prosecution.

    B. separating the patient from the suspected abuser.

    C. the trauma assessment, management, and ensuring the safety of the child.

    D. properly securing the crime scene for investigators.

_____ **2.** A child's developmental stage affects his or her response to injury. As a result:

A. being strapped to a backboard may be considered fun.

B. a paramedic could turn an activity as serious as immobilizing a child's spine on a backboard into a "game."

C. being immobilized on a backboard may be terrifying and anxiety provoking.

D. children should never be strapped or immobilized on a backboard.

_____ **3.** All of the following injury patterns may be more common in pediatric patients EXCEPT:

A. blunt force trauma.   **C.** skull fractures.

B. falls.   **D.** joint dislocations.

_____ **4.** *PAT* is an acronym:

A. developed from a common children's book to help soothe a sick or injured child.

B. developed to remember the proper methods of conducting a hands-on assessment of a child.

C. that stands for *palpating a tender abdomen*.

D. that stands for the *Pediatric Assessment Triangle*.

_____ **5.** One of the best ways to assess a pediatric patient's oxygenation status is to:

A. evaluate the child's respiratory rate.   **C.** auscultate the lungs.

B. evaluate the work of breathing.   **D.** obtain the pulse oximetry.

_____ **6.** Abnormal positioning and retractions are physical signs of increased work of breathing that can easily be assessed without touching the patient. The following are signs of increased work of breathing EXCEPT:

A. the sniffing position.   **C.** retractions.

B. tripoding.   **D.** all of the above.

_____ **7.** A child with an ominous mechanism of injury (MOI) includes a/an:

A. unstable or compromised airway from a motor vehicle crash.

B. isolated extremity fracture from a fall.

C. conscious, alert child who crashed his or her bicycle while wearing a helmet that cracked.

D. skateboarder with an obvious fractured wrist.

_____ **8.** Paramedics may encounter children with special health care needs. These may include:

A. physical, developmental, and learning disabilities.

B. tracheostomy tubes and artificial ventilators.

C. gastrostomy tubes (G-tubes).

D. all of the above.

_____ **9.** The federally funded program that was created more than 20 years ago in an effort to reduce child disability and death caused by severe illness and injury is known as:

A. the Department of Transportation (DOT) curriculum.

B. NHTSA.

C. EMSC.

D. TSA.

_____ **10.** Inserting an oral airway in a child is similar to inserting an airway in an adult EXCEPT:

A. how you determine the proper size.

B. it should not be used in the presence of ingested caustics.

C. it is inserted in an inverted manner, and then flipped over into the correct position.

D. you must take care to avoid injuring the hard palate.

Labeling

Label the following diagram.

On the following diagram, indicate the technique for measuring the distance to insert an NG or OG tube.

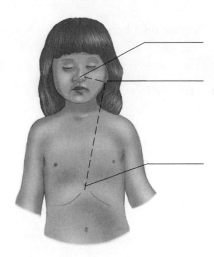

Fill-in-the-Blank

Read each item carefully, and then complete the statement by filling in the missing word(s).

1. A nasopharyngeal (nasal) airway is usually well _____ and is not as likely as the _____ airway to cause vomiting.

2. The _____ - _____ _____ can be used for a child with mild respiratory distress who will not tolerate a facial mask.

3. Bag-mask ventilation is _____ the first step in assisted _____, and it represents definitive _____ _____ for many patients.

4. Potential complications of pediatric intubation include damage to _____ and oral structures, _____ of gastric contents, _____ caused by a vagal response, bradycardia caused by hypoxemia from prolonged attempts, increased intracranial pressure (ICP), and incorrect _____.

5. Because stimulation of the _____ nervous system and _____ can occur during intubation, the paramedic should apply a _____ monitor and a/an _____ _____.

6. The types of shock you may encounter are the same in adults and children: _____, _____, and _____.

7. A pediatric patient with _____ shock will often appear listless or lethargic and may have compensatory _____. The child may appear _____, _____, or _____.

8. Further assessment of a pediatric patient in shock may identify signs of dehydration such as: _____

_____, dry _____ _____ , poor skin _____, _____ capillary refill

with cool extremities.

9. Complications associated with intraosseous infusion may include _____ _____, growth plate

_____, and bone inflammation caused by _____.

10. Cardiogenic shock is _____ in the pediatric population but may be present in children with underlying

_____ heart disease or _____ disturbances.

Identify

In the following case studies, list the chief complaint, vital signs, and pertinent negatives:

1. It's about 3:30 am and you are dispatched priority one for a 2-year-old with difficulty breathing. As you approach the residence, you notice a family member frantically trying to wave you down. You think to yourself that this doesn't look good. You grab your pediatric gear and cardiac monitor and then quickly enter the house. Once inside, you are told that the girl woke the whole household with this terrible barky cough. She is sitting on her mother's lap. The mother states that the child has been irritable for several days with symptoms consistent with an upper respiratory infection, coughing, runny nose, and sneezing. The child has audible stridor, a "seal-like" barking cough, and is conscious and alert. She has an oxygen saturation of 95% on ambient room air. She also has a normal capillary refill. You attempt to take her blood pressure and she begins to get agitated and cling to her mother.

   a. Chief Complaint

   _____

   _____

   _____

   b. Vital Signs

   _____

   _____

   _____

   c. Pertinent Negatives

   _____

   _____

   _____

2. Today is your turn on medivac duty. Medcom dispatches you to intercept a ground ambulance about 25 minutes to the west. As you lift off, you discover that this patient is only 1 week old and was the survivor of a motor vehicle crash involving a fatality. You and your crew arrive on the scene several minutes before the ambulance arrives. The state police are on scene securing the landing zone. They advise you that the patient's mother was holding the baby and both were unrestrained and ejected on impact. The mother suffered fatal injuries. You are thinking the worst and begin to set up your pediatric resuscitation equipment. When the ambulance arrives, you are quickly handed the neonatal trauma patient. The baby has oxygen in place, appears to be wrapped well, and is thoroughly secured with a vacuum splint conforming to his tiny body. The baby appears to be sleeping peacefully and has only a small forehead abrasion. You begin the initial survey as you begin

your flight to the trauma center. The initial assessment indicates an infant with no visible distress. The baby has an intact airway and is breathing at 30 breaths/min, he has an apical pulse rate at 150 beats/min, his skin color appears normal, and the skin is warm and dry. Lung sounds are clear and equal. Oxygen saturation is 96%. Remarkably, there doesn't appear to be any noticeable external bleeding. In fact, the assessment is totally unremarkable. After a "not so routine" mechanism of injury (MOI), the infant is safely delivered to the regional trauma center.

a. Chief Complaint

_____

_____

_____

b. Vital Signs

_____

_____

_____

c. Pertinent Negatives

_____

_____

_____

3. While working in the ALS "fly car," you are dispatched priority one on a mutual assist with a local BLS ambulance. They request that you meet them while they begin the response to the local pediatric emergency department. They state that they are treating a 2½-year-old girl in "status." You arrange a safe place to meet the ambulance and secure your vehicle. As you await their arrival, you prepare your pediatric ALS equipment and begin reviewing protocols. Once on the ambulance, you notice the small patient secured to the cot. Mom is in the front passenger's seat. The child has recently been sick with an upper respiratory infection and low-grade fever. Nothing like this has ever happened before. The child suddenly appeared to go into convulsions after being given oral pediatric acetaminophen for an elevation in her fever. The BLS crew states that the patient was actively seizing on their arrival. They initiated high-flow supplemental oxygen with a pediatric nonrebreathing face mask, requested ALS, and initiated transport. On your arrival, the patient is postictal, with the following vital signs: ashen skin, warm and dry, with a rectal temperature of 100.3°F. The patient responds to pain. Her oxygen saturation is 98%. Pupils are sluggish but equal. The patient has equal bilateral breath sounds. The remainder of the exam is unremarkable. The patient's mother denies any other medications, history, or allergies to medications. She further denies any recent injury or trauma to the child.

a. Chief Complaint

_____

_____

_____

b. Vital Signs

_____

_____

_____

c. Pertinent Negatives

_____

_____

_____

Ambulance Calls

The following case scenarios provide an opportunity to explore the concerns associated with patient management and paramedic care. Read each scenario, and then answer each question.

1. You are called to the scene of a collision in which a 6-year-old child was struck by a car as he darted into the street in front of his home. The child is lying in the street surrounded by a small group of people, including his very distraught parents.

   a. Given the mechanism of injury (MOI), list at least three injuries you must look for in particular in this child.

   (1) _____

   (2) _____

   (3) _____

   b. As you are kneeling beside the injured child, carefully going through the steps of the initial assessment, the child's father (who looks like a pro wrestler) charges over and starts shouting at you: "What the h—do you think you're doing with my kid? Stop messing around and take him to a _hospital_. Can't you see he's hurt bad? He's going to die here while you dingbats muck about." [The father's actual comments are less polite but cannot be quoted verbatim in a workbook.]

   (1) What are your feelings at this moment?

   _____

   _____

   (2) How will you deal with this situation?

   (a) _____

   (b) _____

   (c) _____

   (d) _____

   c. On checking the child's vital signs, you find the following: pulse is 120 beats/min and regular; respirations are 24 breaths/min and unlabored; blood pressure = 90/60 mm Hg. Which of the following conclusions can be drawn from those vital signs?

   (1) The child is going into shock.

   (2) The child has increasing intracranial pressure.

   (3) The vital signs are normal for a child of that age.

   (4) There is probably significant intrathoracic injury.

   (5) There is probably significant intra-abdominal bleeding.

2. You are called around 1:00 am for a child who "can't breathe." A haggard father greets you at the door and tells you that his 2-year-old Tammy has had "a little cold" for a couple of days but otherwise seemed fine. ("It didn't slow her down a bit.") Tonight, however, she began coughing, and the cough kept getting worse. Indeed, even as you are walking toward the child's room, you can hear a loud barking noise. On reaching Tammy's room, you see a very agitated 2-year-old struggling in her mother's lap. Her nostrils are flaring with each inhalation, and there are retractions of her neck muscles. Her lips are bluish. She flails and has a fit of dry coughing as you start to come near. Eventually, you manage to measure a pulse of 160 beats/min and a respiratory rate of 52 breaths/min. When you try to auscultate the child's chest, however, she grabs your stethoscope and yanks it out of your ears.

a. The vital signs are _____ (normal or abnormal?) for a child of this age.

b. The most likely diagnosis is _____.

c. What steps will you take in managing this child?

(1) _____

(2) _____

(3) _____

(4) _____

(5) _____

3. You are called for a 4-month-old infant in respiratory distress. His mother says that he's been "off his feed" for a couple of days and has been sneezing a lot. On examination, you notice that the baby seems to be breathing like a rabbit. The pulse is 180 beats/min, respirations are 60 breaths/min, and blood pressure is 90/60 mm Hg. There is diffuse wheezing throughout the chest.

a. The vital signs are _____ (normal or abnormal?) for a child of this age.

b. The most likely diagnosis is _____.

c. What steps will you take in managing this child?

(1) _____

(2) _____

(3) _____

(4) _____

(5) _____

(6) _____

4. You are called for a 2½-year-old having difficulty breathing. The mother says that she left little Bobby playing quietly in his room, and when she returned half an hour later, she found him in severe respiratory distress. She thinks he's had a slight respiratory infection, nothing serious. "You know, it's just one runny nose after another all winter with them. Each one gives it to the others, and I've got five little ones—so I can't always keep track of who has a runny nose."

You find Bobby in severe respiratory distress. He makes high-pitched squeaks when he tries to inhale, and his eyes look like they are popping out of his head. His lips are blue. You place the back of your hand on his forehead and note that the skin does not feel abnormally warm.

a. The most likely diagnosis is _____.

b. What steps will you take in managing this child?

(1) _____

(2) _____

(3) _____

(4) _____

(5) _____

(6) _____

(7) _____

c. As you are in the middle of treating this child's respiratory problem, he becomes pulseless and apneic. What is the depth and rate of chest compressions that you must perform?

_____

_____

d. Where will you check for a pulse?

_____

e. You find that the pulse is absent. What is the correct compression point for external chest compressions?

_____

_____

f. The monitor shows ventricular fibrillation. Assuming that the child weighs 12 kg, what is the defibrillation dosage?

_____ joules

g. Which drugs may be given by intraosseous infusion if you can't get an IV line established right away?

_____

_____

5. You are called to see a 4-year-old who is "very sick." His mother says that he was fine until a few hours ago when he began complaining of a sore throat. Since then, he would not eat or drink anything, and he is very feverish. You find the child sitting very still, bolt upright in bed, with his chin thrust forward. He does not reply to your questions, but only nods or shakes his head slightly. Saliva is dribbling out of the corners of his mouth. His skin feels very hot. His pulse is 140 beats/min, respirations are 40 breaths/min and quiet, blood pressure is 90/60 mm Hg. The chest is clear.

a. The vital signs are _____ (normal or abnormal?) for a child of this age.

b. The most likely diagnosis is _____.

c. What steps will you take in managing this child?

(1) _____

(2) _____

(3) _____

(4) _____

(5) _____

d. What is the special danger threatening this child?

_____

_____

_____

_____

6. You are called to a field about 6 miles outside of town where a 6-year-old child in the first-grade nature study class is having difficulty breathing. The teacher says that she noticed him lagging behind the others several times during the morning, and finally she found him sitting by himself under a tree, struggling to breathe. You find the child still sitting under the tree, but apparently dozing. It is difficult to wake him, and when he does open his eyes, he just stares at you blankly. When you ask him whether he has taken any medicine today, he just shakes his head and seems to doze again.

On examination, the child's pulse is 160 beats/min and somewhat weak, respirations are 52 breaths/min and shallow, and blood pressure is 90/60 mm Hg on exhalation and 50 systolic during inhalation. The lips look bluish. There is retraction of the neck muscles. The chest does not seem to move with respiration, and it sounds like an empty barrel when you tap on it. You can hardly hear any breath sounds at all. On the child's wrist is a MedicAlert bracelet inscribed "asthmatic."

a. List at least five signs that suggest this child is having a very serious asthmatic attack.

(1) _____

(2) _____

(3) _____

(4) _____

(5) _____

b.   List the steps you would take in managing this case.

(1) _____

(2) _____

(3) _____

(4) _____

(5) _____

(6) _____

7. The very same evening, you are called to see a child who is "short of breath." The child is a known asthmatic.

a. List five questions you would ask the child and his parents in taking the history.

(1) _____

(2) _____

(3) _____

(4) _____

(5) _____

b. Your protocol calls for administering albuterol for an acute asthmatic attack.

(1) What are the relevant *contraindications* to albuterol?

_____

(2) What are the possible adverse *side effects* of albuterol?

_____

_____

(3) What is the correct *dosage,* and how is the drug administered?

_____

_____

8. You are called to a downtown apartment for a "very sick baby." A frightened-looking young mother greets you at the door and hurries you into the bedroom, where a baby is lying very still in its crib. You observe at once that the baby's color is grayish and that it is not breathing. When you touch the baby to open the airway, you can feel that the skin is cold. Describe what you will do from this point on.

_____

_____

_____

_____

_____

_____

_____

_____

_____

9. You are called for a 2-year-old child who is "having a fit." En route to the call, you review in your mind the possible causes of seizures in children.

a. List five causes of seizures in children.

(1) _____

(2) _____

(3) _____

(4) _____

(5) _____

b. List five questions you should ask in taking the child's history.

(1) _____

(2) _____

(3) _____

(4) _____

(5) _____

c. List five things you would look for in particular in examining the child.

(1) _____

(2) _____

(3) _____

(4) _____

(5) _____

d. You learn that the child has never had a seizure before. On examining him, you find that he is no longer seizing but is still somewhat drowsy. His skin is very hot, so you take an axillary temperature and get a reading of 39°C (102.2°F). The pupils are equal and reactive. The neck is supple. The chest is clear. Describe how you would manage this case.

(1) _____

(2) _____

10. You are summoned to a local high school where a 14-year-old girl is having a seizure. The school nurse tells you that the child has never had a seizure in school before. This seizure came on while the girl was in the auditorium watching a movie. The seizure lasted about 5 minutes. One of the teachers then carried the girl to the nurse's office. The nurse was in the middle of trying to contact the girl's mother when the child had another grand mal seizure. Now, as you are speaking with the nurse, you witness a third grand mal seizure that lasts about 6 minutes.

a. List the steps in treating this patient.

_____

_____

_____

_____

b. What drug is used in the emergency treatment of repeated seizures and what are its contraindications?

_____

_____

c. What are the possible adverse side effects?

_____

_____

_____

11. You are called to attend to a 10-month-old baby who sustained burns to the foot when he "stepped on a cigarette." Something about the story sounds fishy to you, and you find yourself on the alert for evidence that the child has been abused.

a. What's "fishy" about the story?

_____

_____

_____

b. List ten possible clues that might substantiate your suspicion that a child has been abused.

(1) _____

(2) _____

(3) _____

(4) _____

(5) _____

(6) _____

(7) _____

(8) _____

(9) _____

(10) _____

c. By the time you finish examining the child, you are privately convinced that the baby was deliberately burned and that, furthermore, he has been burned and beaten in the past. How should you manage this case?

(1) _____

(2) _____

(3) _____

(4) _____

(5) _____

d. Suppose the child's parent refuses to allow the child to be transported to the hospital? What should you do then?

(1) _____

(2) _____

(3) _____

12. You are called to treat an 18-month-old baby who fell off a second-floor balcony to the ground 5 meters (about 15 feet) below. On examination, you find the baby conscious but drowsy. Vital signs are a pulse of 80 beats/min and regular, respirations are 16 breaths/min, and blood pressure is 100/70 mm Hg. There is a bruise on the left forehead. The pupils are equal and reactive to light. The point of maximal impulse (PMI) is in the midclavicular line. Breath sounds are equal bilaterally. The abdomen does not appear distended. The baby is moving all extremities. List the steps in the prehospital management of this case.

a. _____

b. _____

c. _____

d. _____

e. _____

f. _____

13. You are called to the scene of a motor vehicle collision on the interstate highway in which a car jumped the median divider and plowed head-on into an oncoming vehicle. Among the injured are two children, both backseat passengers in the vehicle that was hit. Both children have been removed from the wrecked car by well-meaning bystanders.

a. The first child is about 4 years old and is lying listlessly on the ground. His skin feels cool. His pulse is 160 beats/min and difficult to palpate, his respirations are 48 breaths/min, and his blood pressure is 90/60 mm Hg on both inhalation and exhalation. You find no signs of head injury. The pupils are equal and reactive. The neck veins are not distended. The PMI is in the midclavicular line. There are no bruises on the chest. Breath sounds are impossible to hear in all the noise. There is a seat belt mark across the anterior abdomen, which looks somewhat distended. Capillary refill takes 3 seconds. The right arm appears broken. List the steps in the prehospital management of this case.

(1) _____

(2) _____

(3) _____

(4) _____

(5) _____

(6) _____

(7) _____

b. The second child looks to be about 2 years old and is gasping for breath. The upper airway seems clear, but not much air is moving in and out of the chest. The lips are bluish. The trachea seems to be slanting to the left. It is impossible to auscultate breath sounds in all the noise at the scene. The PMI is in the anterior axillary line. The abdomen looks slightly distended but not bruised. List the steps in the prehospital management of this case.

(1) _____

(2) _____

(3) _____

(4) _____

(5) _____

(6) _____

(7) _____

(8) _____

14. You are called to the scene of a smoky house fire just as one of the firefighters is emerging from the building carrying a baby. "He was in the thick of it," the firefighter tells you. "Out cold when I found him." The baby still seems very drowsy.

   a. Should this infant be intubated? Why or why not?

   _____

   _____

   _____

   _____

   b. List five indications for the immediate intubation of an infant or small child who has been in a fire.

   (1) _____

   (2) _____

   (3) _____

   (4) _____

   (5) _____

15. You are all settled in to watch a football game on your day off when a neighbor comes running in, carrying her lethargic 2-year-old. "Johnny's choking on peanuts!" she wails.
     "Did what?" you ask, not really wanting to know the answer.
     "He's choking. Help, do something, he's turning blue!"

   a. What is the recommended method to relieve a severe airway obstruction in a conscious child? _____

   b. List the steps you would take to achieve this.

   (1) _____

   (2) _____

   (3) _____

   (4) _____

   (5) _____

   (6) _____

True/False

If you believe the statement to be more true than false, write the letter "T" in the space provided. If you believe the statement to be more false than true, write the letter "F."

_____ **1.** A child who is seriously ill or injured will always be agitated and showing clear signs of distress.

_____ **2.** A sunken anterior fontanelle in an infant suggests meningitis or a head injury.

_____ **3.** Neonates are nose breathers, so nasal congestion may compromise their breathing.

_____ **4.** Grunting is a sign of respiratory distress in infants.

_____ **5.** An infant falling from a height is most likely to sustain injury to the head.

_____ **6.** The method of choice for opening the airway of a small child who has been struck by a car is the head tilt–chin lift method.

_____ **7.** To insert an oropharyngeal airway in a small child, introduce the airway tip-upward, and then rotate it 180° and slide it into place.

_____ **8.** Hypotension is an early response to blood loss in infants and small children.

_____ **9.** The first step in assembling the equipment for pediatric intubation is to check the cuff on the endotracheal tube you have selected.

_____ **10.** A straight blade is preferred for pediatric intubation.

_____ **11.** In intubating infants, the laryngoscope blade is slipped beneath the epiglottis, to lift it up, rather than into the vallecula.

_____ **12.** The narrowest point in an infant's airway is the opening between the vocal cords.

_____ **13.** Initial management begins with removal of burning clothing and support of the ABCs.

_____ **14.** Pediatric trauma victims must have a rigid cervical collar in place prior to transport.

_____ **15.** Sinus tachycardia, a pulse rate higher than normal for age, is common in children.

Short Answer

Complete this section with short written answers using the space provided.

1. List six signs suggestive of hypovolemic shock in infants and small children.

a. _____

b. _____

c. _____

d. _____

e. _____

f. _____

2. Upon completing the initial assessment of any seriously injured person, of any age, the paramedic must make a decision whether to transport at once or to proceed to the focused history and physical exam. List ten indications for immediate transport ("load-and-go") of injured infants and children.

a. _____

b. _____

c. _____

d. _____

e. _____

f. _____

g. _____

h. _____

i. _____

j. _____

Word Find

Hidden in the following grid are 12 words or phrases related to what you have studied in this chapter. Find the hidden words in the grid below. Then use the words from the grid to answer the following questions (some words may be used to answer more than one question).

```
O K Q F T M R S P J R N G B V I I Q W B J W K Z I D K Y
D E Z H G K N Y M S G V R W S Y Y L B W P H L I Q E A G
I E M A F I E X H G B W Z U X C H Z B O F O R C A E B M
E Z Z O F V U H U L Z I C H Q I O R D X V F Z L I U I H
N H U F R H Q M Y R N J J B L Q T O Z A D E C B C F P X
P S I E D D I H B P Z P Q G W S F X A G Z T K M G P D P
T N E V E G N I N E T A E R H T E F I L T N E R A P P A
G G O P P I H Y N L Y A N J U Y S J K J Y Z H T J U H L
H E B W D U C X S L M U M O H V Y N N T X P D C C L N M
P H G U Q S E Q T Y M E L B S K O V I M Z C J M K X E R
A V I P N W T P U T B P A A I L V D R N O T H X Y H B R
Q L C H U C Y E T O O A H C G N I L T T O M D Y E K Z Y
Q Z V A D P B T B M G V B W R G W A W S J L C T P F V U
R M S F L J W E X P Z D T N I O V J C T L T K R H N J Y
E Z W F D W O C B K R O I R E P C G J M T H X E C E X S
C M H Y Q S L H K J H B L M U K D Y M O V N A G A J G Y
U U T R K A B I D L L A N E O N A T A L P E R I O D U D
T Y I Z L S B A Y C H D X G X A N H U N M U T R F T S P
N W O Q R O C L I C P V X G U Z R Y S U O K R L P L Q R
U E P R O B Q L U U R K P V X Y V O F B X S Y T R L K U
Y W N J R R M N O G N L G C X B Q Q D K G W I O G N G E
G X D V T J C R A E J L E H N W O J Q I K J Z S I C Q D
O E F H S Z C K G K I F K P E M L D Y K R E Q L H E J Z
V X U X U B R T E N J L U R F D G D S L J T Z U C L Q H
Q V B U L A Z S P X P G B Q I S B R N M W C S R N U B J
L Z X V M A V B U D O D E S C C C Q B X P S P M O R F Y
A P C U O A X N X L M B M G P O Z K U O P V R N H E B K
I A V H G L D X B E N D L H R P P G Y Q D E S W R G Q H
```

1. _____ _____ _____ is the term used for pediatric patients who have been subjected to violent, whiplash-type shaking.

2. The childhood viral disease characterized by edema of the upper airways with barking cough, difficult breathing, and stridor is called the _____.

3. While assessing a patient with _____ _____, a paramedic should suspect meningitis.

4. Paramedics will often find pediatric patients with respiratory distress in the _____ position. This is also the optimal position for intubation.

5. _____ is a condition often found with pediatric patients who have inadequate circulation.

6. Children with partial airway obstructions caused by disease or a foreign body may sometimes emit a harsh high-pitched sound called _____.

7. Placing a face mask over a child may be anxiety provoking. Oftentimes, an effective technique for delivering oxygen is via the _____ - _____ _____.

8. _____ spots are characterized by small purplish, nonblanching spots on the skin.

9. A rattling-type abnormal respiratory sound is called _____.

10. Newborns and neonates often exhibit signs of _____, a cyanosis of the extremities.

11. The first month of a newborn's life is defined as the _____ _____.

12. An ALT or _____ _____ - _____ _____ is often characterized as a sudden serious episode of color change, tone, or apnea that requires mouth-to-mouth resuscitation or vigorous stimulation.

Fill-in-the-Table
Fill in the missing parts of the table.

1. In examining an injured infant or child, you must know exactly what you're looking for so that each second spent on the physical exam is well invested. In the following table, indicate what in particular you would be looking for as you examine each part of the body mentioned.

Body Area	What I Am Looking for in Particular
Head	
Neck	
Chest	
Abdomen	
Extremities	

2. Normal Respiratory Rate by Age

Normal Respiratory Rate by Age	
Age	Respiratory Rate (breaths/min)
Infant	
Toddler	
Preschool-age child	
School-age child	
Adolescent	

3. Normal Pulse Rates for Age

Normal Pulse Rates for Age	
Age	Pulse Rate (beats/min)
Infant	
Toddler	
Preschool-age child	
School-age child	
Adolescent	

4. Normal Blood Pressure for Age

Age	Minimal Systolic Blood Pressure (mm Hg)
Normal Blood Pressure for Age	
Infant	
Toddler	
Preschool-age child	
School-age child	
Adolescent	

Problem Solving

Practice your calculation skills by solving the following math problems.

1. For children 1 to 10 years old, one would calculate the lower limit of acceptable blood pressure for age using the following formula:

Minimal systolic blood pressure = 80 + (2 × age in years)

a. You are evaluating a pediatric trauma patient. His age is 6. What would you estimate a normal systolic blood pressure to be?

_____

b. This patient is a 10-year-old asthmatic. What would you estimate a normal systolic blood pressure to be?

_____

c. On arrival, you have an unconscious pediatric patient. You estimate his age to be 5 or 6 years. What would normal blood pressure be for a patient this age?

_____

2. One would calculate the endotracheal tube size for a child older than one year as follows:

$$\frac{(Age + 16)}{4} = \text{Size of ET tube (in mm)}$$

a. Calculate the appropriate ET tube size of a 6-year-old child.

_____

b. Calculate the appropriate ET tube size of a 9-year-old child.

_____

Skill Drills

Test your knowledge of pediatric dose calculations by completing the following.

1. You have been called to the scene for a 4-year-old child who is unconscious and unresponsive after being shocked by an electrical outlet. He is also pulseless and apneic.

a. He weighs 40 pounds. Appropriate two-person BLS is in progress on your arrival. You attach the patient to your defibrillator/monitor and notice ventricular fibrillation. What energy setting would you use to administer defibrillations?

_____

b. How much energy should be used on subsequent defibrillations?

_____

2. You have now been called to the scene for a 6-year-old girl who has severe anaphylaxis after ingesting peanuts at the ball game. The child is anxious, and she has an increased work of breathing, and poor circulation. She weighs 60 lb.

a. As the paramedic in charge, you decide that among all your other treatment priorities this patient requires epinephrine. How will you administer this drug and at what dose?

_____

_____

b. This patient further requires the administration of diphenhydramine (Benadryl). How will you administer this drug and at what dose?

_____

_____

c. Fortunately, your patient is beginning to improve, but she's still wheezing. What drug would you consider and at what dose?

_____

_____

3. Test your knowledge of skill drills by filling in the correct words in the photo captions.

One-Rescuer Bag-Mask Ventilation for a Child

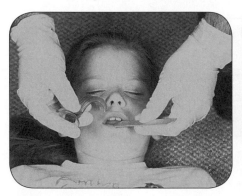

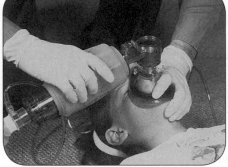

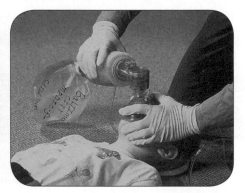

Step 1 Open the _____, and _____ the appropriate airway adjunct.

Step 2 Hold the _____ on the patient's face with a one-handed _____ _____ _____ - _____ technique (E-C clamp). Ensure a good _____ - _____ - _____ seal while maintaining the airway.

Step 3 _____ at a rate of _____ _____ for children. Allow adequate time for exhalation.

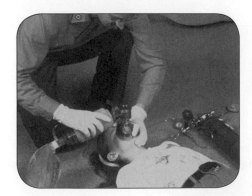

Step 4 Assess effectiveness of ventilation by assessing _____ rise and fall of the _____ .

4. Test your knowledge of this skill drill by placing the photos below in the correct order. Number the first step with a "1," the second step with a "2," etc.

Performing Chest Compressions on a Child

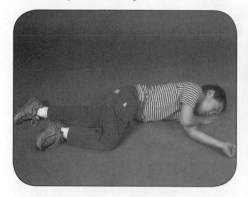

Reassess breathing and pulse after 2 minutes and at 2-minute intervals thereafter. If the child resumes effective breathing, place him or her in the recovery position.

_____

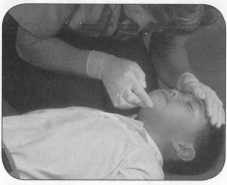

Place the child on a firm surface, and use one hand to maintain the head tilt-chin lift.

_____

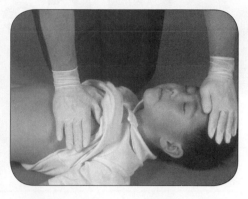

Coordinate compression with ventilation in a 30:2 ratio, pausing for ventilation.

_____

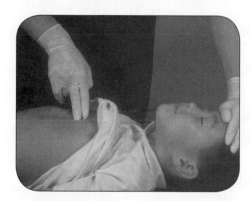

Place the heel of your hand over the middle of the sternum (between the nipples); avoid compression of the xiphoid process.

_____

CHAPTER

42 Geriatrics

Matching

Match each of definitions in the left column to the appropriate term in the right column.

_____ 1. A tendency to constancy or stability in the body's internal milieu

_____ 2. The assessment and treatment of disease in someone 65 years or older

_____ 3. A chronic deterioration of mental functions

_____ 4. The number of pacemaker cells in the sinoatrial node decreases dramatically as a person ages

_____ 5. These lose their flexibility and may be further immobilized by arthritic changes

_____ 6. Immobility and consolidation of a vertebral joint

_____ 7. A decrease in bone mass and density

_____ 8. Not a normal part of aging and can lead to skin irritation, skin breakdown, and urinary tract infections

_____ 9. Progressive hearing loss, particularly in the high frequencies, along with lessened ability to discriminate between a particular sound and background noise

_____ 10. An acute confusional state characterized by global impairment of thinking, perception, judgment, and memory

_____ 11. When the inside wall of the artery tears and allows blood to collect between the arterial wall layers

A. Spondylosis

B. Aortic dissection

C. Delirium

D. Musculoskeletal system

E. Dementia

F. Presbycusis

G. Incontinence

H. Homeostasis

I. Cardiovascular system

J. Geriatrics

K. Osteoporosis

Multiple Choice

Read each item carefully, and then select the best response.

_____ 1. Geriatrics is the assessment and treatment of disease in someone _____ years or older.

    A. 55   **C.** 75

    B. 65   **D.** None of the above

_____ **2.** A 35-year-old is aging just as fast as an 85-year-old, but the older person exhibits the cumulative results of a _____ process.

    A. longer   **C.** degenerative

    B. shorter   **D.** cumulative

_____ **3.** Over time, cardiac output declines, mostly as a result of a/an _____ stroke volume.

    A. increasing   **C.** decreasing

    B. strengthening   **D.** weakening

_____ **4.** Musculoskeletal changes, such as _____, may also affect pulmonary function by limiting lung volume and maximal inspiratory pressure.

    A. kyphosis   **C.** decreased bone mass

    B. osteoporosis   **D.** arthritis

_____ **5.** Incontinence is not a normal part of aging and can lead to:

    A. skin irritation.   **C.** urinary tract infections.

    B. skin breakdown.   **D.** all of the above.

_____ **6.** _____ enables us to maintain postural stability by using a variety of receptors in the joints and information provided by the eyes. As these mechanisms fail with age, people become less steady on their feet, and the tendency to fall increases markedly.

    A. Balance   **C.** Proprioception

    B. Posture   **D.** Homeostasis

_____ **7.** Elderly patients are much more vulnerable to the following temperature stresses EXCEPT:

    A. heat exhaustion.   **C.** the absence of a febrile response to illness.

    B. hypothermia.   **D.** hormonal temperature effects.

_____ **8.** Chronic obstructive pulmonary disease (COPD) includes all of the following EXCEPT:

    A. chronic asthma.   **C.** emphysema.

    B. chronic bronchitis.   **D.** diuretic intolerant edema.

_____ **9.** The extent of bone loss that a person undergoes is influenced by numerous factors, including:

    A. genetics, smoking, and level of activity.   **C.** age, skin, and diet.

    B. age, sex, and genetics.   **D.** smoking, age, and skin.

_____ **10.** Some patients fear that mentioning a symptom will lead to a diagnosis or treatment that will jeopardize their independence. "If I mention those pains in my stomach," the older person may reason, "_____"

    A. "they'll put me in that nursing home to die."

    B. "I'll be okay; besides, if I die they'll fight over the money."

    C. "I can't afford another hospitalization and more prescriptions."

    D. "they'll put me in the hospital, and I may never come out of that place again."

Labeling

Label the following diagrams with the correct terms.

1. Label the portions of the lower gastrointestinal (GI) system that are hemorrhaging.

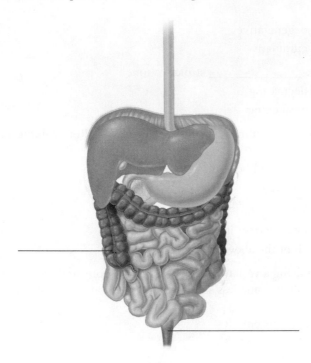

2. Label the portions of the upper GI system that are hemorrhaging.

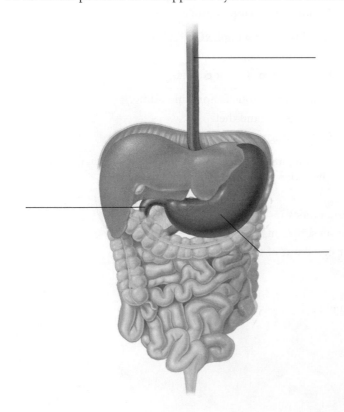

Fill-in-the-Blank

Read each item carefully, and then complete the statement by filling in the missing word(s).

1. _____ people constitute an ever-increasing proportion of patients in the health care system, particularly the _____ care sector.

2. There is a widespread tendency to attribute genuine disease symptoms to "_____ _____ _____" and to neglect their treatment.

3. The heart _____ with age, probably in response to the chronically increased afterload imposed by stiffened blood vessels.

4. A person's _____ capacity also undergoes significant _____ with age, largely because of decreases in the elasticity of the lungs and in the size and strength of the respiratory muscles.

5. As a person ages, the kidneys shrink in size. This decline in weight results from a loss of functioning _____ _____, which translates into a smaller effective _____ surface.

6. The consequent decrease in _____ may lead to malnutrition. Other changes in the mouth include a reduction in the volume of _____, with a resulting _____ of the mouth.

7. Narrowing of the _____ disks and _____ of the vertebrae contribute to a decrease in _____ as a person ages, along with changes in posture.

8. A hearing-related impairment noted in the elderly population is _____ _____. Onset of symptoms usually occurs in early middle age, with symptoms presenting in _____ that last several _____ at a time.

9. _____ and loss of _____ of the skin are the most visible signs of aging. Wrinkling occurs because the skin becomes thinner, _____, less elastic, and more _____.

10. Heart attack is the major cause of _____ and _____ in people older than 65 years, and its potential for mortality increases significantly after a person reaches _____ years.

Identify

In the following case studies, list the chief complaint, vital signs, and pertinent negatives.

1. On arrival to the Adult Day Care Center, you discover an 84-year-old woman who has "fallen." She normally walks with the assistance of a cane or walker. She is lying on a deeply carpeted floor and is conscious, alert, and complaining of right-sided midthigh pain. The fall didn't appear to be witnessed. Her aid was assisting another client when the fall occurred. Your patient does not have a good recollection of what happened. She denies chest pain, shortness of breath, dizziness, nausea, or vomiting. She also denies tripping and falling. The area appears clear of obstacles, rugs, or other obvious trip hazards. Your physical exam is as previously indicated. You notice some inward rotation and shortening of the extremity. Her pulse is 84 beats/min and very irregular. Her oxygen saturation is 88% on room air. Her blood pressure is 106/86 mm Hg. The patient's skin turgor is poor, with a delayed capillary refill of > 2 seconds. Pupils are Equal And Round, Regular in size, and react to

Light (PEARRL). An echocardiogram (ECG) shows a sinus rhythm with frequent premature ventricular contractions (PVCs) and short runs of ventricular tachycardia.

a. Chief Complaint

_____

_____

_____

b. Vital Signs

_____

_____

_____

c. Pertinent Negatives

_____

_____

_____

2. It's early afternoon on a clear and warm springtime day. You are dispatched to the parking lot of a local supermarket for a reported motor vehicle crash. On arrival, you discover an elderly man who is 92 years old. He is the driver of a vehicle that struck several parked cars. Bystanders state that the patient appears to be either sleeping or unconscious. You find the patient to be conscious but not alert to person, place, time, or purpose. The police identify his home phone number and call it. A pleasant-sounding elderly woman answers and states that her husband left home over an hour ago to pick up some groceries. She states that he has a problem with "sugar" and wonders if he has his hearing aids in place. As you begin examining the patient and taking his history, it becomes obvious that he's not wearing hearing aids. There is minimally detectable damage to the vehicle as well as the vehicles that were struck. The patient was found not to be wearing his seat belt. He does have a medical identification bracelet on and it indicates extensive cardiac and diabetic history. Vital signs indicate a blood glucose level of 66 mg/dL. His pulse rate is 92 beats/min and regular, and blood pressure is 160/72 mm Hg. His skin is warm and moist, his capillary refill is normal, and he has oxygen saturation of 96% on room air. The man is able to maintain his own airway and gag reflex. He was initially assisted with oral glucose by first responders. The patient is becoming increasingly alert and oriented and denies any injury.

a. Chief Complaint

_____

_____

_____

b. Vital Signs

_____

_____

_____

c. Pertinent Negatives

_____

_____

_____

Ambulance Calls

The following case scenarios provide an opportunity to explore the concerns associated with patient management and paramedic care. Read each scenario, and then answer each question.

1. One way to try to ensure that you don't miss anything important in the patient's history is to ask some general screening questions, irrespective of the patient's chief complaint. Suppose an 80-year-old woman has called for an ambulance because she feels "tired and weak." List 10 general screening questions you would ask to assess the status of her major organ systems.

a. _____

b. _____

c. _____

d. _____

e. _____

f. _____

g. _____

h. _____

i. _____

j. _____

2. You are called to the apartment of a 78-year-old woman who fell down.

a. List five questions you would ask in taking the history of the present illness.

(1) _____

(2) _____

(3) _____

(4) _____

(5) _____

b. List the information you should obtain about the patient's past (other) medical history.

(1) _____

(2) _____

(3)_____

(4)_____

c. List six things you would look for in particular in performing the physical examination.

(1) _____

(2)_____

(3)_____

(4)_____

(5)_____

(6)_____

d. While conducting the physical examination, you will of course be alert for signs or symptoms of those injuries to which older people are particularly vulnerable. List three injuries to which elderly patients are more susceptible.

(1) _____

(2)_____

(3)_____

3. You are called to a shopping center where an elderly man tripped on a potted plant and fell, sustaining a minor laceration to his arm. As you are applying a dressing to the laceration, you notice that he seems very listless and depressed. List five factors related to geriatric suicide.

a. _____

b. _____

c. _____

d. _____

e. _____

True/False

The public (and also, regrettably, health care professionals) holds many widespread misconceptions about the elderly and the process of aging that result in inaccurate stereotypes of elderly persons. If you believe the statement to be more true than false, write the letter "T" in the space provided. If you believe the statement to be more false than true, write the letter "F."

_____ 1. The rate of aging is the same in a 35-year-old as it is in an 80-year-old.

_____ 2. Mental deterioration and some degree of dementia are an inevitable part of the aging process.

_____ 3. Elderly people are more likely than younger individuals to seek emergency care for minor, nonserious complaints.

_____ 4. The pain mechanism is often depressed among the elderly.

_____ 5. The possibility of hearing loss increases with age.

_____ **6.** Sweat gland activity increases, hindering the ability to sweat and to regulate heat.

_____ **7.** A specific illness or injury in elderly people is more likely to result in generalized deterioration.

_____ **8.** Cellulitis is an acute inflammation in the skin caused by a viral infection. This condition usually affects the lower extremities.

_____ **9.** Elderly patients must always be placed in a traction splint for a femoral fracture.

_____ **10.** One clue to elder abuse is unexplained injuries that do not fit the stated cause.

Short Answer

Complete this section with short written answers using the space provided.

1. Patients older than 65 years of age account for one third of all ambulance calls today. As the population continues to age, that percentage can be expected to increase. It is therefore important for paramedics to understand the special problems and challenges posed by caring for the elderly. List five characteristics of the elderly that make it particularly challenging to diagnose their problems correctly and provide them with appropriate care.

a. _____

b. _____

c. _____

d. _____

e. _____

2. The process of aging in our society is nearly always accompanied by social and psychological stresses that may have an enormous impact on health. List two potentially stressful changes that tend to occur in a person's life as he or she approaches the "golden age."

a. _____

b. _____

3. The normal aging process produces changes in nearly every organ system of the body. It is important to know what constitutes a _normal_ age-related change so that such a change will not be mistaken for a sign of disease (and, conversely, so that signs of disease will not be disregarded as "just part of getting old"). For each of the following organ systems, list two changes in structure or function that occur as a normal consequence of aging.

a. Cardiovascular

(1) _____

(2) _____

b. Respiratory

(1) _____

(2) _____

c. Renal

(1) _____

(2) _____

d. Digestive

(1) _____

(2) _____

e. Musculoskeletal

(1) _____

(2) _____

f. Nervous

(1) _____

(2) _____

g. Homeostatic

(1) _____

(2) _____

4. In younger patients, the chief complaint often has considerable value in localizing the patient's underlying problem. A middle-aged man suffering a myocardial infarction, for example, will usually complain of pain or discomfort in his chest, while a young person with pneumonia usually will have a cough and a fever. Among the elderly, on the other hand, the response to serious illness tends to be less specific. List four responses to illness common among seriously ill elderly patients.

a. _____

b. _____

c. _____

d. _____

5. Obtaining an accurate history from an elderly patient requires considerable skill because there are a number of obstacles to history taking among the elderly that do not exist when you talk with younger patients. List four obstacles to obtaining a medical history from an elderly person, and indicate what steps you can take to overcome each of them.

a. Obstacle: _____

_____

What I can do to try to overcome the obstacle: _____

_____

b. Obstacle: _____

_____

What I can do to try to overcome the obstacle: _____

_____

c. Obstacle: _____

_____

What I can do to try to overcome the obstacle: _____

_____

d. Obstacle: _____

_____

What I can do to try to overcome the obstacle: _____

_____

6. In a middle-aged patient, the clinical presentation of such conditions as acute myocardial infarction or congestive heart failure is usually straightforward. In an elderly person with the same problem, the clinical presentation may be much less clear-cut. List at least two signs or symptoms that are commonly part of the clinical presentation of acute myocardial infarction and of congestive heart failure in the elderly.

Condition	Possible Signs and Symptoms in the Elderly
Acute myocardial infarction	
Congestive heart failure	

7. One of the most common presenting symptoms among the elderly is an acute confusional state (delirium). List five conditions likely to present as delirium in the elderly.

a. _____

b. _____

c. _____

d. _____

e. _____

8. The best drug for an elderly patient is very often *no* drug because the likelihood of adverse drug reactions increases sharply with advancing age. Emergency medical services (EMS) providers must be careful not to add to the problem by giving elderly patients medications that cause toxic effects. List three drugs used in emergency care, in the prehospital setting, that are especially likely to produce adverse reactions in the elderly.

a. _____

b. _____

c. _____

Crossword Puzzles

Use the clues in the column to complete the puzzle.

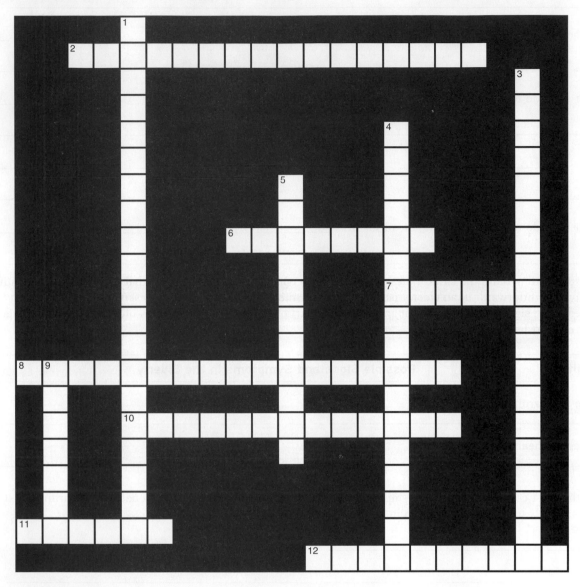

Across

2. Out of touch with reality
6. A disease that produces irreversible brain failure
7. A hot, flushed patient who is also tachycardic and tachypneic may have this
8. These generally remain asymptomatic until they become large or rupture
10. This includes not just talking, but also listening
11. Characterized by black, tarlike stools
12. This includes physical, sexual, emotional, neglect, and financial

Down

1. The death of part of the heart muscle due to the blockage of one of the coronary arteries
3. Characterized by degenerative changes in the cervical spine
4. Characterized by involuntary movements or tremors affecting one or both sides of the body
5. Characterized by vomiting red blood
9. An organization that provides terminal care for patients and support for their families

Fill-in-the-Table

Fill in the missing parts of the table.

Causes of Falls in the Elderly	
Cause	**Clues to Suggest This Cause**
Extrinsic (accidental)	
Intrinsic drop attacks	Sudden fall; patient found on the ground somewhat confused, often temporarily paralyzed and unable to get up; no premonitory symptoms
Postural hypotension	
Dizziness or syncope	Marked bradycardia or tachyarrhythmias
Stroke	
Fracture	Patient felt something snap before falling

CHAPTER

43 Abuse, Neglect, and Assault

Chapter Review

The following exercises provide an opportunity to test your knowledge of this chapter.

Matching

Match the types of abuse to the appropriate description.

_____ **1.** Keeping a person from getting a job

_____ **2.** Making negative comments

_____ **3.** Hitting or kicking

_____ **4.** Performing sex against a person's will

_____ **5.** Playing mind games

A. Physical abuse

B. Emotional abuse

C. Economic abuse

D. Sexual abuse

Indicate which is a profile characteristic of an abused older patient and which is a profile characteristic of a person who abuses elders.

_____ **1.** Socially isolated

_____ **2.** Women

_____ **3.** Poor impulse control

_____ **4.** Exhibits problem behavior

_____ **5.** History of domestic violence

A. Characteristic of an abused older patient

B. Characteristic of a person who abuses elders

Multiple Choice

Read each item carefully, and then select the best response.

_____ **1.** Which type of child abuse has the greatest incidence?

    A. Physical

    B. Sexual

    C. Neglect

    D. Psychological

_____ **2.** Which of the following is NOT a risk factor for child abuse?

    A. Child with disability

    B. Disorganized family structure

    C. Parent was abused

    D. Financial stability

_____ **3.** You are called to the scene of a 4-year-old child injured inside a residence. You enter the house and find the child and a parent. You assess the child and become suspicious about the injury. Your partner interviews the parent. Which of the following is a red flag for child abuse by a caregiver?

A. The caregiver overreacts to the child's condition.

B. The caregiver seems forthcoming about what happened.

C. The caregiver is enraged about care being provided by emergency medical services (EMS).

D. The caregiver seems concerned.

_____ **4.** You have completed a call where there is a high suspicion of child abuse. When you write the prehospital care report (PCR), what type of information is helpful to include for child protective services when they review the report?

A. Subjective

B. Speculative

C. Conjecture

D. Objective

_____ **5.** You are called to a residential neighborhood for an elderly person who has fallen. You are met at the door by a person who says she is the patient's daughter. You enter the room to find the patient, who is extremely dirty, on the floor and observe the house has garbage scattered around. The patient seems scared. Which of the following is NOT a characteristic of an abuser of the elderly?

A. Lives with the victim

B. Older than 50 years

C. Has impulse control

D. Depends on the victim for financial support

_____ **6.** You are on the scene of a domestic dispute. The police have secured the scene, and while you are treating the spouse, she screams out that her husband won't let her get a job. This is considered to be what form of domestic abuse?

A. Emotional

B. Economic

C. Social

D. Physical

_____ **7.** A patient of a sexual assault is often found in which of the following states?

A. Denial

B. Bargaining

C. Guilt

D. Stupor

_____ **8.** At a call to a nursing home for a patient with pneumonia, you observe what may be signs of neglect. What makes a nursing home have an increased risk for abuse?

A. Young staff

B. Large facility (more than 100 beds)

C. Multipurpose (assisted living and high need)

D. Understaffed

_____ **9.** You have been called to a residence where there is a 5-year-old boy who reportedly fell while running and hit his forehead. He has a bruise and an abrasion. While you do an assessment to determine if there are any additional injuries, you notice the boy has numerous bruises of different colors. Which location of bruises on the child would make you most suspicious they might be the result of child abuse?

A. Knees

B. Arms

C. Lower legs

D. Back

_____ **10.** When you handle a nursing home call, certain signs might alert you to abuse. Which of the following is NOT considered a sign of abuse for a nursing home patient?

A. Tied off catheter

B. Undocumented decubitus ulcers

C. Dementia

D. Dangerous use of restraints

Fill-in-the-Blank
Read each item carefully, and then complete the statement by filling in the missing word(s).

1. In the mnemonic CHILD ABUSE, the letters in the word *abuse* stand for:

A: _____

B: _____

U: _____

S: _____

E: _____

2. In most states, the paramedic is a/an _____ reporter in child abuse or neglect cases.

3. _____ neglect refers to the deliberate withholding of companionship, medicine, food, or assistance with mobility.

4. _____ is the simultaneous use of many medications.

5. _____ _____ and _____ are crimes of power, force, and violence.

6. Domestic abuse can take on the following four forms: _____, _____, _____,

and _____.

7. Older people are at an increased risk for abuse in nursing facilities that have a history of providing inadequate care,

are _____, and provide _____ _____ for their employees.

8. When documenting a patient's history on a prehospital care report, record only the _____ facts.

_____ statements made by those on the scene or by the patient should be in quotation marks.

9. _____/glove burns and _____ burns occur when a child is immersed in hot water.

10. Approximately _____% of abused or neglected children who die are younger than 6 years of age.

Identify
In the following case study, list the chief complaint, vital signs, and significance of the assessment findings.

You are called to the scene of a child who is complaining of abdominal pain. When you arrive on scene, you find a 5-year-old girl who keeps saying her stomach hurts. The mother is the only adult on the scene and is almost hysterical, stating that the child is out of control and she can't control her. Your assessment identifies bruising of the abdomen and rigidity. The vial signs are a pulse of 130 beats/min and thready, a blood pressure of 70/40 mm Hg, and respirations of 36 breaths/min.

1. Chief Complaint

_____

_____

_____

2. Vital Signs

_____

_____

_____

3. Significance of the Assessment Findings

_____

_____

_____

Ambulance Calls

The following case scenarios provide an opportunity to explore the concerns associated with patient management and paramedic care. Read each scenario, and then answer each question.

1. You are called to an apartment where a 3-year-old boy is sitting on the couch not saying a word or making eye contact. You are let into the apartment by a man who identifies himself as a friend of the boy's mother and who is watching the child. The child reportedly fell and hit his head. Your partner decides to step aside and use a code to the dispatcher requesting a police officer to the scene. The head injury looks suspicious because of its location. It looks instead like the child did not fall but was pushed into a wall because the bump and abrasion are on the top of the head. Continuing with the assessment, you notice multiple bruises in various stages of healing on the boy's back and buttocks. You are suspicious of what appears to be partly healed burn marks on the palms of the hands. List five red flags indicating that this might be child abuse.

   a. _____

   b. _____

   c. _____

   d. _____

   e. _____

2. A 9-1-1 call is received for an 85-year-old woman who doesn't feel well. When you arrive at the residence, she states that she lives alone. You ask if she has any assistance in the home, and she tells you that her daughter helps out but that she hasn't been by in about a week. She seems sad and says her daughter is the only person who stops by. You look around and see there is very little food and there is garbage on the floors and on the counters. While obtaining a SAMPLE history, you ask about medications and are told that the daughter has not refilled the woman's prescriptions, and the woman missed a doctor's appointment because the daughter failed to drive her. You are concerned your patient is a victim of both active and passive neglect. Give three examples of active neglect and one example of passive neglect.

   a. Active Neglect

   (1) _____

   (2) _____

   (3) _____

   b. Passive Neglect

   (1) _____

3. The police have secured the scene of a domestic fight. You are called into the residence to transport the wife, who has sustained some minor injuries. Your assessment identifies some bruises on the woman's legs and arms from kicking and being hit. While en route to the hospital, the patient shares that her husband is abusive. He reportedly always calls her names and makes negative comments, he undercut her attempt to get a job, and he forces her to have sex when she doesn't want to. Place the types of abuse occurring in this domestic abuse scenario into the appropriate categories.

Physical

_____

Emotional

_____

Economic

_____

Sexual

_____

True/False

If you believe the statement to be more true than false, write the letter "T" in the space provided. If you believe the statement to be more false than true, write the letter "F."

_____ **1.** Of the different types of child abuse, neglect has the highest incidence.

_____ **2.** Neglected children are hard to detect because they are often well nourished, bright, and engaging.

_____ **3.** Most reported occurrences of child abuse are from middle-class families with both parents living in the home.

_____ **4.** In the mnemonic used for assessing child abuse (CHILD ABUSE), the A stands for affect.

_____ **5.** One of the characteristics shared by caregivers of maltreated children includes lack of parenting knowledge.

_____ **6.** Soft-tissue injuries are the most common finding in the physical exam of an abused child.

_____ **7.** Don't bother to observe the scene or household dynamics with a pediatric patient because they yield very little information about identifying potential child abuse.

_____ **8.** The profile of a person who abuses elders includes young adults with good impulse control.

_____ **9.** Passive neglect occurs when an older person is ignored or left alone.

_____ **10.** Polypharmacy means simultaneous use of many medications.

_____ **11.** Battered patients usually will give accurate information about their injuries and seek help.

_____ **12.** Men who are battered may be too humiliated to report the incident.

_____ **13.** Multiple bruises in various stages of healing are not a significant finding when considering child abuse.

_____ **14.** Doughnut burns are common burns in children and not an indicator of potential child abuse.

_____ **15.** It is usually preferable to have a same-gender caregiver assist with the victim of sexual abuse.

Short Answer

Complete this section with short written answers using the space provided.

1. List eight clues that would lead you to suspect that an injured child is the victim of physical abuse.

a. _____

b. _____

c. _____

d. _____

e. _____

f. _____

g. _____

h. _____

Word Find

Hidden in the following grid are 20 words or phrases related to what you have studied in this chapter. Find the hidden words in the grid below. Then use the words from the grid to answer the following questions (some words may be used to answer more than one question).

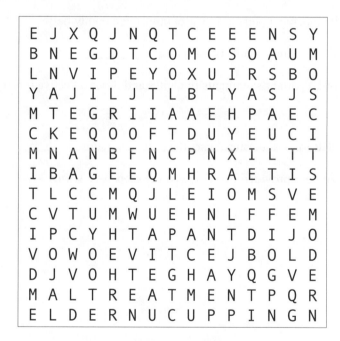

```
E J X Q J N Q T C E E E N S Y
B N E G D T C O M C S O A U M
L N V I P E Y O X U I R S B O
Y A J I L J T L B T Y A S J S
M T E G R I I A A E H P A E C
C K E Q O O F T D U Y E U C I
M N A N B F N C P N X I L T T
I B A G E E Q M H R A E T I S
T L C C M Q J L E I O M S V E
C V T U M W U E H N L F F E M
I P C Y H T A P A N T D I J O
V O W O E V I T C E J B O L D
D J V O H T E G H A Y Q G V E
M A L T R E A T M E N T P Q R
E L D E R N U C U P P I N G N
```

1. Refusal of a caregiver to provide such life necessities, such as; food, shelter or medical care is called _____.

2. Any form of maltreatment that results in harm is called _____.

3. The general term for the action of physical and psychological abuse that causes damage and long term complications to a child is called _____.

4. The 'E' in the mnemonic CHILD ABUSE stands for _____.

5. The 'A' in the mnemonic CHILD ABUSE stands for _____ .

6. A "red flag" for caregiver behavior for child abuse where the individual doesn't seem to care is called _____.

7. A cultural practice of placing warm cups on the skin to pull out illness from the body is called _____.

8. Paramedics required by some states to report suspicious forms of child maltreatment are called _____ reporters.

9. Violence in the home between family members such as a husband and wife is called _____ violence.

10. When an older person is neglected it is referred to as _____ abuse.

11. _____ abuse includes any improper action that injuries or harms a young person or infant.

12. The characteristics of an abused older patient such as women over 75 years old who is socially isolated is called a

_____.

13. _____ abuse includes making negative comments, calling names, or playing mind games.

14. _____ assault is an attack against a person in which there is a rape.

15. Sexual intercourse inflicted forcibly on another person, against their will, is called _____.

16. _____ is unlawfully placing a person in fear of immediate bodily harm.

17. The person who has experienced sexual assault is called the _____.

18. Thorough _____ of all patient statements in quotes and other objective information on the patient care report

(PCR) is crucial.

19. When documenting on the PCR for a domestic abuse, the statements must be _____, nonjudgmental, and exact.

20. Statements that are opinion and are provided by people on the scene of a sexual assault and should be placed in quotes on the

PCR are _____.

Fill-in-the-Table

Fill in the missing parts of the table.

When assessing for possible child abuse, the CHILD ABUSE mnemonic is helpful.

Mnemonic	What the Letter Represents
C	
H	
I	
L	
D	
A	
B	
U	
S	
E	

C H A P T E R

44 Patients With Special Needs

Chapter Review

The following exercises provide an opportunity to test your knowledge of this chapter.

Matching

Match each of the items in the left column to the appropriate definition in the right column.

_____ 1. Emotional/mental impairment

_____ 2. Conductive deafness

_____ 3. Osteoarthritis

_____ 4. Myasthenia gravis

_____ 5. Sensorineural deafness

_____ 6. Obesity

_____ 7. Down syndrome

_____ 8. Aphasia

_____ 9. Hemiplegia

_____ 10. Cerebral palsy

_____ 11. Muscular dystrophy

_____ 12. Poliomyelitis

A. A degenerative joint disease associated with aging

B. Term generally used when someone is 20% to 30% over their ideal weight

C. A highly contagious viral infection that can cause paralysis and death, and that created a serious epidemic in the past but is now prevented in the United States through a vaccine

D. Neuromuscular disorder in which voluntary muscles are poorly controlled

E. Paralysis of one side of the body

F. The loss of the ability to communicate in speech, writing, or signs

G. A curable temporary condition caused by an injury to the eardrum

H. A permanent lack of hearing caused by a lesion or damage to the inner ear

I. Illnesses that cause a person's emotions to become out of control

J. An inherited muscular disease that causes degeneration of the muscle fibers

K. A genetic chromosomal defect that can occur during fetal development and that results in mental retardation as well as presence of certain physical characteristics, such as a round head with a flat occiput and slanted, wide-set eyes

L. An abnormal condition characterized by the chronic fatigability and weakness of muscles, especially in the face and throat, that results from a defect in the conduction of nerve impulses at the nerve junction caused by a lack of acetylcholine

Multiple Choice

Read each item carefully, and then select the best response.

_____ 1. Which of the following would be considered speech impairments?

    A. Articulation disorders   **C.** Fluency disorders

    B. Language disorders   **D.** All of the above

_____ 2. When establishing communication with a patient with speech impairment, the paramedic should do which of the following?

      A. Ask the patient how he or she would be comfortable communicating.

      B. Use an interpreter.

      C. Be patient because communicating is going to take time.

      D. All of the above.

_____ 3. You arrive on the scene to discover that your patient with special needs has a service dog. As a friendly, patient advocate–oriented paramedic, it is okay for you to do which of the following?

      A. Play with the dog.

      B. Take the dog out for a quick game of fetch.

      C. Realize the dog is a working dog and shouldn't be played with without permission.

      D. Treat the dog as part of the patient team.

_____ 4. The different types of paralysis include all of the following EXCEPT:

      A. Hemiplegia   **C.** Myasthenia gravis

      B. Quadriplegia   **D.** Paraplegia

_____ 5. All of the following are helpful tips when moving a morbidly obese patient EXCEPT:

      A. Treat the patient with dignity and respect.

      B. Avoid trying to lift the patient by only one limb, which would risk injury to the person's overtaxed joints.

      C. Follow up on the patient's carefully monitored diet.

      D. Coordinate and communicate all moves to all team members *prior* to starting.

_____ 6. Patients with Down syndrome are at greater risk for which of the following medical conditions?

      A. Hearing and vision problems

      B. Medical complications that affect the cardiovascular, sensory, endocrine, orthopedic, dental, and gastrointestinal systems

      C. Enlarged tongue and dental anomalies that can lead to speech abnormalities

      D. All of the above

_____ 7. As health care providers, you and your team will often be called on to assist a patient who is facing imminent death or terminal illness. Signs of impending death include all of the following EXCEPT:

      A. Decreased orientation

      B. Decreased nutritional status

      C. Bradycardia and tachycardia

      D. The need for performance of ALS skills and cardiopulmonary resuscitation (CPR)

_____ 8. Clues that a patient has a communicable disease include which of the following?

      A. Rashes   **C.** Ill appearance

      B. Coughing   **D.** All of the above

_____ 9. Fears about paying for care should not keep any patient from seeking help. Knowing which of the following facts would potentially help a fearful patient decide to seek treatment/transportation?

      A. Remember—no patient should be refused transport to an emergency care facility based on his or her ability to pay.

      B. Federal laws allow patients to be seen and evaluated when they seek help.

      C. Many hospitals have a mechanism for providing free treatment or treatment at reduced rates for indigent individuals.

      D. All of the above.

_____ **10.** Many disabled patients use service dogs, most notably blind persons. When dealing with working dogs, it is best for the paramedic to do which of the following?

  A. Keep animal treats in response bags to reward positive behavior.

  B. Pet the dog and establish rapport.

  C. Have bystanders restrain the animal because it may become agitated at paramedics.

  D. Don't distract the dog unless the patient gives you permission.

Labeling
Label the following diagrams with the correct terms.

Label the following American Sign Language (ASL) signs with the appropriate meaning.

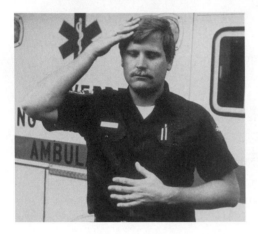
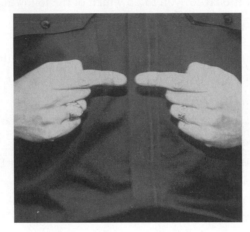
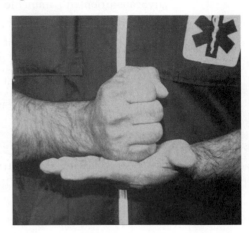

_____   _____   _____

Fill-in-the-Blank
Read each item carefully, and then complete the statement by filling in the missing word(s).

1. Hearing challenges are generally classified into two types: _____ and _____ deafness.

2. Most people who are hearing _____ have learned to use body language, such as hand gestures and _____.

3. Speech may be delayed by _____ or psychosocial factors. For others, it may be altered by _____, illness, or _____ impairment.

4. Signs of voice production _____ include _____, _____, inappropriate pitch, or abnormal nasal _____.

5. A person with visual impairment may feel _____, especially during the chaos of a/an _____. He or she may have learned to use other senses such as _____, touch, and _____ to compensate.

6. Patients with _____ syndrome are usually *extremely* obese. They experience _____, _____, and _____.

7. Two thirds of children born with _____ _____ have congenital heart disease.

8. Paramedics need to be good at listening. Always "listen" carefully to your _____—not just the words spoken, but also heed the patient's _____, facial _____, and body _____.

9. As children grow, symptoms of cerebral palsy may either become _____ or stay the same. Related complications include _____ impairments, hearing and language difficulties, _____, and mental _____.

10. Spina bifida is the most common permanently disabling _____ _____. In this disorder, during the first month of _____, the fetus' spinal _____ does not close properly or completely and vertebrae do not _____.

Identify

In the following case studies, list the chief complaint, the history of present illness, and the other medical history.

1. You have been called to the scene by distraught family members. The patient is becoming increasingly disoriented and appears unresponsive. The patient is exhibiting an irregular breathing pattern with periods of apnea. Some family members have what appears to be a valid prehospital Do Not Resuscitate Order (DNR).

    a. Chief Complaint

    _____

    _____

    _____

    b. History of the Present Illness

    _____

    _____

    _____

    _____

    _____

    c. Other Medical History

    _____

    _____

    _____

    _____

    _____

2. You are responding to a call to an adult group home for adults with disabilities. The nature of the call is for a patient with seizures. On arrival, you are met by staff members who have the patient's complete chart. The patient has a history of Down syndrome and a seizure disorder. The patient is on multiple medications and has been given rectal diazepam (Diastat).

a. Chief Complaint

_____

_____

_____

b. History of the Present Illness

_____

_____

_____

_____

_____

_____

c. Other Medical History

_____

_____

_____

_____

_____

_____

3. Your patient has a chief complaint of fever. The patient's home health aide states that the patient's urine has been cloudy and he's suddenly developed a fever of 101.3°F. He is conscious and alert, but is confined to a wheelchair. He communicates with a writing board. He is a quadriplegic and has a Foley catheter, tracheotomy, colostomy, and feeding tube.

a. Chief Complaint

_____

_____

_____

b. History of the Present Illness

_____

_____

_____

_____

_____

_____

c. Other Medical History

_____

_____

_____

_____

_____

Ambulance Calls

The following case scenarios provide an opportunity to explore the concerns associated with patient management and paramedic care. Read each scenario, and then answer each question.

1. You receive an "Alpha" response for a patient with chronic pain. On arrival, you note the wheelchair ramp in front of the apartment. Once inside you recognize your patient. You have provided care for her in the past. She is 36 years old and is complaining of severe lower back pain and is requesting transportation to the medical center. She is somewhat difficult to interact with. She's not very polite. Despite that, you continue to be professional and initiate care. She has a history of spina bifida and is seated in her motorized wheelchair. She is covered in a blanket.

   a. What can you do to help alleviate her discomfort during transfer from her wheelchair to the cot?

   _____

   _____

   _____

   b. Based on your knowledge of spina bifida, what other medical issues may be present?

   _____

   _____

   _____

2. Tonight you are working a special event at the civic center. It's the concert of a popular country singer. The place is packed. Other than a couple of requests for ice packs and ear plugs, the event has been uneventful. Suddenly, security requests EMS to section 103 for a person having a seizure. Your patient is a 12-year-old girl with her mom. The patient has Down syndrome and a seizure disorder. The seizure is over by the time you arrive, but the patient appears postictal and has a large amount of saliva and snoring-type respirations.

   a. How would you go about treating the patient?

   _____

   _____

   _____

b. What are the characteristic physical features of someone with Down syndrome?

_____

_____

_____

True/False

If you believe the statement to be more true than false, write the letter "T" in the space provided. If you believe the statement to be more false than true, write the letter "F."

_____ **1.** Whatever the source of the challenge, patients with special needs will require you to adapt your assessment and management to accommodate their needs.

_____ **2.** A family member may prove to be a poor teammate.

_____ **3.** Impatience with or interruption of a patient who stutters may frustrate the patient more and cause the stuttering to get worse, making assessment and history taking difficult.

_____ **4.** Patients with a total laryngectomy would receive a stoma and might communicate by burping sounds or by using an electronic or mechanical device.

_____ **5.** Patients with dysphagia rarely have a need for emergency airway interventions.

_____ **6.** A severely disabled person may not have the ability to care for himself or herself, communicate, understand, or respond to their surroundings.

_____ **7.** Patients with mental impairments view all strangers, especially paramedics in uniform, in a friendly and calm manner.

_____ **8.** Cystic fibrosis is a chronic dysfunction of the endocrine system that targets multiple body systems but primarily the respiratory and digestive systems.

_____ **9.** Muscular dystrophy is an acquired muscular disease that causes degeneration of the muscle fibers. In many cases, the destroyed fibers are replaced by fat or connective tissue.

_____ **10.** Patients with myasthenia gravis have facial and throat muscles that could become so weak that the patient suffers an acute onset of respiratory failure. In such a case, you need to intervene immediately with airway management, ventilatory support, and possibly intubation.

Short Answer

Complete this section with short written answers using the space provided.

1. Oftentimes, paramedics treat patients who are hesitant about allowing transport. One of the primary reasons encountered is the financial concern voiced by patients. This is a legitimate patient concern and one that often must be addressed in the prehospital environment.

   a. Describe how you could go about getting a patient with financial concerns to go to the emergency department.

_____

_____

_____

_____

   b. Are there any free clinics in your response area to which you could refer patients?

_____

c. Are you legally and medically allowed to transport to these clinics?

_____

d. Are hospitals required to evaluate the patients you bring them?

_____

_____

2. Many of the patients a paramedic encounters have hearing impairments. Sometimes this impairment is readily noticeable.
   a. What clues would indicate to you that your patient has a hearing impairment?

_____

_____

_____

   b. How would you go about communicating with someone with a hearing impairment?

_____

_____

_____

3. Transporting obese patients can be particularly challenging for paramedic crews. Describe strategies that would be helpful to the patient and the EMS providers.

_____

_____

_____

_____

_____

4. You respond to a car crash. On arrival, you discover a frightened but apparently uninjured rear-seat passenger. Everyone else appears to be out of the car walking around. You discover that the passenger has a visual impairment.
   a. What are some of the causes of visual impairments?

_____

_____

   b. What can paramedics do to alleviate some of the fears felt by patients with visual impairments?

_____

_____

Word Find

Hidden in the following grid are 21 words or phrases related to what you have studied in this chapter. Find the hidden words in the grid below. Then use the words from the grid to answer the following questions (some words may be used to answer more than one of the questions).

```
Y W S Y M Q M D O H A Q L Y D V C S U M M S S P
A T W I K U X E X B U I S K O R S G Y Q E S I O
I K I T S L S X N A E L G S A E S A J C N E T L
G Z Q L F O W C D T A S I E N E S U Y N T N I I
E W C D I S R R U P A T I F L T L V T Y A F R O
L U R V B B I B L L I L A T H P R N T Z L A H M
P D B W U P A A I R A E I E Y M I T B V I E T Y
A T A H L H R S H F D R N L E T F M I X M D R E
R A Z E O B D T I E C I D A L K K F E D P L A L
A M G E E F R P V D A I W Y W N U C W H A A O I
P I S R C A S I L G L R T C S E E W H B I R E T
A H E B R H T N R Q A A G S G T D S Y R R U T I
Q C D N G C H A G F G X T R Y K R Q S F M E S S
O R H D U I V W M K G C T N B C N O C T E N O M
E R S D Q I A P H A S I A P E T V P P D N I B Y
C N N D S S E N L L I L A N I M R E T H T R D Q
Y O D O W N S S Y N D R O M E W P I L R Y O N B
C E T U M U L T I P L E S C L E R O S I S S Z K
L S O W U X O P N A J W A T Q X T P L J Z N S H
B A J D E A T A S C R E K L L S T Y N E V E M S
U W I W S C V W B D V W P K P D H W S H V S N E
A D I F I B A N I P S Z F U S R L K H Y X E Q L
U C P L P E X Z R A I G T M Z I W P S D L Z D L
S V U L O U T K K L N E D L F E Z I H Y B F N U
```

1. The loss of the ability to communicate. _____

2. _____ is a joint inflammation that causes pain, swelling, and a decreased range of motion.

3. A nonprogressive, bilateral, neuromuscular disorder in which voluntary muscles are poorly controlled. It results from developmental brain defects in utero. _____ _____

4. A form of deafness that is temporary and usually curable that is caused by an eardrum injury. _____ _____

5. _____ _____ is a usually fatal disease that targets multiple body systems.

6. _____ _____ is insufficient development of the brain resulting in the inability to learn and socially adapt at the usual rate.

7. Also known as trisomy 21. _____ _____

8. Paramedics should be good listeners when interacting with patients with a/an _____/_____ _____.

9. _____ is the term used to describe a patient with paralysis to one side of the body possibly from a head injury or stroke.

10. A generic term used to describe a variety of illnesses that result in emotional, cognitive, or behavioral dysfunction. _____ _____

11. Two types of _____ _____ are distinguished: relapsing and progressive.

12. _____ _____ is an inherited disease that causes degeneration of the muscle fibers.

13. The first symptoms of _____ _____ usually present as weakness in the eye or eyelid movement.

14. Diseases that often result in public ridicule and affect about 9 million Americans. _____

15. _____ is a degenerative joint disease associated with aging.

16. Paralysis of all four extremities and the trunk of the body. _____

17. This disease is now rare in the United States thanks in part to the Salk and Sabin vaccines. _____

18. Term used to define the paralysis of the lower parts of the body. _____

19. _____ _____ is permanent and may be caused by lesions or damage to the middle ear.

20. _____ _____ is the most common permanently disabling birth defect.

21. Paramedics need to provide supportive care for patients and their families that are dealing with a _____ _____.

Fill-in-the-Table

Fill in the missing parts of the table. A special need is identified in the left column. Paramedics should use the right column to describe a particular patient care need based on the special need identified.

Special Need	Associated Patient Care Need
Speech impairments	
Visual impairments	
Paralysis	
Obesity	
Developmental disabilities	
Pathologic challenges	

CHAPTER

45 Acute Interventions for the Chronic Care Patient

Chapter Review

The following exercises provide an opportunity to test your knowledge of this chapter.

Matching
Match each of the definitions in the left column with the appropriate terms in the right column.

_____ 1. The introduction of either single cytotoxic drugs or combinations of cytotoxic drugs into the body for the purpose of interrupting or eradicating malignant cellular growth

_____ 2. Drawing of air into the lungs; airflow from a region of higher pressure (outside the body) to a region of lower pressure (the lungs); occurs during normal (unassisted) breathing

_____ 3. Discharge that contains pus

_____ 4. The formation of an opening to allow the passage of urine

_____ 5. Large, electrical devices that concentrate the oxygen in ambient air and eliminate other gases

_____ 6. Separation of the edges of a wound

_____ 7. A surgical procedure in which the larynx is removed

_____ 8. Forcing of air into the lungs

_____ 9. Surgical opening into the trachea

_____ 10. Establishment of an opening between the colon and the surface of the body for the purpose of providing drainage of the bowel

A. Purulent exudates

B. Tracheostomy

C. Chemotherapy

D. Oxygen concentrators

E. Dehiscence

F. Laryngectomy

G. Positive-pressure ventilation

H. Colostomy

I. Negative-pressure ventilation

J. Ureterostomy

Multiple Choice
Read each item carefully, and then select the best response.

_____ 1. The philosophy of hospice care began in:

    A. England in the 1960s.

    B. France in the 1950s.

    C. New York City in the 1980s.

    D. Germany in the 1990s.

_____ 2. As you arrive on scene, you observe that the patient has tripped over a bath rug that caught under her walker leg. How does your teachable moment occur?

    A. In assisting the patient when it is appropriate to contact emergency medical services

    B. In educating the family on the benefits of a long-term in-patient facility

C. In assisting the patient and her family to recognize the need to remove scatter rugs

D. In teaching your paramedic intern how to assess long bone injuries

_____ **3.** What is tidal volume?

A. The amount of air inhaled or exhaled during normal, quiet breathing

B. The formation of an opening to allow the passage of urine

C. Chronic deterioration of mental functions

D. A surgical procedure in which the larynx is removed

_____ **4.** Your evaluation of patients receiving home oxygen or support ventilations is no different from evaluation of any other patient EXCEPT:

A. assessing the work of breathing.

B. looking for accessory muscle use.

C. assessing pulse oximetry.

D. measuring the length of oxygen tubing from the oxygen device.

_____ **6.** Home oxygen systems involve:

A. nasal cannulas.

B. oxygen.

C. nasal cannulas and oxygen.

D. small-volume nebulizers.

_____ **7.** To ventilate a patient with a laryngectomy, you should:

A. ventilate through the mouth and nose.

B. use positive-pressure ventilation.

C. seal the nose and ventilate through the mouth.

D. ventilate through the stoma.

_____ **8.** A central venous catheter is used for many types of home care patients, including those receiving:

A. chemotherapy.

B. long-term antibiotic or pain management.

C. high-concentration glucose solutions.

D. all of the above.

_____ **9.** Patients who are chronically ill or fragile may have devices that allow medications and fluids to be infused or body fluids to be removed and monitored. These devices place the patient at increased risk for the following cardiovascular complications EXCEPT:

A. anticoagulation.

B. embolus formation.

C. dehydration.

D. air embolus.

_____ **10.** Catheter dysfunction occurs frequently. This complication can be minimized and treated when the paramedic is aware of preventative measures. These measures may include which of the following?

A. Position the patient in a semi-Fowler's or upright position if tolerated.

B. Inspect and keep the device area clean.

C. Use the device site only for what it was designed for.

D. All of the above.

_____ **11.** What is the name of a surgical opening in the large intestine that is brought to the surface of the abdomen to drain solid waste?

A. Suprapubic catheter

B. Ureterostomy

C. Colostomy

D. Stoma

_____ **12.** Which of the following factors may place patients at the greatest risk for infections?

A. Poor nutritional status

B. Immunosuppression

C. Implanted vascular devices

D. All of the above

_____ **13.** Postpartum depression may be caused by which of the following?
- **A.** A drop in hormone levels following childbirth
- **B.** Pregnant women being treated for depression prior to pregnancy
- **C.** Patients predisposed to fatigue and diabetes
- **D.** None of the above

_____ **14.** Which of the following are legal documents that deal with a patient's medical conditions and desires?
- **A.** Durable power of attorney
- **B.** Living wills
- **C.** Do Not Resuscitate orders
- **D.** All of the above

_____ **15.** Coronary artery disease, acute myocardial infarctions (AMIs), and primary heart muscle weakness may be factors in:
- **A.** an oxygen perfusion mismatch.
- **B.** ineffective preload.
- **C.** congestive heart failure.
- **D.** none of the above.

Fill-in-the-Blank

Read each item carefully, and then complete the statement by filling in the missing word(s).

1. _____ refers to the introduction of either single cytotoxic drugs or combinations of cytotoxic drugs into the body for the purpose of interrupting or eradicating malignant cellular growth.

2. Early dementia can be managed in the _____ _____, but advanced dementia generally requires _____ _____ care.

3. _____ _____ _____ is often not recognized or treated because normal changes during pregnancy such as fatigue, insomnia, strong emotional reactions, and changes in body weight may occur during pregnancy and after pregnancy. These same symptoms may also be signs of depression.

4. Drainage from a wound consists of fluid and cells. _____ _____ is a clear, watery drainage. _____ _____ is pus, which consists of white blood cells, liquefied dead tissue, and bacteria.

5. A/an _____ is a surgical opening in the large intestine that is brought to the surface of the abdomen to drain solid waste.

6. _____ _____ _____ relieve anxiety and the pain of frequent insertion attempts for patients. At the same time, they create potential complications. If a device complication is suspected, the paramedic should not _____ to access the device.

7. Negative-pressure _____ mimic the body's normal method of _____. These devices—which may be called ponchos, turtleshells, or belts—enlarge the chest, dropping _____ _____ below the atmospheric pressure and allowing air to rush in.

8. Some patients use _____ _____, which are large electrical devices that concentrate the oxygen in ambient air and eliminate other gases. Such a system eliminates frequent delivery of oxygen cylinders, is less expensive, and is easy to maintain.

9. According to the Haddon matrix framework, injuries occur in a certain time sequence: the _____-_____ _____, the event phase, and the _____ phase.

10. Premature newborns or those with congenital heart, lung, or _____ problems often require home care, including a/an _____ _____.

11. The body perceives pain as a/an _____. In response, it activates the _____ nervous system, leading to elevated blood pressure, _____, and tachypnea.

12. _____ differs from a/an _____ catheter in that the catheter is surgically placed into the bladder. In the latter case, the ureters remain intact and continue to drain the kidneys into the _____ _____.

Identify

In the following case studies, list the chief complaint, vital signs, and pertinent negatives.

1. You receive a priority 2 call for a conscious alert man who is 36 years old. On arrival, you discover that the patient is wheelchair dependent and his mental status is somewhat confused. The patient's home health aide states the patient is a paraplegic, appears to have a catheter blockage, and is excreting very dark foul-smelling urine. He has a Foley catheter. Your assessment reveals a conscious but not alert patient. The skin is warm and dry, lung sounds include bilateral wheezing, his oxygen saturation is 92%, and he has slightly delayed capillary refill. Patient has a sinus tachycardia on the monitor. His blood pressure is 124/78 mm Hg. The patient's pulse rate is 100 beats/min. PEARRL (Pupils Equal And Round, Regular in size, reactive to Light). Motor neurologic to his upper extremities is equal bilaterally.

   a. Chief Complaint

   _____

   _____

   _____

   b. Vital Signs

   _____

   _____

   _____

   c. Pertinent Negatives

   _____

   _____

   _____

2. You are dispatched to an interfacility transport between an acute care facility and a long-term rehabilitation hospital. Your patient is a 23-year-old woman who is comatose as the result of a motor vehicle crash and subsequent head injury. She has demonstrated very slow but slight neurologic improvement. She is ventilator dependent and is intubated via a partial tracheostomy. She also has a Foley catheter as well as feeding tubes. Prior to accepting the patient for transfer you determine the following: blood pressure is 90/60 mm Hg, pulse is 120 beats/min, oxygen saturation is 89%, skin turgor is poor; the patient's skin is ashen, warm, and dry.

a. Chief Complaint

_____

_____

_____

b. Vital Signs

_____

_____

_____

c. Pertinent Negatives

_____

_____

_____

3. Your Advanced Life Support crew is responding to a priority 1, unresponsive patient. On arrival, you are met by upset family members who state that the patient is "gone." Other family members are cajoling you to come quickly and help. You are presented with a Do Not Resuscitate (DNR) order. You quickly assess the patient while contacting medical control. The patient is unconscious, unresponsive, pulseless, and apneic. The patient appears to be on an extensive array of advanced home care equipment. Once monitored, you discover a paced rhythm with no associated peripheral pulses. The family confirms that the patient has an implanted cardiac pacemaker. Medical control agrees with your decision not to initiate resuscitative efforts.

a. Chief Complaint

_____

_____

b. Vital Signs

_____

_____

_____

c. Pertinent Negatives

_____

_____

_____

Ambulance Calls

The following case scenarios provide an opportunity to explore the concerns associated with patient management and paramedic care. Read each scenario, and then answer each question.

1. You respond to a respiratory distress call for a 28-year-old ventilator-dependent man. The patient is extremely anxious, and he is very cyanotic. His apnea monitor is activated, and he is actively trying to cough. It appears as though his tracheostomy tube is occluded. Describe the steps required to suction and clean the patient's tracheostomy.

   a. _____

   b. _____

   c. _____

   d. _____

   e. _____

   f. _____

   g. _____

   h. _____

   i. _____

2. Your patient is a 51-year-old woman who has breast cancer. She is complaining of exertional dyspnea as well as left-sided chest discomfort and pain in her jaw radiating to her left shoulder. She is on numerous medications and has an extensive history that includes cardiac myopathy, a left-sided mastectomy, and an implanted central venous catheter for blood draws, chemotherapy, and fluid replacement. Assuming your local protocols allow the access of central venous catheters, list the steps necessary for accessing the device and drawing blood.

   a. _____

   b. _____

   c. _____

   d. _____

   e. _____

   f. _____

   g. _____

   h. _____

   i. _____

   j. _____

   k. _____

   l. _____

   m. _____

n. _____

o. _____

3. You are called to the scene of a patient who receives extensive home health care as a result of a neurologic disease. The patient has adapted very well to the home health care environment and has numerous assist devices.

a. Describe several factors to consider as you perform your scene size-up.

(1) _____

(2) _____

(3) _____

(4) _____

(5) _____

b. Describe the factors involved in the focused history and physical exam for the chronic care patient.

(1) _____

(2) _____

(3) _____

c. Describe the factors involved in your patient's detailed physical exam.

(1) _____

(2) _____

(3) _____

(4) _____

True/False

If you believe the statement to be more true than false, write the letter "T" in the space provided. If you believe the statement to be more false than true, write the letter "F."

_____ **1.** In rehabilitation care, the objective is to restore a person with disabilities to his or her maximum potential in several areas.

_____ **2.** Patients generally choose hospice care to save their personal finances in the ever expensive realm of health care.

_____ **3.** Paramedics have a unique opportunity to listen to patients and their families, observe the home care situation, and assist in securing substantial financial resources or reporting to protective agencies.

_____ **4.** When you assess the home health care patient's environment, note whether nutritional support is adequate and whether basic needs such as a reliable, safe heat source, good ventilation, electricity, and water are available.

_____ **5.** To conduct the initial assessment of patients with chronic illness, first gather a general impression. Does the patient appear to be on the point of death? If so, try to troubleshoot the cause and equipment failure involved.

_____ **6.** Observe the scene for signs of unsafe medication administration practices.

_____ **7.** The level of detail required for a physical exam in the home care setting is similar to any other physical exam performed in paramedic practice. The need for a comprehensive examination should be completed on each and every patient regardless of circumstances.

_____ **8.** Cystic fibrosis increases the amount of mucus present in the airway, limiting air flow and reducing diffusion across the pulmonary capillary membrane.

_____ **9.** Some patients may have an implantable pacemaker that delivers synchronized electrical stimulation to three chambers of the heart, enabling the heart to pump blood more efficiently throughout the body.

_____ **10.** Patients who have gastric tubes in place may still be at increased risk for aspiration. To minimize the risk of regurgitation and aspiration, the patient should be upright, at least to 60°, when medication or nutrition is being infused. They should ideally be kept upright for 10 to 15 minutes after feeding.

_____ **11.** Because of the short urethra in the male, men are at greater risk for urinary tract infections than women are. Given the ongoing risk of an infection with an indwelling catheter, urosepsis is one of the likely causes of septic shock in such patients.

_____ **12.** Immobile patients with chronic illnesses are at high risk for skin breakdown, leaving them susceptible to infection. Perform a careful assessment of your patient's skin.

_____ **13.** If the amount of drainage from a wound increases, especially 10 to 15 days after injury, dehiscence is likely.

_____ **14.** The risk of pulmonary embolus is increased in both pregnancy and in the postpartum period. The incidence of thromboembolic disease in pregnancy has been reported to range from 1 case in 200 deliveries to 1 case in 1,400.

_____ **15.** Because of serious time constraints and call volumes, paramedics shouldn't assume the role of health educators.

Short Answer

Complete this section with short written answers using the space provided.

1. Medication administration has several purposes in the home health care setting. Name three of these purposes.

a. _____

b. _____

c. _____

2. Paramedics have a unique opportunity to interact with patients and their families in the home health care setting. List three techniques in which a paramedic may be helpful.

a. _____

b. _____

c. _____

3. List resources that may provide financial support for patients in the home care environment.

a. _____

b. _____

c. _____

d. _____

e. _____

4. Effective means of preventing transmission of microorganisms include:

    a. _____

    b. _____

    c. _____

    d. _____

5. Calls to patients receiving home care sometimes result from:

    a. _____

    b. _____

6. It is important to assess for airway patency in all patients, but it is especially important in patients with artificial airways. What are the most critical steps in improving airway clearance and patency in these patients?

    a. _____

    b. _____

    c. _____

7. List the signs that may be an indication of air embolus.

    a. _____

    b. _____

    c. _____

Fill-in-the-Table

Fill in the missing parts of the table.

    1. Fill in the serious complications associated with vascular access devices.

Serious Complications Associated With Vascular Access Devices	
Complication	**Assessment Findings**
Occlusion	
Catheter thrombosis	Swelling of arm, neck, or shoulder; pain
Sepsis	
Catheter migration	
Catheter breakage	Leaking or bleeding from catheter
Embolism (air)	
Embolism (PICC/midline catheter)	Inadvertent removal with distal portion of catheter missing

Crossword Puzzle

Use the clues below to complete the puzzle.

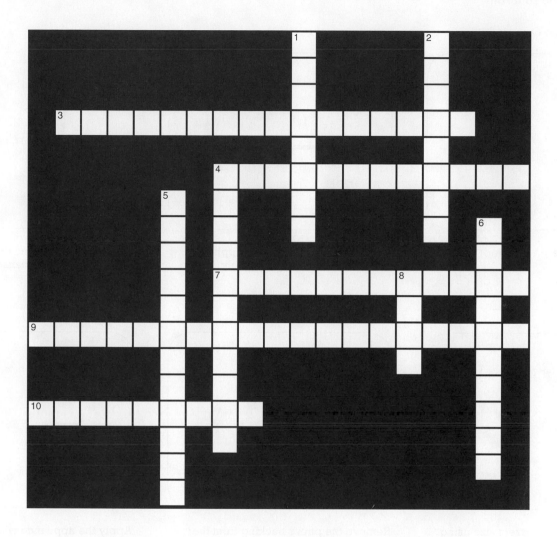

Across

3. Transplant recipients or individuals with human immunodeficiency virus infection

4. Planned surgical procedure in which an opening is placed in the trachea below the cricoid ring

7. A surgical procedure in which the larynx is removed

9. Large electrical devices that concentrate the oxygen in ambient air and eliminate gases

10. Surgical opening in the large intestine that is brought to the surface of the abdomen to drain solid waste

Down

1. From the same Latin root as hospitality

2. A progressive brain disorder with an insidious onset

4. Volume of air breathed in and out during a normal breath

5. A useful tool for identifying injury prevention opportunities

6. The leading cause of maternal death

8. Typically used for sleep apnea

Skill Drills

Test your knowledge of skill drills by placing the following photos in the correct order. Number the first step with a "1," the second step with a "2," and so forth.

1. *Replacing an Ostomy Device*

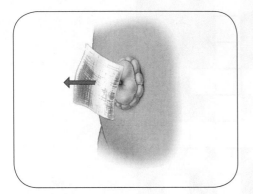

Remove the gauze.

_____

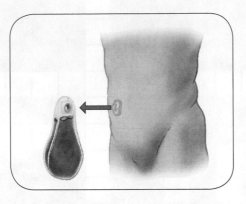

Empty/remove the current appliance and dispose of it appropriately.

_____

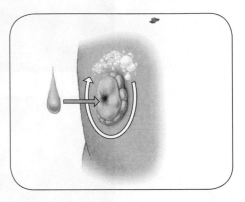

Wash the area around the stoma with soap and water. Cleanse the stoma with water.

_____

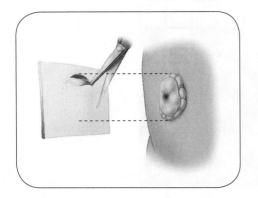

Cut the wafer to the correct size using the patient's measurement tracing.

_____

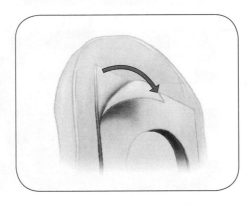

Remove the paper backing from the wafer.

_____

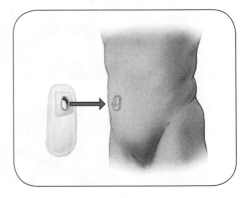

Apply the appliance with the stoma centered in the wafer cutout.

_____

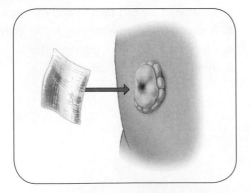

Place a clean gauze pad over the stoma.

_____

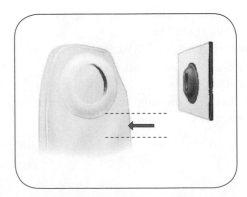

Attach the appliance to the wafer.

_____

Test your knowledge of these skill drills by filling in the correct words in the photo captions.

2. *Catheterizing Adult Male Patient*

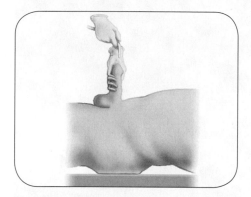

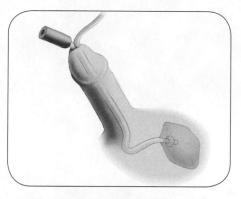

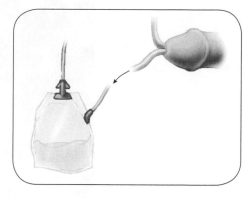

Hold the penis at a _____° angle to the body and insert the catheter.

Insert the catheter until the Y between the drainage port and the _____ port is at the tip of the penis. For a straight catheter, insert approximately _____ inch(es) more.

Allow _____ to drain.

2. *Catheterizing Adult Female Patient*

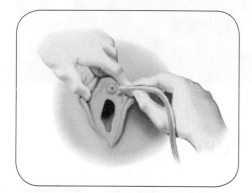

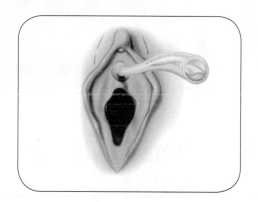

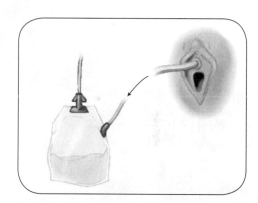

Locate the _____ _____ anterior to the vagina and insert the catheter.

When _____ is evident in the tubing, insert the catheter another _____ to _____ inches.

Allow the urine to _____.

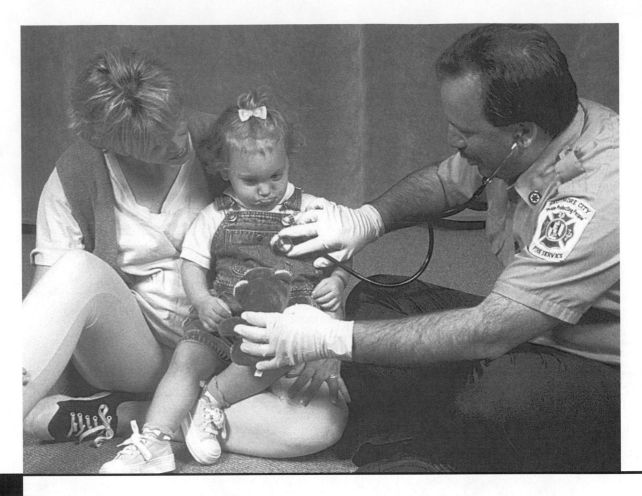

SECTION 6 CASE STUDY

2-Year-Old Female with High Fever

At 1:40 AM, you are dispatched to 311 West Kronkosky Street for a child with high fever. You and your partner proceed to the scene with a response time of approximately 5 minutes.

Upon arriving at the scene at 1:45 AM, you are greeted at the door of the residence by a young female holding her child. She tells you that her daughter has been running a fever, but now she is "not acting right." The child, a 2-year-old female, is crying and very irritable. You perform an initial assessment with the child in her mother's arms.

Initial Assessment

Level of Consciousness	Crying, irritable
Chief Complaint	According to the mother, "Fever and not acting right."
Airway and Breathing	Airway is patent; respirations, increased and unlabored.
Circulation	Radial pulses, rapid and bounding; skin, hot and flushed; capillary refill time, 2 seconds; no gross bleeding

1. What is your initial treatment for this child?

_____

_____

_____

You have completed the appropriate initial treatment for the child. The mother tells you that she is usually easily able to console and calm her daughter by picking her up when she is sick; however, for some reason, the child is not easily consoled this time and actually cries more when she is picked up. You perform a focused history and physical examination with information provided by the mother.

Focused History and Physical Examination

Onset	"She started running a fever about a day and a half ago."
Duration	"She has been sick for the last day and a half."
Associated Symptoms	"She has refused to eat anything for the past day or so. Also, I noticed that she has been grabbing the sides of her head; however, she doesn't seem to move her head, she only moves her eyes. She vomited twice in the last 12 hours."
Evidence of Trauma	No gross signs of trauma; mother denies a history of trauma
Seizures	No seizures were observed.
Fever	Rectal temperature, 102.5°F
Interventions Prior to EMS Arrival	"I gave her 1½ tsp of children's ibuprofen about 30 minutes ago."

2. What is your field impression of this child?

_____

_____

_____

_____

3. What are petechiae and purpura? What do they indicate?

_____

_____

_____

_____

The child remains conscious, but is not resistant to your assessment. You advise the mother that the child should be transported to the emergency department; she agrees. Shortly before departing the scene, you obtain a set of baseline vital signs and a SAMPLE history.

Baseline Vital Signs and SAMPLE History	
Blood Pressure	Not obtained
Pulse	120 beats/min, strong and regular
Respirations	36 breaths/min and regular; adequate depth
Oxygen Saturation	98% (on supplemental oxygen)
Signs and Symptoms	Fever, apparent headache and nuchal rigidity, vomiting, irritability
Allergies	None
Medications	None on a regular basis; ibuprofen 30 minutes ago
Pertinent Past History	Recent runny nose and cough
Last Oral Intake	12 hours prior, but promptly vomited
Events Leading to Illness	Recent URI symptoms, followed by onset of fever and irritability

4. What treatment will you provide to this child en route to the hospital?

_____

_____

_____

_____

You secure the child on the stretcher, place mother on the bench seat, and begin transport. En route, you continue oxygen therapy and continuous monitoring of the child. Your transport time is relatively short, so you perform a quick ongoing assessment of the child and then call your radio report to the receiving facility.

Ongoing Assessment

Level of Consciousness	Conscious, irritable, crying
Airway and Breathing	Airway remains patent; respirations, 34 breaths/min and unlabored
Oxygen Saturation	98% (on supplemental oxygen)
Blood Pressure	Not obtained
Pulse	124 beats/min, strong and regular

You deliver the child to the emergency department. Upon arrival, you note the development of a fine rash to the child's lower extremities. After giving your verbal report to the attending physician, you complete your patient care form and give a copy to the registration clerk. Subsequent assessment and a lumbar puncture (LP) confirm the condition that you suspected. The child is given antibiotics immediately and is admitted to the hospital.

46 Ambulance Operations

Chapter Review

The following exercises provide an opportunity to test your knowledge of this chapter.

Matching

Match each of the numbered items below to the appropriate type of ambulance transport.

Your air ambulance transports to a regional trauma center. Your ground ambulance transports to a community hospital. Choose the correct transportation for your patient.

A. Air ambulance

G. Ground ambulance

_____ **1.** 50-year-old in cardiac arrest

_____ **2.** 8-year-old having an asthma attack

_____ **3.** 22-year-old thrown from a rollover crash

_____ **4.** 44-year-old with amputation of the left hand

_____ **5.** 26-year-old mountain climber that fell approximately 50 feet

_____ **6.** 24-year-old with a breech presentation delivery

_____ **7.** 56-year-old with an active upper gastrointestinal (GI) bleed

_____ **8.** 18-year-old with a broken femur from an all-terrain vehicle (ATV) crash

_____ **9.** 2-year-old drowning victim who fell through ice at the local pond

_____ **10.** 34-year-old with a broken ankle from a football game

Multiple Choice

Read each item carefully, and then select the best response.

_____ **1.** The first ambulances were developed in:

A. 1790.   **C.** 1864.

B. 1860.   **D.** 1937.

_____ **2.** Which of the following should be done at the beginning of each shift?

A. Change the oil in the ambulance.

B. Complete an ambulance equipment/supply checklist.

C. Wash the ambulance.

D. Replace the supplies that were used the day before.

_____ **3.** When leaving the scene, what should you tell family members that are following you to the hospital?
   A. Drive as fast as you can with your flashers on.
   B. Follow the ambulance with your flashers on.
   C. Drive normally and do not follow the ambulance.
   D. Don't come until the doctor has called you.

_____ **4.** What can happen to the grass on the side of the road if you park the ambulance on it?
   A. Nothing.
   B. It can catch fire.
   C. It can die from the fumes of the ambulance.
   D. It can clog up the underside of the ambulance and cause the ambulance to stop running.

_____ **5.** What should you use when backing up an ambulance?
   A. The mirrors
   B. The guidance system that beeps when you are about to run into something
   C. The mirrors and a spotter
   D. Never back up an ambulance; always park so you can leave without backing up

_____ **6.** When did civilian use of rotary-winged aircraft begin?
   A. 1910   **C.** 1973
   B. 1943   **D.** 1985

_____ **7.** How big should the standard landing zone be for a typical helicopter?
   A. 50 × 50 feet   **C.** 100 × 100 feet
   B. 75 × 75 feet   **D.** 100 × 100 yards

_____ **8.** What type of light should you use to mark a landing zone?
   A. A strobe light in each corner of the zone
   B. A strobe light in the center of the zone
   C. A spotlight shining straight up in the center of the zone
   D. Blue flares in the center of the zone

_____ **9.** When should you approach the helicopter after it has landed?
   A. Only after the blades have come to a complete stop
   B. As soon as it touches down
   C. When the pilot or crew on the helicopter signal for you to approach
   D. Never approach; let the crew come to you

_____ **10.** Which of the following is not a key factor in staffing your ambulances?
   A. Unit cost of each run   **C.** Response times
   B. Taxpayer subsidies   **D.** The types of calls you will respond to

Labeling

Label the following diagram with the correct terms.

1. Label the following locations of the landing zone.

        A. where to post guard   **C.** pilot's area of vision

        B. pilot's blind area

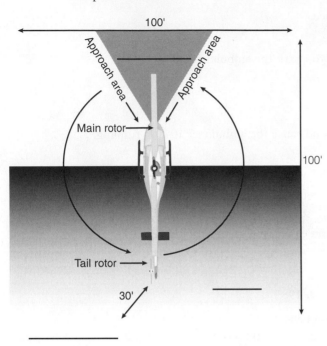

Fill-in-the-Blank

Assume you have been called to the scene of a road crash. Among the equipment listed here, mark an X beside that which you would grab to take along on your first dash from the ambulance to the patient. If any equipment you need has been left off the list, add it at the end and explain why you need it.

One sure way to *waste* time at the scene of a collision (or at any call) is to make a dozen trips back and forth to the ambulance to fetch equipment and supplies that you left behind. Well-organized paramedics take with them everything needed for the initial assessment and first stages of management.

_____ Long-leg air splint		_____ Stethoscope	
_____ Drug box		_____ Flashlight	
_____ Portable suction unit		_____ Triangular bandages	
_____ Oxygen cylinder		_____ Chemical cold packs	
_____ OB kit		_____ Cervical collar	
_____ Pocket mask		_____ Traction splint	
_____ Oropharyngeal airways		_____ Nonrebreathing mask	
_____ Intravenous fluid bags		_____ Long backboard/straps	
_____ Dressing materials		_____ Oral thermometer	
_____ Large-bore IV cannulas		_____ Fire extinguisher	
_____ Head immobilizer		_____ Bed pan	
_____ Self-adhering roller bandage		_____ Heavy-duty scissors	
_____ Selection of board splints		_____ Emesis basin	
_____ Wheeled cot stretcher		_____ Handheld radio	
_____ ECG monitor		_____ Adhesive bandages	
_____ Contact lens remover			

Other equipment that might be needed:

_____

_____

_____

_____

_____

Identify

In the following case study, list the chief complaint, vital signs, and pertinent negatives.

Walt and Dave respond to a two-vehicle crash. Their patient is a 41-year-old woman who tried to avoid a car that crossed the center line on the highway. The sport utility vehicle (SUV) she was driving rolled twice and landed on its wheels. The back portion was struck by the oncoming car. Walt is able to gain access through a back door and performs manual stabilization. Dave begins an assessment on the patient. She is conscious and alert and remembers the entire collision. She is complaining of pain in her left shoulder area. The rapid trauma assessment shows a deformity of the left collarbone and bruising beginning around the seat belt marks. Because of the collarbone, a cervical collar won't fit, and so Dave and Walt immobilize the woman on a backboard, pad the neck and head with towels, and then tape them down. Walt first applies supplemental oxygen and then begins baseline vital signs on the woman. He finds that her breathing is 22 breaths/min and shallow with decreased lung sounds on the left. Her pulse is 114 beats/min, and blood pressure is 132/84 mm Hg. The heart monitor shows sinus tachycardia with a few PVCs every few minutes. The patient can feel her arms and legs and is rating her pain in the shoulder at a 9/10. Her Pupils are Equal And Round, Regular in size, and react to Light (PEARRL). Skin is warm, but to help with shock, Dave turns the heat on in the unit and places a blanket over her. Walt starts an IV, and they monitor her heart and breathing on the way to the trauma center. Walt does a detailed physical exam that turns up a few small scrapes and bruises to her legs. He gets a SAMPLE history just as they pull into the regional trauma center.

a. Chief Complaint

_____

_____

_____

b. Vital Signs

_____

_____

_____

c. Pertinent Negatives

_____

_____

_____

Ambulance Calls

The following case scenarios provide an opportunity to explore the concerns associated with patient management and paramedic care. Read each scenario, and then answer each question.

1. Unit 2 has been dispatched to a new subdivision for a man who fell off a second-story roof. When Cory and Bill arrive, they find a 22-year-old man unconscious lying on a large pile of dirt. Cory and Bill don't really like each other much and neither one is willing to concede to the other. They both sprint to the patient to try and be the "lead" medic on the scene. Neither one of them has bothered to take any equipment. The patient is lying on his back. Cory finally performs C-spine stabilization while Bill starts a rapid trauma assessment, but that is kind of hard because he has no equipment. Bill sends a worker from the scene to get his orange airway bag out of the squad. After the airway bag arrives, oxygen is applied and Bill does a rapid assessment. The patient doesn't seem to have any broken bones, but is still out cold. One of the workers is trying to tell Cory what happened, but Cory won't listen. He lets the worker know that they are "here" now, and they will handle any medical problems. After about 15 minutes of being on scene, Bill finally has to go get a C-collar, backboard, and cot because the construction workers can't seem to find them even with Bill yelling at them. After they get the patient in the unit, they take vital signs, and they both try to grab the airway bag so that they can intubate. After a few seconds of arguing, they decide to do rock, paper, scissors to pick who gets to intubate. Cory wins and succeeds in intubating, and Bill decides to start a couple of IVs. Bill gives Cory a high-five after he sticks a 14-gauge in the left AC. After they get ready to roll, there is a discussion and another rock, paper, scissors contest to decide who is going to drive. Thirty-four minutes after reaching the scene, they are on the road to the closest hospital. Because their patient is starting to posture, they decide to turn around and head for the trauma center, another 15 minutes away.

   a. What should Cory and Bill have done prior to arriving on the scene?

   _____

   _____

   _____

   _____

   _____

   _____

   _____

   b. List six questions you would ask the workers at the scene.

   (1) _____

   (2) _____

   (3) _____

   (4) _____

   (5) _____

   (6) _____

c. Discuss Cory and Bill's transport decision, and what you would have done differently.

_____

_____

_____

_____

_____

_____

_____

_____

_____

_____

2. Jeff and Larry both show up just a few minutes late for their shift. Both of them were up late the night before watching the Monday night football game on TV. They both agree that because they are late and they each have headaches they will skip the morning check of the squad and go straight for the coffee and aspirin. Right away, they get a call for a woman who has fallen in front of the local grocery store. As they climb into the unit and take off, Jeff can hardly keep the squad on the road. It is doing a shimmy and shake down the road. When they arrive at the grocery store, the patient seems to be okay and doesn't want to go anywhere but home. She denies any pain and is alert. She states she just stepped off of the curb wrong and lost her balance. The store manager is the one that insisted on calling for an ambulance. Jeff turns off the squad when they decide this is a no-transport and grabs the paperwork for the patient to sign off on. After getting that all cleared up, they jump back into the squad to leave, but it won't start. They miss two calls while waiting for a tow truck. After they get the squad back to the service station, they are really embarrassed to find they were out of gas, and the shimmy they felt earlier was because of low pressure in a back tire. They finally make it back to the station around noon to a very angry supervisor and a stressed-out crew number 2 who had to cover calls for Jeff and Larry.

a. Why should you check your squad at the beginning of every shift?

_____

_____

_____

_____

b. What visual factors would you check before jumping in and running a call?

_____

_____

_____

_____

True/False

If you believe the statement to be more true than false, write the letter "T" in the space provided. If you believe the statement to be more false than true, write the letter "F."

_____ **1.** The standards for ambulances are determined by the Food and Drug Administration (FDA).

_____ **2.** Original guidelines called for ambulances to be painted orange and white.

_____ **3.** The DOT KKK Standards developed the three main types of ambulances.

_____ **4.** The defibrillator and pulse oximeter do not need to be tested.

_____ **5.** Brake fade is tested before driving the ambulance.

_____ **6.** Commission on Accreditation of Ambulance Services (CAAS) recommends that urban response time should be less than 8 minutes.

_____ **7.** One of the System Status Management (SSM) goals is to have a paramedic in every unit.

_____ **8.** A paramedic should always act as an advocate for the patient.

_____ **9.** Due regard states that if you have your lights and sirens on, you have the right of way and can break the traffic laws.

_____ **10.** Patient cost is a disadvantage of using an air ambulance.

Short Answer

Complete this section with short written answers using the space provided.

Only 1 out of 10 trauma patients is critically injured. But for that 1 patient out of 10, every minute that elapses between the time of injury and arrival at the operating suite reduces the patient's chances of survival. For that reason, all those who deal with the case in its pre–operating room phase must act as efficiently as possible. List three ways that you can save seconds, or minutes, of the "golden hour" without compromising the care of the patient.

1. _____

2. _____

3. _____

Secret Message

Identify the following terms from the clues provided, and then use the letters to decode the secret message!

a. Parking on a roadway at night can be _ _ N _ _ _ O _ _.
16 1   21 11 19   17 6

b. A _ _ N _ _ NG zone should be 100 feet by 100 feet.
2 22   7 9

c. SSM attempts S _ _ _ T _ GIC deployment to minimize response times.
14 23 4   18

d. As a paramedic, you should always act as an A _ _ OCAT _ for your patient.
24 10   20

e. Padded cabinet corners were installed to prevent _ NJU _ _ to the EMT.
13   8 5

f. _ _ EEL bounce is a vibration synchronous with road speed.
3 15

g. Wheel _ OBBLE is a common finding at low speeds.
12

Secret Message

_ _ _ _ _ _ _ _ _ _ _ _ _ _ _ _ _ _ _ _ _ _ _ _.
1 2 3 4 5 6 7 8 9 10 11 12 13 14 15 16 17 18 19 20 21 22 23 24

Fill-in-the-Table

Fill in the missing parts of the table.

1. List the advantages of using an air ambulance.

Advantages of Using an Air Ambulance
■
■
■
■

2. List the disadvantages of using an air ambulance.

Disadvantages of Using an Air Ambulance
■ Weather/environment
■
■ Airspeed limitations
■
■ Terrain
■
■

Skill Drills

Test your knowledge of skill drills by placing the following photos in the correct order. Number the first step with a "1," the second step with a "2," etc.

1. *Loading the patient*

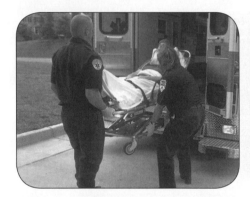

The second paramedic on the side of the cot releases the undercarriage lock and lifts the undercarriage.

_____

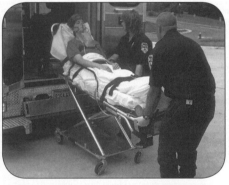

Tilt the head of the cot upward, and place it into the patient compartment with the wheels on the floor.

_____

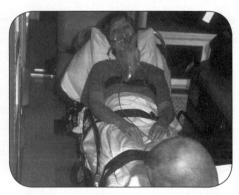

Secure the cot to the brackets mounted in the ambulance.

_____

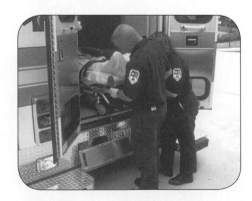

Roll the cot into the back of the ambulance.

_____

2. *Unloading the patient*

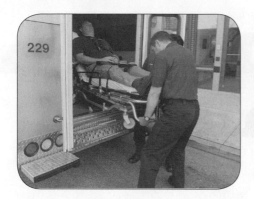

Lifting with your legs, carefully roll the stretcher forward until the undercarriage engages.

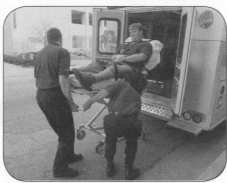

With your partner steadying the stretcher from the side, gently bring the stretcher forward out of the ambulance.

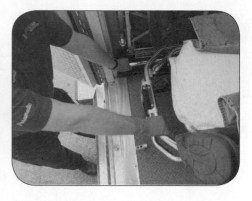

Unlock the head and foot locks.

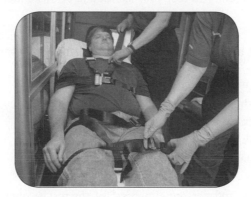

Ensure that the patient is secured to the stretcher.

CHAPTER

47 Medical Incident Command

Chapter Review

The following exercises provide an opportunity to test your knowledge of this chapter.

Matching

Match each of the positions in the right column to the appropriate description in the left column.

_____ **1.** Provides media with clear and understandable information

_____ **2.** Relays information between command and other agencies

_____ **3.** Responsible for food, water, and communications equipment

_____ **4.** Documents expenditures that must be reimbursed

_____ **5.** Counts and prioritizes patients

_____ **6.** Sets up a location for incoming and exiting vehicles and supplies

_____ **7.** Identifies special equipment and personnel needed for the rescue operation

_____ **8.** Works with medical examiners in removal of bodies

_____ **9.** Establishes an area of protection and rest for the rescuers

_____ **10.** Sets up treatment for all priorities of patients

A. Triage officer

B. Logistics section

C. Morgue officer

D. Staging officer

E. Public information officer

F. Treatment officer

G. Finance section

H. Liaison officer

I. Rehabilitation officer

J. Extrication officer

Multiple Choice

Read each item carefully, and then select the best response.

_____ **1.** Critical infrastructure includes all of the following EXCEPT:

    A. the electrical power grid.

    B. the Federal Emergency Management Agency (FEMA).

    C. water and sewage removal.

    D. communication systems.

_____ **2.** A large hazardous material incident would need what kind of command system?

    A. Single command system

    B. Unified command system

    C. Rescue command system

    D. Medical command system

_____ **3.** When sizing up a multiple-casualty incident (MCI) scene, which of the following questions does not fit in scene size-up?

    A. What do I have?

    B. What resources do I need?

    C. Who is coming to help?

    D. What do I need to do?

_____ **4.** What is the triage officer ultimately responsible for?

        A. Triage of every patient   **C.** Counting and prioritizing all patients

        B. Movement of patients to a treatment sector   **D.** Transportation to the hospitals

_____ **5.** Where should the rehabilitation area be located?

        A. As close as possible to the treatment area   **C.** Outside

        B. Next to the media area   **D.** Away from the scene and the media

_____ **6.** What does the _D_ stand for in the IDME mnemonic that applies to triage?

        A. Delayed   **C.** Don't move

        B. Dead   **D.** Decompensated shock

_____ **7.** Which of the following is not a special consideration during triage?

        A. A hysterical and disruptive patient   **C.** Death of a friend

        B. An injured rescue worker   **D.** Hazardous material exposure

_____ **8.** What color triage tag would you give a patient, at an MCI, who is breathing 4 breaths/min after you have opened the person's airway?

        A. Green   **C.** Red

        B. Yellow   **D.** Black

_____ **9.** When arriving on a scene to begin triage, what is a good thing to yell to the patients?

        A. If you can walk, move across the street to the oak tree.

        B. Stay where you are, and we will move all of you.

        C. Everyone just lie still and raise your hand if you think you are okay.

        D. Run for your lives, clear the area as fast as you can.

_____ **10.** What is your number one priority at the scene of an MCI?

        A. Triage of patients   **C.** Treatment of patients

        B. Scene safety   **D.** Setting up the proper sectors

Labeling

Label the following diagrams with the correct terms.

   1. Label the treatment area, triage area, extrication area, and incident area below.

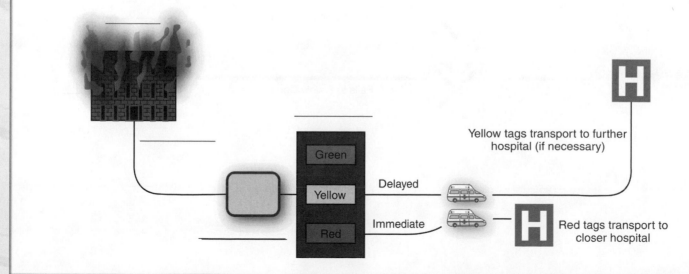

2. The START algorithm. Indicate if the following are:

A. Black/Nonsalvageable

B. Red/Immediate

C. Yellow/Delayed

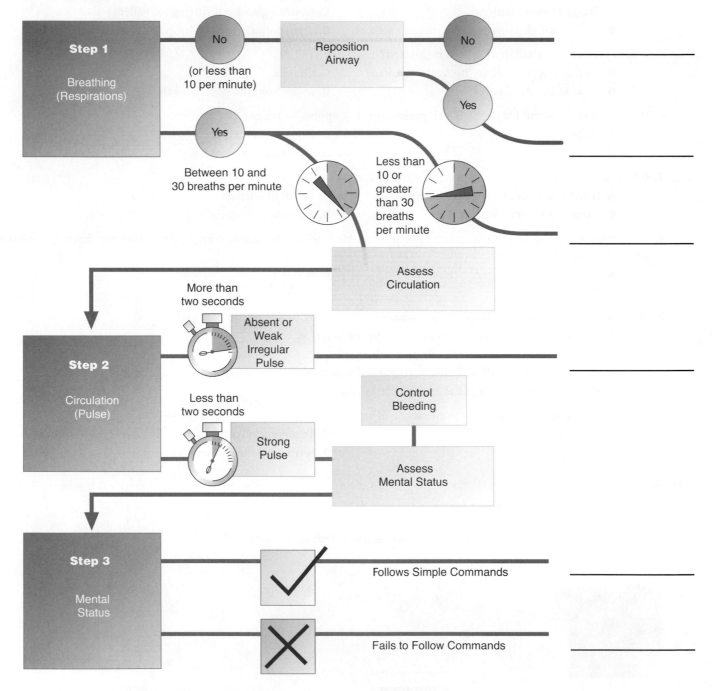

3. The JumpSTART algorithm. Indicate if the following are:

   A. Black/Nonsalvageable

   B. Red/Immediate

   C. Yellow/Delayed

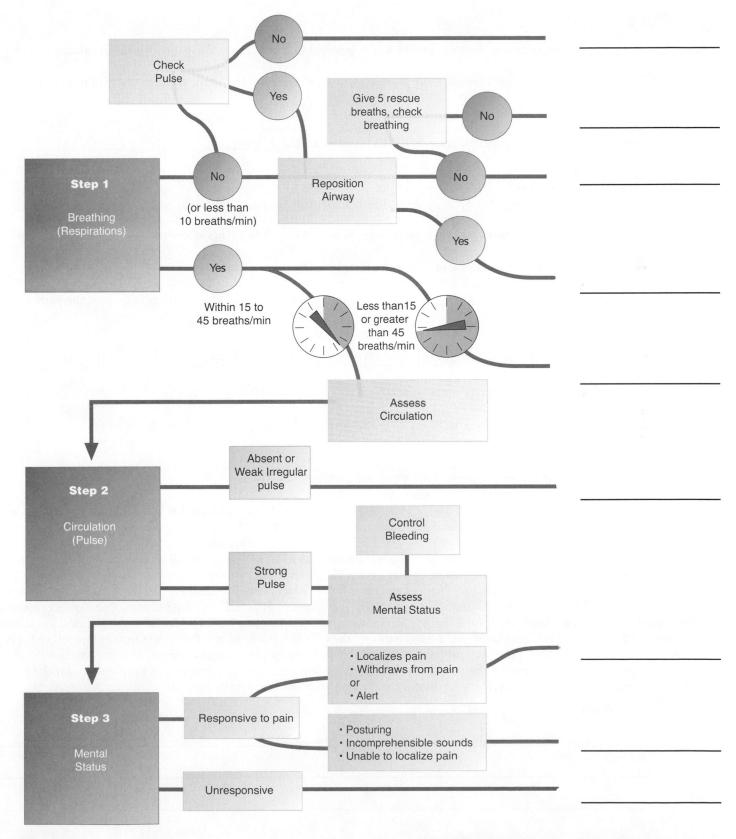

Fill-in-the-Blank

Read each item carefully, and then complete the statement by filling in the missing word(s).

1. A/an _____-_____ _____ is an event in which the number of patients exceeds the resources available to the initial responders.

2. A/an _____ incident is a situation in which it is expected to produce no more patients than are initially present.

3. The _____ section chief is responsible for documenting all expenditures at the incident that will need to be reimbursed.

4. The three officers that will help incident command (IC) the most are the _____, _____, and _____ officers.

5. _____ is a component of the National Incident Management System (NIMS) that establishes measures for all responders to incorporate into their systems in preparation to respond to all incidents at any time.

6. The _____ officer coordinates and distributes patients to the appropriate hospitals.

7. Initial triage done in the field is known as _____, and then the _____ triage is done as the patients are brought to the treatment sector.

8. The *R* in the START triage system stands for _____.

9. _____START was developed for pediatric patients involved in an MCI.

10. The _____ officer is in charge of parking vehicles and collecting supplies to be used at the scene.

Identify

In the following case study, list the chief complaint, vital signs, and pertinent negatives.

You have responded to a blast at a local fertilizer plant. Your patient is a 32-year-old man that is found outside the blast area. He is lying on his side because he has a piece of wood impaled in his left buttock. He is conscious and alert. The wood is sticking out about 6 inches and there is not much blood. He is unable to move because of the wood. Your partner starts the initial assessment and rapid trauma assessment (RTA) as you apply oxygen. RTA shows small nicks and cuts on the man's back and legs, but they are all secondary injuries that are not life-threatening. He says he was knocked to the ground when the explosion occurred. You are taking no chances and place him in a rigid cervical collar even though you won't be able to lay him flat. He is breathing 20 breaths/min, with an oxygen saturation of 97% and clear lung sounds. Pulse is 98 beats/min and regular, and blood pressure is 136/88 mm Hg. The patient rates his pain at a 7/10. His skin is warm and dry. You stabilize the wood in place and place the patient on a backboard and then use pillows to help stabilize him from rolling off of his right side. You get him in the unit, place him on the heart monitor which shows normal sinus rhythm, and then start an IV on him. You give him 5 mg of morphine for the pain because it is really starting to hurt since you moved him. You opt for the regional trauma center even though it is an extra 7 minutes farther away than the community hospital.

1. Chief Complaint

_____

_____

_____

2. Vital Signs

_____

_____

_____

3. Pertinent Negatives

_____

_____

_____

Ambulance Calls

The following case scenarios provide an opportunity to explore the concerns associated with patient management and paramedic care. Read each scenario, and then answer each question.

1. It is a hot, stuffy day in June in your community of 1,600 people. You are on a volunteer rescue squad in your home community and work for a critical care ground transport company in the city 25 miles away. It is your day off and you are enjoying the weather, but there have been tornado watches issued for your area. Later in the afternoon, the weather begins to get a little more serious, and you switch on your radio to get the latest updates. At 4:30 PM sirens go off indicating a tornado in the area, and so you head down to the basement with your kids and the dog. Your wife is at work at the nursing home. Before you know it, it sounds as if a freight train has hit your home. After everything is quiet, you fight your way out of the basement only to see total devastation of what used to be your community. You check with your neighbors to see if they are okay and decide to leave your kids with them. Because your truck is nowhere to be found, you grab a bike lying in the street and head down to the fire department.

Okay, take a little break here and answer a few questions. The fun thing to do is to work in teams and compare notes after you have answered your questions.

a. List 10 things you would like to have in your emergency kit to take with you.

(1) _____

(2) _____

(3) _____

(4) _____

(5) _____

(6) _____

(7) _____

(8) _____

(9) _____

(10) _____

b. There is a lot of damage in the area, and people are gathering in the streets. What are you going to tell them to do as you ride by on your bicycle?

_____

_____

_____

_____

_____

c. What type of hazards can you expect during the 2-mile ride to the fire station?

_____

_____

_____

_____

_____

2. You finally arrive at the fire department as the rest of your crew gathers; there are 24 emergency responders present. It has been estimated that at least 100 homes were destroyed plus the nursing home, which houses 75 patients. This really worries you because you know your wife was there when the storm hit. The firehouse and the high school two blocks away have not been touched by the twister. You have three ambulances and six fire trucks. Emergency management has two pickups, and the sheriff's office has three cars available. Word has gone out to the surrounding communities asking for all the help you can get.

a. Who should take command of this situation, and where should you set up the command post?

_____

_____

b. What type of buildings can be used for an emergency center for the walking wounded and displaced victims of the storm?

_____

_____

3. This is going to be a long night. Power is out all over town. You quickly begin to break into teams to begin searching for patients. There are many injuries at the nursing home as a result of the large number of people who were unable to get underground. You are sent there to work in the treatment center, and you see around 60 people with injuries over the next 6 hours. Your wife has made it through okay with only minor cuts. She is classified as walking wounded and actually pitches in to help with the patients that are worse. It takes 24 hours for all the homes to be searched, and your town suffers three deaths caused by this tornado. Three days later, most of the power has been restored to the houses that are still standing, and things start to calm down around town. There will be cleanup going on for the next few months, and it will take a couple of years to put everything back together. You are thankful that all the agencies in your town, even though they are small, work well together and have prepared for this type of emergency.

a. List some outside agencies in your area that will be able to help you in the first 3 hours of this disaster.

_____

_____

_____

True/False

If you believe the statement to be more true than false, write the letter "T" in the space provided. If you believe the statement to be more false than true, write the letter "F."

_____ **1.** There will never be physicians on the scene of an MCI.

_____ **2.** The planning section solves problems as they arise at an MCI.

_____ **3.** Critical infrastructures include electricity, water, fuel, and communications systems.

_____ **4.** An open incident is where you have not found all the victims.

_____ **5.** Command functions include triage and treatment functions.

_____ **6.** The safety officer has the power to stop all rescue functions.

_____ **7.** The public information officer always keeps close to the command post to keep up on the most current information.

_____ **8.** Face-to-face communications are the best because of infrastructure problems at the scene of an MCI.

_____ **9.** Yellow tag patients are deemed immediate priority patients because they have the best chance of survival.

_____ **10.** The second step in the START process is triage of the nonwalking patients.

Short Answer

Complete this section with short written answers using the space provided.

1. Discuss the first step of the START triage system.

_____

_____

_____

_____

_____

_____

_____

2. Discuss the second step in the START triage system.

_____

_____

_____

_____

_____

_____

_____

3. Why is the JumpSTART triage system needed for a pediatric patient?

_____

_____

_____

_____

4. Why should you participate in the critical incident stress management in the rehabilitation sector?

_____

_____

_____

_____

Crossword Puzzles

Use the clues in the column to complete the puzzle.

Across

4. _____ can overwhelm EMS and community resources.

6. A/an _____ command system is where there is one person in charge.

7. The _____ section chief has responsibility for communication equipment, facilities, food and water, and medical equipment.

8. In March 2004, Homeland Security implemented the _____. (initials)

9. Initials for an event that overwhelms initial responders.

10. A principle of the ICS is to limit the _____ of control of any one individual.

Down

1. The _____ _____ system helps responders to work effectively together.

2. You should have a/an _____ procedure to follow once an incident de-escalates.

3. ICS is designed to control duplication of effort and _____, in which independent decisions about the next actions are made.

5. The number of people that can effectively be supervised by one person is three to _____ people.

Fill-in-the-Table

Fill in the missing parts of the table.

1. MCI Equipment and Supplies

MCI Equipment and Supplies*	
Airway control	PPE (gloves, face shield, HEPA or N-95 mask)
	Rigid tip Yankauer and flexible suction catheters
	LMA, Combitube, ET tubes*
	Tube check, tube restraint, tape, syringes, stylet*
	End-tidal CO_2 device
Breathing	
	Bag-mask device(s) (adult and child), spare masks
	Oxygen delivery devices (nonrebreathing mask, cannula, extension tubing)
	Large-bore IV catheter for thoracic decompression*
Circulation	
	Sphygmomanometer, stethoscope
	Burn dressings, burn sheets, sterile water for irrigation
	1,000 mL bags of normal saline, IV start kits, catheters*
Disability	
	Head beds, wide tape, backboard straps
Exposure	Space blanket to cover patients
	Scissors
Logistic/Command	Sector vests (triage, treatment, transport, staging, command, rescue)
	Pads of paper, pencils, pens, markers
	Assessment cards pod

Note: The items denoted by * could be packaged in an ALS pod.

CHAPTER

48 Terrorism and Weapons of Mass Destruction

Chapter Review

The following exercises provide an opportunity to test your knowledge of this chapter.

Matching

Match each of the items in the right column to the appropriate definition in the left column.

_____ 1. An agent that affects the body's ability to use oxygen

_____ 2. An agent that produces blisters and burns on the skin

_____ 3. The most deadly chemical agents

_____ 4. A germ that requires a living host

_____ 5. A type of hemorrhagic fever

_____ 6. An animal that, once infected, spreads the disease that it is carrying

_____ 7. The amount of time a disease is spread from human to human

_____ 8. Energy that is emitted in the form of rays or particles

_____ 9. Type of protective measure to stop exposure to radiation

_____ 10. Five times more lethal than sarin gas, and has a fruity odor

A. Disease vector

B. Ionizing radiation

C. Vesicant

D. Soman

E. Virus

F. Nerve

G. Rift valley

H. Shielding

I. Metabolic agent

J. Communicability

Multiple Choice

Read each item carefully, and then select the best response.

_____ 1. A virus that has been added to the water supply is called a _____ weapon.

    A. Incendiary   **C.** Biological

    B. Chemical   **D.** Explosive

_____ 2. The Department of Homeland Security rates the current terrorist threats. What does the color orange represent?

    A. General risk of terrorist attack   **C.** No risk of terrorist attack

    B. Severe risk of terrorist attack   **D.** High risk of terrorist attack

_____ 3. A vesicant may produce all of the following, EXCEPT:

    A. seizures.   **C.** stridor.

    B. large blisters.   **D.** irritated eyes.

_____ 4. How long does it take for a patient to begin experiencing the signs and symptoms of sulfur mustard after being exposed?

    A. Immediately   **C.** 4 to 6 hours

    B. 2 to 4 hours   **D.** 6 to 8 hours

_____ **5.** Which of the following agents causes chest tightness, severe cough, and shortness of breath?

    A. Vesicant agent   **C.** Nerve agent

    B. Pulmonary agent   **D.** All of the above

_____ **6.** What does the _S_ stand for in the medical mnemonic DUMBELS?

    A. Salivation   **C.** Stridor

    B. Signs and symptoms   **D.** Seizures

_____ **7.** Which of the following statements correctly identifies a smallpox rash from other types of rashes?

    A. The lesions will be in various stages of healing.

    B. The lesions will all be identical in their development.

    C. The lesions will start on the chest.

    D. The lesions will be different sizes and shapes.

_____ **8.** Which of the following is NOT a route of exposure for the bubonic plague?

    A. Infected fleas   **C.** Waste from infected rodents

    B. Infected rodents   **D.** Infected birds

_____ **9.** What is the most deadly substance known to humans?

    A. Anthrax   **C.** Neurotoxin

    B. Smallpox   **D.** Vesicant

_____ **10.** What is the least harmful form of radiation?

    A. Alpha   **C.** Gamma

    B. Beta   **D.** X-rays

Labeling

Label the correct risk level for each color.

    1. Homeland Security Alert Levels.

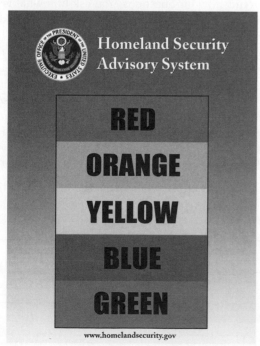

_____

_____

_____

_____

_____

Fill-in-the-Blank

Read each item carefully, and then complete the statement by filling in the missing word(s).

1. _____ _____ _____ _____ is any agent designed to bring about mass death,

   casualties, and massive damage to property.

2. Most of the terrorist acts are _____, meaning the public has no previous knowledge of the attack.

3. Additional explosives set at a site that are intended to injure responders are known as a/an _____ device.

4. _____ _____ _____ is how an agent most effectively enters the body.

5. _____ _____ are the most deadly chemicals developed.

6. G agents were developed by _____ scientists.

7. Bubonic plague infects the _____ system.

8. _____ is a deadly bacterium that lies dormant in a spore.

9. Ricin is made from _____ _____.

10. _____ _____ _____ are strategically placed stockpiles of antibiotics, vaccinations, and other

    medications.

Identify

In the following case study, list the chief complaint, vital signs, and pertinent negatives.

In your private vehicle, you respond to a vehicle crash about 2 miles from your home. Upon arriving at the scene, you see a truck that has rolled. The patient is outside of the truck and bystanders are trying to help him. He is covered in white power that has spilled from the truck. You walk up and take C-spine precautions and start to assess the patient knowing that your squad is about 3 minutes behind you. Jeff is 56 years old and is answering all your questions. You ask him what is in the truck because it is all over him and now you have some on you also. He says it is some kind of chemical he was taking to a local plant. Jeff has some cuts on his arms. As your squad arrives, you yell at everyone to get back and call for the fire department. Unfortunately, you forgot the first rule of scene safety and didn't look around well enough before entering the scene. The chemical is raw organophosphates. You and Jeff get a wonderful water bath from the fire department before anyone can come and help you. Finally, you get Jeff in the squad and find that he is bradycardic with a heart rate of 50 beats/min, and his blood pressure is 98/66 mm Hg. He begins to lose consciousness, respirations are dropping quickly to 9 breaths/min, oxygen saturation is 88%, and he is drooling terribly. You realize that atropine is indicated in organophosphate poisoning. After starting an IV, you give him 2 mg of atropine. You can give up to 5 mg, but you go with the lower dose because of his condition. You have your partner bagging him with 100% oxygen. After what seems like an eternity, he responds well with an increasing heart rate, blood pressure, and respiratory rate. You run code 3 all the way to the hospital. You are evaluated as soon as you get there also to make sure you will be okay.

1. Chief Complaint

   _____

   _____

   _____

2. Vital Signs

_____

_____

_____

3. Pertinent Negatives

_____

_____

_____

Ambulance Calls

The following case scenarios provide an opportunity to explore the concerns associated with patient management and paramedic care. Read each scenario, and then answer each question.

1. You are among the first ambulance personnel to reach the scene of a train derailment involving at least 60 casualties. Authorities on the scene think that this could be an act of terrorism.

   a. As you recall there are five categories of terrorist incidents. They are:

   (1) _____

   (2) _____

   (3) _____

   (4) _____

   (5) _____

   b. You are directed to begin triage of the people trying to get clear of the wreckage. There seems to be a lot of people that are ambulatory, but you are located in a bean field with nothing around you to send the walking wounded toward. There is only one road close by, and it is jammed up with emergency vehicles. What can you do with the ambulatory people?

   _____

   _____

   _____

   _____

   _____

2. You respond to the local swimming pool right before it is scheduled to open. Dispatch says there are several kids coughing and the lifeguards are having a hard time talking on the phone because of coughing spasms. As you arrive, you notice a green haze floating in the air around the pool house. There are about 50 kids standing around waiting for the pool to open.

   a. What is the cause of this green haze?

   _____

   _____

   _____

b. Before you get out of the ambulance, what are you going to do?

_____

_____

_____

_____

c. You have a total of seven kids that are coughing hard, and two lifeguards that are really struggling to breathe. After help arrives, you begin treatment on one of the lifeguards. What type of problems should you expect?

_____

_____

True/False

If you believe the statement to be more true than false, write the letter "T" in the space provided. If you believe the statement to be more false than true, write the letter "F."

_____ **1.** There are suits made for paramedics to shield them from radiation.

_____ **2.** Radiologic material can be found at hospitals, power plants, and colleges.

_____ **3.** Antibiotics will not help with bacteria.

_____ **4.** A virus can live and thrive outside the host body.

_____ **5.** The period of time between being exposed and showing signs and symptoms is known as the incubation period.

_____ **6.** Ebola is a type of hemorrhagic fever.

_____ **7.** Sarin is a vesicant.

_____ **8.** A cyberterrorist's main goal is to scare masses of people through the Internet.

_____ **9.** The Oklahoma City bombing was done by a domestic terrorist.

_____ **10.** The greatest threats to a paramedic during a weapons of mass destruction (WMD) attack are contamination and cross-contamination.

Short Answer

Complete this section with short written answers using the space provided.

1. List three *reactions* sometimes seen in bystanders at a multiple-casualty incident (MCI).

a. _____

b. _____

c. _____

2. As care of the patients proceeds, it is important to fill in pertinent details on each casualty's triage tag. List the information that should be recorded, if it can be obtained, on the triage tag.

a. _____

_____

b. _____

_____

c. _____

_____

d. _____

_____

e. _____

_____

f. _____

_____

Word Find

Hidden in the following grid are 20 words or phrases related to what you have studied in this chapter. Find the hidden words in the grid below. Then use the words from the grid to answer the following questions (some words may be used to answer more than one question).

```
A S N C H L O R I N E B T D E D
I A O S M G V S T C R F I T S I
D L I I D V U I Y O N R A I G S
R I T S C H E A N O T H S E Z S
A V A E G X N C I Y P O N I Y E
C A N M N I H T B S I I U U G M
Y T I E D O A O O M P R K C X I
D I R E R M M H I O L L D H D N
A O U R I B P A R G N W T L X A
R N H R W O X T N H A T I O B T
B E C O N T A C T H A Z A R D I
A A J A N E G A T U M H I I M O
L F G P E V A P O R N W B D S N
X R E O Y C N E T S I S R E P W
O D E F E C A T I O N P Z R A T
T Y Z F T S E T O D I T N A Y Z
```

1. _____ is a term used to describe how long an agent will stay on a surface before it evaporates.

2. Chemical agents can have either a/an _____ or _____ _____.

3. Mustard gas is considered a/an _____.

4. There are no _____ for mustard or phosgene oxime (CX) exposure.

5. The first chemical ever used in warfare was _____.

6. Words for the mnemonic DUMBELS: D_____, U_____, M_____, B_____,

   E_____, L_____ S_____.

7. There are two antidotes for nerve agent exposure in the MARK 1 kits: _____ and 2-PAM _____.

8. Nerve agents are a class of chemical called _____.

9. _____ is a colorless gas that smells like almonds.

10. _____ is the way a terrorist spreads the agent of destruction.

11. A radiologic dispersal device is more commonly known as a/an _____ _____.

Fill-in-the-Table

Fill in the missing parts of the table.

1. Nerve Agents

Nerve Agents						
Name	**Code Name**	**Odor**	**Special Features**	**Onset of Symptoms**	**Volatility**	**Route of Exposure**
Tabun	GA		Easy to manufacture	Immediate		Both contact and vapor hazard
Sarin	GB		Will off-gas while on victim's clothing	Immediate		Primarily respiratory vapor hazard; extremely lethal if skin contact is made
Soman	GD		Ages rapidly, making it difficult to treat	Immediate		Contact with skin; minimal vapor hazard
V agent	VX		Most lethal chemical agent; difficult to decontaminate	Immediate		Contact with skin; no vapor hazard (unless aerosolized)

2. Chemical Agents

Chemical Agents						
Class	**Military Designations**	**Odor**	**Lethality**	**Onset of Symptoms**	**Volatility**	**Primary Route of Exposure**
Nerve agents	Tabun (GA) Sarin (GB) Soman (GD) VX		Most lethal chemical agents can kill within minutes; effects are reversible with antidotes		Moderate (GA, GD) Very high (GB) Low (VX)	Vapor hazard (GB) Both vapor and contact hazard (GA, GD) Contact hazard (VX)
Vesicants	Mustard (H) Lewisite (L) Phosgene oxime (CX)		Causes large blisters to form on victims; may severely damage upper airway if vapors are inhaled; severe intense pain and grayish skin discoloration (L, CX)		Very low (H, L) Moderate (CX)	Primarily contact; with some vapor hazard
Pulmonary agents	Chlorine (CL) Phosgene (CG)		Causes irritation; choking (CL); severe pulmonary edema (CG)		Very high	Vapor hazard
Cyanide agents	Hydrogen cyanide (AC) Cyanogens chloride (CK)		Highly lethal chemical gases; can kill within minutes; effects are reversible with antidotes		Very high	Vapor hazard

CHAPTER

49 Rescue Awareness and Operations

Chapter Review

The following exercises provide an opportunity to test your knowledge of this chapter.

Matching

Match each of the definitions in the left column to the appropriate term in the right column.

_____ **1.** A special litter suited for water rescue

_____ **2.** A pain medication with a contraindication of allergies to aspirin

_____ **3.** The slowing of a person's heart rate caused by drowning in cold water

_____ **4.** A pile of dirt that has been excavated during a trench rescue

_____ **5.** Immersion victims can benefit from this phenomenon

_____ **6.** Pain medication with contraindications for patients who are volume depleted or suffering from severe hypotension

_____ **7.** A climbing technique of controlling the rope as it is fed out to the climbers

_____ **8.** A gas that cannot be detected by your normal senses

_____ **9.** A quick semicontrolled fall with a rope when there is no other means of egress

_____ **10.** A toxic and corrosive chemical with a distinct pungent odor; it is lighter than air

A. Mammalian diving reflex

B. Belay

C. Ammonia

D. Cold protection response

E. Wire Stokes basket

F. Hasty rope slide

G. Carbon monoxide

H. Toradol (ketorolac tromethamine)

I. Morphine

J. Spoil pile

Multiple Choice

Read each item carefully, and then select the best response.

_____ **1.** Which of the following is NOT considered a technical rescue incident?
- **A.** Trench collapse
- **B.** A fender-bender collision
- **C.** Water rescue
- **D.** Wilderness search and rescue

_____ **2.** What is the first priority in a rescue situation?
- **A.** Mobilizing the correct teams
- **B.** Following the golden rule of public service
- **C.** Protecting the patient during the rescue
- **D.** Rescuer safety

_____ **3.** The *A* in the mnemonic FAILURE stands for:
- **A.** additional medical problems not considered.
- **B.** additional patients not accounted for.
- **C.** acclimation to the weather.
- **D.** additional equipment needed.

_____ **4.** You find the entry and rescue teams in the _____ zone(s).

    A. cold   **C.** hot

    B. warm   **D.** warm and hot

_____ **5.** Which of the following is NOT necessary to know when gathering information about a scene BEFORE you arrive?

    A. The road conditions en route to the incident   **C.** Location of the incident

    B. Nature of the incident   **D.** Specific hazard information

_____ **6.** Who is in charge of having all of the utilities shut down at a scene?

    A. Dispatcher   **C.** Police chief

    B. Incident command   **D.** Fire chief

_____ **7.** Which of the following is NOT a technique for calming a patient during a lengthy rescue?

    A. Allowing time for the patient to respond to you

    B. Lying to the patient to keep him or her calm

    C. Being aware of your body language

    D. Making and keeping eye contact with the patient

_____ **8.** On a vehicle, "a post" is:

    A. the post between the front and back seat.   **C.** the post that holds in the windshield.

    B. the post between the middle seat and back seat.   **D.** the post that holds in the back window.

_____ **9.** When you need to stabilize a vehicle, you use a stout piece of lumber that is 4 inches by 4 inches. This is called:

    A. a step block.   **C.** a "C block."

    B. wedging.   **D.** cribbing.

_____ **10.** If you are unable to gain easy access by opening a door to the wrecked vehicle, what is the next best procedure?

    A. Break the windshield   **C.** Peel back the roof

    B. Displace the door   **D.** Break a side window

Labeling

Label the following diagrams with the correct terms.

    1. Label the posts of the vehicle.

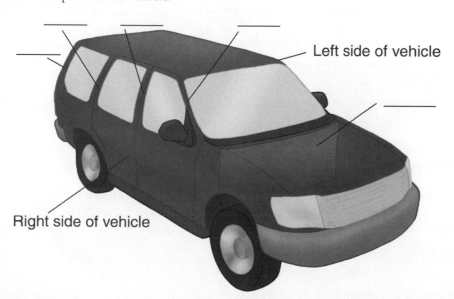

Left side of vehicle

Right side of vehicle

2. Label the following photos with the appropriate type of stabilization technique.
   A. Step blocks
   B. Box crib
   C. Cribbing

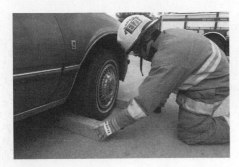   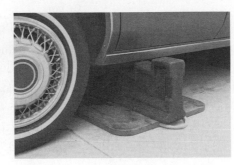   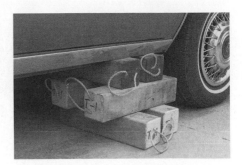

_____   _____   _____

Fill-in-the-Blank

Read each item carefully, and then complete the statement by filling in the missing word(s).

1. Before removing a windshield, you should _____ your patient from flying glass.

2. If the airbag on the driver's side has not deployed during the car crash, it poses a _____ for the driver and the rescuers.

3. When displacing a roof, you should cut the _____ posts and fold back the roof.

4. A/an _____ _____ is a location that is surrounded by a structure that is not designed for continuous occupancy.

5. _____ _____ is a gas that is released when bacteria break down organic material without oxygen. It is flammable, toxic, and colorless.

6. When dealing with an entrapment or trench collapse, the patient is dug out only after _____ has been put in place.

7. If you find yourself being swept away in fast water during a rescue, you should position yourself in the _____-_____ _____.

8. The first thing to do when attempting to help a person during a water rescue is to _____ _____ to the person.

9. When responding to a drowning, you have only a short time before the rescue becomes a/an _____.

10. You respond to a rescue situation where the patient is down a slope that is less than 45°. This is known as a _____-_____ operation.

Chapter 49   Rescue Awareness and Operations

Identify

In the following case study, list the chief complaint, vital signs, and pertinent negatives.

You are called to a vehicle that has rolled down a 75-foot embankment. The special rappelling team responded and has secured your patient on a backboard and placed him in a Stokes basket. They pull the basket up the embankment for you to start working on the patient. He was wearing his seat belt when he lost control of the car and rolled. The patient, Jim, is conscious, but unable to answer any questions except for providing his first name. Your partner applies high-flow supplemental oxygen, and you begin a rapid trauma assessment (RTA) while your partner takes some baseline vitals. Jim has multiple cuts on his face and head, with some blood coming from his left ear. You find instability in the pelvic region and a deformed left arm and collarbone. Jim's blood pressure is 102/68 mm Hg, pulse is thready in the wrist at a rate of 116 beats/min. His oxygen saturation is 96%, and his breathing is shallow at 24 breaths/min. Lungs sounds are slightly diminished on the left side. Jim is cool to the touch and appears very pale. His pupils are equal and round, regular in size, but do not react very quickly to light (PEARRL). You know that Jim needs to be at a regional trauma center, and you call for air medical transport. After hooking up the heart monitor, you find Jim is in sinus tachycardia. Your partner does a halo test on the blood coming from his ear, and it is negative. Jim begins to come around a little more but doesn't remember any of the crash. Your partner starts two large-bore intravenous lines (IVs) with normal saline, while you do a detailed physical exam (DPE). You find some rigidity in the lower abdomen. After you give a quick report to the helicopter personnel, Jim is flown to the closest regional trauma center.

1. Chief Complaint

_____

_____

_____

2. Vital Signs

_____

_____

_____

3. Pertinent Negatives

_____

_____

_____

Ambulance Calls

The following case scenarios provide an opportunity to explore the concerns associated with patient management and paramedic care. Read each scenario, and then answer each question.

1. You and your crew (two other paramedics) are called to the scene of a highway crash just outside of town. Arriving at the scene, you see a late-model sedan "accordioned" against a utility pole. The windshield is shattered. The driver is unconscious, bleeding, and tightly pinned between the steering wheel and the seat. There are no passengers.

    a. List in order the steps you would take. Include details of how you would reach the patient.

    (1) _____

    (2) _____

    (3) _____

    (4) _____

    (5) _____

    (6) _____

    (7) _____

    (8) _____

    b. List the actions you would take after the patient has been transferred to the care of emergency department personnel.

    (1) _____

    (2) _____

True/False

If you believe the statement to be more true than false, write the letter "T" in the space provided. If you believe the statement to be more false than true, write the letter "F."

_____ 1. In an extrication, the primary function of a paramedic is to direct the disentanglement of the patient from the wreckage.

_____ 2. The most efficient access to a patient in a badly damaged vehicle is usually through a window on the passenger side of the vehicle.

_____ 3. Care of the car crash victim should start even before the patient is removed from the vehicle.

_____ 4. The paramedic should use a "hot stick" and wear insulated gloves to remove downed wires that are in contact with a disabled vehicle.

_____ 5. To protect the scene and the rescuers, place a large emergency vehicle at an angle to provide a barrier against oncoming traffic.

_____ 6. A disabled vehicle that is upright on four wheels still needs to be stabilized before anyone enters it to reach the injured inside.

Short Answer

Complete this section with short written answers using the space provided.

1. Discuss the three phases of training that you might receive in technical rescue.

   a. Awareness

_____

_____

   b. Operations

_____

_____

   c. Technician

_____

_____

2. Discuss the five guidelines that are useful when working with a rescue team.

   a. _____

_____

   b. _____

_____

   c. _____

_____

   d. _____

_____

   e. _____

_____

3. What gear is considered minimal for a water rescuer?

_____

_____

_____

4. When breaking glass in an automobile, discuss the differences of the glass in the windows versus the windshield.

_____

_____

_____

Word Find

Hidden in the following grid are 18 words or phrases related to what you have studied in this chapter. Find the hidden words in the grid below. Then use the words from the grid to fill in the table.

```
S P O P E P H R S P R H H E N
S O O P I A L E B E U A A R K
X E O R C N L I V G S N M A X
J R V K T G S I E H I D M L J
N M S O G O R N O R B W E F A
D A H O L D P V I D S I R N U
W G G T W G E O O T K N M Z E
Y Y T E V L B J W D W C Y F T
O A R W R E N C H E H H A V A
L C S K C O H C T S R T T L H
S S R O B O L T C U T T E R D
V N P X S M E G R S L T O M R
R A B W O R C F J H I S C R A
O Z R B K X W D K E K A X E H
O M I B S U G Y C N R E J F I
```

It's been a while since you straightened out the big tin box that houses all your rescue stuff. Eighteen items of rescue gear are jumbled up inside. Locate all your rescue equipment in the box. Make a list of what you've got, and indicate the possible use of each item in a rescue/extrication situation.

Item	Use in a Rescue Situation	Item	Use in a Rescue Situation
1.		10.	
2.		11.	
3.		12.	
4.		13.	
5.		14.	
6.		15.	
7.		16.	
8.		17.	
9.		18.	

Fill-in-the-Table

Fill in the missing parts of the table.

1. Write in the correct statement for the letters for the mnemonic "FAILURE."

F	
A	
I	
L	
U	
R	
E	

Skill Drills

Test your knowledge of skill drills by placing the following photos in the correct order. Number the first step with a "1," the second step with a "2," and so on.

Stabilizing a Suspected Spinal Injury in the Water

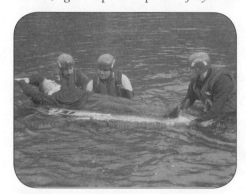

Float a buoyant backboard under the patient.

_____

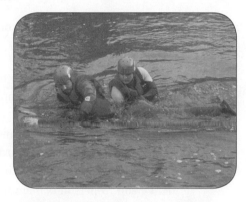

Turn the patient to a supine position in the water by rotating the entire upper half of the body as a single unit.

_____

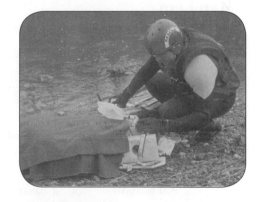

Cover the patient with a blanket and apply oxygen if breathing. Begin cardiopulmonary resuscitation (CPR) if breathing and a pulse are still absent.

_____

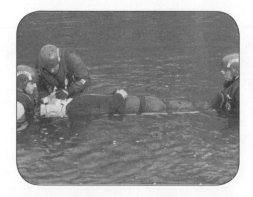

Secure the patient to the backboard.

_____

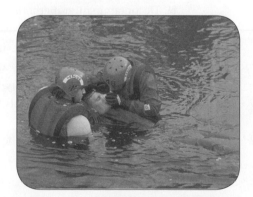

As soon as the patient is turned, begin artificial ventilation using the mouth-to-mouth method or a pocket mask.

_____

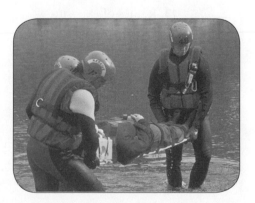

Remove the patient from the water.

_____

CHAPTER

50 Hazardous Materials Incidents

Chapter Review

The following exercises provide an opportunity to test your knowledge of this chapter.

Matching

Match each of the items in the left column to the appropriate definition in the right column.

_____ **1.** Awareness level	**A.** Respirator is mandatory
_____ **2.** OSHA	**B.** Immediately dangerous to life and health
_____ **3.** MSDS	**C.** Dermal, Respiratory, Parenteral, Gastrointestinal
_____ **4.** Rule of thumb	**D.** Air
_____ **5.** Forms of hazardous materials	**E.** Assessment of hazmat team
_____ **6.** NFPA 704	**F.** In-depth information regarding the hazardous material
_____ **7.** Toxicity level	**G.** Depends on the type of hazardous material involved
_____ **8.** Location of greatest hazard	**H.** Person-to-person contamination
_____ **9.** Decontamination	**I.** Most current version should be in every emergency response vehicle
_____ **10.** Dilution, absorption, neutralization, and disposal	**J.** CHEMTREC
	K. Solids, liquids, or gases
_____ **11.** Level D	**L.** Level of hazardous materials protection from turnout gear
_____ **12.** Secondary contamination	**M.** Minimal exposure causes death
_____ **13.** Routes of exposure	**N.** Decontamination methods
_____ **14.** Synergistic effect	**O.** Sets forth training standards
_____ **15.** 800–262–8200	**P.** When two hazardous materials interact
_____ **16.** IDLH	**Q.** Ranks hazardous materials according to health hazard or toxicity levels, fire hazard, reactivity, and special hazards
_____ **17.** Level 4	
_____ **18.** Medical monitoring	**R.** Recognize potential hazards; initiate protective measures
_____ **19.** Vapor density of 1	**S.** Hot zone
_____ **20.** *Emergency Response Guidebook*	**T.** If the entire scene cannot be covered by your thumb, then you are too close

Multiple Choice

Read each item carefully, and then select the best response.

_____ 1. Respiratory exposure to hazardous materials can be all of the following EXCEPT:
  A. efficient.
  C. lethal.
  B. rapid.
  D. parenteral.

_____ 2. As a hazardous liquid is heated or burns it often is converted to a/an:
  A. gas.
  C. diluted nontoxic product.
  B. inert, safe byproduct.
  D. deadly solid.

_____ 3. The threshold limit value (TLV) is the maximum concentration of a toxin to which someone can be exposed in:
  A. 1 hour.
  C. 1 year.
  B. 24 hours.
  D. a 40-hour work week.

_____ 4. Emergency decontamination should be performed:
  A. at each and every hazmat incident.
  B. only if a qualified decontamination team is responding.
  C. only if ordered by the incident commander.
  D. without the need for PPE.

_____ 5. To prepare an ambulance for the transportation of contaminated patients, paramedics should do all of the following, EXCEPT:
  A. remove all necessary equipment, including the cot mattress.
  B. use as much disposable equipment as necessary.
  C. wrap the patient in a plastic barrier.
  D. line the interior of the ambulance with plastic sheets.

_____ 6. A paramedic should have a working knowledge of hazardous materials spills and properly providing care for injured patients. This knowledge should include training to which of the following levels?
  A. Technician
  C. Operations
  B. Awareness
  D. EMS operations

_____ 7. Material Safety Data Sheets (MSDS) provide a considerable amount of useful information to emergency responders. Of the following, which is not provided on the MSDS?
  A. The name of hazardous material
  C. The appropriate mode of transportation
  B. The appropriate first aid measures
  D. The contact information

_____ 8. Hazardous materials teams have many high-tech tools at their disposal. These tools include all of the following, EXCEPT:
  A. CAMEO.
  C. colorimetric devices.
  B. air monitoring equipment
  D. SCBA.

_____ 9. Which of the following steps must be performed by paramedics who discover that a routine-sounding call is a hazardous materials incident?
  A. Isolate the incident as much as possible using the guidelines in the _ERG_.
  B. Remain in the hot zone to evacuate injured patients.
  C. Approach and position your unit downwind from the incident.
  D. Don Level A protection and begin setting up the decontamination corridor.

_____ **10.** Paramedics need to balance the risk/benefit of invasive procedures for hazmat patients because:

    A. IVs may help contamination pass the skin barrier.

    B. PASG/MAST would become contaminated and have to be incinerated.

    C. endotracheal tubes may cause upper airway obstruction as the plastic vaporizes.

    D. there is no known risk; paramedics need to perform patient care as normal.

Fill-in-the-Blank

Read each item carefully, and then complete the statement by filling in the missing word(s).

1. With _____ _____, you may be the first to discover a hazardous materials release.

2. When you first arrive at a call and recognize a hazardous material incident, your most important job will be to identify the _____ _____.

3. "_____ _____ can't save lives."

4. Responding paramedics must gather as much _____ as possible when calling for the hazardous materials team.

5. If you're responding to an incident that involves a _____ vehicle or a/an _____, maintain your high index of suspicion.

6. Other good sources of information for identifying hazardous materials include the _____ _____ _____, which should be carried by the truck driver in the cab, and the _____ or "consist" that is carried by the conductor of a train.

7. There are two basic types of contamination, _____ and _____.

8. _____ _____ is the direct exposure of a patient to a hazardous material.

9. _____ _____ takes place when a hazardous material is transferred to a person from another person or from contaminated objects.

Identify

Respond to the following questions by basing your answers on the Emergency Response Guidebook (ERG) information.

GUIDE 123	**GASES - TOXIC AND/OR CORROSIVE**	**ERG2004**

POTENTIAL HAZARDS

HEALTH
- TOXIC; may be fatal if inhaled or absorbed through skin.
- Vapors may be irritating.
- Contact with gas or liquefied gas may cause burns, severe injury and/or frostbite.
- Fire will produce irritating, corrosive and/or toxic gases.
- Runoff from fire control may cause pollution.

FIRE OR EXPLOSION
- Some may burn, but none ignite readily.
- Vapors from liquefied gas are initially heavier than air and spread along ground.
- Cylinders exposed to fire may vent and release toxic and/or corrosive gas through pressure relief devices.
- Containers may explode when heated.
- Ruptured cylinders may rocket.

PUBLIC SAFETY

- CALL Emergency Response Telephone Number on Shipping Paper first. If Shipping Paper not available or no answer, refer to appropriate telephone number listed on the inside back cover.
- As an immediate precautionary measure, isolate spill or leak area for at least 100 meters (330 feet) in all directions.
- Keep unauthorized personnel away.
- Stay upwind.
- Many gases are heavier than air and will spread along ground and collect in low or confined areas (sewers, basements, tanks).
- Keep out of low areas.
- Ventilate closed spaces before entering.

PROTECTIVE CLOTHING
- Wear positive pressure self-contained breathing apparatus (SCBA).
- Wear chemical protective clothing that is specifically recommended by the manufacturer. It may provide little or no thermal protection.
- Structural firefighters' protective clothing provides limited protection in fire situations ONLY; it is not effective in spill situations where direct contact with the substance is possible.

EVACUATION

Spill
- See the Table of Initial Isolation and Protective Action Distances for highlighted substances. For non-highlighted substances, increase, in the downwind direction, as necessary, the isolation distance shown under "PUBLIC SAFETY".

Fire
- If tank, rail car or tank truck is involved in a fire, ISOLATE for 800 meters (1/2 mile) in all directions; also, consider initial evacuation for 800 meters (1/2 mile) in all directions.

Page 194

1. How dangerous of a substance is this?

_____

_____

_____

2. What type of PPE should you be wearing if you are working in the "inner circle"?

_____

_____

_____

3. Based on the preceding information, what should you do regarding your location and staging area?

_____

_____

_____

4. Identify the four levels of PPE for hazardous materials scenes (A–D) and then indicate their uses.

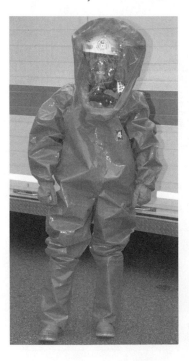
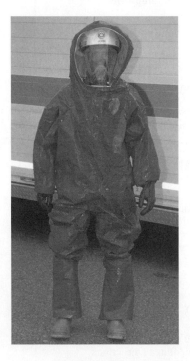
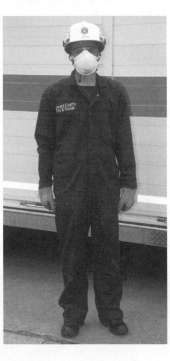
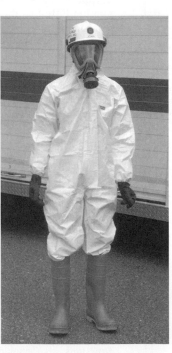

_____   _____   _____   _____

Level A: _____

_____

_____

Level B: _____

_____

_____

_____

Level C: _____

_____

_____

_____

Level D: _____

_____

_____

_____

Ambulance Calls

The following case scenarios provide an opportunity to explore the concerns associated with patient management and paramedic care. Read each scenario, and then answer each question.

1. You are called to the infirmary of a local factory to see an employee who was injured in an unspecified "industrial accident." The plant manager who escorts you in explains, "There was a nasty accident. The valve on the tank of toluene wouldn't close. Jon was splashed in his face. I hope he's OK. He seems to have some trouble breathing. Our hazmat team had to go in and get him, and it took a few minutes for them to suit up and go in."

   Before initiating patient contact, you take out your *Emergency Response Guidebook* and look up the chemical. The *ERG* lists guide number 130. You look up Guide 130. Under Protective Clothing, it lists:

   • Wear positive pressure self-contained breathing apparatus (SCBA).
   • Structural firefighters' protective clothing will only provide limited protection.

   Under Health, it states:

   • May cause toxic effects if inhaled or absorbed through skin.
   • Inhalation or contact with material may irritate or burn skin and eyes.
   • Fire will produce irritating, corrosive, and/or toxic gases.
   • Vapors may cause dizziness or suffocation.
   • Runoff from fire control or dilution water may cause pollution.

   a. Is the scene safe? What immediate precautions should you take to protect yourself and everyone else in the plant? List three considerations for your own immediate safety.

   (1) _____

   (2) _____

   (3) _____

2. You are called to the scene of a railway incident in which the last 5 cars of a 12-car freight train derailed and toppled onto a highway below, crushing motor vehicles beneath them. Before approaching the derailed freight cars and the injured motorists underneath them, you want to make sure those train cars were not carrying a hazardous cargo.

a. List three potential sources of information regarding the nature of the train's cargo.

(1) _____

(2) _____

(3) _____

b. You manage to determine that one of the derailed cars was carrying liquid chlorine, and as a matter of fact, you can already smell chlorine in the air. List the steps you would take at this point (assume that you are in the first public safety vehicle to reach the scene).

(1) _____

(2) _____

(3) _____

(4) _____

True/False

If you believe the statement to be more true than false, write the letter "T" in the space provided. If you believe the statement to be more false than true, write the letter "F."

1. You are called to the scene of a transportation crash in which a truck carrying radioactive waste overturned and caught fire. When you arrive, fire fighters have just extinguished the fire, but there is still a lot of smoke. The driver of the truck is pinned inside the crushed cabin. Indicate which of the following statements about handling this call are true and which are false.

_____ **a.** The ambulance should be parked upwind from the wrecked truck.

_____ **b.** Once the fire is extinguished, the danger of radioactive contamination has passed.

_____ **c.** The ambulance does not need to be decontaminated before the driver transports to the hospital.

_____ **d.** Respiratory exposure can be efficient, rapid, and lethal.

_____ **e.** The Material Safety Data Sheets (MSDS) are helpful in managing hazardous materials.

_____ **f.** The bill of lading describes the contents carried within a vehicle.

2. Indicate which of the following statements regarding hazmat incidents are true and which are false.

_____ **a.** If there are no unusual odors at the scene of a transportation crash, it is safe to assume that hazardous materials are not involved.

_____ **b.** EMS personnel at a hazmat incident may become contaminated with toxic materials by touching a patient who is contaminated.

_____ **c.** In decontaminating a patient exposed to hazmat, one should use a brush to scrub the skin briskly with strong soap and lots of water.

_____ **d.** When decontamination is carried out at the scene, it is unnecessary to notify the receiving hospital that you are bringing in a hazmat case.

_____ **e.** It is preferable that an ambulance team that was not involved in treating and decontaminating the patient be summoned to transport the patient to the hospital.

Short Answer

Complete this section with short written answers using the space provided.

1. The *Emergency Response Guidebook* (ERG) can provide responders with the following information.

   a. _____

   b. _____

   c. _____

2. List other sources of information that may be useful to paramedics responding to a hazardous materials incident.

   a. _____

   b. _____

   c. _____

   d. _____

   e. _____

3. Although it's axiomatic in EMS that you never know what you may find at a call until you reach the scene, nonetheless there are certain types of calls that should start red lights flashing in the back of your brain: ALERT! Possible hazmat call! Listed here are some calls to 9-1-1 during a busy month. Mark an "H" beside those calls that are apt to involve hazardous materials, and indicate what sort of hazardous materials might be involved in each case you marked.

   a. _____ Two-car collision downtown

   _____

   _____

   b. _____ Apartment-house fire

   _____

   _____

   c. _____ Three municipal workers collapsed in a sewer

   _____

   _____

   d. _____ Two police officers injured in a riot

   _____

   _____

   e. _____ Fire in a garden supply store warehouse

   _____

   _____

f. _____ Semitrailer overturned on the interstate

_____

_____

g. _____ Two "men down" on the maintenance staff of the municipal swimming pool

_____

_____

h. _____ Freight train struck car on level crossing

_____

_____

i. _____ Fire in a furniture factory

_____

_____

Crossword Puzzle

Use the clues in the column to complete the puzzle.

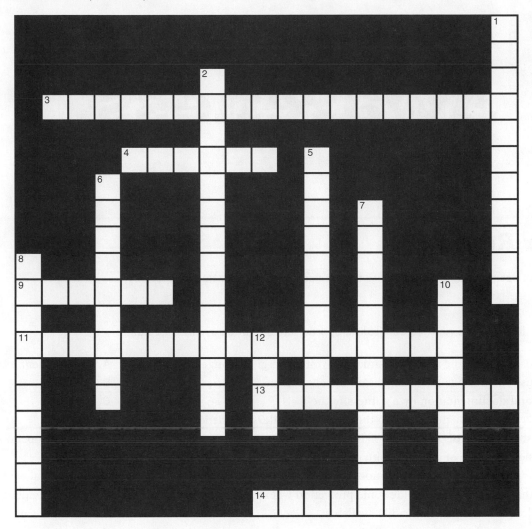

Across

3. Entry of a hazardous material into the bloodstream, either through force of injection or through an open wound
4. Vapor clouds, strange odors, spilled liquids, and multiple victims
9. The highest level of protective suit worn by hazardous materials personnel
11. Two substances interact to produce an overall greater effect than either alone or combined
13. Amount of a hazardous substance sure to cause death
14. Salivation, lacrimation, urination, gastrointestinal activity, and emesis

Down

1. The entire scene should be hidden by a thumb held at arm's length
2. Also known as a topical exposure
5. The longer a hazardous material is in contact with the body or the greater the concentration, the greater the effect will probably be
6. Basic level of hazardous materials training
7. A document carried by drivers of commercial vehicles
8. The temperature at which a vapor can be ignited by a spark
10. Location of the greatest hazard
12. Immediately dangerous to life and health

CHAPTER

51 Crime Scene Awareness

Chapter Review

The following exercises provide an opportunity to test your knowledge of this chapter.

Matching

Match each of the items in the right column to the appropriate definition in the left column.

_____ **1.** At this point during a hostage situation, you are in grave danger because the hostage taker may be extremely nervous

_____ **2.** The oral documentation by a witness of the facts

_____ **3.** The law enforcement should do this before you enter a residence that shows signs of potential violence

_____ **4.** During this stage of a hostage situation, many hostages may begin to develop psychological and emotional problems

_____ **5.** Use this technique to provide some protection when "cover" from a violent situation is not readily available

_____ **6.** Stay 10 to 15 feet away and walk 45° forward of the "A" column when approaching

_____ **7.** This ties a suspect to a crime and includes body materials and objects

_____ **8.** Written measures for dealing with potentially violent incidents

_____ **9.** This is the person riding in the right front seat who makes the approach when two or more paramedics are in a unit that is responding to a motor vehicle crash.

_____ **10.** This is where you stop to look first in the rear and side windows to assess for possible danger when you approach a vehicle (sedan).

A. Concealment technique

B. Capture

C. C column

D. Holding

E. Standard operating procedures (SOP)

F. Testimonial evidence

G. Physical evidence

H. Passenger van

I. Secure the scene

J. Incident commander (IC)

Multiple Choice

Read each item carefully, and then select the best response.

_____ **1.** For maximum safety when arriving at incidents with a single vehicle in which the potential danger is high, your vehicle should be positioned a minimum of how many feet behind the stopped vehicle?

    A. 50   **C.** 25

    B. 15   **D.** 10

_____ **2.** When approaching a passenger vehicle (sedan), you should stop at which column (post) on the vehicle to look in the rear and side windows?

    A. A   **C.** C

    B. B   **D.** D

_____ **3.** When announcing your arrival at the front door of a residence, where should you stand?

    A. To the doorknob side of the door   **C.** In front of the door

    B. To the hinged side of the door   **D.** Ten to 15 feet back from the door

_____ **4.** When you enter a structure, the door you use to enter the building is referred to as the:

    A. tertiary exit.   **C.** primary exit.

    B. secondary exit.   **D.** general exit.

_____ **5.** Which of the following is considered concealment when you are confronted by violence?

    A. Curb   **C.** Utility pole

    B. Depression in the ground   **D.** Shrubbery

_____ **6.** You are dispatched to a residence for a possible sick person. En route to the call, the dispatcher informs you that the caller hung up before all the information could be collected. When you are suspicious that something is not right, prior to announcing your arrival at the door, you should do all the following EXCEPT:

    A. listen for loud noises.   **C.** look through a window for signs of a struggle.

    B. look for neighbors to talk with.   **D.** listen for threatening voices.

_____ **7.** You have entered a residence that you initially thought was safe, but once inside you and your partner are suspicious that there might be trouble. You approach the patient to start the assessment, and your partner starts to look around to see if there is any immediate danger and gather information relevant to providing care. What is this technique called?

    A. Assess and act   **C.** Respond and react

    B. Contact and cover   **D.** Link and look

_____ **8.** In which stage of a hostage situation may hostages begin to develop emotional problems, and the situation calms slightly as police attempt release negotiations?

    A. Surveillance   **C.** Holding

    B. Move   **D.** Resolution

_____ **9.** Which of the following is part of the interview stance and posture that you should use to prepare and control an unexpected attack?

    A. Stand very close to the patient.   **C.** Have your hands clenched.

    B. Stand at a 90° angle to the patient.   **D.** Spread your feet shoulder-width apart.

_____ **10.** You respond to a stabbing. While treating the patient and packaging for transport, you observe some footprints in the patient's blood and you try to work quickly with minimal disruption to the evidence. The footprints are considered:

    A. physical evidence.   **C.** circumstantial evidence.

    B. testimonial evidence.   **D.** substantiated evidence.

Fill-in-the-Blank

Read each item carefully, and then complete the statement by filling in the missing word(s).

1. Becoming completely involved with patient care and failing to see possible physical harm is called _____

   _____.

2. For maximum safety when arriving at an incident with a single vehicle in which the potential for danger is high, position

   your vehicle _____ feet behind the stopped vehicle at a _____ degree angle.

3. When there are two or more paramedics in the unit and you come on the scene of a motor vehicle crash, the person riding

   in the right front seat of the ambulance is the _____ _____.

4. When you approach a van in a situation where safety is a concern, move 10 to 15 feet away from the passenger side,

   and then belly-in and walk parallel until you are approximately 45° forward of the _____ column.

5. When you enter a structure, pick a _____ exit and _____ exit to keep one means of escape accessible

   at all times.

6. To enter a scene where violence is suspected, one technique is for one paramedic to start providing patient care and

   the other to obtain information and warn the partner of the first sign of trouble. This technique is called _____

   and _____.

7. The six stages involved in taking and maintaining hostages are _____ , _____, _____,

   _____, _____ , and _____ .

Identify

In the following case study, list the possible errors in handling scene safety, warning signs of danger, and potential evidence.

You are assigned to respond to a call for an injured person in a residence in a middle-class neighborhood. You are provided no additional information by the dispatcher because the caller hung up before more questions could be asked. You approach the house and hear a loud conversation inside, and without announcing yourself you stand in front of the door and knock. You enter through the front door (primary exit), and without looking around, you ask what is happening. You find a woman on the couch holding her right arm with bruising to the face. She appears to be in considerable pain. Both you and your partner go to the patient and do not pay much attention to the person on the other side of the room who is still arguing with the patient. You see a ceramic object in pieces on the floor and brush it out of the way with your foot as you approach the patient. You start to assess the patient, and your partner cuts and rips through the bloody shirt sleeve to examine the arm. You decide the person standing on the other side of the room is a potential threat and realize that he is between you and the front door. You notice there are a number of tables with drawers and a fire poker in a stand next to the fireplace. Just as you and your partner become anxious about the potential threats, two police officers come through the front door.

1. Errors in Handling Scene Safety

   _____

   _____

   _____

2. Warning Signs of Danger

_____

_____

_____

3. Potential Evidence

_____

_____

_____

_____

Ambulance Calls

The following case scenarios provide an opportunity to explore the concerns associated with patient management and paramedic care. Read each scenario, and then answer each question.

1. You respond to a residence that has previously had calls for domestic violence, but the dispatcher informs you that the information provided was for a medical problem including severe difficulty breathing and no information indicated danger or that responders would be at risk. You are told the police will not arrive for another 5 minutes after you are on the scene. When you arrive at the residence, you are suspicious. What precautions might you take to help ensure that there is no immediate violence that would place you at risk?

_____

_____

_____

2. You and your paramedic partner, who is driving the ambulance, are the first emergency personnel to arrive at the scene where a car ran off the road into a guard rail. When you arrive on the scene, you see no activity around the vehicle, and you see only one person in the driver's seat of the car. You are initially suspicious.

a. How should you park and approach the scene?

_____

b. What precautions should you take to identify the car?

_____

c. Who should be the incident commander?

_____

3. You receive a call for a sick child. You arrive on the scene of the call and someone is outside waiting for you. You are led into the house to find a wheezing pediatric patient who you are told is 7 years old. She is an asthmatic, and her family members report that they can't find her inhaler. You and your partner signal each other to use "contact and cover." You start to treat the patient, and your partner obtains information from the person who met the ambulance. Your partner's observations lead her to believe this residence is a clandestine drug laboratory.

a. What does "contact and cover" mean?

_____

b. What actions should you and your partner take?

_____

c. What are your concerns?

_____

4. Upon arrival at the scene of a shooting, you find a young patient shot in the leg and lying in a pool of blood. You and your partner do a rapid assessment and provide care quickly. The patient is prepared for transport, placed on the stretcher, and loaded into the ambulance. What are your primary concerns when trying to preserve evidence?

_____

_____

_____

_____

_____

_____

True/False

If you believe the statement to be more true than false, write the letter "T" in the space provided. If you believe the statement to be more false than true, write the letter "F."

_____ **1.** Physical evidence is oral documentation by witnesses of facts.

_____ **2.** In a hostage situation, the hostage taker is usually as surprised as the captured person.

_____ **3.** The secondary exit is the door that you use to enter the building.

_____ **4.** When standing at the door to a residence, you should stand on the hinged side of the door.

_____ **5.** When there are two paramedics in an ambulance and you arrive on the scene where a vehicle needs to be checked out, the incident commander (IC) is the driver of the ambulance.

_____ **6.** Some agencies have developed standard operating procedures that guide how to handle potentially violent situations.

_____ **7.** When checking out a vehicle where the back seat is occupied, do not pass the C column until you are sure that it is safe to do so.

_____ **8.** When you arrive at the scene of a single vehicle crash with potential danger, the ambulance should be parked at least 10 feet behind the vehicle.

_____ **9.** To control an unexpected attack, use the interview stance in which you stand at approximately arm's length from the person with your body at a 45° angle.

_____ **10.** Clandestine drug laboratories are not hazardous and present no danger to emergency medical services (EMS) personnel.

Short Answer

Complete this section with short written answers using the space provided.

1. You are on the scene of a call that, because of unsafe circumstances, dictates your retreat to a safe area. After you have backed away from the danger zone and it is safe, what information would you want to provide to the dispatcher?

a. _____

b. _____

c. _____

d. _____

e. _____

2. What three immediate hazards present dangers to emergency responders in regard to a clandestine drug laboratory?

a. _____

b. _____

c. _____

3. When approaching a motor vehicle, a paramedic should always be attentive to impending danger. In which locations in a vehicle could a weapon be concealed?

a. _____

b. _____

c. _____

d. _____

e. _____

f. _____

g. _____

4. When you enter a structure, the primary exit is usually the door you used to enter. What is a secondary exit, and why should it be identified?

_____

_____

_____

_____

5. If paramedics suspect that a situation may become dangerous, a technique of contact and cover can be used. Describe this technique.

_____

_____

_____

_____

6. What is the difference between *cover* and *concealment*?

_____

_____

_____

_____

7. Give three examples each of cover and concealment that you can use when there is danger from a gun.

    a. Cover

        (1) _____

        (2) _____

        (3) _____

    b. Concealment

        (1) _____

        (2) _____

        (3) _____

8. If you are taken hostage by a subject with a gun, what should you assume during the capture stage?

_____

_____

_____

_____

9. You can control an unexpected attack. Always use the interview stance. Describe the specific parts of the stance.

    a. _____

    b. _____

    c. _____

    d. _____

    e. _____

10. There are two general classifications of evidence. Name and provide a brief description of each.

    a. _____

_____

_____

    b. _____

_____

_____

Word Find

Hidden in the following grid are 25 words or phrases related to what you have studied in this chapter. Find the hidden words in the grid below. Then use the words from the grid to answer the following questions (some words may be used to answer more than one question).

```
U E C A P T U R E C L N H E V
K I C R E V O C C L T C A C X
T I R N M S W A T A O Q Z N H
S U R V E I L L A N C E A E O
O R N T U D V M C D G R R L S
H Y O N A B I E K E N E D O T
W O R S E C A V E S I D O I A
E P L A S L T Q E T N N U V G
A M M D M E V I P I R A S B E
P S I E I I R I C N A M C G I
O C N R T N R G S E W M W W O
N T E J C D G P G I L O Q C C
D E F E N S I V E A O C L H L
S E R U D E C O R P I N J A A
Y R A D N O C E S D A N G E R
```

1. A person who is threatening violence or has a weapon that he or she is threatening to use is called a/an _____.

2. When approaching a vehicle after dark, use your vehicle's high _____ and spotlights to light up the exterior and interior of the patient's car.

3. _____ is the stage of a hostage situation when hostages are initially taken, and the perpetrator is trying to gain control.

4. A/an _____ drug lab is one that might be found in a residence and is used to manufacture illegal drugs such as methamphetamine.

5. When two or more paramedics are in a responding unit that approaches from behind a patient's vehicle, the person riding in the right front seat of the ambulance is the incident _____ and makes the approach to the patient's vehicle.

6. When someone hides behind tall grass or shrubbery so that he or she won't be seen in a potentially dangerous situation, this is called _____.

7. A wall or other structure that protects you from a bullet or other projectile is called _____.

8. By assisting the police in maintaining the integrity of a/an _____ scene, you increase the probability that a suspect will be captured and convicted.

9. Your antenna should go up when you encounter a patient whose fists are clenched and who is pacing the room using profane language. You may be in possible _____, and you need to remove yourself and go to a safe place.

10. If violence breaks out while you are on the scene of a call, by knowing some _____ moves you may be able to escape harm and resolve the situation.

11. _____ ties a suspect to a crime and includes objects and impressions.

12. Everything associated with a clandestine lab is _____.

13. The _____ stage of a hostage situation is when those who have been captured start to develop psychological and emotional problems.

14. An individual who is held as a form of human collateral to ensure compliance with demands is called a/an _____.

15. Use a "quick _____" technique to evaluate the advisability of changing locations if you think you are in immediate danger and moving will make it safer.

16. A/an _____ exit is the door used to enter a building.

17. Standard operating _____ are developed by many EMS agencies to guide how to deal with potentially violent situations.

18. A/an _____ exit might be a rear door or an alternate way out, such as a window, in case of an emergency.

19. _____ is the initial stage of a hostage situation where the person who is going to take hostages scopes out the situation.

20. A specially trained unit of the police that handles situations in which there is violence or a potential for violence, such as a hostage situation, is called _____.

21. If you respond to a call, sense danger, and then change to a location that provides better cover, this is considered an evasive _____.

22. Becoming involved in patient care to the point where you are unable to identify possible physical harm is called _____ _____.

23. An event that causes someone to get hurt with a weapon is called _____.

24. _____ signs, such as the sound of people arguing or fighting as you approach a residence, alert you to danger.

25. A/an _____ is an object such as a knife or gun that can be used to harm another individual.

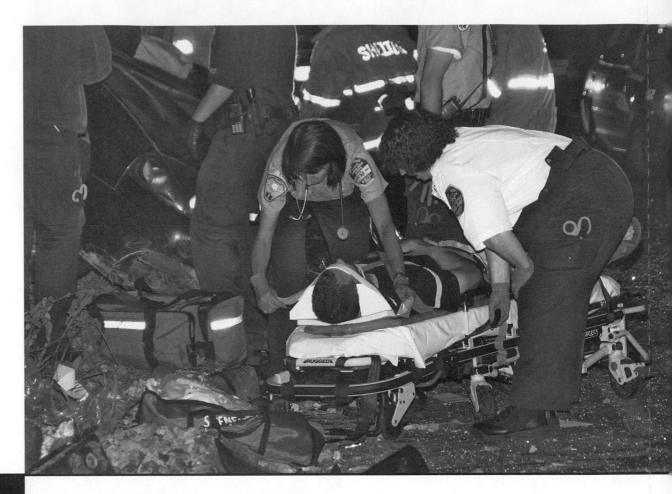

A Mass-Casualty Incident

At 1:30 PM, you are dispatched to 115 Main Street, where a car drove off the road and ran into a building. Dispatch advises you that there are four patients. The police department, fire department, and an additional ambulance are immediately dispatched to the scene. Your response time to the scene is approximately 3 minutes.

Your unit and an engine company arrive at the scene at the same time. Law enforcement is providing traffic control. The second ambulance radios you and advises that their response to the scene will be delayed by 7 minutes. You and your partner triage the four patients. The driver of the car, who refuses EMS care, is being questioned by law enforcement.

Triage Results

Patient 1: 22-year-old conscious, crying female
- Unable to move her legs
- Abrasions to the face and arms
- Respirations, 20 breaths/min and unlabored
- Pulse, 100 beats/min and strong

Patient 2: 60-year-old conscious, restless male
- Abdominal pain
- Wearing a diabetic bracelet
- Respirations, 24 breaths/min and shallow
- Pulse, 110 beats/min weak and irregular

Patient 3: 41-year-old unconscious male
- Large hematoma to the forehead
- Respirations, 8 breaths/min and irregular
- Pulse, 60 beats/min and bounding

Patient 4: 39-year-old conscious and alert female
- Contusion to the forehead
- Pain in left hip
- Respirations, 22 breaths/min and unlabored
- Pulse, 76 beats/min and strong

1. **On the basis of your triage findings, how would you categorize these four patients?**

2. **What are the components of the START triage system?**

You and your partner begin treating the most critically injured patients. You assign fire department personnel, who are certified first responders, to tend to the lesser-injured patients until the second ambulance arrives. You and your partner agree that a third ambulance is needed at the scene.

3. How would you justify the need for a third ambulance?

_____

_____

_____

_____

The second ambulance arrives at the scene, and its crew begins immediate care of the lesser-injured patients. You ask dispatch to notify the local trauma center and advise them of the situation. The dispatcher advises you that the trauma center can accept all four patients.

4. What areas are typically established during a mass-casualty incident?

_____

_____

_____

_____

The third ambulance arrives at the scene as you and your partner depart the scene with patient 3. The second ambulance departs the scene shortly thereafter with patient 2. The two lesser-injured patients are cared for and transported to the trauma center by the third ambulance.

APPENDIX

A Cardiac Life Support Fundamentals

Chapter Review

The following exercises provide an opportunity to test your knowledge of this chapter.

Matching

Match the following phrases to the appropriate age groups as established by the cardiopulmonary resuscitation (CPR) Guidelines 2005:

_____ **1.** Age 1 year to puberty

_____ **2.** Infant at time of birth

_____ **3.** Adolescent and older

_____ **4.** The infant until discharge from initial hospitalization

_____ **5.** Younger than 1 year

A. Newly born

B. Neonates

C. Infant

D. Child

E. Adult

Match the title of the person responsible for assignments of adult resuscitation based on the "model plan" provided in the text:

_____ **6.** Responsible for initial analysis and defibrillation with a signal shock

_____ **7.** Responsible for providing ventilations and ensuring visible chest rise

_____ **8.** Initially responsible for doing high-quality chest compressions

_____ **9.** Brings in the Thumper and works with one of the compressors to transition the patient to mechanical CPR

_____ **10.** Stays in position to relieve the initial compressor

A. Compression 1

B. Compression 2

C. Ventilator

D. Code team leader

E. EMS field supervisor

Multiple Choice

Read each item carefully, and then select the best response.

_____ **1.** Which of the following is at the "base" of the resuscitation pyramid?

    A. Single shock for ventricular fibrillation/ventricular tachycardia

    B. Ventilations

    C. High-quality compressions

    D. Drugs

_____ **2.** With two-rescuer CPR, the health care provider should perform a carotid pulse check for how long?

    A. 5 seconds

    B. 15 seconds

    C. 20 seconds

    D. 30 seconds

_____ **3.** According to *Guidelines 2005*, for the purpose of resuscitation, a neonate is defined as:
      A. the infant at time of birth.
      B. younger than 1 year.
      C. older than 1 year.
      D. the infant until discharge from initial hospitalization.

_____ **4.** When resuscitating a nonbreathing child who has a pulse, the rate for ventilations should be _____ seconds.
      A. 5 to 7
      B. 7 to 8
      C. 3 to 5
      D. 8 to 10

_____ **5.** Where should the pulse check be done for an infant who is suspected of being in cardiac arrest?
      A. Apical   **C.** Radial
      B. Brachial   **D.** Carotid

_____ **6.** Which of the following is *not* one of the indicators of high-quality CPR?
      A. Fast   **C.** Full recoil
      B. Slow   **D.** Hard

_____ **7.** The rate for compressions when doing CPR on an adult is _____ per minute.
      A. 80   **C.** 60
      B. 100   **D.** 120

_____ **8.** Which of the following is a "shockable rhythm" for an adult where defibrillation would be used?
      A. Pulseless electrical activity   **C.** Ventricular tachycardia
      B. Asystole   **D.** Supraventricular tachycardia

_____ **9.** What is the most appropriate way to handle a patient who has an implanted pacemaker and needs to be defibrillated?
      A. Place electrodes over the pacemaker.
      B. Don't defibrillate this patient.
      C. Place electrodes a few inches away from the pacemaker.
      D. Deactivate the pacemaker first before placing electrodes.

_____ **10.** Which one of the following is *not* a role of the code team leader at a resuscitation?
      A. Placing the patient on Thumper   **C.** Talking with Medical Control
      B. Interpreting the electrocardiogram (ECG)   **D.** Keeping track of time

Fill-in-the-Blank

Read each item carefully, and then complete the statement by filling in the missing word(s).

1. Two-rescuer adult CPR provides the cycle of _____ compressions to every _____ breaths, the same as for the single-rescuer technique.

2. Studies of rescuer fatigue show that the person doing the compression tires after about _____ to _____ minutes and the quality of compressions will suffer if the person doing chest compression is not replaced.

3. According to the definitions of age groups in *Guidelines 2005*, in terms of health care, a child is _____ year(s) old to _____.

4. Once an advanced airway has been inserted, the compressions and ventilations are no longer in cycles. Instead, they are _____ with the compressor providing _____ /min and _____ pauses for breaths and the ventilator giving _____ to _____ breaths/min.

5. The two shockable ECG rhythms are _____ _____ and _____ _____ _____.

6. A patient has a transdermal medical patch and needs to be defibrillated. The paramedic should quickly _____ the patch and wipe the chest _____.

7. The vasopressors of choice with initial drug therapy for asystole and pulseless electrical activity (PEA) are either _____ or _____.

8. The _____ _____ _____ is used during CPR and has been shown to enhance the vacuum of the chest during the recoil phase of the compressions.

9. The first and most important way of verifying tube placement with endotracheal intubation is _____ _____ of the tube going through the vocal cords.

10. Many tasks must be performed during resuscitation. This is where _____ and scene choreography help to increase success.

Identify

A successful code relies on high-quality CPR and coordination of interventions. From the following scenario, identify the interventions and insert them (2) as appropriate in the "resuscitation pyramid."

1. You and your paramedic partner are dispatched to a 9-1-1 call for a cardiac arrest. A fire department basic life support (BLS) first response unit is also being sent, and you expect they will be there first because the residence is only a few blocks from their station. You pull up to the house and the fire department personnel are already inside doing CPR. When you walk through the door, you see that the automated external defibrillator (AED) is being attached to the patient. A shock is delivered shortly after you arrive, and CPR is immediately continued. You see that ventilation is being done with a bag-mask device. You verify the rate and see chest rise. Your partner prepares to intubate as you get ready to start an IV. The second defibrillation is delivered and the intubation is now complete and IV initiated. Epinephrine is given and the CPR continues. The next defibrillation returns the patient to a perfusing rhythm. You package and transport. The patient receives bypass surgery and survives to discharge with no neurologic deficit.

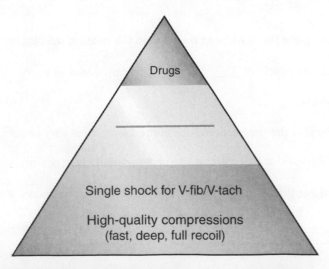

2. When a patient is intubated, it is essential to confirm tube placement. List the techniques used in this case to verify that the endotracheal tube was properly placed according to the American Heart Association (AHA) *Guidelines 2005*.

a. _____

b. _____

c. _____

d. _____

e. _____

f. _____

g. _____

3. When there is a code, members of the team and the code team leader must know their own task as well as the tasks being performed by others. Identify who is performing the following tasks in the preceding scenario:

a. Compressor 1: _____

b. Compressor 2: _____

c. Ventilator: _____

d. Team leader: _____

e. Field supervisor: _____

Ambulance Calls

The following case scenarios provide an opportunity to explore the concerns associated with patient management and paramedic care. Read each scenario, and then answer each question.

1. You are running a code on a patient who has a rhythm on the monitor but no pulse. You determine the patient is in PEA. You think some contributing factors may by causing the patient's problem. You go through the list of *H*s and *T*s. What are you considering to be underlying causes for this cardiac arrest patient? Fill in the following grid.

H		T	
H		T	Tamponade, cardiac
H	Hydrogen ion (acidosis)	T	
H		T	Thrombosis (coronary or pulmonary)
H		T	
H	Hypothermia		

2. All BLS interventions are being delivered appropriately when you and your partner arrive at the scene of a cardiac arrest. You try to intubate the patient, but the patient's anatomy makes it difficult to visualize the cords, and numerous IV attempts fail. While BLS interventions continue, you and your partner decide on alternative ways to better protect the airway using an advanced technique. What alternative method should be used to provide access for drug administration? What are some of the possible alternatives to consider?

_____

_____

---

3. You have been doing cardiac compressions for more than 5 minutes and you're getting tired. You need some relief and all the other units that you would call for backup are committed to other calls.

    a. What alternatives could be used to perform the cardiac compressions?

---

    b. Of the mechanical devices available, does one have an advantage over another?

True/False

If you believe the statement to be more true than false, write the letter "T" in the space provided. If you believe the statement to be more false than true, write the letter "F."

_____ **1.** For high-quality CPR, the compressions should be fast, deep, and allow for partial recoil of the chest.

_____ **2.** If it is a shockable rhythm, administer a single shock, and then CPR should be performed for three (3) cycles before reanalysis of the rhythm.

_____ **3.** Health care providers should perform a carotid pulse check for 5 seconds.

_____ **4.** To make a good mask seal when using a bag-mask device, the "E-C" or "OK" hand position should be used.

_____ **5.** In *Guidelines 2005*, a neonate is defined as an infant from initial hospitalization until discharge.

_____ **6.** With infant CPR, if there is no trauma, you should hyperextend the neck to open the airway using the head tilt-chin lift method.

_____ **7.** After an advanced airway has been inserted during CPR, ventilations should be done at the rate of 8 to 10 breaths/min.

_____ **8.** The two shockable rhythms for defibrillation are ventricular fibrillation and supraventricular tachycardia.

_____ **9.** A patient who has been submerged in water or is soaking wet does not need to be dried off before shocking.

_____ **10.** End-tidal CO_2 should be used as a way to confirm and monitor endotracheal tube placement.

Short Answer

Complete this section with short written answers using the space provided.

1. List the three factors necessary for high-quality compressions with CPR.

    a _____

    b. _____

    c. _____

2. Name the two shockable rhythms for defibrillation.

a. _____

b. _____

3. List three special circumstances that might require special considerations when defibrillating an adult.

a. _____

b. _____

c. _____

4. List five *initial* techniques for verifying successful endotracheal intubation.

a. _____

b. _____

c. _____

d. _____

e. _____

5. List the roles of the code team leader.

a. _____

b. _____

c. _____

d. _____

e. _____

f. _____

g. _____

h. _____

6. List three ways in which the laryngeal mask airway (LMA) and Combitube are similar.

a. _____

b. _____

c. _____

7. What are two devices that can deliver mechanical compressions during CPR?

a. _____

b. _____

Crossword Puzzle

Use the clues in the column to complete the puzzle.

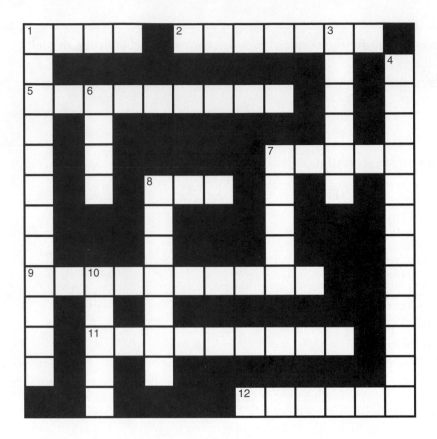

Across

1. High-quality compressions require that they be
   _____ and fast, and allow full chest recoil.

2. Flatline and a nonshockable rhythm is called
   _____.

5. Place electrodes or paddles a few inches from a
   _____ or AICD when defibrillating.

7. The code team member who delivers the shock must always
   first _____ the patient!

8. When assessing the pulse for a patient suspected to be in
   arrest, the carotid artery should be checked for a maximum
   of _____ seconds.

9. The primary method for providing chest compressions
   to an infant with 2 rescuers is to use the two-hands chest
   _____ method.

11. The _____ threshold device will enhance the
    vacuum in the chest, which forms during the chest recoil
    phase of CPR.

12. The initial assessment to determine breathing is to look,
    _____, and feel.

Down

1. One of the "Hs" and "Ts" that contribute to cardiac arrest
   that deals with low blood sugar is _____.

3. The code team _____ is responsible for overall
   timing of the code and reassessment after 2-minute cycles
   of CPR.

4. Ventricular _____ is a shockable rhythm.

6. Another term for a resuscitation is _____.

7. The "_____ of Survival" includes 4 essential
   links: early access, early CPR, early defibrillation, and early
   definitive care.

8. Drug _____ for asystole and PEA includes a
   vasopressor every 3 to 5 minutes.

10. Health care providers define a _____ as 1 year of
    age until signs of puberty.

Rhythm Strips

Practice your rhythm strip analysis skills on the following strips. Identify the following:

A. Asytole   **D.** Normal sinus rhythm

B. Ventricular fibrillation   **E.** Sinus bradycardia

C. Sinus tachycardia

1. _____

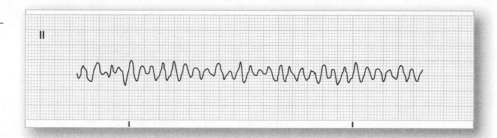

2. _____

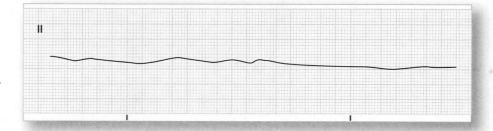

3. _____

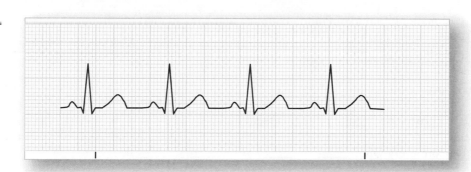

4. _____

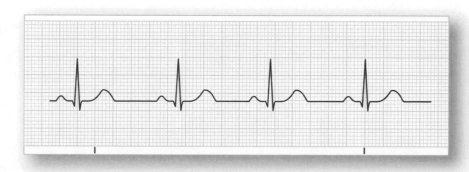

5. _____

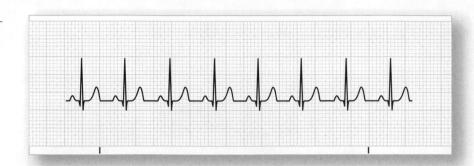

6. You are on standby at a football game when you are called to the bleachers where a man about 60 years old is on the ground and two security officers are performing CPR on him. You observe they are getting chest rise with ventilations and performing quality compressions. You hook up the monitor and apply the defibrillator pads. You have CPR stopped briefly and observe the following rhythm:

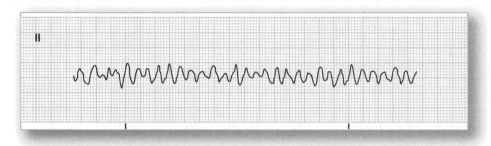

Answer the questions that follow about this ECG strip.

a. RHYTHM: _____ regular _____ irregular

b. RATE: _____ per minute

c. P WAVES: _____ present _____ absent

d. If present, is there a P before every QRS? _____ yes _____ no

e. Is there a QRS after every P? _____ yes _____ no

f. P–R INTERVAL: _____ seconds

g. QRS complexes: _____ normal _____ abnormal

h. Name of rhythm: _____

i. Treatment: _____

Skill Drills

Test your knowledge of skill drills by placing the following photos in the correct order. Number the first step with a "1," the second step with a "2," and so forth.

Single-Rescuer Adult CPR

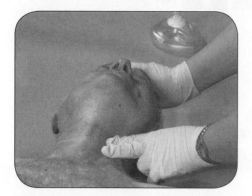

Perform a carotid pulse check (maximum of 10 seconds).

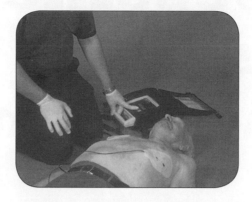

Check the patient's rhythm. If it is shockable, administer a single shock, and then resume CPR immediately for five cycles. Reanalyze the rhythm. If it is not shockable, resume CPR immediately for five cycles.

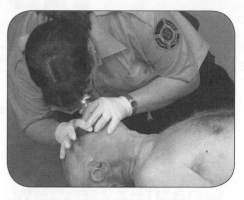

Ventilate two times for 1 second each to achieve visible chest rise. Complete five cycles (approximately 2 minutes) and reassess the patient for a maximum of 10 seconds. If AED has arrived, attach it without interrupting compressions.

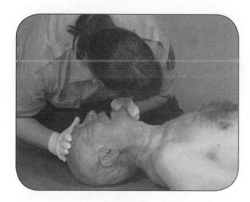

Check for breathing (look, listen, and feel). If no breaths, administer two breaths, each 1 second, achieving visible chest rise.

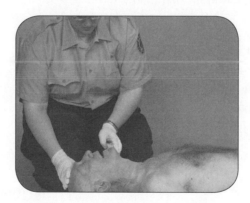

Establish unresponsiveness. Open the airway.

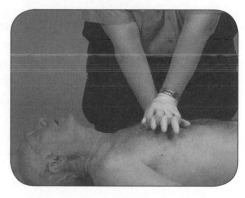

Begin 30 compressions—center of the chest, push hard and fast (rate of 100/min), and allow full chest recoil.

B Assessment-Based Management

Chapter Review

The following exercises provide an opportunity to test your knowledge of this chapter.

Matching

Match each of the items in the right column to the appropriate definition in the left column.

a. Match the type of exams with the descriptions that follow.

_____ **1.** Assesses the Cincinnati Stroke Scale, cranial nerves, and motor function

_____ **2.** Provided for a medical patient that is not responsive

_____ **3.** Includes checking for crowning

_____ **4.** Includes an assessment of lung sounds, pedal edema, and heart sounds

_____ **5.** Provided en route to the emergency department for a trauma patient with specific mechanism of injury (MOI)

A. Rapid physical exam/ assessment

B. Detailed physical exam

C. Neurologic exam

D. Cardiopulmonary (heart/ lungs) exam

E. Obstetric exam

b. Read each item carefully, and then select the best response.

_____ **1.** Classified into two groups: those who are responsive and those who are not

_____ **2.** Physical exam should be this; that is, focused on the body system that the chief complaint and history suggest is the source of problem

_____ **3.** Is crucial to decision making

_____ **4.** The trauma patient without a significant MOI and medical patients who are responsive

_____ **5.** In patient assessment, this is critically important; some experts believe that 80% of medical diagnosis is based solely on this

A. Accurate information

B. Vectored

C. Patient history

D. Medical patients

E. Less rushed approach

Multiple Choice

Read each item carefully, and then select the best response.

_____ **1.** The physical exam "vectors" a focus on the chief complaint and what other criterion to help identify the source of a problem?

    A. Detailed assessment

    B. History

    C. Initial assessment

    D. Physical exam

_____ **2.** Which of the following is NOT part of the objective findings?

    A. ECG
                         C. Blood glucose

    B. SpO_2
                         D. SAMPLE history

_____ **3.** When thinking "scene choreography," the importance of what position cannot be overemphasized?

    A. First responder support
            C. Team leader

    B. Police presence
                  D. Medical Control

_____ **4.** What is the "right stuff" that a paramedic responding to a call must carry?

    A. Packaged equipment being at the patient's side when needed

    B. Only equipment that is the most sophisticated technology

    C. Only advanced life support (ALS) equipment

    D. A radio so needed equipment can be brought to the patient

_____ **5.** Most patients rate a paramedic's quality of care by which of the following?

    A. Assessment skills
                 C. Type of equipment used

    B. Ability to start an IV
               D. People skills

_____ **6.** Which of the following is one of the subclassifications into which a paramedic might group a medical patient?

    A. Significant mechanism of injury (MOI)
      C. Without significant mechanism of injury (MOI)

    B. Not responsive
                    D. Significant chief complaint

_____ **7.** Which of the following is NOT a correct representation for one of the letters in the mnemonic SOAP?

    A. Significant findings
                C. Assessment

    B. Objective information
              D. Plan for treatment

_____ **8.** From which of the following should you NOT allow a distracting injury to divert your attention?

    A. Contacting Medical Control
         C. Determining the mechanism of injury (MOI)

    B. Obtaining a SAMPLE history
        D. Creating an assessment plan

_____ **9.** Which of the following is NOT considered an environmental distracter?

    A. Unruly bystander
                  C. Crowds

    B. High noise level
                 D. Police on the scene

_____ **10.** Pattern recognition and what other factor, based on a lot of field experience, play key roles in the decision-making process of making an accurate assessment?

    A. "Street smarts"
                   C. "Gut instinct"

    B. "People skills"
                  D. "Medical insight"

Fill-in-the-Blank

Read each item carefully, and then complete the statement by filling in the missing word(s).

1. In patient assessment, the _____ is critically important.

2. The physical exam should be "_____"—that is, focused on the body system that the chief complaint and history suggest is the source of the problem.

3. After obtaining _____ information from the patient through interviewing skills (such as SAMPLE), then obtain _____ findings by obtaining vital signs and other parameters.

4. A paramedic's _____ can significantly influence a patient assessment and decision-making abilities.

5. Attempting to prejudge a situation or the patient can lead to _____ _____.

6. _____ _____ include crowds, unruly bystanders, and dangerous situations.

7. The importance of a _____ _____ choreographing the activities of the team at the scene of an emergency cannot be overstated.

8. Medical patients are subclassified into two groups: _____ and _____ _____.

9. Good _____ and excellent _____ _____ go hand in hand.

10. A paramedic responding to emergency calls must carry the "_____ _____"—that is, equipment that is packaged and at the patient's side when the paramedic needs it.

Identify

In the following case study, list the chief complaint, vital signs, and pertinent negatives.

On a call to a motor vehicle crash, you find a 35-year-old man who is unconscious behind the wheel. The scene has been secured by the police, and when you and your partner approach the scene you are told there is only one patient, who is unconscious and appears to be breathing. You notice that the damage to the vehicle seems slight with significant impingement to the passenger's side door where the car hit a guard rail and bounced off. You and your partner start to assess the patient. You check the airway and breathing, and you look for external bleeding while your partner maintains cervical stabilization. There is a smell of alcohol. The airway is open and auscultation identifies air moving in all fields. There is no external bleeding. The patient is responsive to painful stimuli. A check for pulse and sensation identifies a response to both in all extremities. You place the patient on supplemental oxygen and extricate. A set of vital signs is taken: the patient has a pulse of 90 beats/min and regular, respirations are 20 breaths/min and are not labored, blood pressure is 130/90 mm Hg, and oxygen saturation is 98%. Pupils are equal and slightly sluggish, and the abdomen is soft in all four quadrants. The ECG shows normal sinus rhythm, and you start an IV. At the hospital, it is determined that the patient is highly intoxicated and has sustained no significant trauma.

1. Chief Complaint

_____

_____

_____

2. Vital Signs

_____

_____

_____

3. Pertinent Negatives

_____

_____

_____

Ambulance Calls

The following case scenarios provide an opportunity to explore the concerns associated with patient management and paramedic care. Read each scenario, then answer each question.

1. It is 2 AM and you are hoping to lie down for a short nap before the next call. The phone suddenly rings in the on-call room. It is the dispatcher telling you that there is a call at the assisted living center a few blocks away for an 82-year-old woman with difficulty breathing. As you and your partner enter the patient's living room, you find her sitting upright in a chair and you can see she is in respiratory distress. When you ask her questions, she can provide responses with only a few words at a time. You start a rapid physical assessment that includes a cardiopulmonary exam. While you initiate emergency care, such as administering supplemental oxygen, IV, and medications, your partner also tries to get additional subjective information from the patient with assistance from the patient's husband.

   a. What are the components of a cardiopulmonary exam?

      (1) _____

      (2) _____

      (3) _____

   b. What are the two major components of the subjective interview?

      (1) _____

      (2) _____

2. You arrive on the scene of a patient whom you observe from the door to be pale, diaphoretic, and having difficulty breathing. You ask the patient if he has any pain and he responds, "This is the worst chest pain I have ever had. I think I am going to die." You are joined by two first responders and a police officer. As you and your partner start to provide care, the patient goes into cardiac arrest. Immediately, everyone starts to do something, but chaos ensues. This lasts for about 10 seconds until you realize that no good can come from this disorganization and confusion. You stop and tell everyone to freeze. You immediately delegate assignments and monitor the situation to ensure they are done immediately. It works. The patient is quickly defibrillated, oxygenated, and your partner has an IV established rapidly. When you prepare for transport, the patient has a heart rhythm and is responding. What was the critical factor that seems to have made the crucial difference in making this a good outcome? Explain your answer.

   _____

   _____

   _____

   _____

   _____

   _____

3. You and your partner have just finished doing a superb job of assessing and treating a patient with pulmonary edema, and you have packed the patient and are now en route to the hospital. The trip will take approximately 12 minutes. After obtaining another set of vitals, checking the monitor, and asking the patient about changes in breathing effort and pain, you prepare to make a radio report to the receiving hospital, which is also your Medical Control facility. What are the key components of the report and in what format should the report be delivered?

   a. _____

   b. _____

c. _____

d. _____

e. _____

f. _____

g. _____

h. _____

i. _____

True/False

If you believe the statement to be more true than false, write the letter "T" in the space provided. If you believe the statement to be more false than true, write the letter "F."

_____ **1.** In patient assessment, the patient history is of little importance.

_____ **2.** Subjective information includes vital signs and ECG.

_____ **3.** A rapid physical exam and assessment is provided for a medical patient who is not responsive.

_____ **4.** Environmental distracters include unruly bystanders and high noise levels.

_____ **5.** The approach to the patient should not be planned in advance to determine who interviews the patient and who will focus on skills.

_____ **6.** Trauma patients are classified into three groups: conscious, semiconscious, and unconscious.

_____ **7.** For trauma patients without significant MOI, you can take a slightly more comprehensive and less rushed approach.

_____ **8.** A paramedic must have a calm demeanor, look the part, act the part, and have a kind manner.

_____ **9.** Generally, the approach to patient assessment is different for the emergency medical technician—Basic (EMT-B) than for the paramedic.

_____ **10.** The importance of a team leader choreographing the activities of the team at the scene of an emergency cannot be overstated.

Short Answer

Complete this section with short written answers using the space provided.

1. Within the prehospital setting there may be environmental distracters when you are doing an assessment. Give five examples.

a. _____

b. _____

c. _____

d. _____

e. _____

2. Provide a list of essential equipment that a paramedic should bring to the scene for handling circulation assessment and treatment.

a. _____

b. _____

c. _____

d. _____

e. _____

3. What is done during a neurologic exam?

a. _____

b. _____

c. _____

4. What are the two groups into which trauma patients can be subclassified?

a. _____

b. _____

5. A patient who is thought to be "under the influence" and who is acting out, being belligerent, or acting restless may actually have an underlying medical problem or trauma. Give five examples of medical or trauma conditions that could be the underlying cause.

a. _____

b. _____

c. _____

d. _____

e. _____

Word Find

Hidden in the following grid are 25 words or phrases related to what you have studied in this chapter. Find the hidden words in the grid below. Then use the words from the grid to answer the following questions (some words may be used to answer more than one question).

```
U S H M V A M H P C P P X E V
V N Z U M E I Y I L R I D N B
E G C U T S C D O E A E E V H
V S A O T N E T S P C N C I K
I R I O O M E E O I I M I R K
T T R C A P N M S R G A T O D
C Y L R N T E I S D E Y C N E
E W A D A O O R T S H D A M T
J P J T F N C Z A H E Q R E A
B C I E D U T I T T A S P N I
O O P H Y S I C A L I Q S T L
N E V I T C E J B U S V T A E
A C C U R A T E R E D A E L D
L A C I D E M I N I T I A L C
R I G H T A I R W A Y H M A M
```

1. _____ information is critical to your decision making.

2. The physical exam should be _____, that is, focused on the body system that the chief complaint and history suggest is the source of the problem.

3. In the patient assessment, the _____ is critically important.

4. A/an _____ physical exam is provided en route to the ED for a trauma patient with a significant MOI (mechanism of injury).

5. _____ information is obtained from the patient by using your interviewing skills.

6. Pattern recognition and "gut instinct" based on lots of field experience have key roles in the _____ process.

7. _____ findings are obtained from vitals signs, ECG, blood glucose, and so forth.

8. An action _____ for treatment of the patient must consider priority and severity of the patient's condition.

9. Your _____ can significantly influence your assessment and decision-making ability.

10. Attempting to prejudge a situation or patient may lead to _____, also called tunnel vision.

11. Quality management of a patient depends on an accurate medical _____.

12. _____ patients can be difficult to assess.

13. _____ distracters include crowds, unruly bystanders, and violent situations.

14. The importance of a team _____ choreographing the activities of the team at the scene of an emergency cannot be overstated.

15. The _____ concept needs to be reinforced in the classroom with numerous lab scenarios so that members and leaders will be better prepared to respond effectively to emergencies.

16. Carry the "_____ stuff," that is, equipment that is packaged and at the patient's side when you need it.

17. Some of the essential _____ control equipment that should be carried by paramedics includes suction units, laryngoscope blades, and endotracheal tubes.

18. _____ patients can be subclassified into two groups: responsive and not responsive.

19. _____ patients can be subclassified into two groups: significant MOI and those without significant MOI.

20. An effective patient presentation is _____.

21. Good assessment and excellent _____ skills go hand in hand.

22. The first assessment for every patient is the _____ assessment.

23. _____ is critically important, including rotating roles in the classroom and cross-training to assume various assignments that might be performed on the patient care team.

24. When you become a _____, you must leave your attitude and ego at the door!

25. As part of training, a paramedic student practices _____ exams numerous times until the skill is mastered.

Fill-in-the-Table

Fill in the missing parts of the table.

Essential Equipment

Essential Equipment	
Function	**Essential Items**
Airway control	■ PPE (gloves, face shield, and HEPA or N-95 mask) ■ Oral airways, nasal airways ■ Suction unit (electric or manual) ■ ■ LMA, Combitube, ET tubes ■ ■ ■ End-tidal carbon dioxide device
Breathing	■ Pocket mask and one-way valve ■ ■ Oxygen-delivery devices (nonrebreathing mask, cannula, extension tubing) ■ ■ Occlusive dressings ■ ■ Pulse oximeter
Circulation	■ Dressings, bandages, and tape ■ ■ Assessment card and pen ■ ■ AED or manual defibrillator ■ ■ Glucometer ■
Disability and dysrhythmia	■ Rigid collars ■ ■
Exposure	■ ■ Scissors

Section 1: Preparatory

Chapter 1: EMS Systems, Roles, and Responsibilities

Matching

1. C (page 1.17)	**6.** B (page 1.18)
2. D (page 1.17)	**7.** I (page 1.18)
3. A (page 1.17)	**8.** H (page 1.16)
4. F (page 1.17)	**9.** E (page 1.8)
5. G (page 1.18)	**10.** J (page 1.11)

Multiple Choice

1. A (page 1.6)	**6.** D (page 1.12)
2. C (page 1.7)	**7.** C (page 1.9)
3. D (page 1.9)	**8.** B (page 1.6)
4. B (page 1.15)	**9.** C (page 1.8)
5. B (page 1.17)	**10.** C (page 1.9)

Fill-in-the-Blank

1. Mobile Intensive Care Units (pages 1.5, 1.6)

2. Dispatcher (page. 1.8)

3. Reciprocity (page 1.11)

4. Empathy (page 1.12)

5. First priority (page 1.13)

6. Continuous quality improvement (page 1.16)

7. Prospective (page 1.17)

Ambulance Calls

1. a. When you are calling in for an ambulance, you should of course give the name and location of the theater, and possibly the theater number if it is a large multiplex. Always give the patient's chief complaint and current status of the patient, such as if the patient is alert and orientated, and if the person is breathing. Your spouse should also tell the dispatcher that there is a paramedic on scene with the patient, and in some cities the dispatcher might need the paramedic's name.

    b. Any patient that experiences syncope should be seen immediately by a physician. Syncopal episodes can be caused by problems in the heart, neurologic problems, orthostatic hypotension, dehydration, blood loss, medications, and possibly psychiatric problems. It is almost impossible on scene to determine the cause. In this scenario, the patient could have also hurt herself when she fell.

2. a. You should always ensure scene safety for yourself, your patient, and the bystanders involved. This is your number one priority. Make sure the driver has moved the vehicle far enough away from the patient so care can be given. You should also make sure the vehicle is in park and the engine is turned off, with the parking brake set. You can also control the scene by having bystanders block traffic off to the area until law enforcement arrives. (page 1.13)

    b. You should begin treatment by having the EMT-Basic hold C-spine on this trauma patient. You should start with your initial assessment by starting with the ABCs, and then move on to a rapid trauma assessment. After completing the trauma assessment, you determine that the patient has a broken femur and you should apply manual traction on the leg to help stabilize it and control the pain and bleeding until the ambulance arrives.

True/False

1. T (page 1.5)	**6.** F (page 1.13)
2. F (page 1.6)	**7.** T (page 1.16)
3. T (page 1.9)	**8.** F (page 1.17)
4. F (page 1.9)	**9.** F (page 1.14)
5. F (page 1.9)	**10.** T (page 1.13)

Short Answer

1. **a.** Integrity, be open, honest, and truthful with the patients. (page 1.12)
   b. Empathy, understand and identify the feelings of the patients and their families. (page 1.12)
   c. Self-motivation, the internal drive that keeps you compentent in your skills and your professional manners. (page 1.12)
   d. Communication, the ability to express and exchange your ideas, thoughts, and findings on a scene. (page 1.12)
   e. Teamwork and respect, all involved must work together to achieve a common goal—to provide the best possible prehospital care to ensure the overall well-being of the patient. (page 1.12)
   f. Patient advocate, always act in the best interest of your patient. (page 1.12)
   g. Injury prevention, help on the scene by pointing out dangerous situations for the patient in his or her home or surroundings. (page 1.13)
   h. Careful delivery of service, follow protocols and procedures and continuously evaluate your performance. (page 1.13)

2. **a.** Preparation, mentally, physically, and emotionally. (page 1.13)
   b. Response, responding in a safe manner. (page 1.13)
   c. Scene management, safety for yourself, your team, the patient, and bystanders. (page 1.13)
   d. Patient assessment and care, the right assessment and care for all patients. (page 1.13)
   e. Management and disposition, following the protocols, or receiving online medical direction, staying within the scope of your practice. (pages 1.13, 1.14)
   f. Patient transfer, acting as a patient advocate, handing the patient off to the correct person, and providing a report on the patient. (page 1.14)
   g. Documentation, patient care report must always be filled out immediately. (page 1.14)
   h. Return to service, restocking and preparing the unit as quickly as possible for the next call. (page 1.14)

3. Medical control is set up by law as a supervisor for the paramedic. The roles of the medical director are as follows: educating and training personnel (ensuring their competency in the field), participating in selection of new personnel, helping with equipment selection for the field, developing clinical protocols, ensuring a quality improvement program is in place, providing input on patient care, interfacing with the EMS service and other health care agencies, acting as an EMS advocate in the community, and serving as the "medical conscience" of the EMS system. (page 1.15)

4. **a.** Online medical control: allows the paramedic immediate patient care resources. It allows the paramedic to transfer data immediately to the receiving facility for better patient care. (page 1.15)
   b. Protocols: They are a treatment plan for a specific illness or injury. (page 1.15)
   c. Standing orders: A type of protocol that is a written and signed by the medical director that outlines specific directions, permissions, and sometimes prohibitions. (page 1.15)

Crossword Puzzle

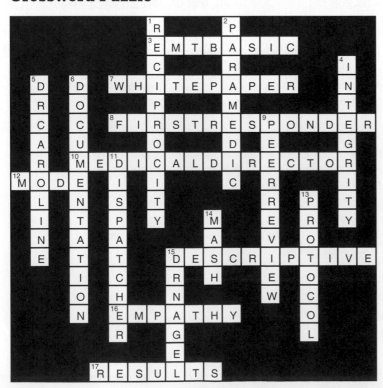

Chapter 2: The Well-Being of the Paramedic

Matching

1. A (page 2.9)   **5.** B (page 2.9)
2. B (page 2.9)   **6.** A (page 2.9)
3. B (page 2.9)   **7.** B (page 2.9)
4. A (page 2.9)

1. A (page 2.10)
2. B (page 2.10)
3. B (page 2.10)

Multiple Choice

1. C (page 2.12)   **6.** D (page 2.12)
2. D (page 2.13)   **7.** D (page 2.11)
3. A (page 2.18)   **8.** C (page 2.10)
4. C (page 2.22)   **9.** A (page 2.12)
5. B (page 2.6)   **10.** B (page 2.14)

Fill-in-the-Blank

1. a. Projection (page 2.12)
   b. Denial (page 2.12)
   c. Conversion hysteria (page 2.13)
   d. Displacement (page 2.12)
2. a. Take care of your own health: (page 2.15)
       Get enough REST.
       Eat a balanced DIET.
       Get regular EXERCISE.
       Treat your body with respect (avoid cigarettes, drugs).
   b. Give yourself some "me" time every day. (page 2.15)
   c. Learn how to relax. (page 2.15)
   d. Do not make unreasonable demands on yourself. (page 2.15)
   e. Do not make unreasonable demands on others. (page 2.15)
   f. Stay in touch with your feelings. (page 2.15)
   g. Learn techniques for shedding stress while on duty. (page 2.15)
   h. Debrief after tough calls. (page 2.15)

Identify

1. Pertinent Negatives (pages 2.4–2.12)
   a. Not sleeping
   b. Too much caffeine
   c. Not exercising
   d. Smoking
   e. Eating too much of the wrong foods
   f. Projecting his negative attitude
2. Stress Reactions (pages 2.11, 2.12)
   a. Projection
   b. Anger

Ambulance Calls

1. a. This is a critical incident for all members of the team. This death of a child is particularly hard on John because of the fact that he also has an infant boy about the same age. He is probably feeling that he is a bad paramedic because the child died, even though every effort was made during the resuscitation. This also might affect his feelings about being a father. (page 2.8)

  b. Paramedics are often under a lot of stress at their job. They can do several things to reduce stress and avoid burnout, such as get enough sleep, eat a balanced diet, and do 30 minutes of aerobic activity three to four times a week. Avoid caffeine, smoking, and recreational drugs. Limit alcohol intake. Make sure that you can devote some time during each day to yourself, and learn to relax with hobbies and social activities. Don't make unreasonable demands on yourself or others. Share your stress by talking or crying. Always debrief after a rough call. (page 2.15, table 2-1)

2. a. You never want to just blurt out that you think that the patient isn't going to make it. Tell the patient that his condition is serious, but you and the hospital team are going to do everything you can for him. Let him talk, and be sympathetic to anything he says. Remember, you might be the last to speak to him, so if he has dying words for his family, make sure to write them down. Make sure that the doctor at the hospital has these words to give to the family when he breaks the news that their loved one has died. (page 2.16)

  b. First, remember that not all dying people will experience all five stages. They may not experience them in "order" either. Encourage the patient to talk about these feelings if possible. (page 2.16)

   (1) Denial. The patient might say things like, "This can't happen to me."

   (2) Anger. Anger might appear as blaming the paramedic, family, or even God. Anger can come in the form of yelling or physical outbursts.

   (3) Bargaining. This can be a patient's way of praying: "Please just let me live long enough to see my family again." They may bargain with you, the doctor, and God.

   (4) Depression. This is characterized by quiet time by the patient, crying, or may be physical contact with anyone close to them, including you.

   (5) Acceptance. The patient may leave the sorrow behind and reflect on his or her life. The patient might want to leave words for the family and to let the family know that it will be okay. Usually, this is the hardest time for the family. The patient doesn't appear to be fighting for life and that sometimes angers family members. Once again, anger is a stage of grief, and the family members will exhibit these feelings also.

True/False

1. F (page 2.4)	**8.** T (page 2.15)
2. T (page 2.6)	**9.** F (page 2.16)
3. F (page 2.7)	**10.** T (page 2.20)
4. F (page 2.9)	**11.** F (page 2.21)
5. T (page 2.10)	**12.** T (page 2.21)
6. F (page 2.12)	**13.** T (page 2.24)
7. F (page 2.13)	**14.** F (page 2.10)

Short Answer

1. a. Cold sweat

  b. Pounding heart

  c. Dry mouth

  d. Feeling "energized" (pages 2.7, 2.8)

2. a. Let the family see the body.

  b. Use the word *dead* instead of euphemisms for the word.

  c. Let the family see your resuscitation efforts.

  d. Give the family some time with the body.

  e. Try to arrange for further support: neighbors, clergy.

  f. Accept the family's right to experience a variety of feelings. (page 2.17)

3. a. Realistic fears

   b. Diffuse anxiety, stemming from a sense of helplessness

   c. Depression

   d. Anger

   e. Confusion (especially in the elderly when they become ill) (pages 2.11, 2.12)

Word Finds

```
O M D F T A C O E T F D I P J E Y A Z
V X E E H N G Y U G I A R A C A I N O
E U M O P Y E O N S A O T N E R G O B
R U O W P R N M P I J I A I E Q J I G
E N T Z X R E L E E C T R T G O S T B
A O I J U A A S C R P I S R B U S C H
T I O B R C L T S E I Y S L A X E A A
I S N A E X I A C I H T O M G M R E S
N U M C O C C R N O S E V F C T S S S
G F E Q N X A Z O M S N D R W K S R L
Y N A L E R T I N G R E S P O N S E E
T O H D E S S E N S S E L P L E H V S
E C D G B R K U H E A D A C H E S O A
I L N M E A I N M O S N I C D W N N T
X A K V B A R G A I N I N G T Z Q E W
N X N O I S S E R G E R F K Z I M A O
A O D I V O R C E L A I N E D F O K R
C W C S C O V A R D E A T H A O C N K
B O I R N N L S N M V Z Z S O R Q Q B
```

 1. Displacement (page 2.12)

 2. Projection (page 2.12)

 3. Stress (page 2.9)

 4. Alerting response (page 2.10)

 5. Denial (page 2.16)

 6. Alarm reaction (page 2.10)

 7. Regression (page 2.12)

 8. Burnout (page 2.14)

 9. Conversion hysteria (page 2.13)

10. a. Death

   b. Divorce

   c. Marriage

   d. Retirement

   e. Job loss

   f. Hassles at work (pages 2.9, 2.10)

11. *Answers may vary.*

   a. Taking exams

   b. Having to deal with angry or aggressive people

   c. Having to meet a deadline

   d. Walking into a room full of strangers

   e. Looking down from a height

12. a. Fear

   b. Anxiety

    c. Helplessness

    d. Depression

    e. Anger

    f. Confusion (pages 2.11, 2.12)

13. a. Denial

    b. Anger

    c. Bargaining

    d. Depression

    e. Acceptance (page 2.16)

14. a. Fatigue

    b. Cynicism

    c. Emotions

    d. Insomnia

    e. Headaches

    f. Overeating (page 2.14)

15. *Students should list two of the following:*

    a. Abuse of drugs or alcohol

    b. Loss of interest in hobbies

    c. Declining physical health

    d. Feeling of tightness in the muscles

    e. Feelings of helplessness and hopelessness (page 2.14)

Problem Solving

    a. 76

    b. 220 − 46 = 174

    c. 174 − 76 = 98 × 0.7 = 69

    d. 69 + 76 = 145 (page 2.5)

Chapter 3: Illness and Injury Prevention

Matching

1. C (page 3.7)
2. A (page 3.6)
3. D (page 3.7)
4. D (page 3.7)
5. A (page 3.6)

6. B (page 3.7)
7. C (page 3.7)
8. A (page 3.6)
9. B (page 3.7)
10. D (page 3.7)

Multiple Choice

1. B (page 3.4)
2. B (page 3.10)
3. C (page 3.11)
4. A (page 3.14)
5. C (page 3.13)

6. D (page 3.12)
7. C (page 3.11)
8. B (page 3.3)
9. C (page 3.4)
10. D (page 3.5)

Fill-in-the-Blank

1. Intervention (page 3.3)
2. Intentional injury (page 3.4)
3. Education, enforcement, engineering/environment, economic incentives (page 3.6, 3.7)
4. Passive interventions (page 3.7)
5. Host, agent, environment (page 3.8)
6. Process objective (page 3.12)
7. Teachable moment (page 3.14)

Identify

Pertinent Negatives:

1. Bath water still standing (page 3.11)
2. Boiling water on stove (page 3.11)
3. Trampoline with no safety net (page 3.11)
4. Knitting needles and scissors left out (page 3.11)

Ambulance Calls

1. **a.** Any time that you are entering a home with the unknown, it is a wise choice to call for law enforcement. As a result of not being able to gain entry, the officer has provided probable cause for breaking the window. This covers the paramedic for unlawful entry. This could also be a potential crime scene, so law enforcement is a must.

   b. When entering a home, you should always carry a radio to contact your team on the outside. A flashlight is also important because finding a light switch in the dark can be hard. Pay attention to the broken glass from the window to prevent an injury to the person entering the home. An old blanket or tarp should be laid inside the window to prevent being cut.

   c. The teachable moment here is done after they determine the patient is okay and doesn't need to be transported. While waiting for the neighbor, Missy and Jake could talk to the patient about how and where to hide an outside key to the home and give the location to the life line personal. Life line services could then let dispatch know where the key is hidden. Also they could construct a list of neighbors with the key to the home. Finally, they could talk to the patient about always taking the cordless phone with him into the bathroom or anytime he is away from a wall phone. (page 3.14)

2. **a.**
   S: Simple. This tape needs to be simple for the children to understand it.

   M: Measurable. They need to have a play phone for the children to practice calling. That way they can see if their video has helped the children understand.

   A: Accurate. All of the information given on the tape and during the practice session should be clear and accurate.

R: Reportable. During the next year, the dispatch center will keep records on the children that use the 9-1-1 system. This allows the following years' programs to change if there is a need.

T: Trackable. After the call, it is evident that the video helped Ryan. Once again this should be reported and the case kept on file. (page 3.11)

b. This video took the scariness away for Ryan. He was able to realize that his mother would not wake up. When he was unable to arouse her, he remembered the 9-1-1 number to call for help. Good job, Larry and Courtney! Part of your job as paramedics is to help the community help themselves.

True/False

1. F (page 3.3)   **6.** T (page 3.11)
2. T (page 3.5)   **7.** T (page 3.12)
3. F (page 3.8)   **8.** F (page 3.11)
4. T (page 3.9)   **9.** T (page 3.13)
5. F (page 3.10)   **10.** F (page 3.14)

Short Answer

1. *Primary injury prevention* is defined as keeping an injury from ever occurring. Example: Removal of small choking hazards such as buttons from a stuffed animal. (page 3.3)

Secondary injury prevention is defined as reducing the effects of an injury that has already happened. Example: Air bags reduce the impact on the person with the steering wheel during a motor vehicle accident. (page 3.3)

2. *Students should list three of the following:*
   a. EMS providers are widely distributed in a population. (page 3.4)
   b. EMS providers reflect the composition of the community. (page 3.4)
   c. In rural communities, EMS providers are sometimes the highest medically trained persons. (page 3.4)
   d. EMS providers can reduce overall injuries as a result of intervention. (page 3.4)
   e. EMS providers are high-profile role models. (page 3.4)
   f. EMS providers are perceived as champions of their patients. (page 3.4)
   g. EMS providers are welcomed to school and organizations for preventative programs. (page 3.4)
   h. EMS providers are perceived as authorities on injuries and illness. (page 3.4)

3. **a.** Education: Education for the public to reduce injuries and illness (page 3.6)
   b. Enforcement: Laws to help curb destructive behaviors (page 3.7)
   c. Engineering/Environment: Changing design of products or spaces to reduce injuries (page 3.7)
   d. Economic Incentives: Provides monetary incentives to reinforce safe behavior (page 3.7)

4. **a.** Host: Child that drowns (page 3.8)
   b. Agent: Drowning (page 3.8)
   c. Environment: The swimming pool (page 3.8)

5. *Students should list three of the following:*
   a. Being male (page 3.10)
   b. Access to firearms (page 3.10)
   c. Alcohol abuse (page 3.10)
   d. History of childhood abuse (page 3.10)
   e. Mental illness (page 3.10)
   f. Poverty (page 3.10)

Crossword Puzzle

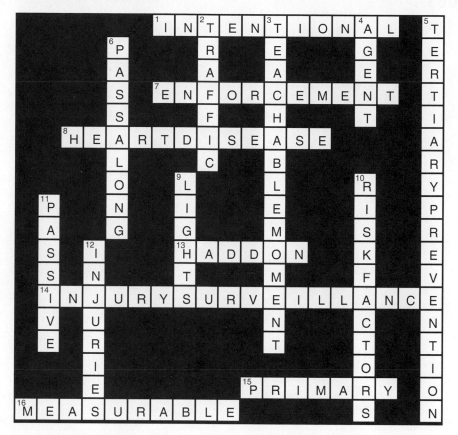

Fill-in-the-Table

What were the top 10 causes of death (in 2002)?
1. Heart disease
2. Cancer
3. Stroke
4. Chronic, lower respiratory disease
5. Unintentional injuries
6. Diabetes
7. Influenza and pneumonia
8. Alzheimer's disease
9. Kidney disease
10. Septicemia

(page 3.6)

Chapter 4: Medical and Legal Issues

Matching

1. A (page 4.14)
2. A (page 4.14)
3. B (page 4.14)
4. A (page 4.14)
5. A (page 4.14)
6. B (page 4.14)

7. B (page 4.5)
8. C (page 4.5)
9. A (page 4.5)
10. D (page 4.5)

Multiple Choice

1. B (page 4.5)
2. C (page 4.5)
3. D (page 4.8)
4. A (page 4.10)
5. D (page 4.12)
6. B (page. 4.14)
7. C (page 4.16)
8. A (page 4.18)
9. C (page 4.20)
10. A (page 4.6)

Fill-in-the-Blank

1. **a.** Informed (page 4.14)
   b. Custodial parent, legal guardian (page 4.14)
2. Plaintiff, defendant (page 4.4)
3. Scope of practice (page 4.7)
4. Advance directive (page 4.12)
5. Emancipated (page 4.14)
6. Person, place, day (page 4.16)
7. **a.** Date and time (page 4.18)
   b. History
   c. Observations
   d. Physical examination
   e. Treatment
   f. Changes

Identify

1. Chief Complaints: Low blood glucose and unconsciousness. Blood glucose levels should be between 80 and 120 mg/dL. This patient's level was 42 mg/dL. He became unconscious at the scene, which gave us implied consent to treat him.
2. Vitals Signs: Oxygen saturation of 97%, respirations of 20 breaths/min, blood glucose 42 mg/dL, blood pressure 132/70 mm Hg, pulse 96 beats/min, lung sounds clear, skin was cool, and pupils were sluggish. After IV and D_{50}, the scenario says vitals were within normal limits and blood glucose returned to a level of 122 mg/dL.
3. Pertinent Negatives: What is NOT wrong with the patient? We look for why the patient became unresponsive. He did not choke, he is not hypoxic, and the medic cannot see any obvious trauma to his head. He has a strong pulse, so we know that he is not in cardiac arrest. He also wakes back up as soon as the D_{50} is given to him. This tells us that the most likely problem was the blood glucose levels. However, the medic should always look into a person becoming unconscious with a very good sample history before being done and letting the patient sign off.

Ambulance Calls

1. **a.** Actions to take: The boy's injury is not life-threatening, nor is it likely to be appreciably aggravated by waiting another hour or so. Tell the school authorities to keep trying to reach the boy's parents and call you back when they have gotten permission to have the boy treated.

b. Provide treatment: This is a classic case of implied consent.

c. Actions to take: Some people would argue that any person who attempts suicide is, by definition, not mentally competent and therefore not able to give informed consent (or informed refusal). But you can't depend on that argument to protect you from a charge of technical assault and battery if you touch the patient or false imprisonment if you take her to the hospital against her will. Ask the boyfriend if the patient is under psychiatric care; if so, perhaps her psychiatrist can be enlisted to help. In states where suicide is a felony, you can call in the police for help. In any event, contact medical command for advice.

d. Actions to take: The best thing to do in this situation is call for police backup. In all probability, this patient will have to be forcibly restrained, and the police are the only ones permitted to authorize that action.

e. Provide treatment: This is a classic case of implied consent.

f. Actions to take: This patient is probably having a heart attack and definitely needs to be in the hospital—but the only legal way to get him there is through patient, sympathetic persuasion. You will need to spend time talking with him, trying to understand his fears, and explaining to him the possible consequence of ignoring his symptoms. If despite your best efforts at persuasion he still refuses treatment and transport, you may not transport him against his will. But be sure to "leave the door open" so that he feels free to call you back later if he should change his mind. (page 4.14)

2. *Students should list three of the following:*

a. Orientation to person, place, and day (page 4.16)

b. Responds to questions appropriately (page 4.16)

c. Absence of signs of mental impairment from alcohol, drugs, head injury, and so on (page 4.16)

d. Evidence that the patient understands the nature of his condition (page 4.16)

e. Evidence that the patient can describe a reasonable plan for follow-up care (page 4.16)

f. Oxygen saturation levels are within normal levels

g. Blood glucose levels are within normal limits

True/False

1. F (page. 4.5)

2. T (page 4.6)

3. T (page 4.7)

4. T (page 4.8)

5. F (page 4.9)

6. T (page 4.10)

7. F (page 4.12)

8. T (page 4.14)

9. F (page 4.14)

10. T (page 4.18)

Short Answer

1. *Students should list three of the following:*

a. Obvious or suspected homicide (page 4.21)

b. Obvious or suspected suicide (page 4.21)

c. Any other violent or unexpected death (page 4.21)

d. Death of a prison inmate (page 4.21)

2. Good Samaritan laws were written to provide immunity from liability to anyone who stops to help at the scene of an emergency. The care provided for is care that is free of charge. Paramedics now have a legal duty to act, which is not covered by the Good Samaritan laws. (page 4.9)

3. a. That harm resulted (page 4.10)

b. That the paramedic had a duty to act (page 4.10)

c. That there was a breach of that duty (page 4.10)

d. That the failure to act appropriately was the proximate cause of the plaintiff's injury (page 4.10)

4. a. Date and times (page 4.18)

b. History (page 4.18)

c. Observations (page 4.18)

d. Physical examination (page 4.18)

e. Treatments (page 4.18)

f. Changes (page 4.18)

5. *Students should list four of the following:*

   a. Child abuse (page 4.20)

   b. Elder abuse (page 4.20)

   c. Injury sustained during commission of a felony (page 4.20)

   d. Drug-related injuries (page 4.20)

   e. Childbirth occurring outside a medical facility (page 4.20)

   f. Rape (page 4.20)

   g. Animal bites (page 4.20)

   h. Certain communicable diseases (page 4.20)

   i. Domestic violence (page 4.20)

6. a. Homicide (page 4.21)

   b. Suicide (page 4.21)

   c. Any other violent or unexpected death (page 4.21)

   d. Death of a prison inmate (page 4.21)

Word Find

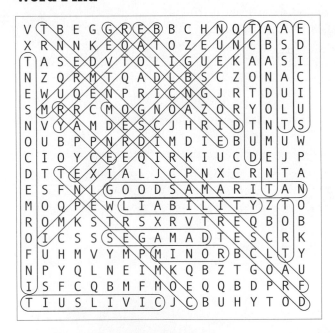

   1. False imprisonment (page 4.5)

   2. Civil suit (page 4.4)

   3. Damages (page 4.4)

   4. Implied consent (page 4.14)

   5. Good Samaritan (page 4.9)

   6. Informed consent, competent (page 4.14)

   7. Liability (page 4.4)

   8. Assault (page 4.5)

   9. Tort (page 4.4)

  10. Abandonment (page 4.12)

  11. Duty to act (page 4.10)

  12. Battery (page 4.5)

  13. Negligence (page 4.10)

  14. Dog bite, rape (page 4.20)

  15. Suicide, murder (page 4.21)

16. Minor (page 4.14)

17. Medical record (page 4.19)

18. Good care (page 4.6)

Secret Messages

a. Abandonment

b. Duty to act

c. Protocol

d. Witness

e. Gag

f. WHO

g. Rh

h. Few

Secret Message: DO WHAT'S BEST FOR THE PATIENT AND YOU WON'T GO WRONG.

Chapter 5: Ethical Issues

Matching

1. M   (page 5.3)
2. E   (page 5.3)
3. UE (page 5.3)
4. E   (page 5.3)
5. UE (page 5.3)

6. M   (page 5.3)
7. UE (page 5.3)
8. UE (page 5.3)
9. M   (page 5.3)
10. UE (page 5.3)

Multiple Choice

1. B (page 5.9)
2. C (page 5.9)
3. C (page 5.8)
4. A (page 5.7)
5. D (page 5.4)

6. B (page 5.3)
7. D (page 5.5)
8. C (page 5.7)
9. B (page 5.10)
10. D (page 5.7)

Fill-in-the-Blank

1. Morals (page 5.3)
2. Patient autonomy (page 5.5)
3. Repeat the order (page 5.6)
4. Do Not Resuscitate Order (page 5.7)
5. Organ donation (page 5.8)
6. Chain of command (page 5.10)
7. Mentor (page 5.10)

Ambulance Calls

1. This is an example of an ethical problem. Ethics are right and wrong, professional behavior, and moral duties. It was unethical for Martin and Linda not to take their call immediately. They are bound by law to respond directly to an emergency. By waiting, they acted in an irresponsible way. (page 5.3)

2. **a.** They wait to finish their food before responding to the call.

   b. Martin states he doesn't want to "babysit" and gives the call to Linda.

   c. Linda uses too large of an IV catheter for this call, just to teach the patient a "lesson" about trying to commit suicide.

   d. Linda's radio report is completely unprofessional.

   e. Linda yells at the patient for being stupid and trying to overdose.

   f. Linda talks about her own "stupid" husband.

   g. Linda tells the patient about intubation as a way to scare the patient.

   h. Martin again makes the comment of babysitting to the patient.

   i. Martin and Linda laugh and joke in the hallways of the ED.

   j. Martin and Linda play rock, paper, and scissors in the ED to decide who will clean the squad instead of both taking part in the cleaning and restocking of the unit.

True/False

1. F (page 5.3)
2. T (page 5.4)
3. T (page 5.5)
4. F (page 5.5)
5. T (page 5.7)

6. F (page 5.7)
7. T (page 5.8)
8. F (page 5.9)
9. T (page 5.10)
10. F (page 5.9)

Short Answer

1. Clearly, each person will have a private code of right and wrong. The paramedic's guiding principle, however it is worded, should be based on overriding concern for the welfare of the patient.

2. This is a very hard situation to handle. The first thing that should be done is to speak directly to the senior paramedic about how offending his or her remarks are. If the remarks continue, it would be time to address this with the chain of command.

3. When responding to code and presented with a DNR order, you must begin to verify the order quickly. Your local protocols will tell you everything you should look for. These are a few of the things that should be on every order: name of patient (confirm with ID that this is the right patient), original signatures of patient and doctor, and dates. Your online medical director will also be able to help you with any questions.

Word Find

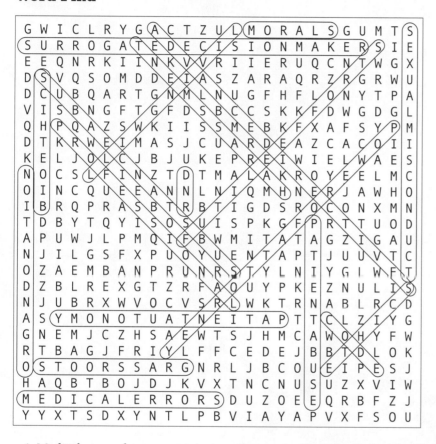

1. Medical errors, harassment, patient abuse, sexual misconduct, substance abuse. (page 5.10)
2. DNR, living will, advance directives (page 5.7)
3. Power of attorney, surrogate decision maker (page 5.7)
4. Organ donation (page 5.8)
5. Grass roots (page 5.10)
6. Professional (page 5.4)
7. Ethics, morals (page 5.3)
8. Bioethics (page 5.3)
9. Code, futile efforts (page 5.8)
10. Patient autonomy, living will (page 5.5)

Chapter 6: Pathophysiology

Matching

(page 6.7)

1. D
2. B
3. A

4. E
5. C

(page 6.27)

6. F
7. B
8. G
9. E

10. A
11. D
12. C

Multiple Choice

1. C (page 6.4)
2. A (page 6.7)
3. D (page 6.8)
4. B (page 6.19)
5. D (page 6.19)

6. D (page 6.20)
7. D (page 6.23)
8. B (page 6.25)
9. C (page 6.27)
10. A (page 6.32)

Labeling

1. The Components of the Organelles of a Cell. (page 6.4)

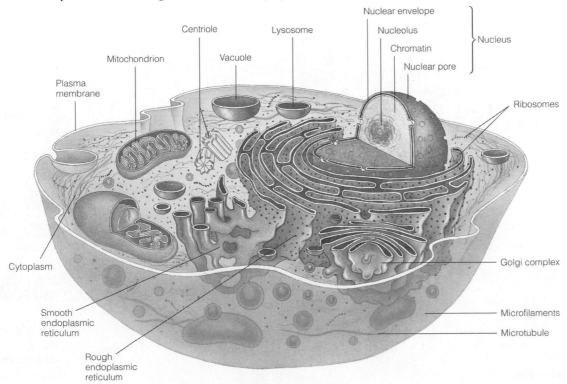

2. Type I Allergic Reaction. (page 6.43)

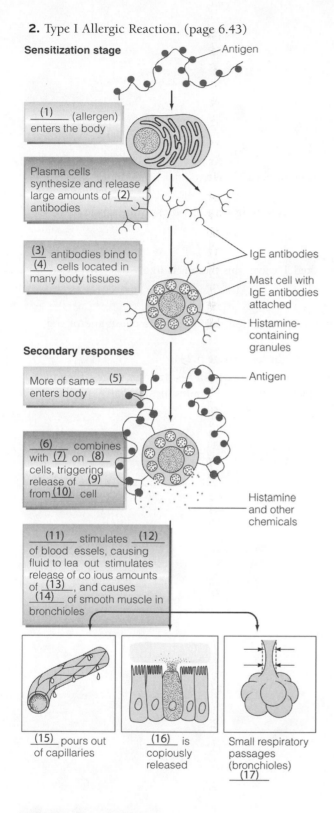

Sensitization stage

Antigen

___(1)___ (allergen) enters the body

Plasma cells synthesize and release large amounts of ___(2)___ antibodies

___(3)___ antibodies bind to ___(4)___ cells located in many body tissues

IgE antibodies

Mast cell with IgE antibodies attached

Histamine-containing granules

Secondary responses

More of same ___(5)___ enters body

Antigen

___(6)___ combines with ___(7)___ on ___(8)___ cells, triggering release of ___(9)___ from ___(10)___ cell

Histamine and other chemicals

___(11)___ stimulates ___(12)___ of blood essels, causing fluid to lea out stimulates release of co ious amounts of ___(13)___, and causes ___(14)___ of smooth muscle in bronchioles

___(15)___ pours out of capillaries

___(16)___ is copiously released

Small respiratory passages (bronchioles) ___(17)___

Fill-in-the-Blank

1. Homeostasis (page 6.5)

2. Adipose tissue (page 6.5)

3. Hyperplasia (page 6.7)

4. Baroreceptors (page 6.10)

5. Oliguria (page 6.11)

6. Hyperkalemia (page 6.12)

7. Buffers (page 6.14)

8. Apoptosis (page 6.18)

9. Multiple organ dysfunction syndrome (page 6.30)

10. Interferon (page 6.40)

Identify

1. Chief complaint: Can't breathe

2. Vital signs: Respirations are 28 breaths/min and shallow. Pulse is 90 beats/min with occasional irregular beats. Blood pressure is 160/90 mm Hg. Oxygen saturation is 90%, and skin is warm and moist.

3. Pertinent Patient history: Chronic obstructive pulmonary disease (COPD), fever, coughing with bloody sputum (page 6.20)

Ambulance Calls

1. a. Based on the angiotensin-converting enzyme (ACE) inhibitor and the peaked T wave, this patient is likely to be hyperkalemic, to have an elevated potassium level.

   b. The immediate treatment is to administer calcium chloride. (page 6.12)

2. a. Crohn's disease affects the gastrointestinal system. It is a chronic inflammatory condition that affects the colon and/or the terminal part of the small intestine.

   b. Symptoms include diarrhea, abdominal pain, nausea, fever, weakness, and weight loss. (page 6.24)

3. Alzheimer's patients might have memory loss and be disorientated to time and day in the early stages. In later stages, they may exhibit restlessness and agitation, and in the final stages of the disease, they may be unable to communicate, may experience urinary and fecal incontinence, and possibly may have seizures. (page 6.25)

True/False

1. T (page 6.4)   **6.** F (page 6.19)

2. T (page 6.5)   **7.** F (page 6.27)

3. F (page 6.7)   **8.** T (page 6.33)

4. T (page 6.10)   **9.** F (page 6.40)

5. F (page 6.14)   **10.** T (page 6.44)

Short Answer

1. a. Urine

   b. Skin and lungs

   c. Feces

   d. Sweat (page 6.8)

2. a. Capillary hydrostatic pressure

   b. Capillary colloidal osmotic pressure

   c. Tissue hydrostatic pressure

   d. Tissue colloidal osmotic pressure (page 6.9)

3. a. Sepsis

   b. Diabetic ketoacidosis

   c. Salicylate poisoning (page 6.14)

4. *Students should provide five of the following:*

   a. Hypoxia

   b. Ischemia

   c. Chemical

   d. Infection

   e. Mechanical (physical damage)

   f. Inflammatory (page 6.15)

5. a. Emphysema

   b. Bronchitis

   c. Sinusitis

   d. Laryngitis

   e. Pneumonia

   f. Asthma (page 6.20)

6. a. Exercise-induced syncope

   b. Syncope associated with chest pain

   c. History of syncope in a close family member (ie, parent, sibling, child)

   d. Syncope associated with startle such as the response to a loud noise (page 6.23)

7. a. Stage 1: Memory loss, lack of spontaneity, disorientation to time and date

   b. Stage 2: Impaired cognitive and abstract thinking, restlessness, agitation, wandering, inability to carry out daily living activities, impaired judgment, and inappropriate social behavior

   c. Stage 3: Indifference to food, inability to communicate, urinary and fecal incontinence, and seizures (page 6.25)

8. a. Basophils

   b. Eosinophils

   c. Neutrophils

   d. Monocytes

   e. Lymphocytes (page 6.32)

9. a. Margination

   b. Activation

   c. Adhesion

   d. Transmigration (diapedesis)

   e. Chemotaxis (page 6.39)

10. a. Alarm

   b. Resistance

   c. Exhaustion (page 6.46)

Crossword

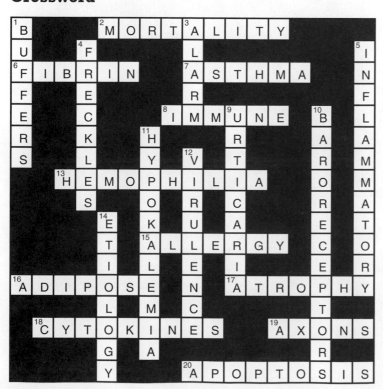

Fill-in-the-Table

1. (page 6.27)

Signs and Symptoms in the Phases of Hypoperfusion

Compensated	Decompensated
■ Agitation, anxiety, restlessness	■ Altered mental status (verbal to unresponsive)
■ Sense of impending doom	■ Hypotension
■ Weak, rapid (thready) pulse	■ Labored or irregular breathing
■ Clammy (cool, moist) skin	■ Thready or absent peripheral pulses
■ Pallor with cyanotic lips	■ Ashen, mottled, or cyanotic skin
■ Shortness of breath	■ Dilated pupils
■ Nausea, vomiting	■ Diminished urine output (oliguria)
■ Delayed capillary refill in infants and children	■ Impending cardiac arrest
■ Thirst	
■ Normal blood pressure	

Chapter 7: Pharmacology

Matching

As important as knowing the correct dosage of a drug is knowing the route(s) by which it is administered and how fast it can be expected to take effect by any given route. The relative speed of onset of action by different routes is as follows (page 7.16):

1. G Intracardiac injection (15 seconds)
2. D Intravenous injection (30–60 seconds)
3. B Endotracheal spray (3 minutes)
4. E Sublingual tablet (3–5 minutes)
5. I Intramuscular injection (10–20 minutes)
6. H Rectal suppository (5–30 minutes, but unpredictable)
7. A Subcutaneous injection (15–30 minutes)
8. F Oral (30–90 minutes)
9. C Topical application (hours to days)

Multiple Choice

1. B (page 7.5)
2. C (page 7.6)
3. D (page 7.8)
4. A (page 7.12)
5. D (page 7.13)
6. D (page 7.15)
7. B (page 7.15)
8. B (page 17.17)
9. C (page 7.20)
10. A (page 7.22)

Labeling

1. Organization of the nervous system. (page 7.11)

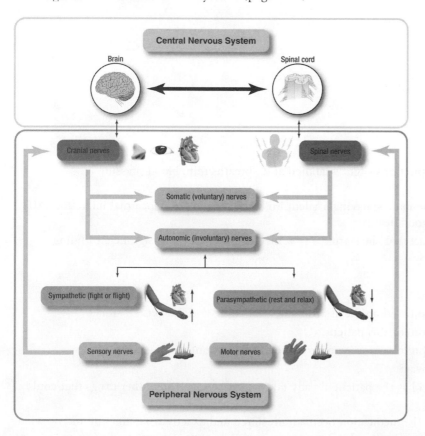

2. Drug sources and examples. (page 7.6)

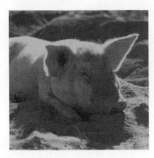
Animals

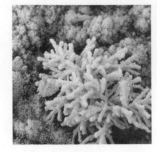
Minerals

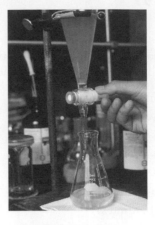
Laboratories

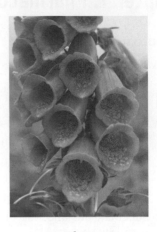
Plants

Fill-in-the-Blank

1. Indications (page 7.23)

2. Contraindications (page 7.24)

3. Antagonists (page 7.24)

4. S = Salivation/sweating
L = lacrimation
U = urination
D = defecation/drooling/diarrhea
G = gastric upset
E = emesis (page 7.26)

5. Alpha-1 (page 7.27)

6. Beta-2 (page 7.27)

7. Diuretic (page 7.28)

8. Chronotropic (page 7.28)

9. Inotropic (page 7.28)

10. Dromotropic (page 7.28)

Identify

1. Chief complaint: Heart palpations

2. Vital signs: Pulse is 60 beats/min, regular and weak, respirations slightly labored at 22 breaths/min; blood pressure is 90/60 mm Hg, and skin is pale.

3. Pertinent negatives: No pain (it should be noted that she may be having a 'silent MI', which means a myocardial infarction (MI) without pain or discomfort), no nausea, and relatively good health.

Note: The information about the patient regarding the fact that she started a new medication might be a significant finding because the patient may be having an iatrogenic response. (page 7.22)

Ambulance Calls

1. a. Right patient—Does this patient meet the criteria and based on the assessment, vital signs, and SAMPLE history?

b. Right medication—Is morphine the correct medication for this patient?

c. Right dose—Based on the patient's weight and your protocols, are you giving the right amount?

d. Right route—Is the drug being given in the optimal way?

e. Right time—Is this drug given when it should be and has the patient already taken or been given any other drugs that could interact?

f. Right documentation and reporting—What time has the medication been administered and exactly what amount and by what route? Because this is a controlled substance, are there any other legal requirements for documentation? (page 7.4)

2. a. Mechanism of medication—active vs. passive transport

  b. Blood flow and medication—effectiveness of the circulatory system (certainly an issue in cardiac arrest)

  c. Surface area—passing through nontargeted cells to reach their intended receptor targets

  d. Medication concentration—concentration of the administered medication

  e. Environmental pH—pH affects the ability of a medication to ionize (The pH of the patient's blood in arrest is a concern.) (page 7.19)

3. a. Age

  b. Weight (the doses for many drugs administered are calculated based on the weight of the patient)

  c. Sex

  d. Environment

  e. Time of administration

  f. Condition of the patient

  g. Genetic factors

  h. Psychologic factors (page 7.21)

True/False

  1. F (page 7.5)   **6.** T (page 7.12)
  2. F (page 7.7)   **7.** F (page 7.14)
  3. T (page 7.10)   **8.** T (page 7.37)
  4. T (page 7.9)   **9.** F (page 7.16)
  5. F (page 7.11)   **10.** T (page 7.17)

Short Answer

1. a. Chemical

  b. Generic

  c. Trade

  d. Official (page 7.5)

2. a. Drug names

  b. Classification

  c. Mechanism of action

  d. Indications

  e. Pharmacokinetics

  f. Side and adverse effects

  g. Route of administration

  h. Drug forms

  i. Doses

  j. Contraindications

  k. Special considerations (page 7.23)

3. a. Glomerular filtration

  b. Tubular secretion

  c. Partial reabsorption (page 7.20)

4. *Students should provide six of these reactions:*

  a. Idiosyncrasy

  b. Tolerance

  c. Cross-tolerance

  d. Tachyphylaxis

  e. Cumulative effect

  f. Summation effect

g. Synergism

h. Potentiation

i. Interference (page 7.22)

5. a. Alpha-1 produces peripheral vasoconstriction, associated with mild bronchoconstriction.

   b. Alpha-2 controls the release of norepinephrine.

   c. Beta-1 increases the heart rate, causes muscles to contract, produces automaticity, and triggers cardiac electrical conduction.

   d. Beta-2 stimulates vasodilation and bronchodilation. (page 7.27)

Word Find

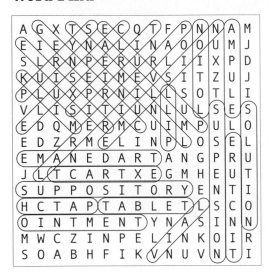

(page 7.15)

1. Preparation of a drug for external use, usually to relieve some discomfort: a **lotion** or **liniment**.

2. Aqueous suspension of an insoluble drug: **milk**.

3. Preparation of a volatile substance dissolved in alcohol: **spirit**.

4. Dilute alcoholic extract of a drug: **tincture**.

5. Drug suspended in sugar and water: **syrup**.

6. Oil distributed in small globules in water: **emulsion**.

7. Drug shaped into a ball or oval, often coated to disguise an unpleasant taste: **pill**.

8. Cylindrical gelatin container enclosing a dose of medication: **capsule**.

9. Resembles question 8, but not made of gelatin and does not separate: **pulvule**.

10. Powdered drug that has been molded or compressed into a small disc: **tablet**.

11. Drug mixed in a firm base that melts at body temperature: **suppository**.

12. Medication impregnated in adhesive that is applied to the surface of the skin: **patch**.

13. Semisolid preparation for external application, usually containing a medicinal substance: **ointment**.

14. Drug suspended in alcohol and flavoring: **elixir**.

15. Concentrated preparation of a drug made by putting the drug into solution and evaporating off the excess solvent to a prescribed standard: **extract**.

16. Liquid containing one or more chemical substances *entirely dissolved*, usually in water: **solution**.

17. Preparation of finely divided drug whose ingredients separate out on standing: **suspension**.

18. Any route of administration other than through the digestive tract: **parenteral**. (page 7.17)

19. Lasix is the **trade name** of the drug whose **generic name** is furosemide. (page 7.5)

Fill-in-the-Table

1. (page 7.16)

Rates of Absorption by Different Routes	
Route of Administration	**Time Until Drug Takes Effect***
Topical	Hours to days
Oral	30–90 min
Rectal	5–30 min (unpredictable)
SC injection	15–30 min
IM injection	10–20 min
Sublingual tablet	3–5 min
Sublingual injection	3 min
Inhalation	3 min
Endotracheal	Unknown; unpredictable
IO	60 s
IV	30–60 s
Intracardiac	15 s
*In a healthy person with normal perfusion.	

2. The Components of a Drug Profile (page 7.23)

Component of Drug Profile	Description
Drug name	Chemical, generic, and trade names with graphic representation
Mechanism of action	How the medication causes the intended effect
Indications	Reason or condition for which medication is given
Pharmacokinetics	How the medication is absorbed or distributed
Side or adverse effects	Undesired effects from the medication
Routes of administration	All the routes by which the drug can be administered
Drug forms	Profiles the various forms and concentration of how the drug is made available for clinical use
Doses	Amount of drug that should be administered for a particular condition
Contraindications	Conditions under which it is inappropriate to administer a particular medication
Special considerations	Contains all the information necessary to safely and effectively administer the medication to pediatric, geriatric, or pregnant patients.

Chapter 8: Vascular Access and Medication Administration

Matching

1. A (page 8.7)   **4.** B (page 8.7)
2. B (page 8.7)   **5.** A (page 8.7)
3. B (page 8.7)   **6.** A (page 8.7)

1. C (page 8.3)   **3.** D (page 8.3)
2. B (page 8.3)   **4.** A (page 8.3)

Multiple Choice

1. C (page 8.3)   **9.** B (page 8.23)
2. B (page 8.4)   **10.** B (page 8.35)
3. D (page 8.8)   **11.** D (page 8.39)
4. B (page 8.9)   **12.** B (page 8.39)
5. B (page 8.13)   **13.** C (page 8.45)
6. C (page 8.15)   **14.** A (page 8.55)
7. A (page 8.20)   **15.** B (page 8.37)
8. C (page 8.21)

Labeling

Common Sites for Intramuscular Injections (page 8.45)

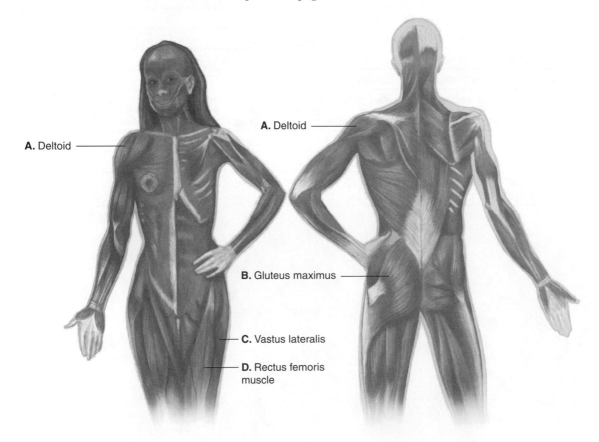

A. Deltoid

A. Deltoid

B. Gluteus maximus

C. Vastus lateralis

D. Rectus femoris muscle

Fill-in-the-Blank

1. Colloid (page 8.8)
2. Crystalloid, saline (page 8.8)
3. hypertonic, hypotonic, isotonic, hypertonic, isotonic, hypotonic (pages 8.7, 8.8)
4. lower, higher, osmosis (page 8.5, 8.6)
5. edema (page 8.6)

Ambulance Calls

Intravenous lines are supposed to help save lives, but they may cause problems (most of which can be prevented!).

1. **a.** *You* are the patient's problem! You weren't keeping an eye on the IV. The 59-year-old man who is suddenly short of breath has most probably developed circulatory overload because his "keep-open" IV became a "runaway IV" and poured an extra liter of fluid into his vascular space in a very short period of time.
   b. What you need to do is slow the IV to keep-open, sit the patient up with his legs dangling, and radio your physician for further instructions. (page 8.22)

2. **a.** The frail old woman probably has very frail veins, and your IV has apparently ruptured the wall of one of those veins and infiltrated.
   b. What you have to do is discontinue the IV, and start a new one at another site, if she really needs it. If not, wait until you reach the ED where a new IV can be inserted under more controlled conditions.
   c. Other things that might cause an IV to slow down include tightening of the clamp, a kink in the tubing, the tip of the catheter resting up against the wall of the vein, flexion at a joint causing the vein to kink, and the IV bottle hung too low. (page 8.19)

3. **a.** When bright red blood comes spurting back in your face, it's a pretty good indication that the vessel you have accidentally cannulated is an artery.
   b. What you need to do is immediately withdraw the catheter and hold firm pressure over the puncture site for at least 5 minutes. (page 8.21)

4. **a.** A painful, red, swollen venipuncture site is a sign of thrombophlebitis.
   b. The treatment is to discontinue the IV, and put a warm compress (hot pack) over the puncture site.
   c. The likelihood of thrombophlebitis can be minimized by:
      (1) Adequate disinfection of the skin before venipuncture
      (2) Wearing sterile gloves to start an IV
      (3) Covering the puncture site with a sterile dressing
      (4) Securing the catheter firmly so it can't wobble around inside the vein (page 8.20)

5. **a.** **Yes**, he is probably seriously injured. The reason for that conclusion is the signs of shock already evident: restlessness; cold, clammy skin; and the thirst itself.
   b. You decide to start an IV with lactated Ringer's, which is a **crystalloid** solution. To calculate the IV rate, you need to recall the equation:

   $$\text{gtt/min} = \frac{\text{Volume to be infused} \times \text{gtt/mL}}{\text{Time of infusion (in minutes)}}$$

   $$= \frac{200 \text{ mL} \times 10 \text{ gtt/mL}}{60 \text{ min}}$$

   = 33.3 gtt/min (for practical purposes, that is 30 gtt/min) (page 8.31)

   c. The steps in troubleshooting an IV are as follows:
      (1) Check the IV fluid.
      (2) Check the administration set.
      (3) Check the height of the IV bag.
      (4) Check the type of catheter used.
      (5) Check the constricting band. (page 8.19)

True/False

1. F (page 8.3)
2. T (page 8.4)
3. F (page 8.4)
4. F (page 8.4)
5. T (page 8.5)
6. F (page 8.5)
7. F (page 8.6)
8. T (page 8.7)
9. F (page 8.8)
10. T (page 8.10)
11. F (page 8.11)
12. F (page 8.12)
13. F (page 8.13)

14. F (page 8.18)
15. T (page 8.19)
16. T (page 8.21)
17. F (page 8.22)
18. T (page 8.23)
19. F (page 8.24)
20. F (page 8.27)
21. T (page 8.28)
22. F (page 8.29)
23. T (page 8.30)
24. T (page 8.32)
25. T (page 8.33)

Short Answer

1. **a.** Allow the arm to hang off the stretcher.
   b. Pat or rub the area.
   c. Apply chemical heat packs for at least 60 seconds. (page 8.15)

2. **a.** The gauge of the needle
   b. The site of the IV
   c. The type of fluid that you are administering
   d. The rate at which the fluid is running (page 8.15)

3. *Students should list three of the following:*
   a. Infiltration: Signs and symptoms are local edema around the site, continued IV flow after occlusion of the vein above the insertion site, and patient complains of tightness and pain around the IV site. (page 8.19)
   b. Thrombophlebitis: Signs and symptoms are tenderness and pain along the vein as well as redness and edema at the site of the venipucture. (page 8.20)
   c. Occlusion: Signs and symptoms are decreasing drip rate or the presence of blood in the tubing or a positional IV. Also if the bag of fluids is empty, it can cause an occlusion by clotting around the site of the IV. (page 8.20)
   d. Vein irritation: Signs and symptoms include the solution tingling, stinging, itching, or burning. If redness develops at the IV site, discontinue the IV and start a new IV with all new equipment and fluids. (page 8.20)
   e. Hematoma: Signs and symptoms are rapid blood pooling below the skin around the IV site, leading to tenderness and pain. Use direct pressure to stop the hematoma. Evaluate the site to see if the IV is good and can be used. If not pull out the IV and apply direct pressure. (page 8.20)
   f. Nerve, tendon, or ligament damage: Signs and symptoms are numbness, tingling, sudden shooting pain. Remove the IV and select a different site. (page 8.21)
   g. Arterial puncture: Signs and symptoms are bright red spurting blood with a much faster flow. Discontinue the site and apply direct pressure to the IV site until the bleeding stops. (page 8.21)

4. **a.** Name of the drug
   b. The dose of the drug
   c. Time the drug was given
   d. The route through which the drug was given (IV, IM, etc.)
   e. Name of the paramedic who gave the drug
   f. The patient's response or lack of expected response to the drug (page 8.34)

Crossword Puzzle

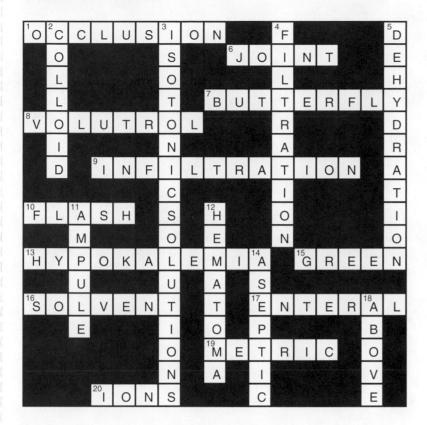

Fill-in-the-Table

Route of Administration	Where on the body does the medication go?
Enteral route	1. Gastrointestinal tract (page 8.35)
Oral	2. By the mouth (page 8.36)
Intradermal	3. Injection into the dermis (page 8.42)
Percutaneous	4. Through the skin and mucous membranes (page 8.50)
Sublingual	5. Under the tongue (page 8.51)
Endotracheal	6. Bagged in through the ET tube (page 8.55)
Buccal	7. Between the cheek and gums (page 8.51)
Transdermal	8. Applied topically (page 8.50)
Intramuscular	9. Injection into the muscle (page 8.44)
Rectal	10. Into the rectal mucosa (page 8.38)
Parenteral	11. Any route other than the gastrointestinal tract (page 8.38)
Subcutaneous	12. Injection between dermis and muscle (page 8.43)
Intravascular	13. Directly into a vein (page 8.45)
Ocular	14. Drop or ointment into the eye (page 8.52)
Aural	15. Into the ear canal (page 8.52)
Inhalation	16. Inhaled into the lungs (page 8.53)
Intranasal	17. Within the nose (page 8.52)

Problem Solving

1. To give the baker 200 mL per hour with a macrodrop set (page 8.27):

$$\text{gtt/min} = \frac{\text{Volume to be infused} \times \text{gtt/mL of administration set}}{\text{Total time of infusion in minutes}}$$

$$= \frac{200 \text{ mL} \times 10 \text{ gtt/mL}}{60 \text{ min}}$$

= approximately 33.3 gtt/min

2. For the patient who needs only a keep-open line (page 8.28):

$$\text{gtt/min} = \frac{30 \text{ mL} \times 60 \text{ gtt/mL}}{60 \text{ min}}$$

= 30 gtt/min

3. This problem, which involves calculating concentrations and flow rates, is not merely a theoretical exercise; it is typical of the calculations you will be making every day in your work as a paramedic, and a slip of the decimal point could kill someone!

a. Your vial of lidocaine contains 50 mL of 4% lidocaine, so by definition it contains (pages 8.30 and 8.31):

$$\frac{4 \text{ g of lidocaine}}{100 \text{ mL}} = \frac{2 \text{ g of lidocaine}}{50 \text{ mL}}$$

b. When you add that 2 g of lidocaine to a volume of 500 mL

$$\frac{2 \text{ g}}{500 \text{ mL}} = \frac{2,000 \text{ mg}}{500 \text{ mL}} = 4 \text{ mg/mL}$$

(Ignore the volume in which the lidocaine was suspended.)

c. If the patient is to receive 2 mg per minute, he must receive

$$\frac{2 \text{ mg/min}}{4 \text{ mg/mL}} = 0.5 \text{ mL/min}$$

d. Thus, the number of drops per minute at which you have to set the infusion is
0.5 mL/min × 60 gtt/mL = 30 gtt/min

4. 12 g × 1,000 mg/g = 12,000 mg (page 8.29)

5. $\dfrac{156 \text{ lb}}{2.2 \text{ lb/kg}}$ = 70.9 kg

Round up to 71 kg (page 8.29)

6. Step 1: 135 ÷ 2 = 67.5
Step 2: 67.5 × 0.10 = 6.75
Round 6.75 to 7
Step 3: 67.5 − 7 = 60.5
Round up to 61
Patient's weight in kilograms for field purposes is 61 kg. (page 8.30)

7. $\dfrac{6 \text{ mg}}{10 \text{ mg/mL}}$ = 0.6 mL (page 8.31)

8. Concentration on hand:

$$\frac{20 \text{ mg}}{10 \text{ mL}} = 2 \text{ mg/mL}$$

Volume you will give:

$$\frac{2 \text{ mg}}{2 \text{ mg/mL}} = 1 \text{ mL}$$

9. (page 8.32)

  a. 10 µg/kg/min × 80 kg = 800 µg/min (desired dose)

  b. $\dfrac{800 \text{ mg (or } 800{,}000 \text{ µg)}}{500 \text{ mL}}$ = 1.6 mg/mL

  c. $1.6 \dfrac{\text{mg}}{\text{mL}} \times 1{,}000 \dfrac{\text{µg}}{\text{mg}}$ = 1,600 µg/mL (page 8.29)

  d. $\dfrac{800 \text{ µg/min}}{1{,}600 \text{ µg/mL}}$ = 0.5 mL/min

  e. $0.5 \dfrac{\text{mL}}{\text{min}} \times 60 \dfrac{\text{gtt}}{\text{mL}}$ = 30 gtt/min

10. (page 8.29)

Microgram (µg)	Milligram (mg)	Gram (g)	Kilogram (kg)
500	0.5	0.0005	0.0000005
1,000,000.0	1,000.0	1.0	0.001
1,000,000,000.0	1,000,000.0	1,000	1.0
1,000.0	1.0	0.001	0.000001
1.0	0.001	0.000001	0.000000001
800,000.0	800.0	0.8	0.0008
15.0	0.015	0.000015	0.000000015

Milliliter (mL)	Deciliter (dL)	Liter (L)
5,000.0	50	5.0
1.0	0.01	0.001
10.0	0.1	0.01
1,000.0	10.0	1.0
250.0	2.5	0.25

11. (page 8.28, 8.30)

Patient's weight in pounds (lb)	Patient's weight (lb) ÷ 2	Weight (lb) ÷ 2 × 10% (move the decimal one place to the left)	Subtract your 10% from the weight ÷ 2	Patient's weight in kilograms (kg)	Patient's weight in lb ÷ 2.2 = patient's weight kilograms (kg)
60 lb	60 ÷ 2 = 30	30 × 10% = 3	30 − 3 = 27	27 kg	27.27 kg
16	8	0.8 (≈ 1)	8 − 1 = 7	7	7.27
138	69	6.9 (≈ 7)	69 − 7 = 62	62	62.72
8	4	0.4 (≈ 0.5)	4 − 0.5 = 3.5	3.5	3.64
250	125	12.5	125 − 12.5 = 112.5	112.5	113.64
36	18	1.8 (≈ 2)	18 − 2 = 16	16	16.36
82	41	4.1 (≈ 4)	41 − 4 = 37	37	37.27
180	90	9.0	90 − 9 = 81	81	81.82
330	165	16.5 (≈ 17)	165 − 17 = 148	148	150

12. (page 8.29) Volume conversions:

1,000 mL NS	500 mL NS	250 mL NS	100 mL NS	50 mL NS
100 g	50 g	25 g	10 g	5 g
1,600 g	800 g	400 g	160 g	80 g
1,000 g	500 g	250 g	100 g	50 g
40 g	20 g	10 g	4 g	2 g
100 g	50 g	25 g	10 g	5 g

13. (page 8.32)

a. $\dfrac{120 \text{ gtt/min}}{60 \text{ gtt/mL}} = 2 \text{ mL/min}$

b. $\dfrac{120 \text{ gtt/min}}{15 \text{ gtt/mL}} = 8 \text{ mL/min}$

c. $\dfrac{120 \text{ gtt/min}}{30 \text{ gtt/mL}} = 4 \text{ mL/min}$

14. (page 8.30) This table is based on the formula: $(F - 32) \times 0.555 = C$

Temp in degrees F	Degrees F - 32	Degrees F - 32 × 0.555	Temp in degrees C
32 F	0	0	0
95	95 - 32 = 63	63 × 0.555 = 34.97	34.97 (approx 35)
98.6	98.6 - 32 = 66.6	66.6 × 0.555 = 36.96	36.96 (approx 37)
101	101 - 32 = 69	69 × 0.555 = 38.3	38.3 (approx 38)
104	104 - 32 = 72	72 × 0.555 = 39.96	39.96 (approx 40)

15. (page 8.31) Determine how much medication is prescribed for your patient by body weight by filling in the table below.

Desired dose	Patient's weight in pounds (lb)	Patient's weight in kilograms (kg)	Medication administered
1 mg/kg lidocaine	90	90 ÷ 2.2 = 40.9 kg (≈ 41 kg)	41 kg × 1 mg lidocaine = 41 mg lidocaine to administer
0.2 mg/kg atropine	30	30 ÷ 2.2 = 13.6	13.6 kg × 0.2 mg atropine = 2.72 mg atropine to administer
0.05 mg/kg lorezapam	180	180 ÷ 2.2 = 81.8	81.8 kg × 0.5 mg = 4.09 mg lorezapam to administer
30 mg/kg methylprednisolone	220	220 ÷ 2.2 = 100	100 kg × 30 mg = 3,000 mg = 3 g methylpred-nisolone to administer
15 mg/kg phenobarbitol	12	12 ÷ 2.2 = 5.5	5.5 kg × 15 mg = 82.5 mg phenobarbitol to administer

16. (page 8.30, 8.31) Base your calculations on volumes replaced at 20 mL/kg of patient body weight.

Patient's weight in pounds (lb)	Patient's weight in kilograms Weight in lb ÷ 2.2 = wt kg or use the "10% trick"	Volume to be infused with first bolus @ 20 mL/kg
60	60 lb ÷ 2.2 = 27 kg	27 kg × 20 mL/kg = 540 mL
80	80 lb ÷ 2.2 = 36 kg	36 kg × 20 mL/kg = 720 mL
100	100 lb ÷ 2.2 = 45 kg	45 kg × 20 mL/kg = 900 mL
125	125 lb ÷ 2.2 = 57 kg	57 kg × 20 mL/kg = 1,140 mL
150	150 lb ÷ 2.2 = 68 kg	68 kg × 20 mL/kg = 1,360 mL
175	175 lb ÷ 2.2 = 80 kg	80 kg × 20 mL/kg = 1,600 mL
190	190 lb ÷ 2.2 = 86 kg	86 kg × 20 mL/kg = 1,720 mL
220	220 lb ÷ 2.2 = 100 kg	100 kg × 20 mL/kg = 2,000 mL (= 2L)
300	300 lb ÷ 2.2 = 136 kg	136 kg × 20 mL/kg = 2,720 mL

17. (page 8.30) Find the weight of the following medications in 1 mL of solution:

 a. 100 mg/10 mL lidocaine = 10 mg/1 mL lidocaine

 b. 1 mg/10 mL epinephrine = 0.1 mg/1 mL epinephrine

 c. 40 mg/14 mL furosemide = 2.9 mg/1 mL furosemide

 d. 6 mg/2 mL adenosine = 3 mg/1 mL adenosine

 e. 20 mg/5 mL diazepam = 4 mg/1 mL diazepam

 f. 10 mg/5 mL naloxone = 2 mg/1 mL naloxone

 g. 2 mg/5 mL albuterol = 0.4 mg/1 mL albuterol

 h. 150 mg/3 mL amiodarone = 50 mg/1 mL amiodarone

 i. 25 g/125 mL activated charcoal = 0.2 g/1 mL activated charcoal = 200 mg/1 mL activated charcoal

18. (page 8.30) Find the weight of the following medications in 1 mL of solution. Follow the example below.

 50% dextrose = 50 g/100 mL = 0.5g/1 mL

 a. 1 % xylocaine = 1 g/100 mL = 0.01 g/1 mL (or 10 mg/mL)

 b. 10% dextrose = 10 g/100 mL = 0.1 g/1 mL (or 100 mg/mL)

 c. 0.5% albuterol = 0.5 g/100 mL = 0.005 g/1 mL (or 5 mg/mL)

 d. 10% calcium chloride = 10 g/100 mL = 0.1 g/1 mL (or 100 mg/mL)

 e. 50% magnesium sulfate = 50 g/100 mL = 0.5 g/1 mL (or 500 mg/mL)

 f. 5% alupent = 5 g/100 mL = 0.05 g/1 mL (or 50 mg/mL)

 g. 0.9% sodium chloride = 0.9 g/100 mL = 0.009 g/1 mL (or 9 mg/mL)

19. (page 8.29, 8.32) Determine the amount of dopamine in *micrograms* (mcg) per milliliter when 800 *milligrams* (mg) of dopamine are added to the following bags of normal saline (NS): (note: 1 mg = 1,000 mcg)

 a. 800 mg/500 mL = 1.6 mg/1 mL = 1,600 µg/1 mL

 b. 800 mg/250 mL = 3.2 mg/1 mL = 3,200 µg/mL

 c. 800 mg/1,000 mL = 0.8 mg/1 mL = 800 µg/mL

 d. 800 mg/100 mL = 8.0 mg/1 mL = 8,000 µg/mL

20. (page 8.31) Desired dose in mg ÷ concentration in mg/1 mL = volume to administer (concentration = the "dose on hand")

 a. Desired dose = 15 mg

 Concentration = 100 mg/20 mL = 5 mg/1 mL

 15 mg ÷ 5 mg/mL = 3 mL of medication will be administered

 b. Desired dose = 3 mg halperidol

 Concentration = 5 mg halperidoL/1 mL

 3 mg ÷ 5 mg/mL = 0.6 mL of halperidol will be administered

c. Desired dose = 750 mg calcium chloride

Concentration = 1,000 mg calcium chloride/10 mL = 100 mg calcium chloride/1 mL

750 mg ÷ 100 mg/mL = 7.5 mL of calcium chloride will be administered

Skill Drills

1. Drawing Medications From an Ampule (page 8.40)

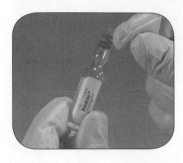

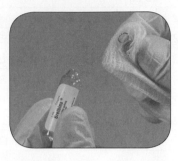

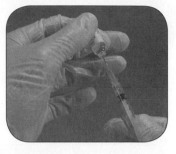

Step 1: Gently tap the stem of the ampule to shake medication into the base.

Step 2: Grip the neck of the ampule using a 4" × 4" gauze pad, and snap the neck off.

Step 3: Without touching the outer sides of the ampule, insert the needle into the medication in the ampule, and draw the solution into the syringe.

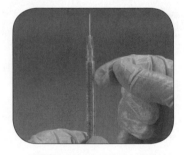

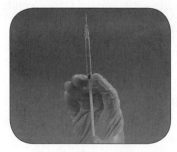

Step 4: Holding the syringe with the needle pointing up, gently tap the barrel to loosen air trapped inside.

Step 5: Gently press on the plunger to dispel any air bubbles, and recap the needle using the one-handed method.

2. Administering a Medication via Small-Volume Nebulizer (page 8.54)

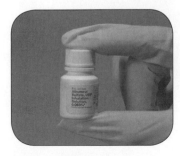

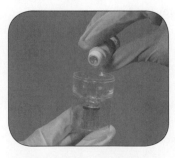

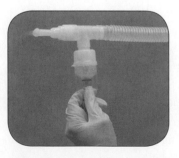

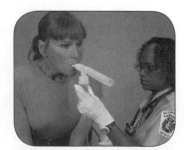

Step 1: Check the medication and the expiration date.

Step 2: Add premixed medication to the bowl of the nebulizer.

Step 3: Connect the T piece with the mouthpiece to the top of the bowl, connect it to the oxygen tubing, and set the flowmeter at 6 L/min.

Step 4: Instruct the patient to breathe as deeply as possible and hold his or her breath for 3 to 5 seconds before exhaling. Monitor the patient for effects.

3. Drawing Medication From a Vial (page 8.41)

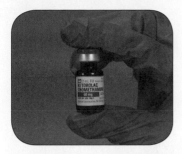

Step 1: Check the medication and its **expiration** date.

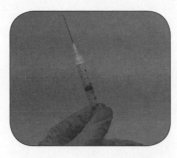

Step 2: Determine the amount of medication needed, and draw that amount of **air** into the syringe.

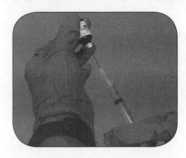

Step 3: Invert the **vial**, and insert the needle through the rubber stopper. Expel the air in the syringe to the vial, and then withdraw the amount of medication needed.

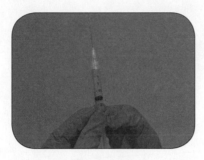

Step 4: Withdraw the **needle**, and expel any air in the syringe.

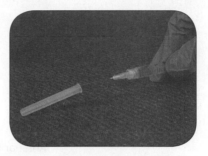

Step 5: Recap the needle using the **one-handed** method.

Chapter 9: Human Development

Matching

(pages 9.4, 9.15)

1. C
2. I
3. F
4. B
5. E

6. J
7. A
8. D
9. G
10. H

Multiple Choice

1. D (page 9.4)
2. B (page 9.3)
3. D (page 9.4)
4. B (page 9.6)
5. C (page 9.12)

6. D (page 9.12)
7. A (page 9.13)
8. A (page 9.12)
9. B (page 9.11)
10. C (page 9.9)

Labeling

1. The fontanelles. (page 9.6)

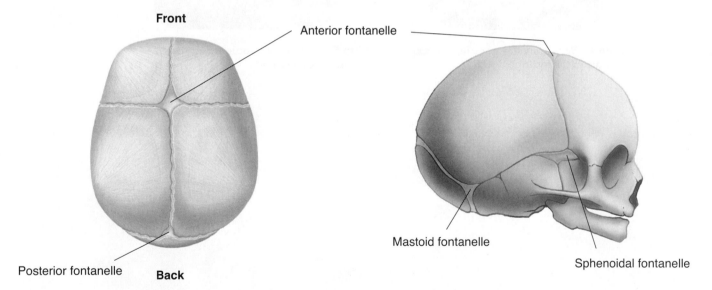

Front

Anterior fontanelle

Posterior fontanelle   **Back**

Mastoid fontanelle

Sphenoidal fontanelle

Fill-in-the-Blank

1. Foramen ovale (page 9.4)
2. Palmar grasp (page 9.4)
3. Fontanelles (page 9.4)
4. Growth plates (page 9.5)
5. Bonding (page 9.6)
6. Trust; mistrust; routine (page 9.7)
7. Aneurysm (page 9.11)
8. Mesenteries (page 9.12)
9. Terminal drop hypothesis (page 9.13)
10. Increases; decreases (page 9.12)

Identify

1. Chief complaint: Fell and hip hurts a great deal
2. Vital signs: Pulse 90 beats/min and thready; respirations 24 breaths/min and shallow; and blood pressure 100/70 mm Hg.
3. SAMPLE history:
   Signs/Symptoms: Externally rotated foot, discoloration, and a great deal of pain
   Allergies: None
   Medications: Medications for congestive heart failure
   Pertinent Medical History: Congestive heart failure, past smoker, and heart attack last year
   Last Oral Intake: Ate breakfast a few hours ago
   Event: Tripped and fell (pages 9.11, 9.12)

Ambulance Calls

1.

Reflex	How to Test	Appropriate Response
a. Moro reflex	Startle the infant (clap your hands once near child).	Infant opens arms wide and spreads fingers; Seems to grab at things.
b. Palmar grasp	Place an object—a finger—in the infant's palm.	The child should grasp your finger
c. Rooting reflex	Touch the infant's cheek.	Infant should turn head toward the touch
d. Sucking reflex	Stroke the infant's lips.	Infant should respond as if preparing to feed

(page 9.4)

2. **a.** The patient is considered a late adult. It is not uncommon to have visual issues that make it difficult for her to get around and that may also contribute to trauma such as a low fall. She may not be able to read small print such as that found on a prescription medical container, and she may not be focusing well.

   In addition, she may have some hearing loss that makes it difficult for her to hold a conversation and be understood, potentially leading to confusion and inaccurate responses to questions. (pages 9.11–9.13)

   b. While going through body systems, be concerned about cardiac-related issues and aneurysms when addressing cardiovascular issues. She may have a cardiac history and diminished cardiac output as a result of her age. Her body may not be able to compensate with rapid blood pressure changes, so vital signs are important and you must consider asking if she gets dizzy when she sits up or stands. A cardiac event is always a consideration even if there are no overt signs present. When considering respiratory issues, be aware of elderly persons' diminished ability to clear secretions and the fact that she may have diminished lung capacity, which can mean low air exchange. Ask yourself whether there are any signs of respiratory distress in this patient. Because stagnant air can remain in the lungs, hypercarbia is a concern. When considering renal and gastric issues, ask about pain and discomfort as well as bowel and urinary habits. The renal and gastrointestinal systems become less efficient with age, causing an inability to properly process fluids, nutrients, and electrolytes. The nervous system should be addressed. Elderly people have slower motor and sensory responses, which can place them at risk for injury. Slow bleeds into the brain may initially appear with subtle signs. If there is a concern, perform a stroke assessment. (pages 9.11–9.13)

3. **a.** Privacy is an issue among adolescents. Therefore, with both her mother and girlfriend in the room, asking if she is pregnant is inappropriate. Your partner should have waited until there was no family or friends present before asking this question. If the opportunity does present itself before reaching the emergency department, let the staff know. (pages 9.9–9.10)

   b. Palpitation of the abdomen must be done in a way that respects the patient's privacy and if possible by a paramedic of the same gender as the patient. It may have been appropriate to wait until the patient was loaded into the ambulance to perform this assessment. (pages 9.9–9.10)

True/False

1. T (page 9.4)
2. F (page 9.4)
3. F (page 9.4)
4. T (page 9.7)
5. F (pages 9.8–9.9)
6. T (page 9.11)
7. T (page 9.12)
8. F (page 9.13)
9. T (page 9.12)
10. F (page 9.12)

Short Answer

1. **a.** Moro reflex
   b. Palmar grasp
   c. Rooting reflex
   d. Sucking reflex (page 9.4)
2. **a.** Cholesterol
   b. Calcium (page 9.11)
3. **a.** Decreased ability to clear secretions
   b. Decreased cough reflex
   c. Decreased gag reflex
   d. Cilia diminish with age
   e. Innervation of airway structures decreases, resulting in decreasing sensation. (page 9.12)
4. **a.** Diminished visual acuity
   b. Visual distortions
   c. Harder for the eye to focus
   d. Peripheral field is narrower
   e. Hearing loss (page 9.13)
5. **a.** Gastrointestinal distress
   b. Upper respiratory tract infection (page 9.7)
6. **a.** Control
   b. Following rules
   c. Competitiveness (page 9.8)
7. **a.** Loss of respiratory muscle mass
   b. Increased stiffness of the thoracic cage
   c. Decreased surface area available for air exchange (page 9.12)

Crossword Puzzle

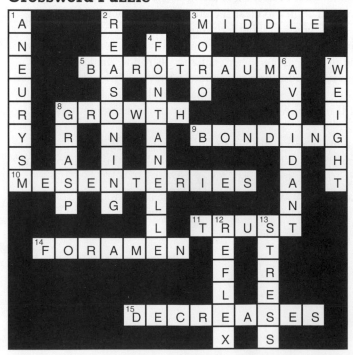

Fill-in-the-Table

1. Secondary sexual characteristics

Male Characteristics	Female Characteristics
Enlargement of external organs	Breasts and thighs increase in size
Pubic and ancillary hair begins to appear	Menstruation begins (can begin younger than teenage years)
Voice changes	Acne occurs
Acne occurs	Release of follicle stimulating hormone and luteinizing hormone (both of which increase estrogen and progesterone production)

(page 9.9)

2.

Vital Signs at Various Ages				
Age	Pulse Rate (beats/min)	Respirations (breaths/min)	Blood Pressure (mm Hg)	Temperature (°F)
Newborn (0 to 1 month)	90 to 180	30 to 60	50 to 70	98 to 100
Infant (1 month to 1 year)	100 to 160	25 to 50	70 to 95	96.8 to 99.6
Toddler (1 to 3 years)	90 to 150	20 to 30	80 to 100	96.8 to 99.6
Preschool age (3 to 6 years)	80 to 140	20 to 25	80 to 100	98.6
School age (6 to 12 years)	70 to 120	15 to 20	80 to 110	98.6
Adolescent (12 to 18 years)	60 to 100	12 to 16	90 to 110	98.6
Early adult (19 to 40 years)	70	12 to 20	90 to 140	98.6
Middle adult (41 to 60 years)	70	12 to 20	90 to 140	98.6
Late adult (61 and older)	Depends on health	Depends on health	Depends on health	98.6

(page 9.4)

Chapter 10: Patient Communication

Matching

(page 10.8)

1. O	**6.** C
2. O	**7.** C
3. C	**8.** O
4. C	**9.** C
5. O	**10.** C

Multiple Choice

1. D (page 10.4)	**6.** C (page 10.8)
2. A (page 10.5)	**7.** A (page 10.10)
3. B (page 10.6)	**8.** B (page 10.11)
4. B (page 10.7)	**9.** D (page 10.14)
5. C (page 10.8)	**10.** B (page 10.14)

Fill-in-the-Blank

1. Service (page 10.3)
2. Communication (page 10.4)
3. Calm (page 10.5)
4. Inflection (page 10.5)
5. Six (page 10.6)
6. Open-ended question (page 10.8)
7. Neutral (page 10.10)
8. Police (page 10.12)
9. Toys (page 10.12)
10. Respect (page 10.13)

Identify

1. Chief complaint: Unresponsiveness and difficulty breathing. She does not respond to the sternal rub, but does still have a gag reflex.
2. Vital signs: Blood pressure is 46/- mm Hg with respirations of 30 breaths/min and shallow. Oxygen saturation is 80% (hypoxic), and she has an irregular pulse of 36 beats/min. Skin is cool and she has mottling on her.
3. Pertinent negatives: Because of the home health nurse and the DNR, you do not attach a ECG monitor, and you do not provide any measures to this patient.

Ambulance Calls

1. There is no single correct answer to the dilemma posed in this question: How do you reply to a patient when he asks, "Am I going to die?" However, there are some general guidelines (page 10.9):
   - Do not try to minimize the seriousness of the patient's situation. Most patients who are near death *know* at least that they are in serious condition. If you are merrily chirping, "There, there, everything is going to be fine," the patient will simply assume that (a) you don't understand the situation, or (b) it is forbidden for him to speak to you honestly about his fears. Those are *not* the messages you want to convey!
   - Do not, on the other hand, take away all hope. As long as a person is alive, there is hope for him.

   In the situation described, therefore, you might say something like this: "Sir, your situation is very serious, but we have an excellent rescue team here, with the best medical backup, and we're going to do everything we can to save your life." Also let the patient know that you are willing to listen to what he has to say, to transmit any messages he has for other people, and so forth.

2. In the case of the diabetic patient, you have to remember the patient can become violent. You should begin to talk calmly to the patient. Tell her your name and reassure her you are there to help her. Take a nonaggressive stance, but be wary of the patient. Explain to the patient that you want to test her blood glucose level, start an IV, and give her glucose through the IV. If the patient is fighting you, you may need to use law enforcement to subdue the patient. As soon as you get the patient's glucose levels to normal, she will calm down and thank you (page 10.9)!

3. **a.** You should have asked if there is anybody able to translate for the patient and the family in the area.

   b. Explain to the translator why the candles must be blown out before using the oxygen. You may ask for permission first; if it is not granted, move the woman before applying the oxygen.

   c. The student's "rock out" sign has made her feel that the devil has just arrived in her bedroom. Along with you using the red pen to write her name, she now feels you are both associated with the devil.

   d. Your translator can help keep the woman and her family calm and make your transition to her caregiver much easier. You should have the translator explain *everything* that you are doing *before* you do it. Most important is to take the translator to the hospital with you to continue care and keep the patient calm on the way to the hospital. (page 10.13)

True/False

1. T (page 10.4)   **6.** T (page 10.7)

2. F (page 10.5)   **7.** T (page 10.8)

3. F (page 10.5)   **8.** F (page 10.9)

4. F (page 10.6)   **9.** F (page 10.10)

5. T (page 10.6)   **10.** T (page 10.12)

Short Answer

1. There are three types of questions:

   a. Open-ended questions are designed to draw the answer out in the patient's own words. They help start a dialogue with the patient so that the interviewer can get a solid idea of the problems the patient is having.

   b. Closed-ended questions are used more to get specific answers to questions. The answers should be one or two words. These questions can sometimes be answered with a yes or a no.

   c. The third type is a payoff question. These questions can reveal a lot of the subsurface problems of the patient. It gets down to the core of the patient's problems. (page 10.8)

2. *Students should provide three of the following:*

   a. Therapeutic smile is one of the best ways to tell your patient to calm down. By smiling, you can put the patient at ease, and it will help you keep your calm.

   b. Direct eye contact is an easy way to let your patients know that you are there for them. It helps to reassure your patients that they are number one as you take care of them.

   c. Touch is a wonderful way to put people at ease when you respond to their medical emergencies. Always use a reassuring touch in a neutral area of the patient's body, such as an arm or shoulder. Simply holding a person's hand when he or she is scared is a wonderful way of calming the person.

   d. Gentleness is a quality of touch.

   e. An open body posture will put your patient at ease. Standing above the patient or with your arms crossed sends the wrong message to your patients.

   f. A pleasant demeanor is needed when dealing with patients. People need to know they are with someone who is safe and cares about them. (pages 10.10, 10.11)

3. When dealing with a hostile patient or a patient who is agitated such as the psychiatric patient, your first responsibility is to protect your own safety and the safety of your crew and bystanders. Use an open stance and a calm voice to try and talk the patient down. If you cannot get the patient to relax and accept help, you will have to call law enforcement to subdue your patient. (page 10.12)

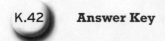

Crossword Puzzle

¹E		²M	O	D	E	S	³T	
Y							O	
E		⁴W		⁵B	O	D	Y	⁶N
C		E		E			S	O
⁷T	O	O	L		⁸R			N
N		⁹C	L	O	S	E	D	V
T		O		W		S		E
A		M			P		R	
¹⁰C	L	E	N	C	H	E	D	B
T				C			A	
	¹¹N	E	U	T	R	A	L	

Section 1 Case Study: Answers and Summary

1. What is the appropriate order of initial management for this patient?

Management for the critically injured patient is based on what is going to kill the patient first. In most cases, airway management takes priority over all else; however, this is not always the case. The following represents the appropriate order of initial management for *this* patient:

■ **Bleeding control**
- The bright red blood spurting from the injury behind the patient's knee suggests a severed or partially severed popliteal artery. If not immediately controlled, severe arterial bleeding can result in death within a matter of minutes.
  - In the case of *this particular patient*, bleeding control takes priority over airway management. Because the patient is screaming in pain, he obviously has a patent airway.

■ **100% supplemental oxygen**
- The patient's respirations, although increased, are producing adequate tidal volume. Therefore, 100% oxygen via nonrebreathing mask is appropriate.
  - This patient is displaying signs of shock (ie, restlessness, tachycardia, diaphoresis). Therefore, 100% supplemental oxygen should be administered as soon as possible.

Monitor the patient for signs of inadequate breathing (eg, shallow depth, decreased mental status) and be prepared to provide ventilatory assistance.

■ **Shock management**
- Elevate the patient's legs 6 to 12 inches.
  - Elevation of the legs will not only help control bleeding from the lower extremity wound, but will facilitate venous return to the right side of the heart (increased preload), increasing cardiac output, and maintaining perfusion to the vital organs of the body.
- Thermal management
  - Place a blanket on the patient to help maintain body temperature. Patients in shock do not have enough oxygen needed to produce energy and maintain body temperature.
  - Hypothermia interferes with the body's clotting mechanisms and may worsen the patient's bleeding.

2. How will you manage the continued bleeding from the patient's injury?

Initial management for severe bleeding involves applying direct pressure to the wound and elevating the extremity above the level of the heart. Direct pressure and elevation are typically performed simultaneously, and, in the majority of cases, adequately controls the bleeding **(Figure 1-1)**. A pressure dressing should then be applied over the wound to maintain constant pressure **(Figure 1-2)**. If bleeding continues, place additional dressings over the pressure dressing. The site should be closely monitored for signs of continued bleeding, as evidenced by blood soaking through the pressure dressing. The popliteal fossa is a difficult place to secure an adequate pressure dressing. Be prepared to proceed to the next step in bleeding control should direct pressure fail.

There are occasions when, despite the application of direct pressure, elevation, and pressure dressings, the wound continues to bleed. This is common when large arteries (eg, femoral, radial, popliteal) are damaged or in areas of the body where maintenance of adequate pressure is difficult (eg, popliteal fossa). If, despite initial bleeding control measures, the wound continues to bleed, apply pressure to a proximal arterial pressure point while maintaining direct pressure and elevation **(Figure 1-3)**. Because your patient's injury involves bleeding from the popliteal artery behind the knee, the appropriate proximal arterial pressure point would be the femoral artery. **Figure 1-4** illustrates the major arterial pressure points of the body.

It should be noted that continuing to apply additional dressings to a severely bleeding wound will prove ineffective. Although the blood is contained within the additional dressings, the patient is still losing blood externally. If pressure application at a pressure point proximal to the site of bleeding is ineffective, apply a tourniquet to the extremity

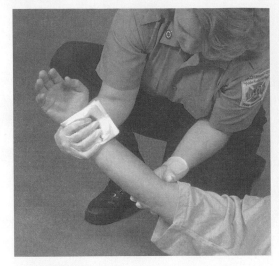 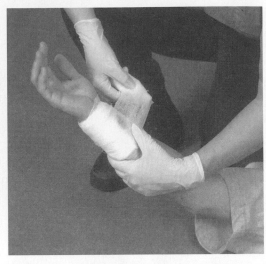

■ **Figure 1-1** Direct pressure and elevation should be performed simultaneously to control severe bleeding.

■ **Figure 1-2** Apply a pressure dressing to the wound to maintain constant pressure.

proximal to the site of bleeding. This may not be possible if the bleeding is coming from the proximal humerus or proximal thigh—two locations where application of a tourniquet proximal will not be feasible because of the shoulder and hip, respectively. However, for bleeding at the level of the elbow or distal in the upper extremity or at the level of the knee and distal in the lower extremity (as in the current situation), correct tourniquet application is almost always an effective means of controlling bleeding.

Another method for controlling severe bleeding if initial methods fail is to remove all dressings, locate the site of the bleeding, and apply digital (finger) pressure directly to the site. Some EMS system protocols allow the paramedic to clamp the bleeding vessel with a pair of hemostats. In general, this method is less effective than applying pressure to a pressure point and is very difficult to effectively accomplish in the prehospital environment.

In the worst-case scenario, when all attempts to control bleeding fail, immediately transport the patient to the closest hospital while continuing bleeding control efforts en route.

IV therapy would clearly be of no benefit to the patient with severe, uncontrolled bleeding. Remember to focus your efforts on treating what will kill the patient *first*.

3. What is the appropriate IV fluid resuscitation regimen for this patient?

The goal of IV therapy in the shock trauma patient is to maintain adequate perfusion, regardless of whether the patient is bleeding internally or externally. Optimally, lost blood should be replaced with blood. However, because blood must be refrigerated, typed and cross-matched and has a short shelf life, it is not practical for use in the prehospital setting.

Crystalloid solutions, such as normal saline or lactated ringers, are more practical for use in the prehospital setting than blood. They are well-balanced solutions that closely resemble the electrolyte concentration of plasma. Additionally, they are less expensive and have a longer shelf life than blood.

As previously discussed in other case studies within this book, IV therapy for the patient with internal bleeding should be somewhat conservative, infusing just enough IV fluid to maintain adequate perfusion (eg, good mental status, systolic blood pressure of 90 mm Hg). Because internal bleeding cannot be controlled in the prehospital setting, rapid IV fluid infusions may interfere with the body's hemostatic processes, thus resulting in increased internal hemorrhage and deterioration of the patient's condition.

External bleeding, however, can be controlled in the prehospital setting; therefore, IV fluid resuscitation in the hypotensive patient should be more aggressive. After you have controlled all external bleeding and you have no reason to suspect internal hemorrhage, infuse 1,000 mL of a crystalloid solution and then reassess the patient. Continue to administer

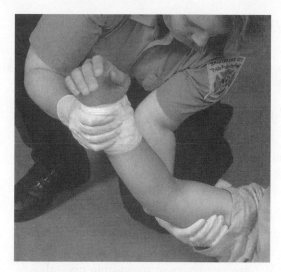

■ **Figure 1-3** If, despite initial efforts to control bleeding, the wound continues to bleed, apply pressure to a proximal arterial pressure point while maintaining direct pressure and elevation.

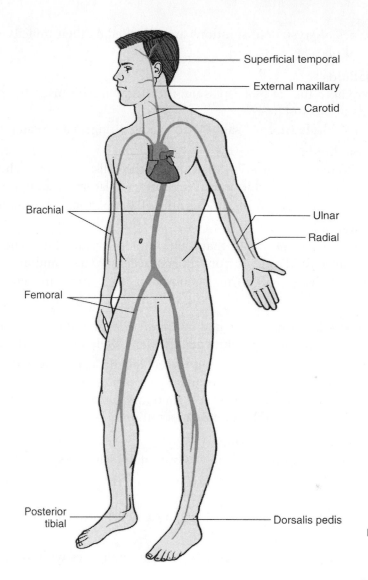

Superficial temporal

External maxillary

Carotid

Brachial

Ulnar

Radial

Femoral

Posterior tibial

Dorsalis pedis

■ **Figure 1-4** Arterial pressure point locations

fluid boluses as needed until you have stabilized the patient's blood pressure at 90 mm Hg and/or systemic perfusion has improved (eg, improved mental status, stronger peripheral pulses).

Because two-thirds of crystalloid solutions leave the intravascular space within 1 hour after administration, you must administer 3 mL of crystalloid solution for every 1 mL of estimated blood loss.

Crystalloid solutions improve tissue perfusion by increasing circulating volume and facilitating the transport of oxygen-carrying red blood cells that remain in the vascular space; however, they do not carry oxygen themselves. Additionally, because excessive crystalloid administration may result in hemodilution of the blood, administration of more than 3 liters in the prehospital setting should be reserved for situations where perfusion cannot be maintained by any other means.

The paramedic should follow locally established protocols or contact medical control as needed regarding IV fluid resuscitation for the shock patient.

4. What is the difference between crystalloid and colloid solutions?

Crystalloid solutions, which are the primary solutions used for prehospital fluid resuscitation, contain electrolytes and water. However, because crystalloids lack proteins and larger molecules, their presence in the vascular space, once administered, is of relatively short duration. Furthermore, crystalloids, unlike whole blood, do not have the ability to carry oxygen.

The three main types of crystalloid solutions are classified by their tonicity (number of particles per unit volume) relative to that of blood plasma:

- **Isotonic crystalloids**
  - Tonicity is equal to that of blood plasma; therefore, in a normally hydrated patient, they will not cause a significant shift in fluids or electrolytes.
  - 0.9% sodium chloride (normal saline) and lactated ringers are examples of isotonic crystalloids.

- **Hypertonic crystalloids**
  - Has a higher solute concentration than that of the cells; therefore, when administered to a normally hydrated patient, they cause fluid to shift out of the intracellular space and into the extracellular space.
  - 50% dextrose in water ($D_{50}W$) is an example of a hypertonic crystalloid.

- **Hypotonic crystalloids**
  - Has a lower solute concentration than that of the cells; therefore, when administered to a normally hydrated patient, they cause fluid to shift from the extracellular space and into the intracellular space.
  - 0.45% sodium chloride (half normal saline) and 5% dextrose in water (D_5W) are examples of hypotonic crystalloids.

As previously discussed, normal saline and lactated ringers are the most commonly used IV crystalloids in the prehospital setting because of their ability to immediately and rapidly expand circulating volume.

Colloid solutions contain large proteins and molecules that cannot pass through the capillary membrane; therefore, relative to crystalloids, they remain in the vascular space for a longer period of time. Additionally, the osmotic properties of colloids attract water into the vascular space; therefore, a small amount of colloid can significantly increase intravascular volume. The following are examples of colloid solutions:

- **Plasmanate (plasma protein fraction)**
  - The principle protein in plasmanate is albumin, which is suspended in a saline solution.

- **Dextran**
  - Not a protein; however, it contains large sugar molecules with osmotic properties similar to that of albumin.

- **Hetastarch (Hespan)**
  - Similar to dextran in that it contains large sugar molecules with osmotic properties similar to those of proteins

- **Salt-poor albumin**
  - Contains only human albumin. Each gram of albumin administered causes retention of approximately 18 mL of water in the vascular space.

Although colloids maintain vascular volume better than crystalloids, their use in the prehospital setting is not practical. Colloids have a short shelf life, are costly, and have specific storage requirements, attributes that make them more suitable for the hospital setting. Like crystalloids, the colloids listed do not have the ability to carry oxygen.

5. What is the purpose of performing a detailed physical examination?

The detailed physical examination (**Table 1-1**) is a comprehensive head-to-toe examination that is performed on patients who are either critically injured or unconscious. It encompasses all of the components of the initial and rapid assessments; however, it is more in-depth, methodical, and takes more time to perform.

The purpose of the detailed physical examination is to detect injuries or conditions that were either not evident during earlier assessments or that did not require immediate emergency care.

With critically ill or injured patients, you will seldom have time to perform this time-consuming examination because you will often be preoccupied performing ongoing assessments and rendering emergency treatment. If, while en route to the hospital, the patient's condition deteriorates, you should immediately repeat an initial assessment and address any newly developed life-threatening conditions. Because this may occur several times throughout transport, you will likely not have time to perform a detailed physical examination.

Table 1-1   Detailed Physical Examination

Head
- Inspect and palpate the cranium for bleeding, pain, deformities, or instability.
- Inspect and palpate the facial bones for pain, deformities, or instability.
- Inspect the ears, nose, and mouth for drainage or potential obstructions.
- Inspect the pupils for size, shape, equality, and reactivity to light.

Neck
- Assess the position of the trachea (eg, midline or deviated).
- Inspect the jugular veins for distention.
- Palpate the cervical spine for pain or deformities.

Chest
- Inspect the chest for symmetry, paradoxical movement, retractions, and bruising.
- Palpate the chest for pain, crepitus, or instability.
- Auscultate breaths sounds bilaterally.
  - Determine if breath sounds are equal on both sides of the chest.
  - Note any abnormal breath sounds, such as wheezing, rales, or rhonchi.

Abdomen/pelvis
- Inspect the abdomen for bruising and distention.
- Palpate four quadrants of the abdomen for pain, guarding, rigidity, or masses.
- Palpate the painful area last.
- Palpate the pelvis for pain, crepitus, or instability.
  - Gently push in and down on the iliac crests.
  - Never rock the pelvis back and forth.
  - Do not repalpate the pelvis if it was unstable or painful during previous assessment.

Lower extremities
- Inspect and palpate for pain, crepitus, and deformities.
- Assess gross motor and sensory functions and distal pulses.

Upper extremities
- Inspect and palpate for pain, crepitus, and deformities.
- Assess gross motor and sensory functions and distal pulses.

Posterior
- Inspect and palpate the posterior thorax for pain or deformities.
- Inspect and palpate the lumbar region and buttocks for pain or deformities.
  - Because the patient will often be immobilized on a spine board, you will usually not be able to inspect the posterior in the detailed physical examination.
  - Assessment of the posterior should be performed when you log-roll the patient to place them on the spine board.

If, however, your transport time to the hospital is lengthy and you have addressed all life-threatening injuries or conditions, a detailed physical examination should be performed.

It is most appropriate to perform a detailed physical examination of your patient in the back of the ambulance while en route to the hospital. Remaining at the scene to perform a thorough examination on a critically ill or injured patient would clearly delay definitive care and increase the possibility of a poor patient outcome.

Summary

During the initial assessment of your patient, all airway, breathing, and circulation problems must be immediately corrected. Invasive procedures, such as IV therapy or intubation, are of no value to the patient if there is uncontrolled bleeding or a nonpatent airway.

The patient in this case study had an obviously patent airway; however, he had an uncontrolled arterial hemorrhage. Therefore, controlling the bleeding had priority over applying oxygen. If, however, sufficient help was available (eg, first responder, law enforcement), then bleeding control and oxygen therapy could have been accomplished simultaneously. Remember that the order in which you manage your patient's injuries or condition is based on what will be the *most rapidly* fatal. A severe, uncontrolled arterial hemorrhage will kill the patient before you can even prefill the reservoir of a nonrebreathing mask!

Once a patent airway has been established and all external bleeding has been controlled, the patient should be rapidly assessed for signs of shock. If signs of shock are present, immediately transport the patient and perform all interventions, such as IV therapy and cardiac monitoring, en route to the hospital.

In addition to 100% oxygen and thermal management, shock caused by external blood loss should be treated with aggressive IV infusions of an isotonic crystalloid solution (eg, normal saline, lactated ringers). The goal of IV therapy is to maintain adequate perfusion (eg, systolic blood pressure of 90 mm Hg, improved mental status). Because crystalloid solutions quickly leave the vascular space, you must infuse 3 mL for each 1 mL of estimated blood loss. Because excessive crystalloids may hemodilute the blood, more than 3 liters should not be administered in the prehospital setting unless absolutely necessary to maintain perfusion.

Continually monitor the patient en route to the hospital and be prepared to infuse additional IV fluids for blood pressure maintenance, assist ventilations for inadequate breathing, or perform CPR if the patient develops cardiac arrest.

Section 2: Airway
Chapter 11: Airway Management and Ventilation

Matching

1. B (page 11.20)	**11.** T (page 11.52)
2. A (page 11.21)	**12.** C (page 11.98)
3. A (page 11.21)	**13.** E (page 11.44)
4. B (page 11.20)	**14.** A (page 11.38)
5. T (page 11.52)	**15.** C (page 11.41)
6. C (page 11.98)	**16.** A (page 11.38)
7. T (page 11.52)	**17.** D, E (pages 11.42, 11.44)
8. N (page 11.52)	**18.** B (page 11.38)
9. N (page 11.52)	**19.** C, D (pages 11.41, 11.42)
10. T (page 11.52)	**20.** B (page 11.38)

Multiple Choice

1. C (page 11.8)	**9.** C (page 11.12)
2. A (page 11.20)	**10.** D (page 11.18)
3. D (page 11.38)	**11.** C (page 11.85)
4. B (page 11.52)	**12.** D (page 11.85)
5. B (page 11.87)	**13.** C (page 11.85)
6. D (page 11.94)	**14.** A (page 11.88)
7. A (page 11.102)	**15.** B (page 11.90)
8. B (page 11.10)	

Labeling

1. Parts of the larynx (page 11.8)

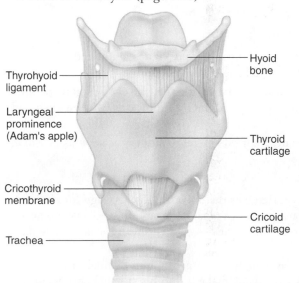

2. The child's epiglottis and surrounding structures (page 11.10)

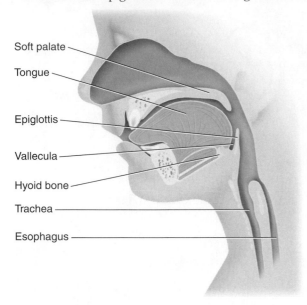

Soft palate
Tongue
Epiglottis
Vallecula
Hyoid bone
Trachea
Esophagus

Fill-in-the-Blank

1. Hypoxemia, preoxygenation (page 11.54)
2. Sniffing (page 11.55)
3. 30 (page 11.59)
4. Rise, carbon dioxide (page 11.13)
   fall, oxygen (page 11.13)
5. Stroke, alcohol consumption (page 11.24)
6. Whistle-tip, tonsil-tip (page 11.30)
7. Facing the roof of the mouth (page 11.32)
8. Preoxygenate (page 11.54)

Identify

1. Chief complaint: Choking
2. Vital signs: Respirations are 28 breaths/min and shallow. Decreased right-side lung sounds. Pulse is 98 beats/min and regular. Blood pressure is 128/86 mm Hg. Skin is blue and cool. Oxygen saturation is 88% and the patient is confused.
3. Pertinent negatives: The patient has clear lung sounds on the left, which suggest to the paramedic that the cap has gone down the right mainstem. Because there are sounds on the right, you know that only a portion of the right lung has been blocked and the cap must be stuck in the bronchial tree.

   There is nothing other than oxygen and a fast ride that you can give this patient! He needs to get to surgery as soon as possible.

Ambulance Calls

1. **a.** 2. The patient described in this question is showing classic signs of **choking**. He gives the universal distress sign for choking (clutches his neck), staggers, and falls—all without making a sound. The reason he isn't making a sound is because no air is moving past his vocal cords, which means that his upper airway is completely obstructed—and *that* means *he is going to die if you don't act at once*! (page 11.24)

   b. 2. The most urgent priority is to try to expel the foreign body from his airway, which means giving him manual thrusts. There's no reason to pump his stomach (answer 1) because his problem is what *didn't* make it into his stomach, not what did! Clearly, he is not in any shape to gargle with salt water (answer 3), and neither would it help him if he could. At the moment, he doesn't need epinephrine (answer 4), although he may need it very soon, if his airway obstruction is not relieved and he suffers cardiac arrest as a consequence. And he certainly doesn't need a sedative such as diazepam (Valium) (answer 5); he's already sedated quite enough by his hypoxemia. (What's hypoxemia? Check the glossary if you don't remember.) Both this question and the one preceding illustrate why it's not a good idea to try to grab a quick dinner while you're on duty. Caroline's

Law of Dining on Duty states: If you are going to get called to a cardiac arrest during your shift, the call is going to come at the precise moment that the pizza you ordered comes out of the oven. (page 11.26)

2. a. 5. When your friend starts to choke on his hot dog, as evidenced by his paroxysm of violent coughing, the *first* thing you should do is **encourage him to keep coughing** (answer 5). A cough generates air flows of gale-force velocity—far more powerful than anything you could generate artificially by, for example, using manual thrusts (answer 3). Sticking your finger in the mouth of a panicky, choking person (answer 2) is a good way to lose a finger; and reaching blindly into the throat with *any* instrument, let alone barbecue tongs (answer 4), is as likely to produce a rather messy tonsillectomy as it is to snare a wayward hot dog. There's no point in trying to ventilate your friend artificially (answer 1); he's still got some air exchange by his own efforts, and blowing into his mouth may just force the hot dog farther down his airway. (page 11.27)

b. 3. When coughing fails to expel the foreign object and your friend becomes completely obstructed (as evidenced by his aphonia), *that* is the time to give the Heimlich maneuver (answer 3). He's still conscious, so the finger sweep (answer 2) and head tilt (answer 1) are still inappropriate. The barbecue tongs (answer 4) are *always* inappropriate. And there's no point now in encouraging him to keep coughing (answer 5); if he *could* cough, he would. (page 11.26)

c. When the Heimlich maneuver does not work and your friend becomes unconscious, your next steps should be as follows:

   (1) Open his mouth (tongue-jaw lift), and perform a quick finger sweep to remove any accessible obstructing material.

   (2) Then try to open the airway by head tilt–chin lift.

   (3) Attempt to ventilate mouth-to-mouth.

   (4) If you cannot force air past the obstruction, give abdominal thrusts until the foreign body is expelled from the victim's airway *or* just do cardiopulmonary resuscitation (CPR) chest compressions. (page 11.26)

d. When the paramedics arrive with all their gear, you finally have the means to take definitive action. At that point, you should take the following steps:

   (1) Try to visualize the obstructing material by direct laryngoscopy, snare it with a Magill forceps or strong suction under direct vision, and remove it.

   (2) Open the patient's airway by head tilt–chin lift. See if he is breathing.

   (3) If he is not breathing, give artificial ventilation with supplemental oxygen. (page 11.27)

3. Probably this body builder has a short, very muscular neck, which is a classic situation for a difficult intubation.

a. When the cords won't come into view, ask your partner to apply downward pressure on the cricoid cartilage.

b. That maneuver also accomplishes another useful thing, namely, it helps prevent passive regurgitation. (page 11.47)

c. When you've finally got the tube in, you need to verify its position. To do so, ventilate through the tube and

   (1) Look to see if the chest rises with each ventilation.

   (2) Listen for breath sounds on both sides of the chest with each ventilation. (page 11.59)

4. Nasotracheal intubation doesn't always go smoothly, and one needs to be prepared to spend a little time getting it right.

a. You can tell that the tip is moving toward the glottis by

   (1) Putting your ear over the tube and hearing and feeling the movement of air through the tube.

   (2) Seeing misting inside the tube (from condensation of the patient's breath).

b. When the bleeps from the monitor start getting farther and farther apart, it means that the patient's heart is slowing down (ie, she is developing bradycardia).

c. You must immediately

   (1) Stop advancing the tube.

   (2) Attach the tube to an oxygen source.

   (3) Give atropine, 0.5 mg IV, to speed up the patient's heart. (You will learn a lot more about atropine and its actions in Chapter 27; don't panic if you don't understand at this point why it is being administered.) The passive backflow of gastric contents from the stomach up the esophagus and into the throat is called regurgitation, and it is *not* a good thing. (page 11.68)

d. As you try again to advance the tube, you notice gastric contents creeping up the back of the patient's throat, a process called regurgitation. Regurgitation is dangerous because the gastric contents—which may include stomach acids along with the triple cheeseburger the patient had for lunch—are prone, once they have reached the laryngopharynx, to get sucked down the trachea and into the lungs (a process called aspiration).

e. The lungs don't like gastric acid and triple cheeseburgers; they respond by developing a chemical pneumonia, sometimes serious enough to be fatal.

f. If you see gastric contents creeping up the back of the patient's throat as you are intubating, immediately ask your partner to apply cricoid pressure, which will squeeze the esophagus shut between the cricoid cartilage and the cervical vertebrae and thereby prevent any more material from ascending into the pharynx.

g. The tip of the endotracheal tube should be advanced through the vocal cords at the beginning of inhalation, when the cords are open most widely.

5. a. 31 minutes.

b. The oxygen is going to run out before you get back.

$$\text{Duration of flow} = \frac{(\text{Gauge pressure} - 200 \text{ psi}) \times C}{\text{Flow rate}}$$

$$= \frac{(800 \text{ psi} - 200 \text{ psi}) \times 0.26}{5 \text{ L/min}}$$

Only if you let the cylinder run down all the way to zero will you manage to squeeze 40 minutes' worth of oxygen out of it, but you will have to make sure you keep up your pace as you trudge through the woods carrying the stretcher. If you are starting to drag, you'd better decrease the flow rate to the nasal cannula to about 4 L/min. And *next time,* make sure you take a *full* oxygen cylinder with you! (page 11.35)

6. **(1)** Seeing the patient's chest rise and fall with each breath you give

(2) Feeling the compliance of the patient's lungs in your own lungs

(3) Hearing and feeling air escape through the patient's mouth during his passive exhalation (page 11.40)

7. a. To minimize gastric distention during artificial ventilation, you need to

(1) Keep the patient's airway fully open.

(2) Avoid excessive ventilation volumes. Blow in only that volume of air needed to make the chest rise.

(3) Use cricoid pressure to prevent air from going down the esophagus. (page 11.47)

b. When the patient's belly starts to distend despite your best efforts, reposition his head to try to improve the airway and pay more attention to the ventilation volumes. Do not, at that point, take any action to try to relieve the gastric distention. (page 11.47)

c. When, however, the patient's gastric distention begins to interfere seriously with your ability to get any air into his lungs, you will have to attempt to decompress the stomach. It will not be a pleasant job. Roll the patient quickly to his side, facing away from you, and press firmly over his epigastrium. He will probably regurgitate, perhaps massively, so be prepared to sweep his mouth free of vomitus before you roll him back supine.

If you answered either of those "What should you do?" questions with the phrase, "Call an ambulance!" give yourself an extra point. Unless you want to spend the night doing CPR all by yourself in the movie theater, you should send someone for help at the very outset. (page 11.48)

8. The advantages of the pocket mask over other devices for giving artificial ventilation include

(1) Its immediate availability (assuming you remember to carry it in your pocket).

(2) Its adaptability; it can be deployed with or without supplemental oxygen.

(3) Its potential to be used as a simple face mask if the patient resumes breathing.

(4) Its effectiveness; it is much easier to maintain a good seal with a pocket mask (and therefore deliver good volumes) than it is with a bag-mask device. (page 11.40)

9. The patient in congestive heart failure has fluid in his alveoli, and for that reason a portion of his cardiac output is not picking up any oxygen as it passes through the lungs (a situation called *shunt*). It is not surprising, therefore, that his oxygen saturation is reduced.

a. 3. The SaO_2 reading of 86% is abnormally low. A normal reading would be between 97% and 99% on room air. There's no reason to suspect an artifact (erroneous reading) because the reading is quite consistent with the patient's clinical presentation.

b. The measure you need to take immediately when you see a reading like that (or, even without a pulse oximeter, when you see a patient in respiratory distress) is to administer oxygen. (What would be the best device for administering supplemental oxygen to this patient?)

c. Possible sources of an erroneous reading in this patient include the following (students will list three sources):

(1) Bright ambient light may be interfering with the reading. Cover the sensor with a towel or aluminum foil if you suspect that's the problem.

(2) Check if the patient is moving. The oximeter may confuse patient motion for a pulse.

(3) The sensor may be picking up venous pulsations. Move it to a different finger or to the ear lobe and recheck.

(4) If it's cold in the ambulance and the patient's peripheral blood vessels constrict as a consequence, the resulting **poor** perfusion of the extremities may lead to false oximetry readings. (page 11.19)

10. Probably the primary indication for using an end-tidal carbon dioxide monitor is to check the placement of an endotracheal tube in a *spontaneously breathing, normally perfused patient.*

   a. In the case described, you can conclude that the tracheal tube is in the esophagus. If the tube were in the trachea, as it's supposed to be, the carbon dioxide concentration of the exhaled gas ought to be at least 2%, translating into a tan or yellow color on the sensor.

   b. The action you should take right away is to deflate the cuff and remove the tracheal tube. Preoxygenate the patient before you make another attempt to intubate. (page 11.60)

11. **a.** The person breathing quietly 12 breaths/min with a tidal volume of approximately 500 mL has a minute volume as follows:

   Minute volume = Respiratory rate × Tidal volume

   = 12 breaths/min × 500 mL/breath

   = **6,000 mL/min** (6 L)

   b. After the crash, when paralysis of the respiratory muscles prevents the person from taking deep breaths (and respiratory distress and fear prompt him to increase his respiratory rate), the minute volume changes as follows:

   Minute volume = Respiratory rate × Tidal volume

   = 20 breaths/min × 200 mL/breath

   = **4,000 mL/min**

   c. The situation is much more serious than it might seem from a 33% reduction in minute volume. A person whose tidal volume is so small is doing little more than moving his dead space back and forth (do you remember what dead space is?), so there is little true alveolar ventilation and therefore little carbon dioxide removal.

   Because carbon dioxide will not be removed efficiently, the level of carbon dioxide in the blood will rise, and the arterial PCO_2 will rise, by definition a situation of hypoventilation.

   d. As a result, the patient's pH will **fall**, reflecting the increased acidity of his blood.

   e. The resulting derangement in his acid–base balance is called a **respiratory acidosis**—"acidosis" because the pH is lower than normal, "respiratory" because the source of the problem is in the respiratory system (the failure to breathe deeply enough).

   f. The treatment required in the acute situation is to assist the patient's ventilations to improve the tidal volume and flush out some of that excess carbon dioxide. (page 11.11)

12. Next time you have to go up four flights of steps, you'll probably remember to take a full E cylinder, not a half-empty D cylinder.

$$\text{Duration of flow} = \frac{(\text{Gauge pressure} - 200 \text{ psi}) \times C}{\text{Flow rate}}$$

$$= \frac{(900 \text{ psi} - 200 \text{ psi}) \times 0.16 \text{ L/psi}}{10 \text{ L/min}}$$

$$= \textbf{11 minutes}$$

(page 11.35)

13. In this question about a head-injured patient, you had to review both some respiratory physiology along with the pathophysiology of head injury.

   a. If the patient's respiratory rate is 8 per minute and his tidal volume is 500 mL, his minute volume is calculated as follows:

   Minute Volume = Tidal volume × Respiratory rate

   = 500 mL/breath × 8 breaths/min

   = **4,000 mL/min** (4 L/min)

   b. That minute volume is **smaller** than normal. (Normal is around 6 L/min.)

   c. Therefore, you can conclude that the patient's arterial PCO_2 will tend to **increase**, so his pH will **decrease**. The net effect will be an acid–base disorder called a **respiratory acidosis**. The way you can help correct that abnormality is to **assist the patient's ventilations**. This will thereby increase his minute volume (which will blow off more carbon dioxide). (page 11.11)

14. Hypercarbia occurs when a person is not moving enough air in and out of his lungs to remove the carbon dioxide being produced by metabolism.

   a. Hypercarbia can be caused by

   (1) Diabetic ketoacidosis (increased CO_2 production)

   (2) Narcotic overdose (decreased respiratory rate)

(3) Spine injury (decreased tidal volume)

(4) Rib fracture (decreased tidal volume—because it *hurts* to take breaths of normal volume)

b. The way to help normalize the PCO_2 of a hypercarbic patient is to increase his minute volume, that is, to assist his ventilations so that his tidal volume is larger (and perhaps give an extra breath here and there, to increase his respiratory rate as well). (page 11.15).

16. a. *Students will list six of the following conditions that can cause hypoxemia:*

(1) Pulmonary edema

(2) Pneumonia

(3) Drowning

(4) Chest trauma

(5) Airway obstruction

(6) Pneumothorax

(7) Inhalation of smoke or toxic fumes

(8) Respiratory arrest

b. The treatment for hypoxemia is to give supplemental oxygen! That may sound obvious, but it is truly remarkable how many hypoxemic patients arrive at the emergency room by ambulance *without* oxygen being administered. *Don't be stingy with oxygen!*

c. A compound whose pH is *less* than 7.0 is called an **acid**, whereas a compound whose pH is *greater* than 7.0 is called a **base**.

d. An **electrolyte** is a substance that dissociates into charged components in water. A positively charged molecule, such as Na^+, is a **cation**, whereas a negatively charged molecule, such as Cl^-, is called an **anion**.

e. The most important component of the red blood cell, or **erythrocyte**, is an iron-containing protein called **hemoglobin**, which binds oxygen in the lungs and releases oxygen in the tissues. When that protein is not saturated with oxygen, it imparts a bluish color to the blood, which is reflected in a bluish color of the skin called **cyanosis**.

f. When there is failure of tissue perfusion for any reason, the resulting state is called **shock**. One way that state can come about is if there is cardiac standstill or **asystole**. However that state of inadequate tissue perfusion occurs, one of the immediate results is that the body cells, unable to obtain enough oxygen, switch to **anaerobic** metabolism. (page 11.16)

True/False

One of the most important things to remember about suctioning is that *suctioning removes air as well as liquids.*

1. T (page 11.30)   **4.** T (page11.30)

2. T (page 11.31)   **5.** F (page 11.31)

3. F (page 11.30)

Short Answer

1. *Students will list four of the following:*

a. The tongue

b. A foreign body

c. Swelling (edema)

d. Trauma to the face or neck

e. Aspirated vomitus (page 11.25)

2. a. Provides a secure airway.

b. Protects the airway from aspiration.

c. A T tube enables delivery of aerosolized drugs directly into the lung for rapid absorption into the bloodstream. (page 11.52)

3. a. Respiratory failure

b. Apnea

c. Inability of patient to protect own airway (page 11.52)

4. a. Accidental intubation of the esophagus

b. This complication can be *avoided* by

(1) Positioning the patient correctly for intubation

(2) Seeing the tube pass through the vocal cords

(3) Checking for breath sounds over both lungs after intubation and epigastrium

c. If it does occur, intubation of the esophagus can be *detected* by

(1) Gurgling noises over the epigastrium during ventilation

(2) Absence of breath sounds over the lungs during ventilation

(3) Failure of the patient to "pink up" on ventilation

Once detected, accidental intubation of the esophagus can be *corrected* by immediately withdrawing the tracheal tube and ventilating the patient with a bag-mask device. No further attempt to intubate the patient should be made until the patient has been reoxygenated for at least 3 minutes.

d. Accidental intubation of a bronchus (usually the right main bronchus)

e. Can be avoided by stopping as soon as the cuff passes the vocal cords.

f. If it does occur, bronchial intubation can be *detected* by absence of breath sounds over one lung (usually the left).

Once detected, bronchial intubation can be *corrected* by deflating the cuff, and then slowly drawing the tube back until breath sounds become audible in both lungs. Then, reinflate the cuff and mark the tube at the teeth. (page 11.52)

5. The principal hazard of using a neuromuscular blocker is that it converts a breathing patient with some sort of airway into a nonbreathing patient without any airway—so if you are unable to intubate within 30 seconds and you have trouble maintaining an airway manually, the patient will need a surgical airway urgently. (page 11.94)

6. a. Minute volume = Tidal volume × Respiratory rate

= 500 mL/breath × 12 breaths/min = **6,000 mL** (6 L)

b. The minute volume will *decrease* if

(1) The tidal volume is decreased (shallow breaths, as in spinal cord injury), or

(2) The respiratory rate slows (as in heroin overdose)

c. If the minute volume does decrease, the arterial blood gases will show a rise in PCO_2 because carbon dioxide will not be removed efficiently and so will accumulate in the blood. (Unless a person stops breathing altogether, or very nearly so, decreases in minute volume do not affect the *oxygenation* of the blood as dramatically.) (page 11.11)

7. *Students will list six indications.*

a. Pulmonary edema

b. Pneumonia

c. Drowning

d. Chest trauma

e. Airway obstruction

f. Pneumothorax

g. Inhalation of smoke or toxic fumes

h. Respiratory arrest (page 11.14)

8. *Students will list four signs of acute respiratory insufficiency.*

a. Tachypnea (rapid breathing)

b. Hyperpnea (abnormally deep breathing)

c. Use of accessory muscles to breathe

d. Nasal flaring

e. Cyanosis (bluish tinge to the lips and nail beds)

f. If you mentioned dyspnea—a *feeling* of shortness of breath—that's all right, but technically speaking, dyspnea is a symptom, not a sign. (page 11.16)

9. *Students will list six safety precautions.* Safety precautions around oxygen cylinders include the following:

a. No smoking!

b. No grease.

c. Keep out of extreme heat.

d. Use the right valve.

e. Keep all valves closed when not in use.

f. Keep cylinders firmly secured.

g. Keep your face and body to the side of the cylinder. (page 11.35)

10. *Students will list six causes.* The causes of respiratory arrest include

    a. Airway obstruction by the tongue in an unconscious person

    b. Choking

    c. Laryngeal edema

    d. Respiratory center depression (drugs, head injury)

    e. Stroke

    f. Electric shock

    g. Primary cardiac arrest (page 11.24)

11. **a.** LOOK at the chest to see if it rises and falls.

    b. LISTEN over the nose and mouth for the sound of air flow.

    c. FEEL with your cheek over the nose and mouth for the movement of air. (page 11.19)

12. A person who has suffered respiratory arrest will need **controlled** ventilation.

13. In *controlled* ventilation, the rescuer has to breathe for the patient. In *assisted* ventilation, by contrast, the patient *is* breathing spontaneously, and the rescuer simply boosts the tidal volume.

14. With *any* form of artificial ventilation, the primary objective is to normalize the PCO_2 by moving air in and out of the lungs. Controlled ventilation also aims to supply oxygen to the alveoli.

15. This was, in fact, a rather unfair question, for at this point in the course you are not yet familiar enough with specific emergencies to be able to know when the pulse oximeter would be most useful. In general, any time you have a patient whose state of oxygenation may be in jeopardy, the pulse oximeter can help you keep tabs on things (students will list three situations):

    a. A patient with trauma to the chest, in whom pneumothorax or hemothorax (or both) may interfere with oxygenation

    b. A patient in pulmonary edema, who has a large shunt because of fluid in his alveoli

    c. A patient undergoing tracheal intubation

    d. A patient undergoing suctioning

    e. A patient having a severe asthma attack or deterioration of chronic lung disease

    f. A drowning victim (page 11.18)

16. The spine-injured patient with weakness or partial paralysis of the respiratory muscles does not have the strength to inhale deeply. Thus, his tidal volume will be smaller than normal, so his minute volume will also **decrease**, leading to an **increase** in his arterial PCO_2. (page 11.11)

17. **a. (1)** Aphonia

    (2) Universal distress signal (clutching the throat)

    (3) Dusky or cyanotic skin

    (4) Exaggerated or ineffectual breathing movements (page 11.25)

    b. The steps of treating a conscious choking victim are as follows:

    (1) Determine if obstruction is complete (can he talk?). If not, encourage him to cough.

    (2) But *if obstruction is complete:* use the Heimlich maneuver.

    (3) Keep repeating steps 1 and 2 until successful or until victim loses consciousness. (page 11.25)

18. Wow, when don't you give oxygen? Oxygen helps patients more than anything. It is your number one drug to use!

    a. Shock

    b. Severe pain

    c. Respiratory distress

    d. Partial airway obstruction

    e. Any time the patient is intubated

    f. Asthma patients

    g. Any time patient is confused

    h. Stroke patients

    i. Any type of trauma

    Of course, this is a partial list and just about anything will go for this question!

19. There are many signs of respiratory distress. *Always* give oxygen to the patient in respiratory distress.

    a. Shallow or labored breathing

   b. Retractions of the intercostal muscles

   c. Cyanosis

   d. Wheezing or stridor (page 11.25)

20. Endotracheal intubation is indicated when:

   a. Patient has no gag reflex and is unconscious.

   b. Patient is in cardiac arrest.

   c. Patient is unable to protect own airway. (page 11.52)

21. For the patient found in *respiratory acidosis* (the heroin overdose), the treatment is to assist ventilations to improve the minute volume and blow off the excess CO_2. (page 11.13)

Word Find

1. Imagine you are an oxygen molecule floating past someone's face, minding your own business, just as that person is starting to take a deep breath. As his **diaphragm** and **intercostals** contract, the volume of his chest increases, so the pressure inside the chest (intrathoracic pressure) decreases. As a consequence, air is sucked in through the **nares**, and you are swept along with it.

   After having a shower and completing a security check in the nasal hairs, you enter the **pharynx**. You then proceed down the **larynx**, through the **glottis**, and into the **trachea**. (Had you gone down the esophagus instead, you would eventually have been expelled from the stomach as part of a **burp**.) Moving a little farther, you find yourself at a crossroads, called the **carina**, where you can either take a left turn into the left **bronchus** or a right turn into the right **bronchus**. You choose the straighter, shorter path, to the **right**. The airway in which you are traveling branches many times into smaller and smaller **bronchioles**, until finally you reach a tiny sac at the end of the road, an **alveolus**. There you find the first opportunity to cross a membrane into a capillary and board a red blood cell for the journey to peripheral tissues. (Up to this point in your journey, you have been traveling only in **dead space**, that is, the part of the airway where gas exchange does not take place.)

   Some of your friends who started the journey with you did not make it as far as you did. One of them accidentally tickled the throat on his way down the airway and got expelled with gale force by a **cough**, which is the airway's most powerful mechanism for eliminating foreign material. Another of your colleagues found himself recruited into a hiccup, also known as **singultus**.

   Yet another friend of yours made the journey all the way down the airway only to find the air spaces at the end of the line collapsed, a situation called **atelectasis**. It had come about when a little bleb on the surface of the lung ruptured, allowing air to enter the space between the visceral and parietal **pleura**, and thereby creating a small **pneumothorax**. The net effect was that blood reaching the collapsed alveoli could not pick up any **oxygen** like yourself, but rather had to return to the left heart as if it had never passed through the lungs at all, a situation called **shunt**. If a very large proportion of alveoli are nonfunctional (eg, collapsed, filled with fluids), a large part of the blood circulating through the lungs will be similarly affected, and the person's arterial PO_2 will fall below normal (ie, below about 60 mm Hg), a condition known as **hypoxemia**.

   Sometimes scattered alveoli collapse simply because a person doesn't take deep enough breaths to keep all his alveoli inflated. The body therefore has a mechanism to help periodically pop open collapsed alveoli, and that is to **sigh**. Do so now, before you proceed to the next question. (pages 11.6 and 11.7)

2. The exchange of gases among the tissues, lungs, and atmosphere is called **respiration**. The movement of air in and out of the lungs (more specifically, the flushing of **carbon dioxide** out of the lungs by breathing) is called **ventilation**, and its effectiveness is determined by the volume of air inhaled or exhaled each minute, that is, the **minute volume** (= respiratory rate × **tidal volume**). If that volume of air inhaled each minute is *less* than normal, the arterial PCO_2 **rises**, and the blood gases show **hypercarbia** (excess CO_2 in the blood). We call that situation **hypoventilation**, that is, breathing that is insufficient to remove excess CO_2 from the body. The most extreme example occurs when a person is not breathing at all (respiratory arrest, or **apnea**).

On the other hand, when someone breathes very deeply or very rapidly (or both), his PCO_2 will fall; that is, he will develop **hypocarbia**. We refer to that situation—when excessive breathing lowers the PCO_2 below about 35 mm Hg—as **hyperventilation**. (pages 11.14–11.16)

Fill-in-the-Table

1. Knowing *when* to deploy a piece of equipment is just as important as knowing *how* to deploy it.

	Oropharyngeal Airway	**Nasopharyngeal Airway**
Use for:	Deeply unconscious patient who has no gag reflex, especially if being ventilated by bag-mask device Bite-block for intubated patient	Patient with an altered mental status
Do not use for:	Patient with intact gag reflex	Patient with trauma to the nose Suspected basilar skull fracture (blood or clear fluid draining from nose)

(page 11.32)

2.

Device	**Flow Rate**	**Oxygen Delivered**
Nasal cannula	1–6 L/min	24%–44%
Nonrebreathing mask	15 L/min	24%–44%
Bag-mask device with reservoir	15 L/min – flush	Nearly 100%

(page 11.38)

3. Every piece of equipment in the ambulance has its indications and sometimes contraindications. You need to be aware of both.

Adjunct	**Indicated for:**	**Do not use in:**
Oropharyngeal airway	Airway maintenance in deeply unconscious, breathing patient To improve effectiveness of bag-mask ventilation	Patient who is not deeply unconscious Severe trauma in the mouth Any patient with intact gag reflex
Combitube	Cardiac arrest when it is not feasible to intubate the trachea Patient who has swallowed corrosives	Patient who is not deeply unconscious
LMA	Cardiac arrest when it is not feasible to intubate the trachea	Patient who has food in his stomach and may aspirate
Endotracheal intubation	Cardiac arrest Deep coma Absent gag reflex Imminent danger of upper airway obstruction (eg, respiratory burns)	Patients with intact gag reflex or likelihood of laryngospasm

(pages 11.32, 11.52–53, 11.85, 11.88–90)

Skill Drills

1. *Nasogastric Tube Insertion in a Conscious Patient* (page 11.50)

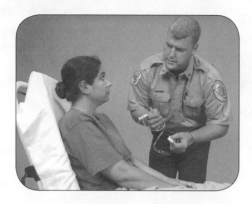

Step 1: Explain the procedure to the patient, and oxygenate the patient if necessary. Ensure that the patient's head is in a neutral position and suppress the gag reflex with a topical anesthetic spray.

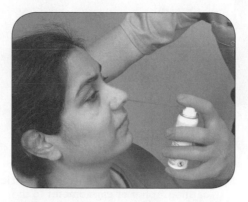

Step 2: Constrict the blood vessels in the nares with a topical alpha agonist.

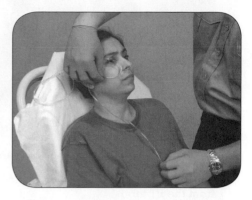

Step 3: Measure the tube for the correct depth of insertion (nose to ear to xiphoid process.)

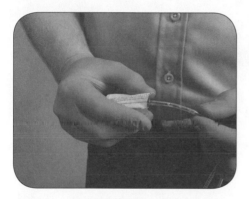

Step 4: Lubricate the tube with a water-soluble gel.

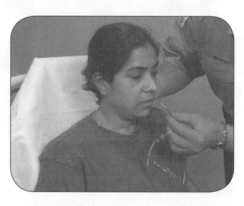

Step 5: Advance the tube gently along the nasal floor.

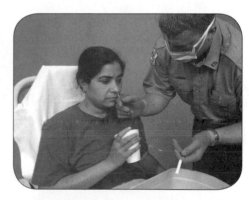

Step 6: Encourage the patient to swallow or drink to facilitate passage of the tube.

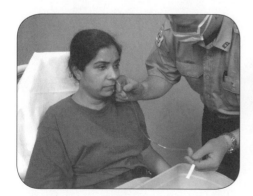

Step 7: Advance the tube into the stomach.

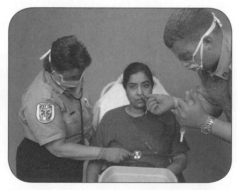

Step 8: Confirm proper placement: auscultate over the epigastrium while injecting 30 to 50 mL of air and/or observe for gastric contents in the tube. There should be no reflux around the tube.

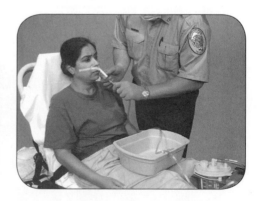

Step 9: Apply suction to the tube to aspirate the gastric contents, and secure the tube in place.

2. *Using Colorimetric Capriography for Carbion Dioxide Detection* (page 11.61)

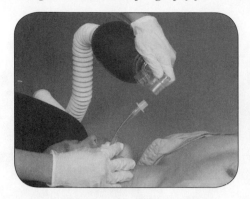

Step 1: Detach the ventilation device from the ET tube.

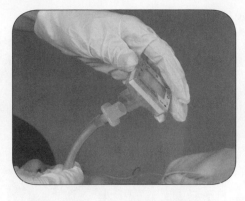

Step 2: Attach an in-line colorimetric capnographer or capnometer to the proximal adapter of the ET tube.

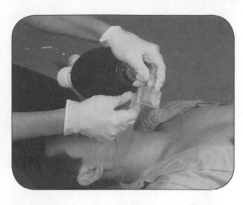

Step 3: Reattach the ventilation device to the ET tube, and resume ventilations.

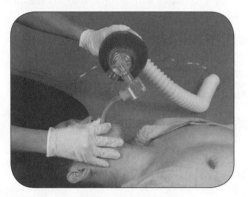

Step 4: Monitor the device for appropriate reading (appropriate color change or digital reading).

Section 2 Case Study: Answers and Summary

1. What initial management is indicated for this patient?

- Positive pressure ventilations (bag-valve-mask device or pocket-mask device)
  - This patient has multiple signs of inadequate breathing, including confusion, rapid and labored respirations, inability to speak in full sentences, and perioral cyanosis.
  - Tidal volume is needed and can only be provided with the use of positive pressure ventilatory support.
  - Consider placing a nasopharyngeal airway if the patient's level of consciousness further decreases.

2. What is your interpretation of this cardiac rhythm?

The cardiac rhythm depicted is *atrial fibrillation*, which is characterized by an irregularly irregular rhythm and the absence of discernable P waves (**Figure 2-1**).

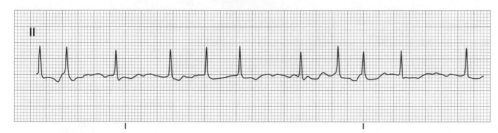

■ **Figure 2-1** Your patient's cardiac rhythm.

Atrial fibrillation is caused by multiple ectopic foci in the atria that discharge in a chaotic fashion. Many of the impulses are blocked at the AV junction, while others are allowed to pass through. This randomized impulse passage through the AV junction causes the ventricular rhythm in atrial fibrillation to be irregularly irregular.

Atrial fibrillation is often seen with conditions such as congestive heart failure and COPD (eg, emphysema) and is commonly caused by pulmonary hypertension with subsequent atrial dilation.

3. What is your field impression of this patient?

This patient is suffering from an *acute exacerbation of emphysema* and is quickly approaching complete respiratory failure. The following assessment findings support this field impression:

- History of emphysema, no doubt attributed to his history of cigarette smoking, is characterized by the barrel-shaped appearance of his chest.
- Recent flu-like symptoms, which indicate a possible respiratory tract infection, the most common precursor to acute exacerbation of COPD.
- Temperature of 101.5° F, which confirms the presence of an infection.
- Acute worsening of his shortness of breath, which is classic in COPD exacerbation following an acute respiratory tract infection.

Emphysema falls within a myriad of conditions collectively called COPD. Other forms of COPD include chronic bronchitis, and, to a lesser degree, asthma, which is more of an episodic disease rather than a chronic one.

Emphysema is a progressive, irreversible pulmonary disease that is most often attributed to a history of long-term cigarette smoking or repeated exposure to other toxic substances. The incidence of emphysema is much higher in men than in women.

Emphysema results in gradual destruction of the alveolar walls due to a loss of pulmonary surfactant, which decreases the surface area of the alveolar membrane and interferes with gas exchange in the lungs. Additionally, the number of pulmonary capillaries decreases, which increases the resistance to pulmonary blood flow. This process ultimately

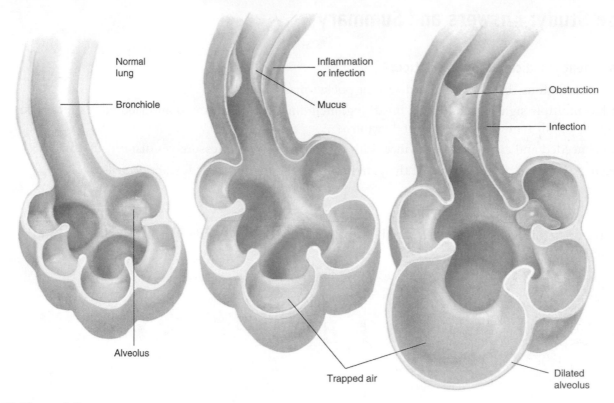

Normal lung

Bronchiole

Alveolus

Inflammation or infection

Mucus

Trapped air

Obstruction

Infection

Dilated alveolus

■ **Figure 2-2** Pulmonary infections in already damaged airways.

causes pulmonary hypertension, which may lead to right-sided heart failure (cor pulmonale). Because the right side of the heart must pump against a high-pressure gradient, atrial dilation may occur, thus resulting in atrial fibrillation.

Emphysema also weakens the walls of the small bronchioles, which, in combination with alveolar wall destruction, decreases the ability of the lungs to effectively recoil during exhalation. This causes air to become trapped in the lungs, giving the person's chest a characteristic barrel-shaped appearance. Frequent pulmonary infections further the degree of air trapping because of inflammation and mucous production within the bronchioles (**Figure 2-2**).

The destruction of lung tissue causes the alveoli to collapse (atelectasis). The patient attempts to compensate for this by breathing through pursed lips, thus creating an effect similar to that of positive-end expiratory pressure (PEEP).

As the degenerative process of emphysema continues, the partial pressure of oxygen in the arterial blood (PaO_2) decreases and remains chronically low. This stimulates red blood cell production, perhaps even to excessive levels (polycythemia), which would explain why the patient's skin remains pink (pink puffer) despite inadequate pulmonary gas exchange. The presence of cyanosis, therefore, would indicate severe hypoxia in patients with emphysema, more so than if it were present in an otherwise healthy person.

Patients with COPD tend to retain carbon dioxide and, therefore, have a chronically elevated partial pressure of arterial carbon dioxide ($PaCO_2$). Chemoreceptors that monitor the levels of oxygen in carbon dioxide in the body eventually become accustomed to this, and the respiratory center in the brain (medulla oblongata) stops using increased $PaCO_2$ levels to regulate breathing, as it does in an otherwise healthy person. This activates a mechanism called the hypoxic drive, which increases breathing stimulation when PaO_2 levels fall and inhibits breathing stimulation when PaO_2 levels increase. In rare cases, the administration of high-concentration oxygen, which can quickly increase PaO_2 levels, may cause the chemoreceptors to stop stimulating the respiratory centers, resulting in hypoventilation or even apnea. If this occurs, simply assist the patient's ventilations. Never withhold oxygen from a hypoxic patient, even in the face of this potential, although highly uncommon, threat.

Patients with emphysema are predisposed to lower respiratory tract infections such as pneumonia because of their diminished ability to effectively expel secretions from the lungs. In addition, hypoxia-related cardiac dysrhythmias may occur.

Patients with emphysema and COPD in general learn to live with their chronic illness on a daily basis and grow accustomed to the normal respiratory distress and physical limitations that accompany it. When they call EMS, something has changed for the worst.

The signs and symptoms of emphysema are summarized in **Table 2-1**.

Table 2-1 Signs and Symptoms of Emphysema

Barrel-chest appearance	Pink skin color
Nonproductive cough	Wheezing and rhonchi
Severe exertional dyspnea	Pursed-lip breathing (prolonged inspiration)

4. Are the patient's vital signs and SAMPLE history consistent with your field impression?

The patient's vital signs do not reinforce a field impression of COPD exacerbation as much as his medical history does. In particular, the recent flu-like symptoms that preceded an acute exacerbation of his respiratory distress make this a classic case.

Because this patient takes numerous medications, each of which is used to treat different conditions, it would be worthwhile to briefly review each of them.

- Albuterol (Ventolin, Proventil)
  - Selective beta2-agonist that dilates the bronchioles and is thus used to treat diseases associated with bronchiole constriction and/or inflammation, such as asthma, emphysema, and bronchitis
- Lanoxin (Digoxin, Digitalis)
  - A cardiac glycoside that is used for, among other conditions, ventricular rate control in patients with chronic atrial fibrillation
- Warfarin (Coumadin)
  - An anticoagulant commonly prescribed as prophylactic therapy to patients with atrial fibrillation who are prone to developing microemboli (small clots) when blood stagnates in the poorly contracting atria
- Methyldopa (Aldomet)
  - A centrally acting antiadrenergic used in the treatment of hypertension. Its active metabolite, alpha-methylnorepinephrine, lowers the blood pressure by stimulating central inhibitory alpha-adrenergic receptors and reducing plasma levels of renin. Renin is a proteolytic enzyme of the kidney that plays a major role in the release of angiotensin, a potent vasoconstrictor.

5. What specific treatment is required for this patient's condition?

■ Endotracheal intubation

- If the paramedic has difficulty providing effective ventilations utilizing basic means (bag-valve-mask device, pocket-mask device), endotracheal intubation should be performed to facilitate administration of 100% oxygen directly into the patient's lungs and more definitively protect the patient's airway.
- As evidenced by the patient's falling oxygen saturation level and markedly diminished level of consciousness, it is clear that bag-valve-mask ventilation is not providing adequate oxygenation.
- Because of the patient's already diminished level of consciousness, a hypnotic-sedative drug (Versed, Etomidate) may be all that is required in order to facilitate intubation. If, however, sedation alone is not effective, a neuromuscular blocker (paralytic) may be needed to perform rapid sequence intubation (RSI).
  - When inducing paralysis with medications, succinylcholine (Anectine) is the preferred initial agent to use. Succinylcholine has a duration of action of only 3 to 5 minutes, which means that if intubation is unsuccessful, you will not have to ventilate the patient with a BVM device for a prolonged period of time. Succinylcholine does, however, depolarize potassium ions, which produces muscular fasciculations (generalized muscle

twitching). Therefore, use of a nondepolarizing paralytic, such as vecuronium (Norcuron) in a premedication, or priming, dose prior to inducing full neuromuscular blockade with succinylcholine is advisable. Once intubation is *successfully performed and confirmed,* neuromuscular blockade can be maintained with a longer-acting paralytic, especially if your transport time is going to be prolonged. Again, vecuronium, which has a 45-minute duration of action, would be an appropriate drug to use.

- Follow locally established protocols regarding the use and doses of neuromuscular blockers for RSI.

■ **Pharmacologic interventions**

- *Aerosolized bronchodilators* can be administered endotracheally with a small-volume inline nebulizer. The following medications can be given alone, or in combination:
  - Selective beta2-adrenergic agonists, such as albuterol (Ventolin, Proventil), metaproterenol (Alupent), or isoetharine (Bronkosol)
  - Anticholinergic bronchodilators such as ipratropium (Atrovent)
    – When used in combination with beta agonists, the beta agonist must be administered first, followed by a 5-minute interval prior to administering Atrovent.
  - Aerosolized bronchodilators, because of their rapid onset of action (3 to 5 minutes), would be the preferred initial pharmacologic intervention because of the severity of the patient's condition. The significant bronchoconstriction, which is impairing effective positive pressure ventilation in this patient, must be reversed as soon as possible. Follow locally established protocols regarding the dose of endotracheally administered bronchodilators.
- *Intravenous glucosteroids*
  - Methylprednisolone (Solu-Medrol): Reduces acute and chronic inflammation and potentiates the relaxation of bronchiole smooth muscle caused by beta-adrenergic agonists.
    – Solu-Medrol has an onset of action of approximately 1 to 2 hours. The adult dose varies, and usually ranges from 40 to 125 mg IV.

The goal in treating patients with acute COPD decompensation—or any lower airway disorder for that matter—is to correct hypoxemia and to relieve the bronchoconstriction that is causing the hypoxemia. These actions will prevent respiratory failure and subsequent cardiac arrest.

Administration of 100% supplemental oxygen is the first and most important intervention. Oxygen may be given with a nonrebreathing mask or via positive pressure ventilatory support if the patient's respiratory effort is inadequate.

Medications, administered either by aerosol or IV or both, are needed to relax the smooth muscles of the lower airways, thus improving ventilation and facilitating oxygenation.

6. Is further treatment required for this patient?

By improving this patient's oxygenation status, his level of consciousness has improved, and he is now resisting the endotracheal tube. Because of the potential for vomiting and aspiration following removal of the endotracheal tube and the possibility that his condition could worsen, he should remain intubated. Extubation in the field (unless done by the patient) is not commonly performed. For patient comfort and to prevent field extubation by the patient, consider administering additional doses of a long-acting paralytic (eg, Norcuron) and/or keep the patient sedated with the appropriate medications (Versed, Valium).

Although his oxygen saturation of 92% is slightly low, it may be as good as it gets for this chronically ill patient, and is still better than 81%! Continue to monitor his ventilatory status, oxygen saturation, and electrocardiogram. He is still prone to cardiac dysrhythmias.

7. Are there any special considerations for this patient?

As previously mentioned, patients with COPD have chronically low PaO_2 levels and are stimulated to breathe based on these levels (hypoxic drive).

If high concentrations of oxygen are administered, the respiratory centers in the brain may be fooled into thinking that the patient is adequately oxygenated and will therefore send messages to the respiratory muscles to decrease the rate and strength of breathing. Oxygen-induced hypoventilation or apnea occurs in less than 3% to 5% of patients with COPD. Should this rare event occur, simply provide positive pressure ventilatory support. Never withhold oxygen from a hypoxic patient!

Summary

When patients with chronic respiratory disease call EMS, a significant change has occurred in their condition. Otherwise your assistance would not have been requested.

Due to the nature of their illness, patients with COPD typically have a baseline respiratory distress; however, they cannot live with *severe* hypoxia any better than a healthy person would.

An acute lower respiratory tract infection, such as pneumonia, in which the patient cannot effectively expel secretions from their lungs, is the most common precursor to exacerbation of COPD. The mucous production and bronchiole inflammation that accompany many respiratory infections only worsens the patient's hypoxia.

You must perform a careful, systematic assessment of the patient and provide the appropriate treatment in a timely manner. It is critical that you recognize the difference between an adequately and inadequately breathing patient.

Prehospital care focuses on ensuring adequate oxygenation and ventilation and pharmacologically reversing bronchoconstriction. Definitive care includes treating the underlying cause of the exacerbation, which usually involves antibiotics to treat the underlying infection. If the patient begins to show signs of respiratory failure, such as a rapidly falling oxygen saturation level or decreasing level of consciousness, use sedating agents and neuromuscular blocking medications to intubate the patient without delay.

Section 3: Patient Assessment
Chapter 12: Patient History

Matching

(page 12.14)

1. A	**8.** A
2. A	**9.** A
3. B	**10.** A
4. A	**11.** A
5. A	**12.** A
6. B	**13.** A
7. B	

Multiple Choice

1. B (page 12.9)	**6.** D (page 12.17)
2. C (page 12.11)	**7.** C (page 12.17)
3. A (page 12.13)	**8.** B (page 12.20)
4. D (page 12.15)	**9.** A (page 12.18, 12.19)
5. B (page 12.16)	**10.** C (page 12.20)

Labeling

1. S	**5.** NS
2. NS	**6.** S
3. S	**7.** S
4. NS	**8.** NS

Fill-in-the-Blank

1. Field diagnosis (page 12.6)

2. Introduce yourself (page 12.7)

3. Present illness (page 12.8)

4. Eye level (page 12.10)

5. Face to face (page 12.20)

6. Empathy (page 12.12)

7. Reflection (page 12.11)

8. HIPPA (page 12.9)

9. Medical history (page 12.10)

10. Orderly, systematic (page 12.4)

Ambulance Calls

1. Accident scenes like the one pictured in this question are fairly characteristic of those you will actually encounter in your work. You can learn a lot from the scene and the people there if you know what to look for and what to ask.

    a. The potential sources of information about what happened to the patient at the scene are:

        (1) The scene itself

        (2) The patient

        (3) The bystanders at the bus stop and perhaps in the diner

        (4) Any medical identification devices the patient might be carrying

b. From observing the scene, you can tell that

   (1) The driver was driving somewhat erratically.

   (2) Something caused him to swerve off the road (perhaps he saw something in the road or thought he saw something).

   (3) The driver was conscious when he went off the road (he was able to apply the brakes).

   (4) Massive forces were involved in the accident (enough to break the telephone pole).

   (5) The driver struck his head against the windshield.

c. It is necessary to take a history

   (1) To find out what happened. *Why* did he swerve off the road? Did something cross his path? Did he suddenly feel ill?

   (2) To find out what hurts, that is, to start searching for his most serious injuries.

   (3) To find out whether he has any underlying medical problems that might complicate his care. If, for example, he is taking anticoagulant drugs (drugs that interfere with blood clotting) after a previous heart attack, he could lose a great deal of blood from what might otherwise be a fairly minor wound.

   (4) To gather information that might otherwise be unavailable to the hospital staff, such as data on the mechanisms of injury.

d. Before you start taking the history, you need to

   (1) Clear your mind of any preconceived ideas about the patient (eg, "He must have been drunk.").

   (2) Introduce yourself, and explain your role.

   (3) Find out the patient's name.

   (4) Try to position yourself at the patient's level—lean over or crouch down near the car window.

   (5) Initiate some physical contact, for example, put a hand on the patient's shoulder and instruct him not to move until you have examined him.

True/False

1. T (page 12.14)   **6.** T (page 12.17)

2. F (page 12.16)   **7.** T (page 12.17)

3. F (page 12.15)   **8.** F (page 12.6)

4. T (page 12.16)   **9.** F (page 12.10)

5. T (page 12.16)   **10.** T (page 12. 11)

Short Answer

1. a. In eliciting the history of the present illness from a patient whose chief complaint is "pain in my gut," one would want to know at least the following:

   (1) Did anything in particular provoke the pain? What brought it on? Does anything make it worse? Does anything make it better?

   (2) What is the quality of the pain? What is it like?

   (3) Does the pain radiate anywhere? Where is it precisely?

   (4) How severe is the pain?

   (5) What was the timing of the pain; that is, when did it come on? Has it been there constantly since, or does it come and go?

   (6) Are there any associated symptoms, such as nausea, vomiting, diarrhea, constipation? (page 12.8)

b. In inquiring about the patient's *other medical history,* you need to find out the following:

   (1) Does he have any major underlying medical problems? One way to find out is to ask, "Are you presently under a doctor's care for any condition?"

   (2) Does he take any medications regularly?

   (3) Does he have any allergies?

   (4) Does he have a family doctor, or does he go regularly to a particular hospital? (page 12.14)

2. In taking the history of a head-injured patient, you need to find out the following. *Students should provide five of the following:*

   a. The circumstances of the accident: How did the injury occur? What were the mechanisms of injury?

   b. Whether the patient lost consciousness at any point. If so, when? For how long?

   c. Whether the patient vomited.

   d. What the patient's current symptoms are (assuming he is conscious and can tell you).

e. Whether the patient has ingested drugs or alcohol within the past few hours.

f. Whether the patient has any significant underlying illnesses. (page 12.8)

3. The four questions you need to answer in making your survey of the scene are the following:

a. Is it safe for me to approach the victim(s)?

b. Is there any hazard to the patient?

c. Am I going to need any help?

d. Do I need any special equipment to reach the patient?

If you do *not* ask and answer those questions at every incident scene, your career as a paramedic may be very short indeed, for you will not notice the downed high-tension line draped over the car, or the little trail of fire creeping toward the vehicle, or the bus about to plow into the disabled vehicle that is still in the middle of the road. (page 12.7)

4. Possible sources of information about what happened to the patient include the following:

a. The patient himself (the most important source if the patient is conscious)

b. Bystanders or family

c. The scene (mechanisms of injury)

d. Medical identification devices (page 12.7)

Word Find

Signs

1. Halitosis
2. Swelling
3. Pallor
4. Cyanosis
5. Jaundice
6. Tachypnea
7. Bruise
8. Distended neck veins
9. Hypotension
10. Stridor
11. Fever
12. Wheezing
13. Rash
14. Black eye
15. Burp
16. Apnea
17. Dilated pupils

Symptoms

1. Sore throat
2. Nausea
3. Pain
4. Headache
5. Dizzy spell
6. Dyspnea
7. Chest pain
8. Fatigue
9. Indigestion
10. Heartburn
11. Earache
12. Hunger
13. Thirst
14. Stomachache
15. Itch
16. Cramps
17. The blahs

Were you able to sort out symptoms from signs? One way to do so is to consider that you can take a history (ie, elicit all the patient's *symptoms*) over the telephone, without ever seeing the patient. On the other hand, you can observe all of the patient's *signs* even if the patient cannot communicate.

Fill-in-the-Table

1. (page 12.12)

Layman's Lingo	EMS Lingo
My sugars	I'm a diabetic
Fell out	Had a syncopal episode
Has the fits	History of seizures
Water pills	Furosemide (Lasix)

Chapter 13: Physical Examination

Matching

Observing the condition of the patient's skin can give you a great deal of information about his or her cardiovascular status, state of oxygenation, and level of stress. (page 13.11)

1. B   **3.** C
2. D   **4.** A

The funny little noises issuing from a patient's airway and lungs can be very informative. (pages 13.22–13.23)

1. D   **4.** B
2. E   **5.** C
3. A

Spotting abnormal physical signs is only part of physical assessment; the other part is drawing the correct conclusions from those signs.

1. I   **10.** S
2. J, M   **11.** O
3. D, O, U   **12.** C
4. A, G, V   **13.** R
5. T   **14.** F
6. J, L   **15.** Q
7. N, C   **16.** H
8. K, L   **17.** E
9. B   **18.** P

Multiple Choice

1. D (page 13.4)   **6.** A (page 13.31)
2. B (page 13.8)   **7.** B (page 13.36)
3. A (page 13.9)   **8.** C (page 13.25)
4. C (page 13.10)   **9.** D (page 13.41)
5. C (page 13.12)   **10.** C (page 13.12)

Labeling

1. Nine regions of the abdomen (page 13.27)

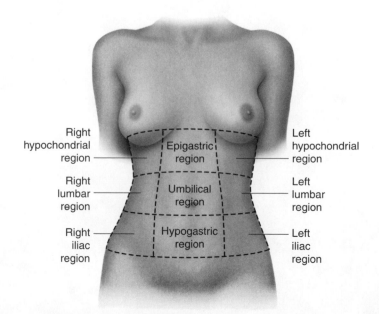

Right hypochondrial region

Epigastric region

Left hypochondrial region

Right lumbar region

Umbilical region

Left lumbar region

Right iliac region

Hypogastric region

Left iliac region

2. Lymphatic system (page 13.35)

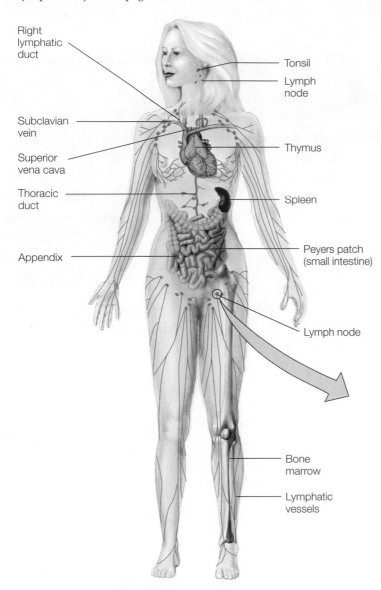

Right
lymphatic
duct

Tonsil

Lymph
node

Subclavian
vein

Thymus

Superior
vena cava

Thoracic
duct

Spleen

Appendix

Peyers patch
(small intestine)

Lymph node

Bone
marrow

Lymphatic
vessels

Fill-in-the-Blank

1. Vital signs (page 13.6)

2. Ophthalmoscope (page 13.9)

3. Skin (page 13.11)

4. Midsized, dilate, constrict (page 13.14)

5. Pulmonary evaluation (page 13.20)

6. Low wheezes (page 13.22)

7. Systole, diastole (page 13.24)

8. Relevant history (page 13.27)

9. Ascites (page 13.29)

10. Intraperitoneal, extraperitoneal (page 13.27)

Identify

1. Chief complaint: Pain in abdomen
2. Vital signs: Alert; skin pale, cool; lungs clear; respirations 20 breaths/min; oxygen saturation is 98%. Blood pressure is 100/78 mm Hg; sinus tachycardia; bounding pulse at 112 beats/min. Pain is 8 on a scale of 1 to 10. Guarding in abdomen.
3. Pertinent negatives: No period for 5 weeks, no vaginal bleeding, no allergies or medications. Two normal births.

Ambulance Calls

   a. **(1)** How far did Jake fall?

      (2) Did he lose consciousness or did they see a change in mental status before the emergency medical technicians (EMTs) arrived?

      (3) Has he vomited or been nauseated?

      (4) Did he move at all since the fall?

      (5) Does he have any allergies or take any medications?

      (6) Has he ever had any injuries before?

   b. Suction, inspect the mouth and nose, check for cerebrospinal fluid (CSF), and apply oxygen.

   c. No, because it is a high break, and his level of consciousness is okay, the splint should have been in place before placing him on the backboard to avoid any more injury to the arm.

   d. Because there is nothing sticking out, cover it with an occlusive dressing, and be very careful when placing him on the backboard.

   e. Jake could have a punctured lung or damaged spinal cord. There is no way of knowing what structures the nail has entered. Check lung sounds often to make sure needle decompression is not needed.

   f. Do a detailed physical exam to discover and treat any secondary injuries.

   g. Jake could have head injuries, punctured lungs, spinal injuries, and blunt force trauma to his abdomen. Remember what organs are in this region and how they can bleed.

True/False

1. F (page 13.44)	**6.** F (page 13.34)
2. T (page 13.43)	**7.** F (page 13.32)
3. T (page 13.43)	**8.** T (page 13.30)
4. F (page 13.39)	**9.** T (page 13.26)
5. T (page 13.36)	**10.** F (page 13.6)

Short Answer

1. Physical assessment is all about looking for *signs* of illness or injury, irrespective of what the patient may or may not have told you. In assessing the patient's general appearance, take note of the following:

   a. The position in which the patient is found

   b. The patient's level of consciousness/mental status

   c. The patient's behavior and degree of distress

   d. Any obvious wounds or deformities

   e. The skin CTC (color, temperature, condition) (page 13.10)

2. In assessing a patient's level of consciousness, you want to use quantifiable measurements, that is, measurements that can be replicated by others. Thus, you must observe and describe the patient's level of consciousness in terms of specific responses to specific stimuli. In the case of the patient described here, you would ask questions such as, "What is your full name? date of birth? address? Do you know where you are? Do you know today's date?" and record the answers. You would also record whether the speech was in any way slurred or garbled. (page 13.10)

3. The particular numbers you obtained in measuring a classmate's vital signs will, of course, differ. But in reporting your results, you should have mentioned not only the numbers but also the other salient characteristics of the vital signs. For example:

   a. Temperature: 98°F orally

      Pulse: 80 beats/min, full, and regular

      Respirations: 16 breaths/min, regular, unlabored

      Blood pressure: 120/80 mm Hg

In general, when assessing the vital signs, pay attention to the following:

Vital Signs

- Temperature (usually estimated only)
- Pulse
  1. Rate
  2. Force
  3. Rhythm (regular or irregular)
- Respirations
  1. Rate
  2. Rhythm
  3. Ease
  4. Depth
  5. Abnormal noises
  6. Abnormal breath odors
- Blood pressure

   b. An *alternative method for measuring the blood pressure* is by palpation of the radial pulse. Inflate the blood pressure cuff above the estimated systolic pressure. Keep a finger on the radial pulse as you slowly deflate the cuff. The point at which you begin to feel a radial pulse is the systolic blood pressure (the needle on the pressure gauge should start to bounce at that point as well).(page 13.6)

   c. The reason for not removing your fingers from the radial pulse when counting the respirations is to give the patient the impression you are still counting the pulse. As soon as a person becomes aware that his or her breathing is under scrutiny, it becomes very difficult to breathe naturally, and the respiratory rate may change. Thus, it's preferable that the patient not know you are counting his or her breaths. (page 13.7)

4. You can often obtain an extraordinary amount of information from the patient's vital signs. Indeed, some experts in prehospital care argue that there is no need for the paramedic to gather any data about the patient *other than* the vital signs because they provide enough information to decide whether the patient's condition warrants urgent treatment and transport.

Pulse = 120 beats/min, thready, and regular
Respirations = 20 breaths/min, shallow, slightly labored
Blood pressure = 72 mm Hg systolic (by palpation)

   a. The vital signs are **abnormal.**

   b. The pulse is very rapid (tachycardia) and weak, the respirations are at the upper limit of normal (tachypnea) and shallow, and the blood pressure is low (severe hypotension).

   c. These vital signs are typical of hypovolemic shock, and few if any other conditions produce this picture. For confirmation, examine the skin (what would you expect the skin to show in shock?), consider the mechanisms of injury, and so on.

5. Pulse = 72 beats/min, full, and regular
Respirations = 4 breaths/min and snoring
Blood pressure = 110/70 mm Hg

   a. These vital signs are **abnormal.**

   b. The respirations are extremely slow! (The snoring indicates that the airway is also partially obstructed by the tongue, which can happen only in deep sleep or coma.)

   c. From the vital signs only, you can conclude that something has depressed the patient's respirations.

   d. Given the additional information that his pupils are extremely constricted, you could reasonably assume that the most likely cause of the patient's respiratory depression is an overdose of a narcotic drug.

6. Pulse = 60 beats/min, full, slightly irregular
Respirations = 30 breaths/min and deep; no unusual odors on the breath
Blood pressure = 200/140 mm Hg

   a. These vital signs are **abnormal.**

   b. The pulse is borderline, the respirations are abnormally rapid (tachypnea) and deep (hyperpnea), and the blood pressure is extremely high (severe hypertension).

   c. As discussed in a later chapter, this constellation of vital signs is apt to be present in any condition—medical or traumatic—that produces swelling of the brain (cerebral edema).

   d. The finding of unequal pupils serves to substantiate the assumption that the patient has cerebral edema from some cause.

7. Pulse = 56 beats/min, full, and regular

Respirations = 12 breaths/min and unlabored

Blood pressure = 120/65 mm Hg

This set of vital signs underscores the importance of knowing the context in which the vitals were obtained.

    a. They may be normal or **abnormal.**

    b. If they were taken from an Olympic athlete at rest, they are undoubtedly normal. If they were taken from a middle-aged man suffering chest pain, you would tend to be very concerned about a pulse of 56 beats/min.

    c. You would say the patient had a bradycardia and very probably give him atropine to speed up his heart.

8. Signs of skull fracture include the following:

    a. Ecchymoses behind the ears (Battle's sign)

    b. Ecchymoses around the eyes ("raccoon's eyes")

    c. Leakage of clear fluid (CSF) or blood from the nose or ears

    d. Obvious depression in the skull

Crossword Puzzles

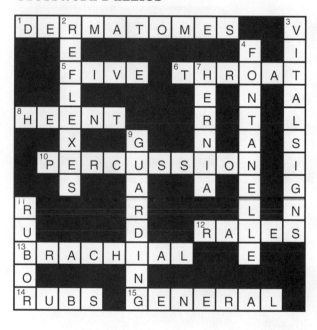

Fill-in-the-Table

1.

Body Region	Trauma Patient	Medical Patient
Head	**Bleeding, scalp depression;** blood or fluid draining from the ears or nose; **eye movements; pupillary signs;** blood, vomitus, or foreign **material in mouth; blue lips**	Facial **asymmetry; icterus; pupillary signs; pallor** of the conjunctivae; **cyanosis** of the lips
Neck	**Tracheal deviation, tenderness, deformity, jugular distention**	**Jugular distention**
Chest	**Bruises, asymmetry, unequal breath sounds**	**Abnormal shape,** abnormal **breath sounds**
Abdomen	**Distention, masses, ecchymoses,** presence of **bowel sounds, rigidity**	**Distention, bowel sounds, tenderness, rigidity**
Back	**Bruises, wounds, spinal tenderness**	Edema
Extremities	**Deformity, bruises, movement, sensation, capillary refill**	**Edema,** equality of **pulses, strength, sensation**

(page 13.13)

2. When you assess an injured patient from head to toe, it helps to know what you are looking for! (page 13.13)

Body Region	What I Will Be Looking for in Particular (in addition to DCAP-BTLS)
Head	Deformity, lacerations, CSF leak, Battle's sign, maxillofacial injury
Neck	Open wounds, subcutaneous emphysema, tracheal deviation, jugular distention, bruises over cervical spine
Chest	Bruises, open wounds, instability, inequality of breath sounds, dullness or hyperresonance
Abdomen	Contusions, open wounds, evisceration, distention, rigidity, cough rebound
Extremities	Deformity, swelling, ecchymoses, pulses, movement, sensation
Back/buttocks	DCAP-BTLS

Skill Drills

1. Examining the Nervous System (page 13.41)

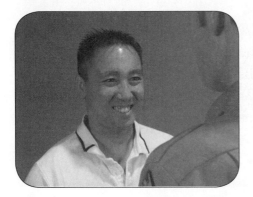

Step 1: Evaluate cranial nerve function.

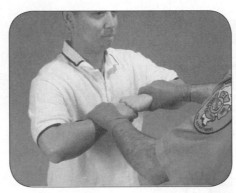

Step 2: Evaluate the patient's neuro-muscular status by checking muscle strength against resistance.

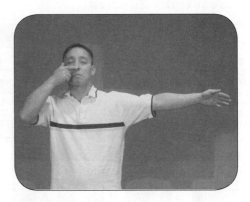

Step 3: Evaluate the patient's coordination by performing the finger-to-nose test using alternating hands.

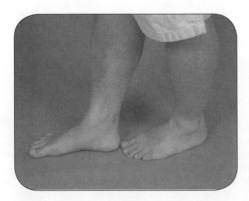

Step 4: If appropriate, test the patient's gait and balance by having the patient walk heel-to-toe or perform the heel-to-shin stance.

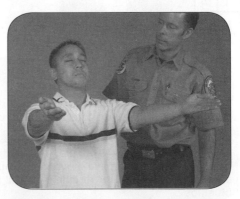

Step 5: Perform the pronator drift test by asking the patient to close his or her eyes and hold both arms out in front of the body.

2. Examining the Chest (page 13.21)

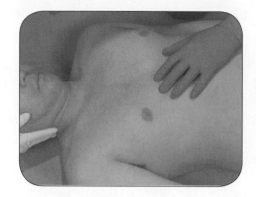

Step 1: Inspect the chest for any obvious DCAP-BTLS.

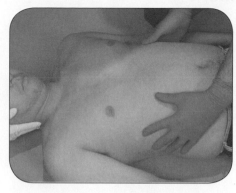

Step 2: Note the shape of the chest.

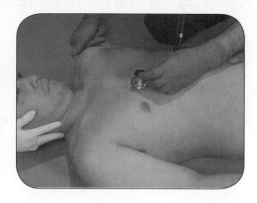

Step 3: Auscultate the lung fields, noting any abnormal lung sounds.

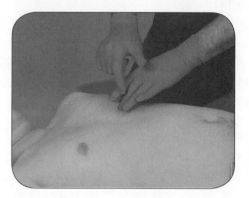

Step 4: Percuss the chest to detect any abnormalities.

Chapter 14: Patient Assessment

Matching

1.

(1) E (page 14.7)   **(7)** K (page 14.31)

(2) C (page 14.9)   **(8)** D (page 14.9)

(3) I (page 14.7)   **(9)** L (page 14.16)

(4) J (page 14.12)   **(10)** G (page 14.18)

(5) F (page 14.12)   **(11)** B (page 14.18)

(6) A (page 14.17)   **(12)** H (page 14.21)

2.

(1) C (page 14.12)   **(4)** B (page 14.14)

(2) E (page 14.12)   **(5)** D (page 14.14)

(3) A (page 14.13)

Multiple Choice

1. A (page 14.4)   **6.** C (page 14.14)

2. C (page 14.4)   **7.** D (page 14.18)

3. D (page 14.7)   **8.** D (page 14.21)

4. A (page 14.8)   **9.** C (page 14.27)

5. C (page 14.11)   **10.** A (page 14.12)

Labeling

1. Mechanisms of Injury and Evaluating Responsiveness (page 14.15)

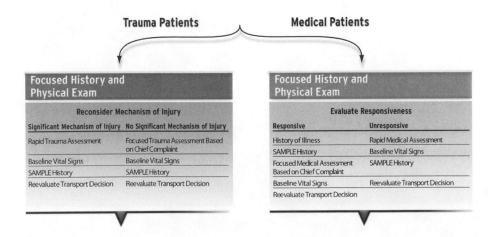

Fill-in-the-Blank

1. Safety, team members (page 14.7)

2. Paranoid, emotionally unstable, armed (page 14.8)

3. Predict, injuries, severity (page 14.9)

4. Initial assessment, life threats (page 14.11)

5. Health, childhood, adult, surgeries, hospitalizations (page 14.16)

6. Respiratory, early, often (page 14.17)

7. Orthostatic, blood pressure, supine, sitting (page 14.17)

8. Multiple, vehicles, traffic, hazardous (page 14.7)

Identify

1. **a.** Patient: Trauma

   b. Mechanism of injury (MOI): Motor vehicle collision, may be high speed, unrestrained passenger, ejected

   c. Transport decision: Immediate because of serious MOI, decreased LOC, and bleeding

2. **a.** Patient: Trauma and medical

   b. MOI: Fall, or it was a medical condition such as a cerebral vascular accident (CVA) or transient ischemic attack (TIA) that caused the fall. Are her poor neurologic symptoms a result of the fall? Probably this was a fall caused by a stroke. The key here would be the hemiparesis.

   c. LOC: Conscious but not alert

   d. Transport decision: This patient requires a complete focused history and physical exam prior to treatment and transport. She may have a number of factors that include head injury, hypoglycemia, cervical spine injury, stroke, and uncontrolled atrial fibrillation, to name a few. This patient needs to have her ABCs secured as well as transport on a long backboard and cardiac monitoring. What's not clear is what occurred first. Both medical and traumatic issues must be taken care of. This patient would also benefit from a facility that is capable of providing trauma and stroke care in a timely manner.

3. **a.** Patient: Medical

   b. LOC: Unconscious, snoring respirations

   c. Transport decision: Delayed, but definitely transport. This sounds somewhat like a typical hypoglycemic patient. You have the tools, training, and medications to reverse his hypoglycemic state with IVs and IV glucose.

Ambulance Calls

1. The patient described in this question fits the description of a "patient found unconscious after trauma." That is, this patient must be presumed to have suffered spinal cord injury.

   a. Therefore, to open the airway, you must use a method that does not involve any extension of the head or neck, such as jaw thrust, jaw lift, or chin lift with the head in neutral position. At the earliest opportunity, it is necessary to intubate the trachea to maintain the airway and protect against aspiration.

   b. As soon as you discover that the patient's breathing is inadequate, you must assist ventilations with a bag-mask device and 100% supplemental oxygen. If the patient is unconscious, it is a good bet that he has a head injury, and he must not therefore be allowed to become hypercarbic. (Why?) Aim to keep his ventilatory rate around 20 breaths/min, with good tidal volumes.

   c. The most likely (but not the sole) explanation of the patient's vital signs and skin condition—normal pulse, hypotension, and warm skin—is neurogenic shock.

   d. The remaining steps in his treatment will include:

      (1) Immobilization on a backboard.

      (2) Starting an IV (preferably while already en route to the hospital) with normal saline. The rate at which you run the IV may be problematic: Shock requires fluids; head injury is best treated by fluid restriction. The patient seems to have both problems. Let the base physician decide what to do about it.

2. By the time you have finished carrying out the initial assessment, you should at least be able to determine your transport decision and therefore if a patient requires immediate transport ("load-and-go" situation) or there is time to carry out some stabilizing measures at the scene.

   a. C.   A 62-year-old driver of a car hit from the side. The door on the driver's side is smashed in. The patient is conscious, in respiratory distress. The left chest is bruised, tender, and does not move symmetrically on respiration. The skin is warm. Pulse is 92 beats/min and slightly irregular, respirations are 30 breaths/min and shallow, and blood pressure is 136/82 mm Hg.

   A flail chest is considered a critical injury because it can lead rapidly to hypoxia.

   b. Steps to be taken at the scene:

      (1) Establish an airway (cervical spine precautions).

      (2) Administer oxygen.

      (3) Stabilize the flail segment with a pillow.

      (4) Immobilize the patient on a long backboard.

      (5) Communicate with medical command or receiving hospital.

c. Steps to be taken en route:

  (1) Detailed physical exam.

  (2) Large-bore IV with fluids.

  (3) Recheck vital and neurologic signs every 5 minutes.

  (4) Be alert for development of tension pneumothorax.

3. Dealing with the unconscious "drunk" is the scenario in which mistakes are most frequently made both in the field and in the emergency department.

  a. *(Students will list five causes.)*

    (1) Alcohol

    (2) Epilepsy

    (3) Insulin overdose (ie, hypoglycemia)

    (4) Overdose with depressant drugs

    (5) Uremia

    (6)*Trauma (the most likely cause in this case)

    (7) Infection (eg, meningitis)

    (8) Psychogenic

    (9) Stroke

  b. This patient must be assumed to have head trauma. He has signs of increasing intracranial pressure (high blood pressure, slow pulse, unequal pupils). Furthermore, he has no wallet, suggesting that he was mugged and robbed. The steps in treating a patient with head trauma are as follows *(students will list seven of the following)*:

    (1) Open the airway with cervical spine precautions. Intubate the trachea as soon as possible because the patient is deeply unconscious and cannot protect his airway.

    (2) Administer supplemental oxygen. If the respiratory rate falls, assist ventilations to maintain a respiratory rate of 20 breaths/min.

    (3) Start an IV to keep a vein open in case you have to administer medications in a hurry.

    (4) As long as you are not absolutely sure of the cause of this patient's coma, check blood glucose. Treat hypoglycemia if present. A trial dose of Narcan (naloxone) may also be helpful in the event of a narcotic overdose.

    (5) Immobilize the patient on a backboard.

    (6) Do not allow the patient to become overheated.

    (7) Monitor cardiac rhythm and vital signs.

    (8) Be prepared to deal with seizures.

    (9) Notify the receiving hospital of a likely head injury and the possible need for neurosurgical intervention.

    (10) Transport to a hospital that has neurosurgical capability.

True/False

1. F (page 14.5)   **7.** T (page 14.13)

2. T (page 14.7)   **8.** F (page 14.16)

3. F (page 14.8)   **9.** T (page 14.17)

4. T (page 14.9)   **10.** T (page 14.17)

5. T (page 14.11)   **11.** F (page 14.27)

6. F (page 14.12)   **12.** T (page 14.31)

Short Answer

1. The initial assessment focuses on the identification and management of life-threatening problems. You should also be able to identify and initially treat threats to the ABCs.

As part of the general impression of your patient, you should ask yourself, "How sick is my patient?"

Treat life threats as you find them, but also decide what additional care is needed and what needs to be done on scene versus en route.

As you move into the focused history and physical exam of a trauma patient, quickly revisit all of the information from your initial assessment, including reconsidering the mechanism of injury (MOI). Collectively, these data may help you identify patients who need to be priority transports to the trauma center. (pages 14.11, 14.21)

2. Priorities of management are, in fact, essential in every type of patient care, but nowhere are they more essential than in emergency care of the ill and injured outside the hospital. The reason is that in the uncontrolled and often chaotic environment of the prehospital setting, *it is easy to forget what to do first* if you don't have a set of priorities that you know by heart. Furthermore, when dealing with the *critically* ill and injured, it is *essential to detect and correct life-threatening conditions as quickly as possible;* a fixed set of priorities enables the rescuer to address the more important problems first and the less important problems later. (pages 14.5, 14.11)

Crossword Puzzle

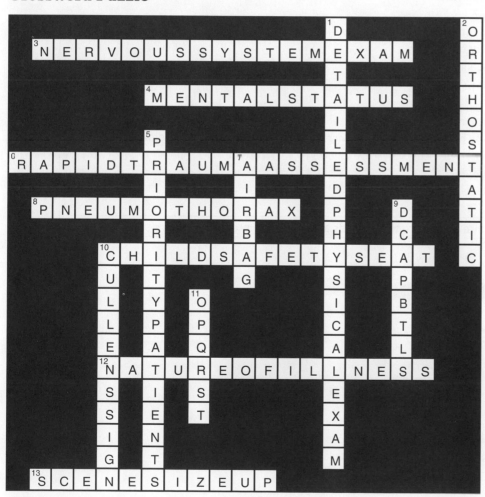

Fill-in-the-Table

1. In conducting the initial assessment of the injured patient, it is good to keep in mind that basically only two things can kill a person fast: hypoxia and exsanguination. What you will be looking for are conditions that can rapidly bring about hypoxia or exsanguination. (page 14.31)

Step	What I Would Look for at This Step
Mental status	A Alert to verbal stimuli V responsive to verbal stimuli P responsive to painful stimuli Unresponsive
Airway	Severe facial trauma Mouth: foreign materials, blood, vomitus, broken teeth Neck: Deformity or open wound over the larynx (Open the airway.)
Breathing	Is breathing present? Signs of respiratory distress Rate and depth of respirations Is the trachea midline? By inspection: bruises, open wounds, deformity, flail chest By palpation: instability of rib cage By auscultation: inequality of breath sounds By percussion: dullness or hyperresonance (Assist ventilations, as needed.)
Circulation	Skin condition: warmth, moisture, color Pulses: rate and quality of carotid pulse; presence or absence of femoral and radial Neck veins distended? Capillary refill time Sources of external bleeding (Control bleeding.)
Transport decision	Does the patient require immediate transport as a result of the preceding factors and MOI?

2. (page 14.13)

Inspection of the Skin	
Skin Color	**Possible Cause**
Red	Fever Hypertension Allergic reactions Carbon monoxide poisoning
White (pallor)	Excessive blood loss Fright
Blue (cyanosis)	Hypoxemia Peripheral vasoconstriction from cold or shock
Mottled	Cardiovascular embarrassment (as in shock)

Skill Drills

1. *The Rapid Trauma Assessment* (page 14.23)

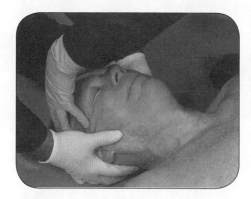

Step 1: Inspect and palpate the skull.

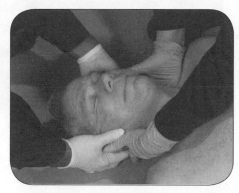

Step 2: Palpate down the posterior cervical spine.

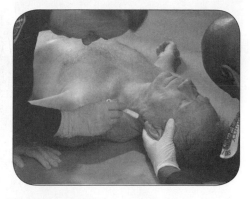

Step 3: Look in and behind the patient's ears.

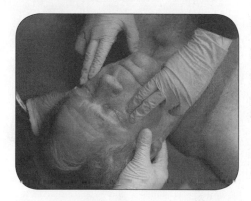

Step 4: Check the pupils, and quickly palpate the orbits.

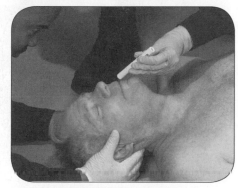

Step 5: Inspect the nose.

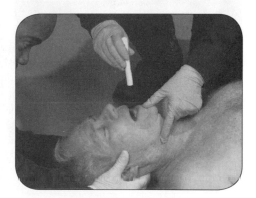

Step 6: Assess the mouth.

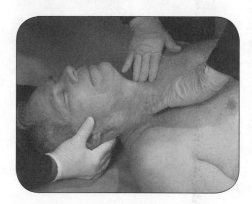

Step 7: Assess the neck.

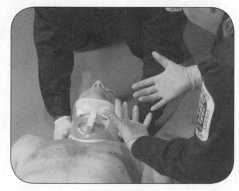

Step 8: Check your gloves for any signs of bleeding. Place a properly sized rigid cervical collar.

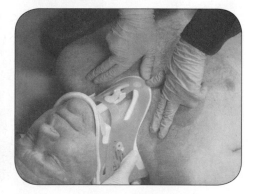

Step 9: Inspect and palpate the chest.

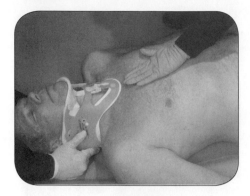

Step 10: Assess for a flail chest or fractured sternum.

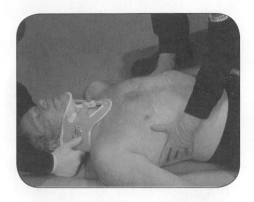

Step 11: Assess for fractured ribs or a flail chest.

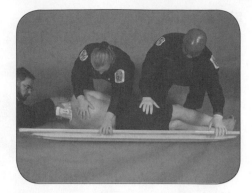

Step 12: If you log roll the patient to a backboard, examine and palpate the thoracic and lumbar spine.

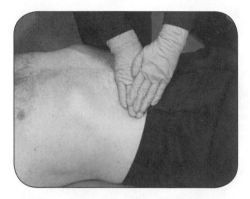

Step 13: Inspect and palpate all four quadrants of the abdomen.

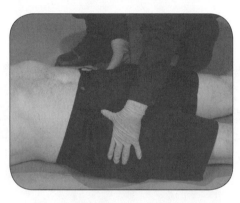

Step 14: Assess the pelvic girdle.

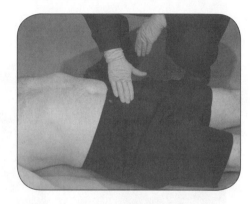

Step 15: Palpate over the bladder.

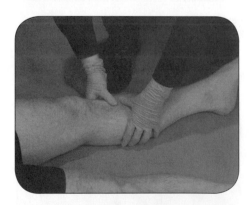

Step 16: Inspect and palpate both lower extremities from hip to ankle.

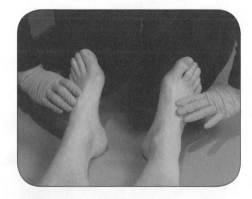

Step 17: Simultaneously assess pedal pulses.

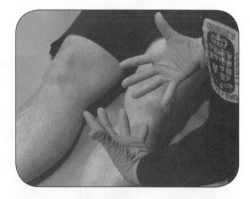

Step 18: Check your gloves for blood.

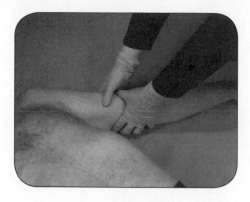

Step 19: Inspect and palpate the arms, and assess pulse, motor function, and sensation.

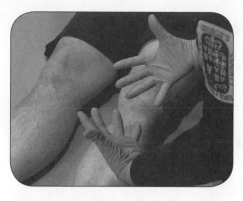

Step 20: Check your gloves for blood.

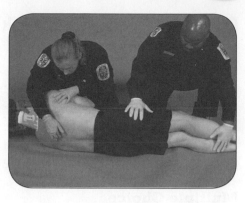

Step 21: Inspect and palpate the back.

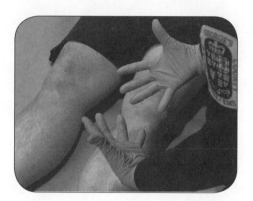

Step 22: Check your gloves for blood.

Chapter 15: Critical Thinking and Clinical Decision Making

Matching

1. A (page 15.5)	**6.** B (page 15.5)
2. B (page 15.5)	**7.** A (page 15.5)
3. A (page 15.5)	**8.** B (page 15.5)
4. A (page 15.5)	**9.** A (page 15.5)
5. B (page 15.5)	**10.** B (page 15.5)

Multiple Choice

1. C (page 15.4)	**6.** D (page 15.11)
2. B (page 15.6)	**7.** C (page 15.11)
3. D (page 15.7)	**8.** B (page 15.4)
4. A (page 15.9)	**9.** A (page 15.6)
5. B (pages 15.11–15.13)	**10.** C (page 15.5)

Fill-in-the-Blank

1. Gathering (page 15.3)
2. Protocols (page 15.5)
3. Think, work (page 15.5)
4. Concept formation (page 15.6)
5. Critical life threats (page 15.6)
6. Working diagnosis (page 15.8)
7. Variables (page 15.10)
8. Trends (page 15.12)

Identify

1. Chief complaint: general malaise.
2. Vital signs: Blood sugar is 110 mg/dL, blood pressure is 160/100 mm Hg. The ECG is normal sinus rhythm with some slight ST-segment depression, with a pulse of 92 beats/min and regular. Oxygen saturation is 97%, lungs clear, and respirations are 18 breaths/min. Skin is warm and dry, and she is PEARRL and alert.
3. Pertinent negatives: After the intervention of the IV at TKO and the nitroglycerin paste the blood pressure drops to 120/70 mm Hg.

Ambulance Call

1. **a.** The little girl in this scenario is unable to tell you her name or where she is. This tells you that she is only a V, or verbal response, using the AVPU scale. She will respond but is not oriented to person, place, or day. She is classified as having an altered mental status and is a priority patient from the start.
   b. You can treat this child under implied consent. Because she has a severe life threat, you can assume the parents would want life-saving treatment to be provided for their daughter.
   c. The vital signs are suggesting that the intracranial pressure is rising. Blood pressure is high for this child's age, and the pulse and respirations are dropping. This tells the paramedics they better be moving toward a regional trauma center as fast and as safely as they can.
   d. The major concern here is to keep a patent airway and provide supplemental oxygen for this patient. Because the patient is breathing under 8 breaths/min and her oxygen saturation is 88%, you know that she is hypoxic. She needs an advanced airway to be inserted as soon as possible, and she may be a candidate for RSI if she continues to have a gag reflex.
2. **a.** Use the highest point or even stand on a car hood (not the one that crashed) and have someone honk the horn until you get the attention of the people around you. Identify yourself and ask the crowd if anyone has medical training. Then, identify a bystander for crowd control. Also designate someone to move down the line of cars and have the person move to the road's shoulder so that emergency vehicles can get through.

b. Everything the locals have is needed! Gain use of a cell phone to communicate with dispatch. Identify yourself and the fact that you are incident command until someone arrives to take over for you. Jaws of Life will be needed and any medical helicopters and ALS units around. Try to get the number of injured patients to the dispatcher as soon as possible. When using the Jaws of Life, a fire truck should be present, so try to get the area cleared of vehicles that were not involved in the collision.

c. You will start to triage the occupants of the two vehicles. That way when help arrives you can direct them to the most critical of patients. Always remember that your safety and the bystanders' safety comes first.

True/False

1. T (page 15.3) **5.** F (page 15.6)

2. T (page 15.4) **6.** T (page 15.8)

3. F (page 15.5) **7.** F (page 15.10)

4. F (page 15.6) **8.** T (page 15.11)

Short Answer

1. a. Read the Scene: As a paramedic, you must ensure your safety and the safety of your crew, patient, and bystanders. Scene safety is first! You will also use your scene to give you clues to the patient's condition. Weather and mechanism of injury (MOI) are also something to look for when reading your scene.

b. Read the Patient: This is where you are deciding if your patient is sick or not sick. You will be observing, talking to, and touching your patient in this phase. You will also be looking for any life threats and taking baseline vital signs.

c. React: Always address any life threats first and handle them as they come up in your assessment. At this time, you will begin to think about your working diagnosis.

d. Reevaluate: Always check your interventions to make sure they are helping your patient. You will also be checking to make sure you have gathered all the information on your patient at this time. You will be watching for any other problems to pop up at this time.

e. Revise the Plan: Once you have begun your treatment, you may realize that your "drunken" patient is really a patient who is having a diabetic emergency. So your treatment plan will have to be revised at this time to properly treat your patient.

f. Review Your Performance: After your call is over, you should do an informal review to see where you can improve your patient care. Sometimes this can be a formal process. It always helps to talk to your team members about each call and learn something from every call you run. (page 15.11)

2. When gathering information, start by asking all the questions you are taught to ask. Start with the chief complaint, SAMPLE history, OPQRST, and all of the mnemonics that you are taught to use. The good paramedic will be able to use open- and closed-ended questions. Frequently, there will be circumstances that will make it hard to gather a good history. Your patient may be unconscious with no family members present to answer questions. There may be a language barrier, or the patient may be unable to speak clearly or hear your questions clearly. You will need to look at the scene around you to help gather information about your patient. You will often need to look at the patient's body position or facial expression. These clues will help you gather information fast about your patient.

When evaluating the information that you have gathered, you must begin to ask if your information is pertinent to the patient's current condition. This is the point where you begin to formulate and enact your treatment plan for the patient. Remember, you must constantly reevaluate your patient and your treatments.

Synthesizing your information goes hand in hand with the evaluation process. This process takes you a little deeper into understanding the disease process or what organ systems have been affected by trauma. This helps you to prepare for any upcoming problems the patient may face. A thinking paramedic will be able to put all the information together and treat the patient in the best way possible. (page 15.3)

Word Find

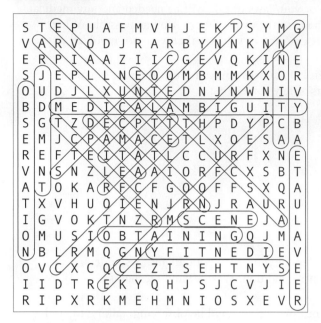

1. Scene, evaluate (page 15.4)
2. Critical thinking (page 15.7)
3. Data, concepts, action (page 15.10)
4. Reflect, performance (page 15.8)
5. Obtaining, auscultate (page 15.11)
6. Synthesize (page 15.4)
7. Identify, medical ambiguity (page 15.10)
8. React, reevaluate (page 15.11)
9. Observations (page 15.7)
10. Implement, judgment (page 15.5)
11. Application (page 15.8)

Chapter 16: Communications and Documentation

Matching

(page 16.4)

1. F	**14.** C
2. C	**15.** B
3. B	**16.** F
4. E	**17.** E
5. G	**18.** D
6. A	**19.** C
7. F	**20.** D
8. D	**21.** B
9. H	**22.** G
10. B	**23.** B
11. E	**24.** H
12. F	**25.** B
13. F	**26.** F

27. In rearranging the sentences into the correct sequence for presentation, there may be some variation in the order of sentences within a given category (eg, the sentences that make up the "history of the present illness," which you labeled B); but all sentences from category B should precede those from category C, which should precede those from category D, and so forth. (page 16.14)

HISTORY

A. Chief Complaint

 (1) 6   The patient is a 51-year-old man with chest pain.

B. History of the Present Illness

 (2) 3   The pain came on while he was watching television.

 (3) 25   He describes the pain as squeezing.

 (4) 23   The pain radiates down his left arm.

 (5) 10   Nothing seemed to make the pain better or worse.

 (6) 15   He also felt nauseated.

 (7) 21   He denies any shortness of breath.

C. Other Medical History

 (8) 19   He is under the care of Dr. Tums for an ulcer.

 (9) 14   The patient takes Maalox (alumina/magnesia) and cimetidine (Tagamet) regularly.

 (10) 2   The patient is allergic to penicillin.

PHYSICAL ASSESSMENT

D. General Appearance

 (11) 18   He was sitting in a chair and appeared to be frightened.

 (12) 20   He was alert and oriented to person, place, and day.

 (13) 8   His skin was pale, cold, and sweaty (diaphoretic).

E. Vital Signs

 (14) 11   The pulse was 52 beats/min and full, with an occasional premature beat.

 (15) 17   His respirations were 20 breaths/min. and unlabored.

 (16) 4   The blood pressure was 190/110 mm Hg.

F. Head-to-Toe Examination

 (17) 13   There was no cyanosis of the lips.

 (18) 12   The neck veins were not distended.

 (19) 7   The chest was clear.

 (20) 26   Lung sounds were clear.

(21) 16   His abdomen was soft and nontender.

(22) 1   There was no pedal edema.

TREATMENT

(23) 5   He was given supplemental oxygen by nasal cannula at 4 L/min.

(24) 22   An IV was started with D₅W to a KVO rate.

CONDITION DURING TRANSPORT

(25) 9   The patient was transported in a semi-Fowler's position.

(26) 24   The blood pressure came down to 170/90 mm Hg during transport.

Question: What do you think is wrong with this patient? Should anything else have been done that was not done?

Now that you've had some practice, this second exercise should be a little easier than the first.

28. F	**38.** G
29. E	**39.** B
30. B	**40.** F
31. C, B	**41.** G
32. F	**42.** F
33. D	**43.** H
34. G	**44.** F
35. A	**45.** F
36. E	**46.** F
37. D	

47. The following shows the sentences rearranged into the correct sequence for presentation:

HISTORY

A. Chief Complaint

(1) 35   The patient is a middle-aged man who was struck by a car while crossing the street.

B. History of the Present Illness

(2) 39   He apparently staggered into the street without looking, as if he were drunk.

(3) 30   Bystanders say that the car that hit him was traveling very fast.

(4) 31   He has a MedicAlert bracelet that says he is a diabetic.

C. Other Medical History

(Apparently none is available; the MedicAlert bracelet could have been listed here, as previously noted.)

PHYSICAL ASSESSMENT

D. General Appearance

(5) 37   The patient was unconscious and did not withdraw from painful stimuli.

(6) 33   His skin is pale, cool, and moist.

E. Vital Signs

(7) 29   The pulse was 92 beats/min, somewhat weak, and regular.

(8) 36   Respirations were 30 breaths/min, deep, and noisy; blood pressure was 160/110 mm Hg.

F. Head-to-Toe Examination

(9) 32   There is a bruise on the left forehead.

(10) 44   There was no blood or fluid draining from his nose or ears.

(11) 42   The pupils were equal, midposition, and reactive to light.

(12) 40   The chest wall was stable, and breath sounds were equal bilaterally.

(13) 45   His abdomen was soft.

(14) 28   The right leg was severely angulated at the mid-femur.

(15) 46   The dorsalis pedis pulses were equal.

G. Treatment

   16. 38   An oropharyngeal airway was inserted, and supplemental oxygen was given by nasal cannula at 4 L/min.

   17. 41   We put the right leg in a traction splint.

   18. 34   He was secured to a long backboard.

H. Condition during Transport

   19. 43   There was no change in his condition during transport.

      Question: What are the likely possible causes of this patient's coma?

Different types of radios or wavebands have different capabilities and are assigned by the FCC for different purposes.

48. U (page 16.6)   **52.** V   (page 16.6)

49. V (page 16.6)   **53.** U   (page 16.6)

50. C (page 16.8)   **54.** U, V, C   (pages 16.6–16.8)

51. C (page 16.8)

55. In taking a history and carrying out a physical examination, you go to a lot of trouble to obtain important information about the patient. It would be a shame if that information was lost because you couldn't communicate it properly. (page 16.14)

AGE, SEX, AND CHIEF COMPLAINT

   (1) F The patient is a 60-year-old woman who collapsed in the bathroom while sitting on the toilet.

A. History of the Present Illness

   (2) J She was apparently well until this morning.

   (3) D Her daughter says that the patient complained of a severe headache before she collapsed.

B. Past Medical History

   (4) B The patient has a history of high blood pressure. (In fact, this is really part of the history of the present illness, if you know what the patient's problem is! She seems to have had a hemorrhagic stroke, so her high blood pressure is one of the predisposing factors.)

   (5) L She was hospitalized 6 years ago for an AMI.

   (6) H The patient's medications include nitroglycerin and Aldomet (methyldopa).

PHYSICAL ASSESSMENT

C. State of Consciousness

   (7) E The patient was still conscious when we arrived, but she rapidly lost consciousness.

D. Vital Signs

   (8) A Pulse is 50 beats/min and regular, respirations are 36 breaths/min and deep, and blood pressure is 180/126 mm Hg.

E. Head-to-Toe Survey

   (9) I Her left pupil is larger than the right and doesn't react to light.

   (10) K Her neck is somewhat stiff.

   (11) C The deep tendon reflexes are hyperactive.

TREATMENT GIVEN SO FAR

   (12) G We are administering oxygen at 4 L/min by nasal cannula.

Multiple Choice

   1. C (page 16.4)   **6.** D (page 16.7)

   2. C (page 16.5)   **7.** A (page 16.18)

   3. D (page 16.7)   **8.** C (page 16.9)

   4. C (page 16.7)   **9.** C (page 16.21)

   5. C (page 16.8)   **10.** D (page 16.21)

Fill-in-the-Blank

   The order of answers given will vary.

   1. The person calling for help needs to be able to talk with the **dispatcher.** The best technical means of establishing that link is **landline (telephone).**

2. The **dispatcher** needs to be able to talk with the **paramedics** or other rescuers. The best technical means of establishing that link is a **two-way radio,** although a pager will suffice for dispatch.

3. The **dispatcher** needs to be able to talk with **other agencies,** such as police, fire, utility companies, and civil defense. The best technical means of establishing that link is **landline (telephone).**

4. The **paramedics** need to be able to talk with **medical command.** The best technical means of establishing that link is **radio or cellular telephone.**

5. The **paramedics** need to be able to talk with the **receiving hospital.** The best technical means of establishing that link is **radio or cellular telephone.**

6. The **area hospitals** need to be able to talk with **one another.** The best technical means of establishing that link is **landline with radio backup.** (page 16.5)

Identify

1. Chief Complaint: Chest Pain

2. History of the Present Illness: The pain was "squeezing" in character, radiated to the left shoulder and jaw, and had been present for 2 hours. The pain was accompanied by increasing difficulty in breathing.

3. Other Medical History: He is known to be a heart patient.

4. General Appearance: The patient was sitting bolt upright; he appeared alert and apprehensive and was in moderate respiratory distress, breathing shallowly 30 breaths/min.

5. Vital Signs: Respiratory rate 30 breaths/min. Pulse was 130 beats/min, weak and regular and blood pressure 200/90 mm Hg.

6. Head-to-Toe Exam: His neck veins were distended to the angle of the jaw at 45 degrees. Wet crackles were heard at both lung bases, and auscultation of the heart revealed a gallop rhythm. The abdomen was not distended. There was a 1+ presacral and ankle edema.

7. Treatment Given: The patient was given oxygen by nasal cannula at 6 L/min and transported to Montefiore Hospital in a semi-sitting position.

8. Pertinent Negatives: The abdomen was not distended; the patient denied nausea, vomiting, sweating, or palpitations.

Ambulance Calls

1. Just about everything was wrong with the transmission quoted!

   a. The unit being called should be mentioned first. So, it should have been, "County Hospital, Medic 12."

   b. It was unnecessarily wordy, wasting a lot of time. ("Be advised that . . ." or "Please 10-9 your message.")

   c. The patient's name was mentioned on the air, along with an abbreviation that a layperson could easily misunderstand. To compound the offense, the paramedic spelled out the initials of the chief complaint in nonstandard phonetic alphabet, using insulting words to do so.

   d. The paramedic was apparently trying to be funny. He may have thought the whole thing was a laugh a minute, but Maggie Jones might be forgiven if she didn't think so. Making insulting references to the patient ("well endowed with adipose tissue") or to the other party on the radio ("Are you deaf or something?") is highly unprofessional and simply reflects on the immaturity of the speaker.

   e. The report of the patient's findings was not given in any sort of standard format. As a result, the people at County Hospital had to waste a lot of time trying to drag the important information out of the paramedics.

   f. Words that are poorly heard by radio, such as "yes," were used.

   g. The paramedic did not repeat back the medication orders to make sure he had received them correctly.

   h. The radio was used for nonmedical communications. ("Pop a few doughnuts into the microwave.") (page 16.10)

2. The best way to find out just how difficult the dispatcher's job can be is to step into that job for a few hours. The information you need to try to obtain from the hysterical caller reporting an accident is as follows:

   - What is the exact location of the incident?

   - What is the telephone number from which the caller is phoning?

   - At this point, dispatch the (first) ambulance. ("Unspecified accident at such-and-such address. Details will follow.")

   - What is the nature of the accident (eg, explosion, road accident, train derailment, building collapse)?

   - How many victims are there?

   - Are there any hazards at the scene, specifically:

     (a) Traffic hazards

   (b) Fire

   (c) Spills

   (d) Downed electrical wires

- If it is a *transport* accident (motor vehicles, train):

   (a) How many vehicles are involved?

   (b) Is it possible to determine what cargoes the vehicles are carrying?

Contact the responding vehicle with additional information. Dispatch additional vehicles and contact other agencies as needed. (page 16.15)

True/False

1. F (page 16.16)   **6.** F (page 16.9)

2. F (page 16.16)   **7.** T (page 16.10)

3. T (page 16.20)   **8.** F (page 16.12)

4. T (page 16.6)   **9.** T (page 16.13)

5. T (page 16.7)   **10.** F (page 16.14)

Short Answer

1. a. Besides the standard information regarding the patient's medical history and physical findings, the trip sheet should contain a record of the times (time the call was received, time the ambulance departed, time the ambulance reached the scene, and so on).

   b. Such a record is important to enable evaluation of such things as response times or how much time is being spent at the scene. (page 16.16)

2. Two reasons for making sure that your trip sheets are accurate and complete are

   a. For the benefit of the patient, whose subsequent care may depend on the information that you have (or have not) provided.

   b. For your own benefit, if the case should ever become a subject for court proceedings. The trip sheet reflects on the person who wrote it. If your trip sheet is sloppy and incomplete, a court would not be unjustified in wondering whether the care you gave the patient was also sloppy and incomplete. (page 16.17)

3. Most radio communications systems require a basic minimum of components. (page 16.9)

Component	Function
Base station	Dispatch and coordination area
Mobile transceiver	Communications with ambulances
Portable transceiver	Communications with paramedics when they are out of their vehicle
Repeater	To extend the range of low-power transceivers
Remote consoles in hospitals	To allow communications with receiving hospitals
Landline/cellular backup	To extend the user network

4. The job of the dispatcher includes the following duties. *Students should list four of the following:*

   a. Extracting information from panicky callers.

   b. Directing the right emergency vehicle to the right address.

   c. Giving advice and first-aid instructions by telephone to distraught people.

   d. Coordinating the response of different agencies to an emergency.

   e. Monitoring field communications to determine if help is needed.

   f. Keeping written records of data such as response times. (page 16.16)

5. An EMS communications system has to provide for at least the following linkages (*Students will draw a diagram):*

   a. Citizen to dispatch center

   b. Dispatch center to ambulances

   c. Dispatch center to hospitals

   d. Dispatch center to medical control

   e. Dispatch center to other services

f. Ambulance to hospitals

g. Paramedic to medical control (page 16.5)

6. TELEMETRY DISPATCHER: Go ahead, Medic 785, you are clear to transmit with MD 802 from Saint Peter's Hospital on Med channel 2.

MEDIC 785: MD 802, this is Medic 785 on med 2. How do you read?

MD 802: Medic 785, this is MD 802. You are loud and clear; proceed with your transmission.

MEDIC 785: I am treating a 58-year-old man who is in moderate distress with a chief complaint of chest pain. He states it came on suddenly while shoveling snow. He describes the pain as crushing under his breastbone and which radiates down his left arm. The pain is a 10 on 10, and he has had the pain for about 15 minutes. The patient states he has no prior history and denies any shortness of breath. He has an allergy to Novocain and takes three aspirins daily as well as 10 mg of Lipitor. He states he has a history of hypertension and high cholesterol with CAD in his family. His last oral intake was lunch 3 hours ago and the 162 mg of chewable aspirin the dispatcher advised him to take prior to our arrival. The events leading up to the incident involved shoveling heavy snow.

Physical exam reveals some crackles at the based of both lungs, not JVD or pedal edema.

His vital signs are respirations of 20 breaths/min. and regular, pulse of 110 beats/min., strong and regular, and a blood pressure of 146/82 mm Hg. His oxygen saturation is 96% on a nonrebreathing mask and his ECG is sinus tachycardia with no ectopy, but the 12-lead shows ST-segment elevation in V_3 and V_4 (possible anterior wall MI).

We are treating him as a rule-out MI and have administered morphine, oxygen. Nitroglycerin and aspirin were self-administered. We are currently transporting and our plan is to continue monitoring him and go through the rest of the fibrinolytic checklist. What's your pleasure on 5 mg of Metoprolol?

MD 802: Medic 785, go ahead with the Metoprolol, and I will alert the cath lab staff right away.

MEDIC 785: Received. Our ETA is 20 minutes.

Secret Messages

Radio communications, even those that take place by cellular telephone, are not private, so think before you open your mouth.

a. Duplex
b. Noisy
c. Biotelemetry
d. Repeater
e. Hertz
f. Band
g. Ring
h. Ask
i. November
j. Goofs
k. Main
l. Any

Secret Message: BEFORE YOU START SPEAKING ON THE RADIO, REMEMBER: ANYONE MAY BE LISTENING.

Fill-in-the-Table

A	Alpha	J	Juliette	S	Sierra
B	Bravo	K	Kilo	T	Tango
C	Charlie	L	Lima	U	Uniform
D	Delta	M	Mike	V	Victor
E	Echo	N	November	W	Whiskey
F	Foxtrot	O	Oscar	X	X-ray
G	Golf	P	Papa	Y	Yankee
H	Hotel	Q	Quebec	Z	Zebra
I	India	R	Romeo		

(page 16.11)

Section 3 Case Study: Answers and Summary

1. What are common contributing factors to falls in the elderly?

Falls are a common cause of injury in elderly patients and can result in serious problems. According to the American Geriatric Society, fall-related injuries are a leading cause of accidental death in the elderly. Additionally, 50 percent of falls result in lesser injuries (eg, soft tissue trauma), which may not be life-threatening, but can have a profound impact on the patient's quality of life. Children and young adults have a higher incidence of falls than the elderly; however, unlike the elderly, their injuries are not associated with a high mortality rate.

Falls in the elderly are caused by intrinsic (patient related) factors, extrinsic (environmental) factors, or a combination of both (multifactorial). Extrinsic factors include torn or loose rugs, poor lighting, furniture obstructions, wet floors, and high steps on stairways.

Intrinsic factors may be age related or the result of an acute or prior medical condition. Age-related changes include impaired balance and coordination (gait impairment), decreased muscle and bone strength, impaired vision and depth perception, and decreased proprioception (perception of body position and movement).

Common acute medical conditions include myocardial infarction, stroke, hypoglycemia, and infection with associated dehydration. Prior medical illnesses, such as stroke, cataracts, and Parkinson's disease, can impair the elderly patient's balance and coordination, leading to falls.

The use of certain medications can also predispose the elderly patient to falls. These medications include anxiolytics such as temazepam (Restoril) and diazepam (Valium), antidepressants such as amitriptyline (Elavil) and paroxetine (Paxil), and antihypertensives such as propranolol (Inderal) and metoprolol (Lopressor). Medication-related falls are often the result of nervous system impairment, drug-to-drug interaction, or inadvertent overdose. Many elderly patients take multiple medications (polypharmacy) for different medical conditions, and it is often impossible to determine how one drug will interact with another.

The cause of falls in the elderly is often multifactorial. An over-medicated patient may trip on a loose rug or fall down steps or the patient may experience a syncopal episode and strike their head on an end table as they fall. **Table 3-1** summarizes the factors that commonly contribute to falls in the elderly.

Through a careful and systematic assessment of the patient, the paramedic must attempt to determine the cause of the patient's fall. In many cases, a fall may be the only presenting sign of an acute illness. Unfortunately, the patient's fall may be the result of physical abuse, which should be suspected when the injury sustained does not coincide with the mechanism described.

Table 3-1   Contributing Factors to Falls in the Elderly

Extrinsic factors
- Torn or loose rugs
- Poor lighting
- Furniture obstructions
- Wet floors
- High steps on stairways

Intrinsic factors
- Age-related changes
  - Impaired balance and coordination
  - Decreased muscle and bone strength
  - Impaired vision or depth perception
  - Impaired proprioception
- Acute medical conditions
  - Myocardial infarction
  - Stroke
  - Hypoglycemia
  - Infection and dehydration
- Prior medical conditions
  - Stroke
  - Cataracts
  - Parkinson's disease
  - Medications (polypharmacy)

Multifactorial
- Fall during a syncopal episode
- Overmedication with resultant fall

2. What are some common causes of altered mental status in the elderly?

You should assume that any alteration in mental status is abnormal until proven otherwise, regardless of the patient's age. Advanced age does not automatically equate to an altered mental status. Elderly patients are frequently capable of highly creative and productive thought processes.

By the time a person reaches the age of 80, brain size has decreased by approximately 10 percent; however, this decrease in brain size does not affect the person's intelligence. The following slight changes, however, which are not present in all patients, are commonly associated with the aging process:

- Forgetfulness
- Psychomotor slowing
- Decreased reaction time
- Difficulty remembering recent events

When assessing an elderly patient with altered mental status, you must first determine the patient's baseline mental status. According to the neighbor, your patient is normally well oriented. This confirms the presence of a new onset in altered mentation.

Elderly patients are predisposed to several neurological disorders that can produce alterations in mentation. It may not be possible to determine the exact cause in the prehospital setting, which is why these patients should be evaluated in the emergency department. **Table 3-2** lists some of the more common causes of altered mental status in the elderly.

Table 3-2   Common Causes of Altered Mental Status in the Elderly

Cerebrovascular disorders
- Transient ischemic attack
- Stroke

Cardiovascular disorders
- Acute myocardial infarction
- Cardiac dysrhythmias

Postictal phase following a seizure

Medication reactions
- Interactions between multiple drugs
- Underdose or overdose

Infections/Sepsis
- Pneumonia
- Urinary tract infection

Electrolyte disturbances and dehydration

Nutritional deficiencies
- Hypoglycemia
- Deficiency of vitamin B12 (cobalamin)

Thermoregulatory dysfunction
- Hypo- or hyperthermia

Structural abnormalities
- Dementia
- Brain tumor
- Subdural hematoma

Approximately 15 percent of Americans over the age of 65 experience varying degrees of dementia. Dementia is defined as a progressive, irreversible impairment of cognitive function. Alzheimer's disease, a common cause of dementia, is a degenerative disease of the brain that results in impaired memory, thinking, and behavior. Approximately 4.5 million Americans are affected by Alzheimer's disease. Brain tumors, which typically grow slowly, are another possible cause of dementia.

Table 3-3   Common Causes of Delirium
Acute myocardial infarction or stroke
Drug overdose
Emotional disturbances
Hypoxia
Sepsis
Seizures
Dehydration
Endocrine disorders • Hyper- or hypothyroidism • Hyper- or hypoglycemia
Intracranial hemorrhage • Subdural hematoma

In the prehospital setting, dementia is often difficult to differentiate from delirium, especially in the absence of a friend or family member who is familiar with the patient's normal mental state. Unlike dementia, delirium is characterized by an acute onset of cognitive impairment and is frequently caused by a life-threatening medical condition **(Table 3-3)**. Delirium can be reversed if the underlying cause is rapidly identified and promptly treated.

Once it has been established that the altered mental status is a new onset, the paramedic should carefully and systematically assess the patient in an attempt to identify and treat the underlying cause. Routine actions include evaluating for signs of trauma, obtaining a blood glucose reading, and considering the administration of naloxone (Narcan) if a drug overdose is suspected.

Again, do not become complacent and assume that an altered mental status in the elderly patient is simply the result of advanced age.

3. What is kyphosis? How will you immobilize this patient's spine and hip?

Kyphosis is an exaggerated curvature (concave ventral) of the spine that results in a rounded or hunched back **(Figure 3-1)**. Kyphosis can occur for many reasons and at any age; however, in the elderly, it is most commonly caused by osteoporosis. As the bones of the spine weaken and thin, they begin to deteriorate and compress. This results in

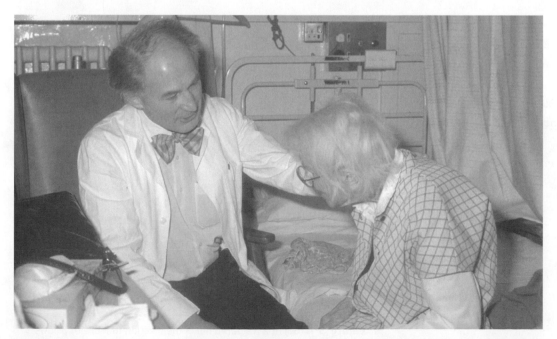

■ **Figure 3-1** Kyphosis is an exaggerated curvature of the spine that results in a rounded or hunched back.

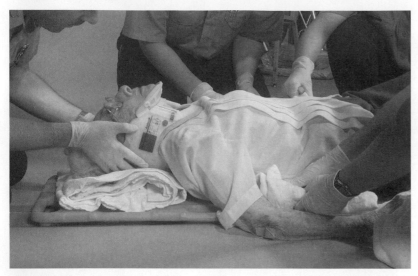

■ **Figure 3-2** Support the head and upper back of the kyphotic patient with pillows and blankets.

deformation of the spine, most commonly in the upper thoracic region.

Because of the age-related deterioration of bone structure (eg, osteoporosis), fractures of the spine can occur with even minor mechanisms of injury. Therefore, spinal immobilization of this patient is clearly necessary.

Immobilizing this patient's kyphotic spine will require modification of the spinal immobilization technique. Additionally, as evidenced by the lateral rotation and shortening of her left leg, you should suspect and treat this patient for a hip fracture.

When immobilizing the spine of kyphotic patients, several pillows or blankets may be required to provide support to the head and upper back **(Figure 3-2)**. Padding of these areas is necessary to provide support, because the kyphotic patient's back will not completely conform to the spine board.

Hip fractures are actually fractures of the proximal portion of the femur near or at the site of articulation with the acetabulum **(Figure 3-3)**. Commonly, fractures of the proximal femur can occur in between the femoral head and the trochanteric region (femoral neck fractures), in between the greater and lesser trochanters (intertrochanteric), or below the lesser trochanter (subtrochanteric).

Hip fractures are commonly splinted by placing pillows or other padding under the injured extremity to support the fracture site in the deformed position **(Figure 3-4)**. Splinting the extremity in the position in which it was found will minimize the risk of further injury as well as reduce the patient's pain.

A long spine board or an orthopedic (scoop) stretcher can be used to immobilize a fractured hip. These devices will allow the patient and the splinting material to be properly secured. Traction splints are not recommended for immobilizing hip

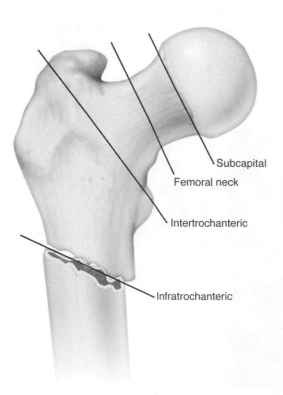

Subcapital
Femoral neck
Intertrochanteric
Infratrochanteric

■ **Figure 3-3** Common hip fracture locations

■ **Figure 3-4** Splint a fractured hip in the position found with pillows and blankets.

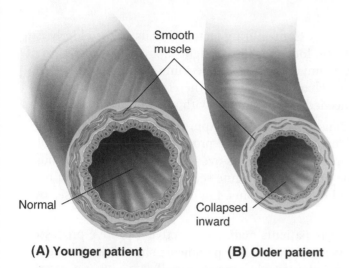

Smooth
muscle

Normal

Collapsed
inward

(A) Younger patient   **(B) Older patient**

■ **Figure 3-5** (A.) Healthy muscle in the younger patient's airway
helps maintain the open airway during the pressures of inhalation.
(B.) Muscle weakening with age can lead to airway collapse.

fractures. Because it is not possible to determine the exact location of the fracture in the prehospital setting, it is not possible to accurately assess the integrity of the pelvis. If the fracture involves the pelvis, applying a traction splint could actually be detrimental and result in further displacement and potentially injury. Furthermore, the risk of injury to the skin and other soft tissues with the application of traction splints in the elderly is potentially higher. Thus, the use of these devices in elderly hip fracture patients should be avoided unless alternatives are inadequate or otherwise inappropriate.

4. How does aging affect the body's ability to compensate for shock?

Even at rest, the aging body's physiologic functions are diminished. Therefore, the ability of the elderly person to effectively compensate for a low cardiac output, hypoxia, and shock is markedly diminished. The respiratory, nervous, and cardiovascular systems are the key body systems that compensate during shock; therefore, age-related changes that occur with each of these systems will be discussed.

The aging process adversely affects ventilatory function, thus impairing the elderly person's ability to compensate for hypoxia. Smooth muscles of the lower airway weaken with age. When increases in tidal volume are needed (eg, hypoxia, shock), the patient attempts to breath deeply; however, the walls of the lower airway collapse. This reduces tidal volume **(Figure 3-5)**.

Loss of respiratory muscle mass, increases in the stiffness of the thoracic cage, and a decreased surface area available for air exchange contribute to a decrease in vital capacity (volume of air exchanged after maximal inhalation and exhalation) of up to 50 percent. Decreased vital capacity causes an increase in residual volume, which is the amount of air remaining in the lungs following a maximal exhalation. This leaves more stagnant air in the alveoli, which impairs effective gas exchange.

With aging, the body's chemoreceptors become less sensitive. Chemoreceptors, which are located in the aortic arch, sense changes in arterial oxygen and carbon dioxide and send signals to the brainstem to regulate breathing accordingly. Additionally, nerve impulse transmission from the brainstem to the diaphragm and the nerves of the intercostal muscles is decreased. The net effect is a decreased ability to quickly increase respirations in response to conditions that cause hypoxia (ie, shock).

The cardiovascular system undergoes, to varying degrees, age-related deterioration that decreases its ability to compensate for shock. The vasculature loses its elasticity, which causes an increase in systolic blood pressure and afterload (the force that the heart must pump against). As a result, the wall of the left ventricle becomes enlarged (hypertrophy) and thickens. The myocardium also loses its ability to effectively stretch (Frank-Starling effect), thus decreasing ventricular filling and contractility. Hypertrophy of the mitral and tricuspid valves also occurs, which impedes blood flow into and out of the heart. These myocardial changes cause a natural decrease in stroke volume and cardiac output. Furthermore, the ability to increase cardiac output to meet increased demands of the body is decreased.

Baroreceptors, which are located in the aortic arch and carotid sinus, become less sensitive to changes in blood volume with age. These receptors, which sense changes in arterial blood pressure, send messages to the adrenal glands, causing them to secrete the hormones epinephrine and norepinephrine, which causes increases in heart rate, myocardial contractility, and blood pressure. The heart's response to epinephrine and norepinephrine decreases with age; therefore, the elderly person is less able to quickly and effectively compensate for blood loss and decreases in blood volume.

Due to age-related decreases in elastin and collagen in the vascular walls, blood vessel elasticity can be reduced by as much as 70 percent in the elderly person. Therefore, compensation in shock is significantly reduced because the peripheral vasculature must be able to constrict and dilate accordingly to maintain blood pressure and adequate perfusion.

Summary

Falls are a leading cause of accidental death in patients over the age of 65. Contributing factors to falls in the elderly can be intrinsic (eg, age-related changes, acute or prior illness), extrinsic (eg, loose rugs, poor lighting), or a combination of both. When assessing the elderly patient who has fallen, the paramedic must attempt to determine the cause of the fall. Because of osteoporosis, spinal fractures can occur with even minor mechanisms of injury; therefore, the elderly patient who has fallen should be immobilized, with modifications made as needed for the patient with a kyphotic spine.

Hip fractures account for nearly 30 percent of orthopedic hospital admissions each year. Approximately 80 percent of hip fractures occur in women and are most frequently seen in the elderly. The elderly are prone to fractures because of osteoporosis, which makes the bones very fragile. Approximately 20 percent of patients over the age of 65 who are hospitalized for a hip fracture die within the first 6 months following the injury. In the acute setting, death following a hip fracture is usually caused by pneumonia, myocardial infarction, or pulmonary embolus. Long-term, common causes of death include pulmonary embolus and sepsis.

Mental status changes do not occur in all patients with age. Many elderly patients maintain effective cognitive processes. Any change in mentation must be assumed to be abnormal until proven otherwise. The paramedic should determine, by talking with friends or family members, whether the patient's mental status has changed, and, if so, to what degree. Common causes of altered mental status in the elderly include, among others, hypoglycemia, medication-related issues, and stroke. Any patient with an altered mental status should be given supplemental oxygen or assisted ventilations as needed.

Age-related changes reduce the elderly person's ability to quickly and effectively compensate for hemodynamic compromise (eg, blood loss). The muscles of the respiratory system weaken, and the chemoreceptors become less sensitive to changes in oxygen and carbon dioxide levels in the blood. Due to hypertrophy and thickening of the ventricular myocardium, stroke volume decreases, resulting in a decreased cardiac output, both at rest and in times of increased demand. Blood vessel elasticity decreases, making the peripheral vasculature less able to constrict and dilate in response to the body's demands.

Section 4: Trauma

Chapter 17: Trauma Systems and Mechanism of Injury

Matching

1. C (page 17.17)
2. B (page 17.16)
3. D (page 17.20)
4. A (page 17.17)
5. B (page 17.16)

6. A–D (pages 17.16, 17.17, 17.20)
7. A   (page 17.12)
8. A   (page 17.15)
9. A, B (pages 17.13, 17.15, 17.16)
10. A, B (pages 17.13, 17.14)

Multiple Choice

1. A (page 17.7)
2. C (page 17.9)
3. B (page 17.13)
4. B (page 17.20)
5. A (page 17.24)

6. D (page 17.26)
7. D (page 17.22)
8. D (page 17.6)
9. A (page 17.7)
10. A (page 17.16)

Labeling

(page 17.24)

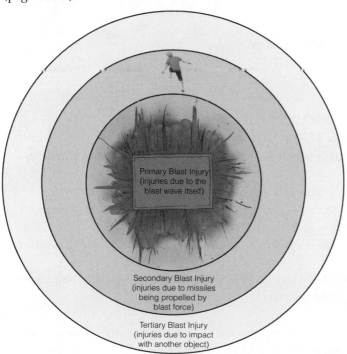

Fill-in-the-Blank

1. Geriatric patients (page 17.18)
2. Anatomic, penetration (page 17.22)
3. Arterial air embolism (page 17.26)

4. a. Height

   b. Position

   c. Surface

   d. Physical Condition

   e. Area (page 17.21)

5. Cervical, neck (page 17.18)

Identify

1. a. Mechanism of injury: Rollover motor vehicle crash

   b. Chief complaint: Pain to radius/ulna, neck pain

   c. Vital signs: Pulse 110 beats/min regular, respiration 16 breaths/min unlabored, blood pressure 106/96 mm Hg, skin ashen

   d. Pertinent negatives: Denies LOC

2. a. Mechanism of injury (MOI): High-speed motorcycle vs. guardrail crash

   b. Chief complaint: Hurts all over

   c. Vital signs: Conscious and alert, skin ashen and diaphoretic, no palpable blood pressure, > 2-second capillary refill, respiration 28 breaths/min

   d. Pertinent negatives: None

3. a. Mechanism of injury (MOI): Possible fall, TIA, cardiac

   b. Chief complaint: Per patient, none; staff states she fell and has pain to hip

   c. Vital signs: Pulse 58 beats/min and irregular, blood pressure 158/110 mm Hg, skin cool/dry, normal capillary refill

   d. Pertinent negatives: Denies chest pain, shortness of breath, neck or back pain

Ambulance Calls

1. Evaluate the MOI and examine the trauma scene for evidence of high-energy trauma.

   a. Speed (page 17.6)

   b. Restrained vs. airbag deployment (page 17.14)

   c. Loss of consciousness (page 17.7)

   d. Physical damage to pole and vehicle, and any intrusion into the vehicle? (page 17.7)

   e. Patient's chief complaint (page 17.7) f. Detailed physical exam (page 17.7)

2. a. Height: The distance that he jumped. This will determine the speed at which he fell and therefore the force of impact with which he hit the ground.

   Position: How he landed. This will tell you what part(s) of the body absorbed the greatest amount of kinetic energy.

   Area: The area over which the impact is distributed—the larger the area of contact at the time of the impact, the greater dissipation of the force and the lesser the peak pressures generated.

   Surface: What kind of surface he landed on. A pile of hay has a lot more give than a concrete sidewalk. The more the surface can "give," the less the falling body will have to deform.

   Physical condition: The physical condition of the patient before the fall. Does he have any underlying physical problems, such as an ulcer or an enlarged spleen, that might predispose him to certain injuries?

   b. Spine, legs, pelvis (page 17.21)

3. Children tend to fall head first, so head injuries are common in children as are injuries to the wrists and upper extremities when the child attempts to break the fall. The surface on which the child falls is very important. (page 17.21)

4. a. Call the police.

   b. (1) The type of firearm used

   (2) Velocity of the projectile

   (3) Physical design of the projectile

   (4) The distance to the target from the muzzle of the firearm

   (5) The type of tissue that is struck (page 17.22)

5. Explosions produce several different mechanisms of injury, and one needs to anticipate each type; otherwise, it is easy to miss the less obvious injuries.

a. Primary blast injury: body damage caused by the explosion

b. Secondary blast injury: damage from being struck by flying debris

c. Tertiary blast injury: patient being hurled against a stationary object

d. Miscellaneous blast injury: burns from hot gases or structural collapse (page 17.24)

6.

Tissues at Risk	Evidence
1. Tympanic membrane	Blood in the ear
2. Pulmonary blast injury	Tight feeling in chest
3. Arterial air embolism	Blurry vision

True/False

1. T (page 17.5)

2. F (page 17.8)

3. F (page 17.8)

4. T (page 17.11)

5. T (page 17.16)

6. F (page 17.18)

7. T (page 17.14)

8. T (pages 17.24, 17.25)

9. D (page 17.7)

10. A (page 17.12)

Short Answer

1. In this question, you are asked to consider the forces involved when a 2,000-lb automobile traveling at 20 mph strikes a pedestrian.

a. Some of the kinetic energy of the vehicle will remain energy of motion, assuming the vehicle keeps moving. (If the driver hits the brakes, the friction of the brakes will transform that kinetic energy into heat.) Some energy will be absorbed by the vehicle in the deformation of the bumper or hood and the remainder will be absorbed by the pedestrian who has been struck by the vehicle.

b. Had the vehicle weighed 6,000 lb instead of 2,000 lb, that is, had its weight (mass) been tripled, its kinetic energy at any given speed would also have tripled, according to the kinetic energy equation: $KE = \frac{m}{2} \times v^2$

c. Had the vehicle been traveling at 60 mph instead of 20 mph, that is, had its velocity been tripled, its kinetic energy would have been increased 9 times because kinetic energy increases as the *square* of the velocity. That is why it is nearly impossible for a pedestrian to survive an impact with a vehicle, even a relatively small vehicle, going faster than about 40 mph—the kinetic energies become overwhelming. (pages 17.10–17.11)

2. When a car traveling at 50 mph slams into a concrete wall, three distinct collisions take place:

a. Collision 1 is between the *automobile* and the concrete wall. Because the automobile is both more mobile and more deformable than the concrete wall, the majority of the kinetic energy is absorbed by the automobile in its rebound off the wall and deformity of the front end.

b. Collision 2 is between the *occupant* and the automobile. In that collision, some of the kinetic energy is absorbed by the automobile (eg, in denting the dashboard), but the larger proportion is absorbed by the occupant.

c. Collision 3 is between the internal *organs* of the occupant and the restraining walls of the person's body (eg, the skull, the chest cage, the pelvic girdle). The majority of the kinetic energy in that collision is absorbed by the internal organs. (pages 17.10–17.11)

3. When you arrive at the accident scene, a close inspection of the scene and of the damaged vehicle(s) can provide extremely important information—information that will enable the doctors who take over the patient's care to detect and manage the patient's problems much more expeditiously. Indeed, what you observe (or fail to observe) about the accident scene could make the difference between life and death for the patient—so keep your eyes open, report what you have observed to the base physician, and record your findings on the patient's trip sheet. (page 17.15)

a. Deformed dashboard

  (1) Ruptured spleen, liver, bowel, diaphragm

  (2) Fractured patella

  (3) Dislocated knee

  (4) Femoral fracture

  (5) Dislocated hip

    b. Deformed steering column

        (1) Sternal or rib fracture

        (2) Flail chest

        (3) Myocardial contusion

        (4) Pericardial tamponade

        (5) Pneumothorax or hemothorax

        (6) Exsanguinations from aortic tear

    c. Cracked windshield

        (1) Brain injury

        (2) Scalp, facial cuts

        (3) Cervical spine injury

        (4) Tracheal injury

    d. Door smashed in

        (1) Fractured hip

        (2) Fractured iliac wing

4. *Students should provide six of the following:*

    a. Facial injuries

    b. Soft tissue neck trauma

    c. Larynx and tracheal trauma

    d. Fractured sternum

    e. Myocardial contusion

    f. Pericardial tamponade

    g. Pulmonary contusion

    h. Hemothorax, rib fracture

    i. Flail chest

    j. Ruptured aorta

    k. Intra-abdominal injuries (page 17.16)

Word Find

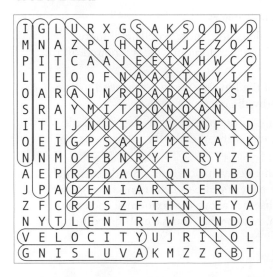

    1. Shearing (page 17.12)

    2. Avulsing (page 17.12)

    3. Blunt trauma (page 17.12)

    4. Lateral impact (page 17.16)

    5. Down-and-under (page 17.14)

6. Up-and-over (page 17.14)

7. Restrained (page 17.14)

8. Unrestrained (page 17.14)

9. Head-on (page 17.11)

10. Penetrating (page 17.11)

11. Entry wound (page 17.23)

12. Implosion (page 17.23)

13. Kinetics (page 17.6)

14. Tympanic (page 17.25)

15. Velocity (page 17.6)

Fill-in-the-Table

1.

Key Elements for Trauma Centers		
Level	**Definition**	**Key Elements**
Level I	A comprehensive regional resource that is a tertiary care facility. Capable of providing total care for every aspect of injury—from prevention through rehabilitation.	1. 24-hour in-house coverage by general surgeons 2. Availability of care in specialties such as orthopaedic surgery, neurosurgery, anesthesiology, emergency medicine, radiology, internal medicine, and critical care 3. Should also include cardiac, hand, pediatric, and microvascular surgery and hemodialysis 4. Provides leadership in prevention, public education, and continuing education of trauma team members 5. Committed to continued improvement through a comprehensive quality assessment program and organized research to help direct new innovations in trauma care
Level II	Able to initiate definitive care for all injured patients.	1. 24-hour immediate coverage by general surgeons 2. Availability of orthopaedic surgery, neurosurgery, anesthesiology, emergency medicine, radiology, and critical care 3. Tertiary care needs such as cardiac surgery, hemodialysis, and microvascular surgery may be referred to a Level I trauma center 4. Committed to trauma prevention and continuing education of trauma team members 5. Provides continued improvement in trauma care through a comprehensive quality assessment program
Level III	Has demonstrated the ability to provide prompt assessment, resuscitation, and stabilization of injured patients and emergency operations.	1. 24-hour immediate coverage by emergency medicine physicians and prompt availability of general surgeons and anesthesiologists 2. Program dedicated to continued improvement in trauma care through a comprehensive quality assessment program 3. Has developed transfer agreements for patients requiring more comprehensive care at a Level I or Level II trauma center 4. Committed to continuing education of nursing and allied health personnel or the trauma team 5. Must be involved with prevention and have an active outreach program for its referring communities 6. Also dedicated to improving trauma care through a comprehensive quality assessment program
Level IV	Has demonstrated the ability to provide Advanced Trauma Life Support (ATLS) before transfer of patients to a higher level trauma center.	1. Include basic emergency department facilities to implement ATLS protocols and 24-hour laboratory coverage 2. Transfer to higher level trauma centers follows the guidelines outlined in formal transfer agreements 3. Committed to continued improvement of these trauma care activities through a formal quality assessment program 4. Involved in prevention, outreach, and education within its community

(page 17.8)

2.

<table>
<tr><td>**"Ring" of Chest Injuries From Impacting the Steering Wheel or Dashboard**</td></tr>
<tr><td>

- Facial injuries
- Soft-tissue neck trauma
- Larynx and tracheal trauma
- Fractured sternum
- Myocardial contusion
- Pericardial tamponade
- Pulmonary contusion
- Hemothorax, rib fractures
- Flail chest
- Ruptured aorta
- Intra-abdominal injuries

</td></tr>
</table>

(page 17.16)

Problem Solving

1. $KE = \dfrac{(200 + 120)}{2} \times 50^2 = 400,000$

2. $KE = \dfrac{120}{2} \times 50^2 = 150,000$ (page 17.10)

Chapter 18: Bleeding and Shock

Matching

1. G (page 18.4)
2. D (page 18.6)
3. J (page 18.10)
4. F (page 18.10)
5. I (page 18.11)

6. B (page 18.15)
7. A (page 18.16)
8. H (page 18.22)
9. C (page 18.27)
10. E (page 18.27)

Multiple Choice

1. B (page 18.5)
2. C (page 18.6)
3. C (page 18.8)
4. D (page 18.9)
5. D (page 18.10)

6. A (page 18.10)
7. B (page 18.12)
8. C (page 18.18)
9. D (page 18.26)
10. B (page 18.7)

Labeling

1. The Cardiovasuclar System (page 18.6)

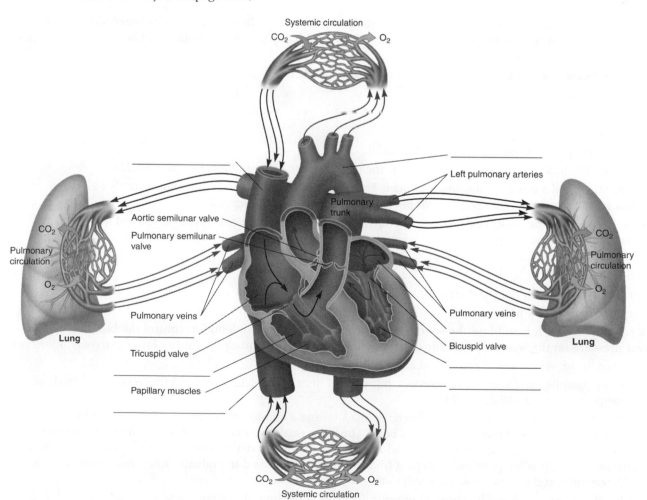

Fill-in-the-Blank

1. PASG or MAST (page 18.12)
2. Hemoglobin (page 18.6)
3. Perfusion (page 18.7)
4. Hemostatis (page 18.9)
5. Melena (page 18.10)
6. Epistaxis (page 18.11)
7. Hypoperfusion (page 18.15)
8. Baroreceptors (page 18.16)
9. Central, peripheral (page 18.17)
10. Multiple-organ dysfunctional syndrome (MODS) (page 18.20)
11. Pulse pressure (page 18.21)
12. Compensated, decompensated, irreversible (pages 18.21–18.22)
13. Normal saline (page 18.25)
14. Anaphylactic (page 18.28)
15. Crystalloids (page 18.27)

Identify

1. Chief complaint: Chest pain
2. Vitals signs: Sinus bradycardia rate of 52 beats/min, crackles in the base of the lungs. Respirations are 24 breaths/min, blood pressure is 80/56 mm Hg, skin is diaphoretic and clammy. Patient is alert with oxygen administration and he is PEARRL (Pupils Equal and Round, Regular in size, react to light).
3. Pertinent negatives: No pulse at wrist, no ectopy on 12-lead echocardiogram (ECG)

Ambulance Calls

1. In assessing the state of perfusion:
    a. You can judge *peripheral* perfusion by checking capillary refill.
    b. The best indicator in the field of *perfusion of vital organs* is the patient's state of consciousness. (page 18.23)
2. You are called to a bar to attend a bleeding, unconscious man. The place is full of noise and confusion—unruly customers, police, curiosity seekers. *This is the time to remember the priorities of the initial assessment:* A-B-C.
    First, before you even enter that bar, make certain that the police have the situation under control. (If you did not include that step in your answer, you do not get *any* points for your answer and, furthermore, you are a very poor risk for life insurance!) *Look first to your own safety,* remember?
    a. Open the patient's **airway**.
    b. Check whether he is **breathing**. If not, start artificial ventilation.
    c. Check whether he has a **pulse**. If he does not have a pulse, start external chest compressions.
    d. Cut away the patient's trouser leg, and **find the source of his bleeding**. When you've found it, **control the bleeding by applying direct pressure on the wound**, preferably over a sterile dressing. Check quickly for other lower extremity injuries.
    e. **Transfer the patient** to the vehicle (he should be on a backboard by now).
    f. **Get under way** to the hospital, and **start an intravenous infusion** en route. Complete your rapid trauma or rapid medical assessment as time permits. (pages 18.22–18.24)
3. One rainy day, a car bomb was detonated in front of a foreign consulate, and a number of bystanders were injured by flying debris, including jagged pieces of metal torn from the car's body. The first casualty you come upon is bleeding from multiple sites, including a deep gash on the right side of the neck and a laceration that has partially severed the right leg at the groin. The leg laceration is gushing blood; it is too proximal to benefit from a tourniquet. It's hard to evaluate skin condition in the rain. Pulse is around 100 beats/min and somewhat weak; respirations are 30 breaths/min.
    This patient earns his "load-and-go" status by virtue of uncontrollable bleeding from the femoral artery.
    a. Steps to be taken at the scene:
        (1) Seal the open wound of the neck.

(2) Administer supplemental oxygen.

(3) Try at least to slow the bleeding from the groin by using pressure dressings and pressure points.

(4) Communicate with Medical Control or the receiving hospital.

b. Steps to be taken en route:

(1) Start two large-bore IVs with rapid infusion of fluids.

(2) Complete a detailed physical exam.

(3) Recheck vital and neurologic signs every 5 minutes. (pages 18.11, 18.14, 18.15)

4. A second casualty from the car bombing, a young man, was sideswiped by a piece of flying debris, which made a clean 14-inch incision straight across his abdomen. He is conscious and in moderate distress. Pulse is 104 beats/min and regular, respirations are 28 breaths/min and slightly labored, and blood pressure is 104/70 mm Hg. What looks to be a major portion of the patient's intestines are outside the abdomen.

Abdominal evisceration is certainly an attention-getter, but it does *not* pose an immediate threat to life.

a. Steps to be taken at the scene:

(1) Administer supplemental oxygen.

(2) Complete the detailed physical exam.

(3) Cover the eviscerated organs with sterile dressings soaked in sterile saline and an occlusive dressing.

b. Steps to be taken en route:

(1) Communicate with Medical Control or the receiving hospital.

(2) Start a large-bore IV with ***<what goes here?>***

(3) Recheck vital and neurologic signs every 5 minutes. (pages 18.11, 18.24–18.25)

5. A third casualty from the car bombing is another young man in considerable respiratory distress. There is a 2-inch-wide hole in his right chest through which you can hear air being sucked on inhalation. His skin is warm. His pulse is 108 beats/min and regular; respirations are 30 breaths/min and gasping; blood pressure is 112/64 mm Hg.

An open chest wound is considered a critical injury because it prevents adequate ventilation of the lungs.

a. Steps to be taken at the scene:

(1) Seal off the sucking chest wound with an occlusive dressing taped on three sides.

(2) Administer supplemental oxygen; assist ventilations as needed.

(3) Communicate with Medical Control or the receiving hospital.

b. Steps to be taken en route:

(1) Complete a detailed physical exam.

(2) Start an IV with fluids.

(3) Recheck vital and neurologic signs every 5 minutes. (pages 18.11, 18.24–18.25)

6. Your initial assessment (IA) has not given you much information regarding *where* precisely this patient has been injured, but the IA *has* given you unmistakable evidence that the patient is in shock (restlessness, profuse sweating). Don't be fooled by the slow pulse—bradycardia occurs sometimes with intra-abdominal bleeding. And *don't wait for the blood pressure to fall before you decide that the patient is in shock*!

a. Steps to be taken at the scene:

(1) Manually stabilize the head/neck and apply a cervical collar.

(2) Administer supplemental oxygen.

(3) Conduct the rapid trauma assessment.

(4) Immobilize the patient on a long backboard.

(5) Prepare for rapid transport to the appropriate facility.

b. Steps to be taken en route:

(1) Complete a detailed physical exam.

(2) Start two large-bore IVs and run a fluid challenge.

(3) Communicate with Medical Command or the receiving hospital.

(4) Conduct an ongoing assessment, rechecking vital and neurologic signs every 5 minutes. (pages 18.11, 18.24–18.25)

True/False

1. F (page 18.22)
2. T (page 18.15)
3. F (page 18.26)
4. T (page 18.19)
5. T (page 18.5)

6. F (page 18.6)
7. T (page 18.8)
8. T (page 18.9)
9. F (page 18.11)
10. T (page 18.14)

Short Answer

1. Three components are required for a functioning regulatory system:

   a. A functioning pump: the heart

   b. Adequate fluid volume: the blood and body fluids

   c. An intact system of tubing capable of reflex adjustments (constriction and dilation) in response to changes in pump output and fluid volume: the blood vessels (page 18.4)

2. Causes of hemorrhagic shock include (*students should provide four of the following*):

   a. External bleeding

   b. Blunt chest trauma

   c. Blunt abdominal trauma

   d. Fractures of the pelvis or femur

   e. Ruptured ectopic pregnancy

   f. Bleeding ulcer (pages 18.18–18.20)

3. Knowing the mechanisms that produce signs and symptoms makes it much easier to remember those symptoms and signs. (*Students will provide four of the following.*) (page 18.21)

Sign or Symptom	Mechanism That Causes the Sign or Symptom
a. Restlessness	Possibly hypoxemia
b. Cold, clammy, pale skin	Peripheral vasoconstriction, the body's attempt to shunt blood away from the "nonvital" periphery to more vital internal organs (like the brain)
c. Weak, rapid pulse	The pulse is weak because (a) the volume is reduced and (b) the arteries are narrowed. It is rapid because the body has to cycle the remaining red blood cells faster to furnish the same amount of oxygen (each red blood cell must make more trips).
d. Rapid breathing	When not enough oxygen is reaching the brain, the brain stem sends signals to the respiratory muscles to increase the minute volume. One way to do that is to increase the respiratory *rate*. (What is another way?)
e. Confusion	When the brain isn't being perfused adequately, it can't think straight.

4. It is absolutely essential that a paramedic be able to recognize the signs of shock. That is why we keep coming back to them. Symptoms and signs of shock include (*students should provide six of the following*):

   a. Restlessness and anxiety

   b. Thirst

   c. Nausea, sometimes with vomiting

   d. Cold, clammy, pale, or mottled skin

   e. Weak, rapid pulse

   f. Rapid, shallow breathing

   g. Changes in the state of consciousness/mental status

   h. Fall in blood pressure (page 18.21)

5. *Students should provide six symptoms and signs of dehydration.*

   a. Loss of appetite

   b. Nausea

   c. Vomiting

   d. Fainting

    e. Poor skin turgor

    f. Shrunken, furrowed tongue (page 18.18)

6. List five methods for the control of external hemorrhage.

    a. Apply direct pressure over the wound.

    b. Elevate the injury above the level of the heart.

    c. Apply a pressure dressing.

    d. Apply pressure at the appropriate pressure point.

    e. Apply a tourniquet. (page 18.11)

Word Find

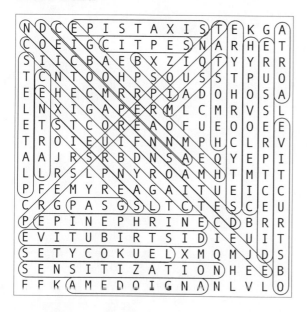

  1. Aorta (page 18.5)

  2. Ejection fraction (page 18.5)

  3. Leukocytes (page 18.6)

  4. Erythrocytes (page 18.6)

  5. Platelets (page 18.7)

  6. External (page 18.8)

  7. Hemorrhage (page 18.8)

  8. Body substance isolation (BSI) (page 18.10)

  9. Epistaxis (page 18.11)

10. Direct pressure (page 18.11)

11. Pressure point (page 18.11)

12. Hemostat (page 18.11)

13. Military anti-shock trousers (MAST); pneumatic anti-shock garment (PASG) (page 18.12)

14. Cardiogenic (page 18.15)

15. Epinephrine (page 18.17)

16. Obstructive (page 18.17)

17. Hypovolemic (page 18.17)

18. Central (page 18.17)

19. Distributive (page 18.18)

20. Septic (page 18.18)

21. Sepsis (page 18.18)

22. Sensitization (page 18.19)

23. Angioedema (page 18.19)
24. Anaerobic (page 18.30)
25. Decompensated (page 18.22)

Fill-in-the-Table

1. Compensated versus Decompensated Hypoperfusion (page 18.21)

Compensated Versus Decompensated Hypoperfusion

Compensated Hypoperfusion	Decompensated Hypoperfusion
■ Agitation, anxiety, restlessness	■ Altered mental status (verbal to unresponsive)
■ _____	■ _____
■ _____	■ Labored or irregular breathing
■ _____	■ Thready or absent peripheral pulses
■ _____	■ _____
■ Nausea, vomiting	■ _____
■ Delayed capillary refill in infants and children	■ _____
■ Thirst	■ _____
■ _____	■ _____
	■ Impending cardiac arrest

Skill Drills

1. *Treating Shock* (page 18.25)

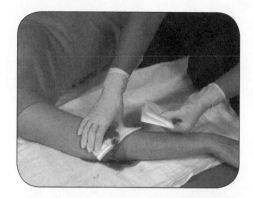

Step 1: Keep the patient supine, open the airway, and check breathing and pulse. Give high-flow supplemental oxygen, and assist ventilations if needed.

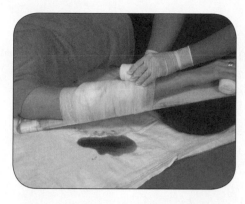

Step 2: Control obvious external bleeding.

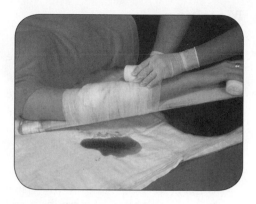

Step 3: Splint broken bones or joint injuries.

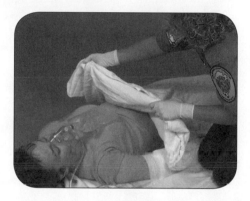

Step 4: Place blankets under and over the patient.

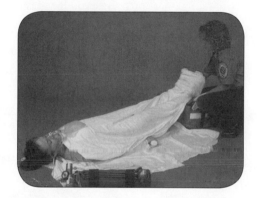

Step 5: If no fractures are suspected, elevate the legs 12 inches. Insert an intravenous (IV) line, and administer warm fluid en route to the emergency department (ED). Insert an IV line at the scene only if transport of the patient is delayed (such as if the patient is pinned).

Chapter 19: Soft-Tissue Injury

Matching

1. L (page 19.4)
2. F (page 19.18)
3. Q (page 19.7)
4. O (page 19.12)
5. M (page 19.9)
6. P (page 19.8)
7. J (page 19.19)
8. I (page 19.5)
9. K (page 19.11)
10. N (page 19.20)

11. T (page 19.7)
12. H (page 19.14)
13. S (page 19.7)
14. E (page 19.6)
15. C (page 19.9)
16. A (page 19.8)
17. R (page 19.13)
18. G (page 19.7)
19. D (page 19.9)
20. B (page 19.5)

Multiple Choice

1. C (page 19.12)
2. B (page 19.18)
3. D (page 19.22)
4. D (page 19.26)
5. A (page 19.14)

6. C (page 19.8)
7. C (page 19.9)
8. C (page 19.18)
9. D (page 19.24)
10. D (page 19.8)

Labeling

1. (page 19.5)

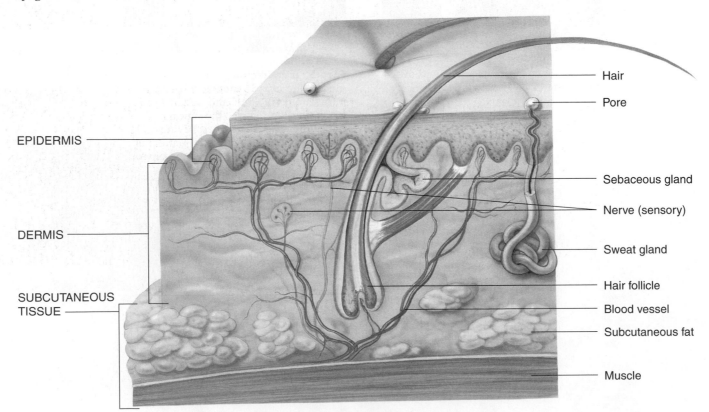

EPIDERMIS

DERMIS

SUBCUTANEOUS TISSUE

Hair

Pore

Sebaceous gland

Nerve (sensory)

Sweat gland

Hair follicle

Blood vessel

Subcutaneous fat

Muscle

2. (pages 19.10, 19.11)

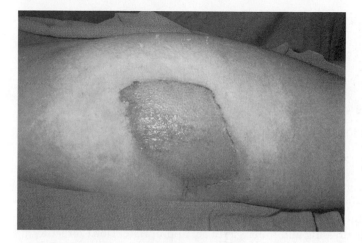

a. Abrasion

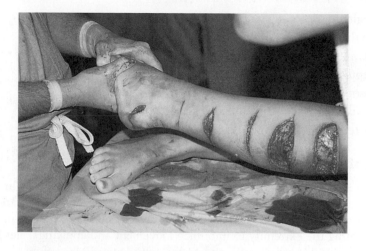

b. Laceration

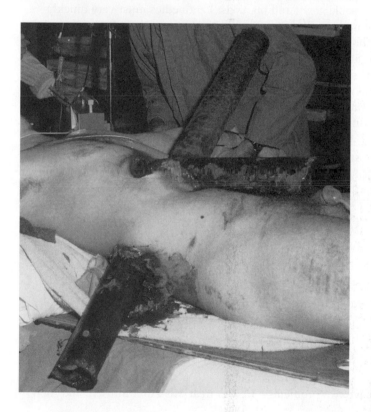

c. Puncture Wound/Impaled Object

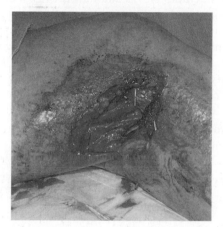

d. Avulsion

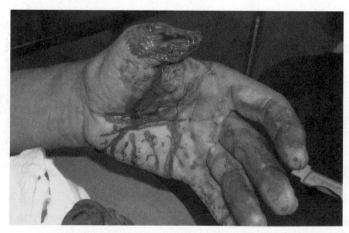

e. Amputation

Fill-in-the-Blank

1. Degloving, debridement (page 19.8)
2. Erythema, pus, warmth, edema, local discomfort (page 19.8)
3. Toxin, contractions, bones (page 19.9)
4. Depth, structures (page 19.10)
5. Vasoconstriction (page 19.11)
6. Police, safe, secondary, killed (page 19.14)
7. Bacteria, limited (page 19.18)

Identify

1. The injury described appears to be a laceration with moderately uncontrolled bleeding. Even though this appears to be an isolated injury a thorough rapid initial assessment is warranted. Treatment would generally include bleeding control. Usually, this can be completed with direct pressure. Sometimes elevation of the extremity and a pressure point is required. Perhaps splinting the extremity to minimize movement and applying a sterile dressing and roller gauze are appropriate. Don't forget to check distal capillary refill and motor neurologic (PMS) before and after bandaging. (page 19.10)

2. This sounds like a classical amputation. Of immediate concern is stopping the bleeding. This will require the paramedic to don PPE, which at the very least includes gloves and may include a disposable gown and blankets. Paramedics must very quickly prepare bulky trauma dressings and be prepared for the potential of uncontrolled bleeding. Bleeding control is often self-limiting in this type of situation. However, if it isn't controlled, methods such as direct pressure, elevation, and use of pressure points may be required. It may be necessary to maintain these steps all the way to the hospital. If necessary, request additional resources. Once bleeding is controlled, begin treating the patient for shock with high-flow oxygen and IV fluid replacement. It's also beneficial as soon as practical to have the patient lay down with his feet elevated. Doing so on your cot enables you to initiate transport immediately. With adequate vital signs, pain medication may also be in order. Above all, don't forget about the amputated fingers. Follow local protocols regarding wet or dry dressings and placing the parts on ice. (page 19.10)

3. This patient has suffered from some type of puncture or stab wound. In her combative state she might not realize how serious the injury could be. As a paramedic you realize that she might have suffered a hemo- or pneumothorax. You rapidly treat the obvious wound with an occlusive dressing and immediately prepare for transportation with high-flow oxygen. You also prepare IVs en route. In a worse-case situation, this patient may require ventilatory assistance and intubation. (page 19.10)

Ambulance Calls

1. **a.** To control the bleeding from Bugsy Butterfingers's left calf, you have several methods available to you:
   (1) Direct manual pressure over the bleeding site (likely to be the most effective)
   (2) Elevation of the bleeding extremity
   (3) Pressure point control, in this case by pressing over the *femoral* artery
   (4) Splinting the left leg
   (5) As a last resort, applying a tourniquet (page 19.19)

   b. If Bugsy's wound had been on the forearm rather than on the leg, pressure over the brachial artery might have helped control the bleeding. (page 19.20)

2. When Frank Fillet accidentally amputates two of his fingers, you have two problems—first to treat Mr. Fillet himself, and then to preserve the amputated parts in optimal condition.

   a. To treat the injury, the first priority is to stop the bleeding. Probably direct pressure will be sufficient because amputations ordinarily do not bleed profusely. Apply lots of fluffed gauze to the stumps of the fingers and bandage the whole hand in a position of function (fingers slightly flexed). The patient will doubtless require a lot of calming down; if you can remain calm, it will help a great deal. (page 19.21)

   b. Once you have taken care of the patient, you can turn your attention to the amputated parts. Rinse the two fingers free of contaminants with cool, sterile saline. Wrap them loosely in saline-moistened sterile gauze. Then, place them in a plastic bag, seal the bag, and place it in a cool container for transport. Do *not* place the amputated part in water or directly on ice! (page 19.21)

3. Bugsy's Butcher Shop is definitely not a healthy workplace. Now poor Hercules Hamburger has also become a casualty—not only of the meat grinder that mangled his hand but also of a "Good Samaritan" who was trying to help. The mistakes made in caring for Hercules include the following:

a. No attempt was made to stop the bleeding by other means, such as direct pressure alone or in combination with pressure point control, splinting, and so on. *A tourniquet is a last resort,* not a first resort!

b. A rope should not be used as a tourniquet, nor should any other narrow materials that can damage underlying tissues.

c. The tourniquet was twisted too tightly. It is virtually never necessary to twist a tourniquet as tight as it will go; the end point is when the bleeding slows sufficiently that it can then be controlled by direct pressure.

d. A tourniquet should never be covered, lest it escape attention. The good Samaritan covered the patient's whole arm in a butcher's apron, perhaps to spare the patient the sight of his mangled extremity. (page 19.21)

4. It is, in fact, rather rare to encounter a patient with an impaled object, but considerable attention is given to the problem in EMT-B and paramedic courses because the consequences of mismanagement could be disastrous.

a. When the impaled object is in the eye, the usual principle applies: Stabilize the impaled object in place. For the eye, the most efficient way to do so is usually with a stack of gauze pads that has a hole in the middle. The gauze pads are passed gently over the impaled object and bandaged in place. If the impaled object is an arrow, as in the present case, it won't be possible to cover it with a paper cup as well. Do not try to shorten the impaled object. Just protect it from being jarred, and be sure to patch the other eye as well, to prevent the injured eye from moving every time the uninjured eye shifts its gaze. (page 19.22)

b. When an object is impaled in the cheek, you have to break the usual rule about not removing an impaled object because it will be impossible to control bleeding inside the mouth as long as the arrow is sticking through the cheek. Therefore, gently pull the arrow out of the cheek. Then, pack the inside of the cheek with sterile gauze, and apply counterpressure with a dressing secured firmly against the outside of the cheek. Keep the patient on his side so that he can more easily spit any blood out of his mouth (instruct him not to swallow blood because blood in the stomach is a stimulus to vomit). (page 19.23)

5. For the man bitten by the Doberman pinscher, the treatment is as follows:

a. Have him stop walking on the injured leg.

b. Clean the wound with lots of soap and water; then, rinse with alcohol (there goes the rest of your gin).

c. Send someone back along the beach to find out details about the dog (eg, name and address of owner), which must be reported to the local health authorities.

d. See that the patient is transported to the hospital for further evaluation of his wound. (page 19.8)

True/False

1. T (page 19.10)   **6.** F (page 19.8)

2. T (page 19.4)   **7.** F (page 19.8)

3. F (page 19.5)   **8.** T (page 19.9)

4. F (page 19.5)   **9.** F (page 19.14)

5. T (page 19.6)   **10.** T (page 19.17)

Short Answer

1. a. It protects underlying tissue from injury.

b. It plays a major role in temperature regulation.

c. It prevents excessive loss of water from the body.

d. It serves as a sense organ for temperature, touch, and pain. (page 19.4)

2. a. Hemostasis

b. Inflammation

c. Epithelialization

d. Neovascularization

e. Collagen synthesis (page 19.6)

3. a. Contusion

b. Ecchymosis

c. Hematoma (page 19.9)

4. a. A body part is trapped for more than 4 hours; then

    b. rhabdomyolysis occurs; then

    c. the trapped body part is freed; and then

    d. by-products of metabolism and harmful products from tissue destruction are released, possibly resulting in cardiac arrest and arrhythmias. (page 19.12)

Word Find

```
E T A X V D T C K S W E F A Q E F N S
C K Y C O T E C Q E C T M O T A E N U
C N L U L G O D E K L E K A S O G O O
H Y R W K Q A S M J H O L C V B I P E
Y U M F M O E P J T B U I A W B W V N
M G U N A A C F Y A N O S D L N E N A
O N X G N T X R U A T C D X S F K A T
S I B J N O E Z R O U J A E H C F V U
I V P G C V Z G M L J P E D L A A J C
S O L A O I E Y A Z F I Y T I A K R B
N L K N N D W R B M G F C V K P P I U
B G G O T Z I N O I S U T N O C O M S
E E A F R Z H O M E O S T A S I S S I
O D Z G A N G R E N E C S F Y R T V E
E X J T C J P S A N B B B J X M F S S
T O I E T S I S Y L O Y M O D B A H R
K O S Y U X K P T H F N B E E C L C K
N J X Z R E D N S K G X N J M E D S I
C H V I E J V G L N M K T L K U M V P
```

  1. Neovascularization (page 19.7)

  2. Contusion (page 19.9)

  3. Rhabdomyolysis (page 19.12)

  4. Erythema (page 19.30)

  5. Degranulate (page 19.5)

  6. Degloving (page 19.11)

  7. Adipose (page 19.6)

  8. Keloid (page 19.8)

  9. Gangrene (page 19.8)

10. Ecchymosis (page 19.9)

11. Homeostasis (page 19.4)

12. Impaled object (page 19.8)

13. Subcutaneous (page 19.29)

14. Fasciotomy (page 19.12)

15. Volkmann contracture (page 19.12)

Skill Drills

1. *Controlling Bleeding From a Soft-Tissue Injury* (page 19.20)

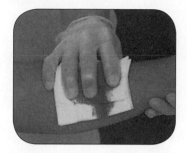 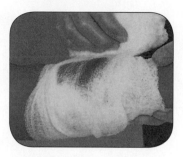 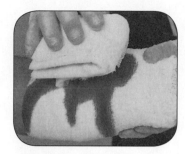 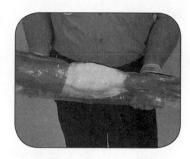

Step 1: Apply direct pressure with a sterile bandage.

Step 2: Maintain pressure with a roller bandage.

Step 3: If bleeding continues, apply second dressing and roller bandage over the first.

Step 4: Splint the extremity.

2. *Applying a Tourniquet* (page 19.22)

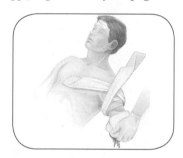 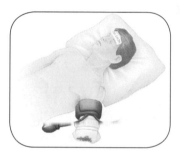 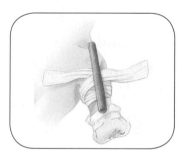

Step 1: Create a 4", multilayered bandage. Wrap the bandage twice around the extremity, just above the bleeding site, and tie a half-knot.

Step 1: (continued) You can also use a blood pressure cuff as an effective tourniquet.

Step 2: Place a stick on top of the half-knot and tie a square knot over the stick.

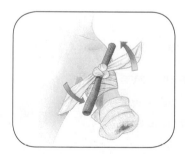 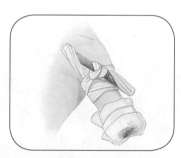

Step 3: Twist the stick until the bleeding stops.

Step 4: Secure the stick so that it will not unwind. Write "TK" and the exact time you applied the tourniquet on a piece of adhesive tape, fasten the tape to the patient's forehead, and notify hospital personnel on arrival.

Chapter 20: Burns

Matching

1. (pages 20.22–20.23)

(1) A		**(5)** B	
(2) A		**(6)** A	
(3) B		**(7)** A	
(4) A		**(8)** A	

2.
- **(1)** D — Put out the fire!
- **(2)** C — Open the airway manually.
- **(3)** A — Administer supplemental oxygen.
- **(4)** H — Intubate the trachea (if there is not a good BLS airway).
- **(5)** F — Pass a nasogastric tube into his stomach.
- **(6)** B — Start an IV.
- **(7)** J — Obtain baseline vital signs.
- **(8)** E — Remove the victim's clothing.
- **(9)** G — Determine the extent and depth of the burn.
- **(10)** I — Cover the burns with sterile dressings.

Multiple Choice

1. D (page 20.12)   **6.** C (page 20.20)
2. B (page 20.13)   **7.** D (page 20.21)
3. A (page 20.16)   **8.** A (page 20.22)
4. C (page 20.16)   **9.** B (page 20.23)
5. B (page 20.18)   **10.** C (page 20.25)

Labeling

1. The skin is the largest organ of the human body and one of the few organs we can easily *see* from the outside of the body. (page 20.5)

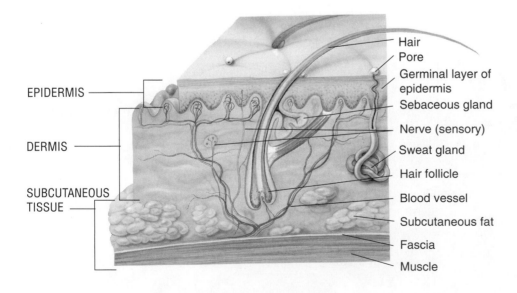

EPIDERMIS

DERMIS

SUBCUTANEOUS TISSUE

Hair
Pore
Germinal layer of epidermis
Sebaceous gland
Nerve (sensory)
Sweat gland
Hair follicle
Blood vessel
Subcutaneous fat
Fascia
Muscle

2. Superficial, partial-thickness, and full-thickness burns (page 20.17)

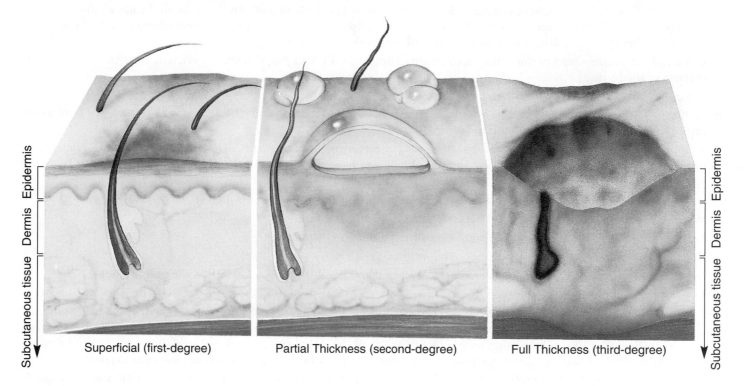

Superficial (first-degree)   Partial Thickness (second-degree)   Full Thickness (third-degree)

Fill-in-the-Blank

1. Skin (page 20.4)

2. Dermis (page 20.6)

3. Scald (page 20.7)

4. Acids, alkalis, bases (page 20.9)

5. Oxidation (page 20.10)

6. Scene is safe (page 20.26)

7. Alpha, beta, gamma (page 20.13)

8. Zone of coagulation (page 20.15)

9. Dry dressing (page 20.23)

10. Decontaminated (page 20.26)

Identify

1. Chief complaint: Woman burned by oil from a hot fryer. Upon arrival, you find her with holes in her jeans on the top of both thighs. She is crying and immediately rates her pain as unbearable.

2. Vital signs: Respirations are 22 breaths/min, oxygen saturation is 97%, lungs are clear, blood pressure is 150/100 mm Hg, pulse is 114 beats/min with sinus tachycardia, skin is cool, pain is 10/10, patient is alert ×3.

3. Pertinent negatives: Airway is open, patient doesn't have any mental deficits, there are no burns other than on the top of her thighs.

Ambulance Calls

1. The patient who jumped from his bedroom window to escape a fire is in grave jeopardy. He is unconscious, so his airway is liable to be obstructed. He may have additional respiratory injury (note the burns to his face), along with head and neck injuries (note the mechanisms of injury). And he almost certainly has at least one broken bone. The steps in treating him are as follows: (page 20.20)

a. Put out the fire in his trousers!

b. Open his airway with cervical spine precautions (ie, chin lift or jaw thrust only).

   c. Administer supplemental oxygen—he's been in a smoky environment.

   d. Intubate the trachea. This patient is unconscious, so his airway is already in jeopardy. In addition, he has almost certainly sustained airway injury—note the singed beard and swollen lips—so don't wait until laryngeal edema closes off his airway altogether. Get the endotracheal tube in while it's still relatively easy to do so.

   e. Cut away the trousers, and perform the rapid trauma assessment. In doing so, you should evaluate the extent, depth, and severity of the burn.

   f. Cover the burns with sterile dressings.

   g. Splint the left leg and any other fractures; immobilize the patient on a backboard. (He fell from 15 feet, so you have to assume until proved otherwise that he injured his spine.)

   h. Start an IV (can be done en route to hospital). Note: The precise point in time at which you start the IV will be determined by the patient's overall condition and the amount of help you have at the scene. If the patient is shocky, start the IV as soon as you've managed the airway.

2. Among the questions you would like answered about the burned patient are the following:

   a. When precisely did the burn occur? (That is, when did the fire break out?)

   b. Was the patient in a closed space with smoke or other products of combustion?

   c. Does the patient have any significant underlying medical problems?

   d. Does the patient take any medications regularly? Had he taken any drugs or alcohol within the past few hours?

   e. Does the patient have any allergies?

You already know the answers to most of the other questions you would usually ask. You can assume that the patient did not lose consciousness while still in the burning building because he managed to jump out the window. You know what he was burned with (flame). And you know that nothing was done until the ambulance arrived. It would, however, be helpful to question the fire personnel regarding toxic products of combustion to which the patient might have been exposed.

3. a. The burn on the right arm is probably **partial thickness (second-degree)** burn. The severe pain virtually rules out a third-degree burn, and the mottling suggests it is more serious than a superficial (first-degree) burn. The appropriate treatment is to **cover the burn with cool, wet, sterile dressings.** If the application of cool dressings is not sufficient to relieve the patient's pain, it may be necessary to give him a small dose of morphine in addition.

   b. The burn on the flank is probably a **superficial (first-degree)** burn, although it could also be partial thickness (it will be impossible to tell for sure until at least another few hours). **Treat it as you would treat a partial-thickness burn** because it might well be one.

   c. The burn on the right leg is probably **full thickness (third-degree)** burn. The leathery appearance, thrombosed veins, and absence of sensation are all characteristic. **Cover the burn with a dry sterile dressing.** (page 20.16)

4. Electric burns can be very deceptive because the extent of injury may not be at all apparent from the burn that is visible on the surface of the body.

   a. The three types of *burns* that may occur from electricity are

     (1) A contact burn, which usually produces a bull's-eye lesion at the point of entry and sometimes also at the point of exit

     (2) A flash burn, an electrothermal injury caused by the arcing of electric current

     (3) A flame burn, which occurs if the electricity ignites a person's clothing or surroundings (page 20.11)

   b. Besides burns, electricity may cause a variety of other injuries or disorders of function, including the following:

     (1) Respiratory arrest

     (2) Cardiac arrest

     (3) Neurologic disorders (seizures, coma, paralysis)

     (4) Kidney damage

     (5) Fractures and dislocations

     (6) Cervical spine injuries (page 20.12)

   c. In dealing with this electrocuted patient lying beside a live cable, you need to take the following steps:

     (1) Secure the scene. Keep all bystanders well back from the live wire. Do not get within reach of the wire if you are not fully trained and fully equipped to deal with power lines. Radio for help, and do not get within range of the wire until it has been inactivated. If you have some creative idea for extricating the patient that does not require your coming within range of the cable (eg, lassoing him and dragging him toward you), you may try such a method, but bear in mind that the patient may have a spinal injury.

(2) As soon as it is safe to approach the patient, ensure that he has an open airway, taking precautions not to hyperextend his neck.

(3) Provide artificial ventilation or cardiopulmonary resuscitation (CPR) as needed.

(4) Administer supplemental oxygen.

(5) If the patient remains unconscious, intubate the trachea (if a BLS airway is not adequate).

(6) Start an IV, and run in lactated Ringer's or normal saline solution as fast as the IV will flow.

(7) Consult the base physician for medication orders.

(8) Cover burns with a sterile dressing.

(9) Splint fractures.

(10) Immobilize the spine on a backboard. (page 20.24)

5. In this question, a young man was rescued unconscious from a house fire.

  a. Signs suggestive of respiratory injury in a burned patient include the following:

    (1) Facial burns

    (2) Singed nasal hairs

    (3) Blistering or redness inside the mouth

    (4) Hoarseness, stridor, or brassy cough

    (5) Sooty sputum

    (6) Wheezing

  b. The first step to take in managing this patient is to *put out the fire* in his clothing!

  c. (1) To calculate the extent of his burns, you need to use a combination of the rule of nines and the rule of palms (page 20.18):

Posterior surface of both legs	18%
Whole left arm	9%
Hand-sized patch of left flank	1%
TOTAL	28%

    (2) Yes, the patient does have a critical burn on at least three counts:

      (a) He has full-thickness burns over more than 10% of his body.

      (b) He has burns of all depths or thicknesses over more than 25% of his body.

      (c) He has burns involving the genitals.

  d. The Parkland formula states that during the *first 8 hours* the patient should receive (page 20.21):

8 mL/hr = ½ × 4 mL/kg body weight × % body surface burned

So for this patient, that means

$$8 \text{ mL/hr} = \text{½} \times 4 \text{ mL} \times 70 \text{ kg} \times 28$$
$$= 3{,}920 \text{ mL}$$

Therefore, during each hour, the patient needs to receive

$$\text{mL/hr} = \frac{3{,}920 \text{ mL}}{8 \text{ hr}}$$

$$= 490 \text{ mL/hr}$$

$$\text{mL/min} = \frac{490 \text{ mL}}{60 \text{ min/hr}}$$

$$= 8 \text{ mL/min}$$

$$\text{gtt/min} = 8 \text{ mL/min} \times 10 \text{ gtt/mL}$$

$$= \textbf{80 gtt/min}$$

  e. (1) The dosage of morphine usually given to an adult in the field is **2 to 5 mg.**

    (2) It is usually given **intravenously** because absorption after intramuscular administration may be erratic if the patient has any perfusion problems.

    (3) Possible *adverse side effects* include the following (Students will list three):

      (a) Hypotension

(b) Bradycardia

(c) Respiratory depression

(d) Nausea and vomiting

6. a. This is a patient who clearly has a serious chest injury. Furthermore, it is a chest injury that is increasing venous pressure. The combination of dyspnea, shock, and distended neck veins is highly suggestive of tension pneumothorax, and so you need to proceed as follows:

b. (1) Administer 100% supplemental oxygen by nonrebreathing mask.

(2) Look for deviation of the trachea, and listen for breath sounds on both sides of the chest. *If breath sounds are unequal:*

(3) Decompress the chest with a 14-gauge cannula in the second intercostal space in the midclavicular line.

(4) Immobilize the patient on a long backboard.

(5) Start transport to a trauma center.

(6) Start at least one large-bore IV en route.

7. The percentage of the patient's body that is burned is (page 20.18):

Entire left leg	18%
Posterior right leg	9%
Left forearm	4%
TOTAL	31%

b. Yes, the patient has a critical burn, for two reasons:

(1) The burn covers more than 25% of the body surface.

(2) The burn involves the genitals.

c. If the pedal pulses are absent in a burned leg, you have to assume that swelling from circumferential burns has cut off the circulation to the foot. If you do not act quickly in such a situation, the patient may lose his leg.

d. What you need to do is cool the burned leg with towels that have been soaked in cold water and transport the patient immediately to the hospital.

True/False

The principles of treating chemical burns do not differ significantly from those of treating thermal burns. In both cases, the first priority is to *put out the fire,* but in a chemical burn, putting out the fire is a more difficult and time-consuming operation.

1. F (page 20.23)		**6.** T (page 20.8)	
2. T (page 20.23)		**7.** F (page 20.8)	
3. F (page 20.9)		**8.** F (page 20.9)	
4. F (page 20.24)		**9.** T (page 20.12)	
5. T (page 20.24)		**10.** F (page 20.14)	

Short Answer

1. a. Rule 1: Never be the tallest object. Stay out of the middle of open fields or open areas.

Don't use ladders, umbrellas, or anything else that makes you taller. Make yourself as small as possible.

b. Rule 2: Never stand under or near the tallest object that is a good conductor. Stay away from trees, metal umbrellas, or towers of any kind.

c. Rule 3: Take shelter in the most substantial structure in which you will be safe if it is hit by lighting. Try to get in an enclosed building if possible. A small metal shed probably would not be a good idea.

d. Rule 4: Avoid touching a good conductor during a lightning storm. This can apply to things inside your home such as the TV, telephone, and computer. (page 20.12)

2. Suspect that a victim of flame burns has suffered respiratory injury if any of the following signs are present (page 20.8):

a. Singed nasal hairs   **d.** Wheezes

b. Stridor   **e.** Brassy cough

c. Sooty sputum   **f.** Hoarseness

3. Injury from a high-voltage electric source or from lightning may produce any of the following (page 20.12):

a. Apnea
f. Delirium
b. Paralysis
g. Exit wound
c. Cardiac arrest
h. Coma
d. Fracture
i. Amnesia
e. Kidney damage
j. Tetany

Word Find

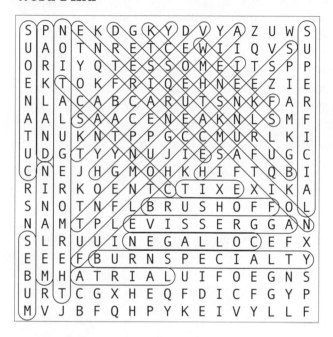

1. Integument (page 20.4)
2. Thermoregulation (page 20.5)
3. Desquamation (page 20.5)
4. Melanin (page 20.5)
5. Collagen (page 20.5)
6. Cutaneous (page 20.5)
7. Sebum (page 20.6)
8. Contact (page 20.7)
9. Burn shock (page 20.8)
10. Vesicant (page 20.10)
11. Atrial (page 20.12)
12. Safety (page 20.14)
13. Hyperemia (page 20.16)
14. Full thickness (page 20.16)
15. Weeks (page 20.20)
16. Parkland (page 20.21)
17. Aggressive (page 20.21)
18. Superficial (page 20.22)
19. Brush off (page 20.23)
20. Flush (page 20.24)
21. Entrance/exit (page 20.25)
22. Burn specialty (page 20.27

Fill-in-the-Table

The Parkland Formula (page 20.21)

Parkland Formula Chart

% Burn	10 kg	20 kg	30 kg	40 kg	50 kg	60 kg	70 kg	80 kg	90 kg	100 kg
10	25	50	75	100	125	150	175	200	225	250
20	50	100	150	200	250	300	350	400	450	500
30	75	150	225	300	375	450	525	600	675	750
40	100	200	300	400	500	600	700	800	900	1,000
50	125	250	375	500	625	750	875	1,000	1,125	1,250
60	150	300	450	600	750	900	1,050	1,200	1,350	1,500
70	175	350	525	700	875	1,050	1,225	1,400	1,575	1,750
80	200	400	600	800	1,000	1,200	1,400	1,600	1,800	2,000
90	225	450	675	900	1,125	1,350	1,575	1,800	2,025	2,250
20 mL/kg	200	400	600	800	1,000	1,200	1,400	1,600	1,800	2,000

This table represents the fluid recommended in the *first hour* (⅛ of the initial 8-hour dose) by the Parkland formula. The final row represents the amount of a 20-mL/kg bolus.

Problem Solving

1. To calculate the patient's fluid needs, first you must assess the extent of his burns. Then, you can calculate the IV rate in the usual fashion.

   a. The percentage of the patient's body that has been burned is calculated as follows (page 20.18):

   Whole right leg   18%
   Anterior left leg   9%
   Anterior trunk   18%
   Whole right arm   9%
   TOTAL   54%

   b. Now you have to calculate the patient's fluid needs. First, you must convert his weight from pounds to kilograms (page 20.21):

   = 70 kg

   Now, according to the Parkland formula, the patient's fluid needs over the first 8 hours will be

   ½ × 4 mL/kg body weight × % of body surface burned

   ½ × 4 mL × 70 kg × 54 = 7,650 mL

   So his fluid needs *per hour* will be

   = 945 mL/hr

   (Practically speaking, that figure can be regarded as equivalent to 1 liter per hour, but you should complete the calculations using the precise figures.)

   Thus, you will need to deliver

   = 15.8 mL/min (ie, **16 mL/min**)

   c. If your infusion set delivers 10 gtt per milliliter, you therefore need to set the rate of the infusion at
   10 gtt/mL × 16 mL/min = **160 gtt/min**

   We included this question to give you a little practice in computing IV rates—just in case you were getting rusty. In this particular case, however, it is an academic exercise only because to deliver the kind of volumes we are talking about—nearly 1 liter per hour—you will have to run the IV wide open, probably under pressure. Usually, when volumes of this sort are required, it makes more sense to start a second and even a third IV line.

   d. For a burned patient, give an intravenous fluid that will remain in the vascular space, such as normal saline or lactated Ringer's solution.

Chapter 21: Head and Face Injuries

Matching

1. C (page 21.34)	**6.** C (page 21.34)
2. A (page 21.33)	**7.** A (page 21.33)
3. B (page 21.33)	**8.** B (page 21.33)
4. D (page 21.33)	**9.** E (page 21.35)
5. C (page 21.34)	**10.** F (page 21.35)

Multiple Choice

1. D (page 21.5)	**9.** C (page 21.31)
2. C (page 21.7)	**10.** D (page 21.32)
3. A (page 21.9)	**11.** B (page 21.33)
4. B (page 21.11)	**12.** B (page 21.35)
5. B (page 21.12)	**13.** C (page 21.36)
6. D (page 21.13)	**14.** D (page 21.37)
7. A (page 21.15)	**15.** A (page 21.38)
8. B (page 21.22)	

Labeling

1. Structures of the Eye (page 21.8)

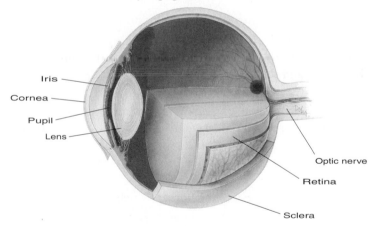

2. Structures of the Anterior Part of the Neck (page 21.11)

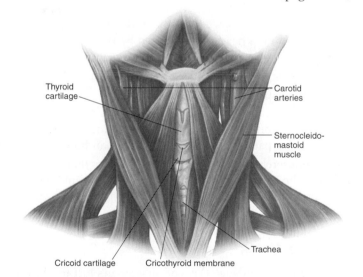

3. Major Regions of the Brain (page 21.12)

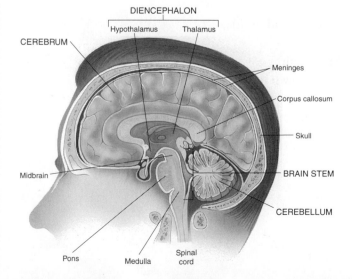

Fill-in-the-Blank

1. Axial (page 21.4)
2. Fontanelles (page 2.5)
3. Blowout (page 21.7)
4. Pupil (page 21.8)
5. Cerebrum (page 21.11)
6. Pons, medulla (page 21.13)
7. Arachnoid (page 21.14)
8. Cervical spine (page 21.16)
9. Airway (page 21.17)
10. Hyphema (page 21.19)
11. Chemicals, heat, light (page 21.19)
12. 20 (page 21.22)
13. Chemical burn (page 21.24)
14. Hour (page 21.26)
15. Occlusive (page 21.28)
16. Coup-contrecoup (page 21.32)
17. Hypertension, Cushing's triad (page 21.32)
18. Epidural (page 21.34)
19. RSI (page 21.39)
20. Body temperature (page 21.39)

Identify

1. Chief complaint: a head injury caused by the rollover and ejection from the vehicle
2. Vital signs: decerebrate posturing, unresponsive, 8 on GCS, respirations are 34 breaths/min and deep, oxygen saturation of 99%, pupils are sluggish, blood pressure is 160/90 mm/Hg, pulse is 72 beats/min, and skin is cool
3. Pertinent negatives: no outward bleeding
4. This girl has an obvious head injury. A trauma center will have a neurosurgeon on hand to treat her. A community hospital would be able only to try and stabilize her and then ship her to a trauma center. She doesn't have that much time. Golden Hour rules that this patient needs surgery within an hour of the incident.
5. She is in decerebrate posturing. This indicates that she already has swelling or bleeding inside the brain that is causing this posture. The pressure is already building on the middle brain stem.
6. The rising blood pressure, slowing heart rate, and the deep, fast respirations are classic Cushing's triad, which indicates a rising intracranial pressure (ICP).

Ambulance Calls

1. If you are able to salvage this young woman's lost tooth, you will have made a friend for life.
   a. Locate the tooth.
   b. Handle the tooth by the crown only. Do not touch the root surface of the tooth.
   c. Rinse the tooth and the empty socket with sterile saline or water (do not allow it to dry).
   d. Carefully place the tooth back in the socket.
   e. Once the tooth is in place, have the patient gently bite down on a gauze roll to maintain pressure against the tooth. (page 21.26)
2. A thorough examination of an injured eye includes assessment of
   a. The orbital rim for ecchymoses, swelling, laceration, and tenderness
   b. The eyelids, for ecchymoses, swelling, and lacerations
   c. The corneas for foreign bodies
   d. The conjunctivae, for redness, foreign bodies, inflammation, and pus

e. The globes for redness, abnormal pigmentation, and lacerations

f. The pupils, for size, shape, equality, and reaction to light (PEARRL)

g. Eye movements in all directions, for evidence of paralysis of gaze or no coordination between the movements of the two eyes

h. Most important of all, visual acuity (page 21.21)

3. a. The principal dangers associated with a laceration of the neck are massive hemorrhage from major blood vessel disruption, airway compromise secondary to soft-tissue swelling, or direct damage to the larynx or trachea. Fatal air embolism is also considered a special danger.

b. Open neck wounds should be sealed with an occlusive dressing immediately. (page 21.27)

4. The mechanisms of injury (MOI) (ie, broken windshield) suggest head trauma, even before you have inspected the patient's head. The patient's suboptimal mental status, his unequal pupils, along with a slow pulse and high blood pressure all add up to rising intracranial pressure (ICP).

a. Steps to be taken at the scene:

(1) Administer supplementary oxygen.

(2) Immobilize the patient on a long backboard. (It may not be easy because the patient may not be cooperative!)

(3) Communicate with medical control or receiving hospital.

b. Steps to be taken en route:

(1) Perform detailed physical exam and ongoing assessment.

(2) Start keep-open IV with normal saline.

(3) Be alert for seizures, vomiting.

(4) Recheck vital and neurologic signs every 5 minutes.

5. In this question about a head-injured patient, you had to review some respiratory physiology along with the pathophysiology of head injury.

a. If the patient's respiratory rate is 8 breaths/min and his tidal volume is 500 mL, his minute volume is calculated as follows:

Minute Volume = Tidal Volume × Respiratory Rate

= 500 mL/breath × 8 breaths/min

= 4,000 mL/min (4 liters/min)

b. That minute volume is less than normal. (Normal is around 6 liters/min)

c. Therefore, you can conclude that the patient's arterial PCO_2 will tend to **increase**, so his pH will **decrease**. The net effect will be an acid–base disorder called a **respiratory acidosis**. The way you can help correct that abnormality is to **assist the patient's ventilations and thereby increase his minute volume (which will blow off more carbon dioxide).**

d. The signs of increasing intracranial pressure (ICP) include the following. *Students will provide five of the following:*

(1) Vomiting

(2) Headache

(3) Altered level of consciousness

(4) Seizures

(5) Hypertension with a widening pulse pressure

(6) Bradycardia

(7) Irregular respirations

(8) Unequal and nonreactive pupil

(9) Coma

(10) Posturing

e. (1) The patient's AVPU rating is P (responds only to painful stimuli).

(2) His score on the Glasgow Coma Scale is 8 points. (page 21.36)

6. It should be clear, after carrying out this exercise, that the Glasgow Coma Scale enables a much more precise description than does the AVPU rating of the patient's level of consciousness.

a. AVPU: somewhere between V and P

GCS: 10

    b. AVPU: V

       GCS: 13

    c. AVPU: somewhere between P and U

       GCS: 5

    d. AVPU: A

       GSC: 15 (page 21.36)

7. In treating the victim of the whiskey bottle, how well did you remember your priorities?

    a. Eliminate the safety hazard. So long as there are tables and chairs being launched into orbit, you and everyone else in the bar are in danger. Try to get all bystanders to leave the premises (call in police help if needed). First priority is scene safety, and then, from a safe distance, see if you can calm the patient. Explain that you are paramedics and that you have come to help him. Such an explanation is often of particular importance in municipalities where paramedics wear uniforms that could be mistaken for police uniforms (a very dangerous practice!).

    b. When you are reasonably certain that it is safe to approach the patient, encourage him to sit down, and examine his scalp by palpating the scalp wound lightly with a gloved finger to make certain that the skull beneath the wound is not fractured.

    c. If there is no evidence of skull fracture, control scalp bleeding by direct manual pressure, and apply a pressure dressing.

    d. Complete the detailed physical exam, and manage any other injuries detected thereby.

True/False

  1. F (page 21.5)   **11.** F (page 21.17)

  2. T (page 21.5)   **12.** T (page 21.19)

  3. F (page. 21.7)   **13.** F (page 21.22)

  4. T (page. 21.9)   **14.** F (page 21.25)

  5. F (page 21.10)   **15.** T (page 21.25)

  6. T (page 21.11)   **16.** T (page 21.28)

  7. T (page 21.12)   **17.** T (page 21.29)

  8. F (page 21.13)   **18.** T (page 21.32)

  9. T (page 21.14)   **19.** F (page 21.33)

10. T (page 21.15)   **20.** T (page 21.35)

Short Answer

  1. a. Closed head injury

     b. Cervical spine injury (page 21.15)

  2. *Students will provide five of the following:*

    a. Swelling of the face

    b. Ecchymoses over the face

    c. Crepitus over a broken bone

    d. Pain to palpation

    e. Instability of the facial bones

    f. Impaired ocular movement

    g. Malocclusion in cases where the jaw is fractured

    h. Visual disturbances

    i. Obvious deformity of the face (eg, flattening of one side) (page 21.15)

Crossword Puzzle

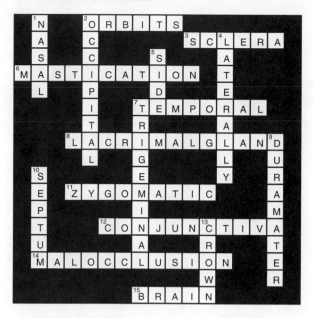

Across:
2. ORBITS
3. SCLERA
6. MASTICATION
7. TEMPORAL
8. LACRIMALGLAND
11. ZYGOMATIC
12. CONJUNCTIVA
14. MALOCCLUSION
15. BRAIN

Down:
1. NASAL
2. OCCIPITAL
4. CAROTENE
5. SDITOR
9. DURAMATER
10. SEPTUM
13. CRANW

Fill-in the Table

1.

Signs and Symptoms of Head Injury
■ Lacerations, **contusions**, or **hematomas** to the scalp
■ **Soft area** or **depression** noted on palpation of the scalp
■ Visible **fractures** or **deformities** of the skull
■ **Battle** sign or **raccoon** eyes
■ CSF **rhinorrhea** or otorrhea
■ Pupillary abnormalities
– **Unequal pupil size**
– **Sluggish or nonreactive pupils**
■ A period of **unresponsiveness**
■ **Confusion** or disorientation
■ Repeatedly asking the same question(s) (**perseveration**)
■ Amnesia (**retrograde** and/or **anterograde**)
■ **Combativeness** or other abnormal behavior
■ Numbness or **tingling** in the **extremities**
■ Loss of **sensation** and/or **motor function**
■ Focal **neurologic deficits**
■ Seizures
■ **Cushing's** triad: **hypertension**, **bradycardia**, and irregular or erratic respirations
■ Dizziness
■ Visual disturbances, **blurred** vision, or **double** vision (diplopia)
■ Seeing "stars"
■ Nausea or **vomiting**
■ Posturing (**decorticate** and/or **decerebrate**)

(page 21.36)

2.

GLASGOW COMA SCALE

Eye Opening

Spontaneous	4	
To Voice	3	
To Pain	2	
None	1	

Verbal Response

Oriented	5	
Confused	4	
Inappropriate Words	3	
Incomprehensible Words	2	
None	1	

Motor Response

Obeys Command	6	
Localizes Pain	5	
Withdraws (pain)	4	
Flexion (pain)	3	
Extension (pain)	2	
None	1	

Glasgow Coma Score Total	**15**	

(page 21.37)

3.

Brain Injury Classification Based on the GCS

- **13 to 15.** Mild traumatic brain injury
- **8 to 12.** Moderate traumatic brain injury
- **3 to 8.** Severe traumatic brain injury

(page 21.37)

Chapter 22: Spine Injuries

Matching

1. B (page 22.16)	**3.** A (page 22.16)
2. C (page 22.9)	**4.** A (page 22.9)

1. D (page 22.9)	**4.** C (page 22.9)
2. A (page 22.8)	**5.** B (page 22.8)
3. F (page 22.9)	**6.** E (page 22.9)

Multiple Choice

1. C (page 22.3)	**6.** C (page 22.17)
2. C (page 22.6)	**7.** D (page 22.20)
3. A (page 22.7)	**8.** A (page 22.21)
4. B (page 22.10)	**9.** B (page 22.25)
5. A (page 22.11)	**10.** D (page 22.15)

Labeling

1. The cervical, thoracic, and lumbar spine areas (page 22.4)

2. The layers of the spinal cord (page 22.6)

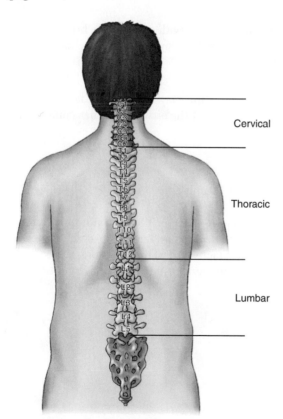

Cervical

Thoracic

Lumbar

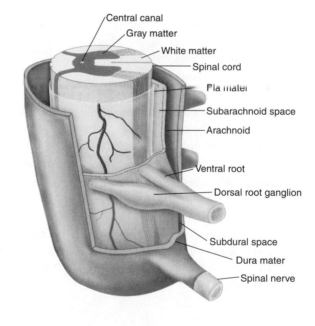

Central canal
Gray matter
White matter
Spinal cord
Pia mater
Subarachnoid space
Arachnoid
Ventral root
Dorsal root ganglion
Subdural space
Dura mater
Spinal nerve

Fill-in-the-Blank

1. Lamina, pedicles (page 22.3)

2. C1, C2 (page 22.4)

3. Brain, spinal cord (page 22.5)

4. Medulla, pons, midbrain (page 22.5)

5. Foramen magnum (page 22.6)

6. Hypothalamus (page 22.7)

7. Complete (page 22.9)

8. Neurogenic shock (page 22.9)

9. Jaw-thrust (page 22.11)

10. Upward, downward (page 22.15)

Identify

1. Chief complaint: Multiple trauma

2. Vital signs: V in AVPU, Glasgow Coma Scale score is 9, cool skin, blood pressure is 100/62 mm/Hg, pulse is 124 beats/min with sinus tachycardia, oxygen saturation is 96%, respirations are 26 breaths/min

3. Pertinent negatives: Lungs are clear, no feeling or response in lower extremities

The chief complaint in this case study is multiple trauma caused by a rollover crash. She is responding to voice and only able to answer what her name is. So, you can call her a V on the AVPU scale and close to a 9 on the GCS scale because of the inability to move her legs. Your patient is hypothermic by touch. Blood pressure is 100/62 mm/Hg, pulse is 124 beats/min with sinus tachycardia on the monitor. Oxygen staturation is 96% but comes up to 98% with 100% oxygen. Her breathing rate is 26 breaths/min and shallow, lungs are clear. The absence of a pulse in either foot could be caused by the hypothermia. She has no feeling or response in her lower extremities. Blood pressure comes up slightly with a warm fluid bolus, which also helps to warm her. Second blood pressure is 108/64 mm/Hg. You did your job by stabilizing her and securing her neck and body to the backboard. The physician later tells you the break was very bad, and there was nothing else you could have done to help her out.

Ambulance Calls

1. a. The bad guy probably has a severe injury to the larynx, such as a laryngeal "fracture," as evidenced by the bruise over his throat, his hoarseness, and his subcutaneous emphysema. Furthermore, given the mechanisms of injury, one has to assume that he has a cervical spine injury as well.

b. The steps of treatment are as follows:

(1) Administer 100% oxygen, and instruct the patient to breathe slowly (rapid inhalation may cause an unstable trachea to collapse inward). It is preferable to avoid intubating the patient in the field, but if the airway becomes compromised further, you may have no choice.

(2) Immobilize the spine by immobilizing the whole patient on a long backboard.

(3) Transport the patient immediately, preferably to a major trauma center.

2. a. The boy has a sensory level around T8 and intact motor function at least from T1 upward. You can assume that his injury is no higher than T8.

b. The boy's hypotension could mean either neurogenic shock or hypovolemic shock. It is very difficult, if not impossible, to distinguish between the two under these circumstances because if the sympathetic nervous system has been disrupted by the spinal cord injury, you will not see the usual signs of shock, such as sweating and tachycardia. Furthermore, the boy's sensory deficit may mask pain from damage to intra-abdominal structures. So, when you encounter shock in such circumstances, you have to *treat it as hypovolemic shock until proved otherwise*.

True/False

1. F (page 22.5)
2. F (page 22.6)
3. T (page 22.7)
4. T (page 22.8)
5. F (page 22.8)
6. F (page 22.9)
7. T (page 22.11)
8. F (page 22.12)
9. F (page 22.14)
10. T (page 22.15)
11. F (page 22.17)
12. T (page 22.18)
13. F (page 22.19)
14. F (page 22.20)
15. F (page 22.23)
16. T (page 22.26)

Short Answer

1. *Students will list eight*

   a. High-velocity crash (> 40 mph) with severe vehicle damage

   b. Unrestrained occupant of moderate- to high-speed motor vehicle crash

   c. Vehicular damage with compartmental intrusion (12 inches) into the patient's seating space

   d. Fall from three times the patient's height

   e. Penetrating trauma near the spine

   f. Ejection from a motor vehicle

   g. Motorcycle crash at greater than 20 mph with separation of driver from bike

   h. Diving injury

   i. Auto–pedestrian or auto–bicycle crash with greater than 5 mph impact

   j. Death of an occupant in the same passenger compartment

   k. Rollover crash (unrestrained) (page 22.10)

2. D Deformity

   C Contusion

   A Abrasion

   P Puncture/penetration

   B Bruising

   T Tenderness

   L Laceration

   S Swelling

   P Pulse

   M Motor

   S Sensory

   (page 22.12)

Word Find

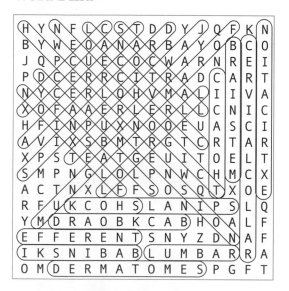

1. Lumbar (page 22.4)

2. Brain stem (page 22.5)

3. Spinal cord (page 22.6)

4. Hyperextension (page 22.8)

5. log roll (page 22.19)

6. Babinski (page 22.15)

7. Neurologic (page 22.12)

8. Cervical collar (page 22.11)

9. DCAP BTLS (page 22.12)

10. Afferent, Efferent (page 22.7)

11. cervical, thoracic, sacrum, coccyx (page 22.3)

12. Jaw thrust (page 22.11)

13. Backboard (page 22.13)

14. Dermatomes (page 22.15)

15. Extrication (page 22.17)

16. Spinal shock (page 22.9)

17. Foramen magnum (page 22.6)

18. Flexion (page 22.8)

19. Shock (page 22.16)

Secret Messages

a. Central nervous (page 22.5)

b. Sympathetic (page 22.7)

c. Spinal shock (page 22.9)

d. Jaw-thrust maneuver (page 22.11)

e. Dermatomes (page 22.15)

f. Four log roll (page 22.17)

The secret message of this lesson is the most important message of the whole chapter:

A NORMAL NEUROLOGIC EXAM DOESN'T RULE OUT A SPINAL INJURY.

Fill-in-the-Table

Landmark Dermatomes			
Nerve Root	**Anatomic Location**	**Nerve Root**	**Anatomic Location**
C2	Occipital protuberance	T10	Umbilicus
C3	Supraclavicular fossa	L1	Inguinal line
C5	Lateral side of antecubital fossa	L2	Mid anterior thigh
C6	Thumb and medial index finger (6-shooter)	L3	Medial aspect of the knee
C7	Middle finger	L5	Dorsum of the foot
C8	Little finger	S1-S3	Back of leg
T2	Apex of axilla	S4-S5	Perianal area
T4	Nipple line		

(page 22.15)

Chapter 23: Thoracic Injuries

Matching

1. D (page 23.22)
2. C (page 23.19)
3. A (page 23.18)
4. B (page 23.18)
5. E (page 23.22)
6. C (page 23.6)
7. B (page 23.6)
8. A (page 23.6)
9. E (page 23.6)
10. D (page 23.6)

Multiple Choice

1. A (page 23.7)
2. C (page 23.9)
3. B (page 23.11)
4. C (page 23.15)
5. D (page 23.22)
6. A (page 23.8)
7. B (page 23.12)
8. C (page 23.18)
9. B (page 23.20)
10. D (page 23.20)

Labeling

1. The Thorax (page 23.4)

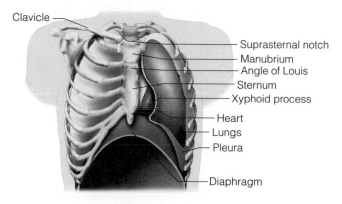

Anterior

Clavicle
Suprasternal notch
Manubrium
Angle of Louis
Sternum
Xyphoid process
Heart
Lungs
Pleura
Diaphragm

Fill-in-the-Blank

1. The mechanisms of injury (MOI), or easily detected injuries, may give clues to the presence of injuries that are harder to find.

If you find:	The patient may have:
1. Steering wheel imprint on anterior chest	Myocardial contusion (page 23.11) Cardiac tamponade (page 23.10) Aortic rupture Pneumothorax or hemothorax (pages 23.8, 23.10) Tracheobronchial injury (page 23.13)
2. Caved-in door on driver's side	Diaphragmatic tear (page 23.12)
3. Fall from a height	Thoracic aortic dissection/transaction (page 23.12) Pulmonary contusion (page 23.10)
4. Bullet entrance wound in fifth left intercostal space	Pericardial tamponade (page 23.10) Injury to liver, spleen, stomach, lungs (look for exit wound)
5. Fracture of ribs 5-7 in a young man	Pulmonary contusion (page 23.10) Pneumothorax and/or hemothorax (pages 23.8, 23.10)
6. Fracture of first and second ribs	Major vascular injury (page 23.12) Hemothorax (page 23.10)

Identify

1. a. Chief complaint: Patient's chest hurts.

b. Physical findings: Patient is verbal, has bruising on the lower chest, diaphoresis, cyanosis dyspnea, equal bilateral breath sounds, tachycardia, weak peripheral pulses, hypotension, and electrical alterans.

c. Signs of Beck's triad: Muffled heart tones, hypotension, and jugular vein distention.

d. The patient most likely has pericardial tamponade. (pages 23.22, 23.23)

2. a. Physical findings: Crackles, vital signs are within normal limits, an ECG shows ischemic changes, and no other signs of hypovolemia.

b. Spaulding effect: You believe that the pressure waves generated by the blunt trauma disrupted the capillary-alveolar membrane.
Inertial effects: The tissues accelerated and decelerated at different rates causing a tear.
Implosion: The pressure created by the trauma compresses the gases within the lung.

c. Do not run the IV wide open. If the mechanism of injury (MOI) suggests pulmonary contusion, be stingy with IV fluids unless there are signs of shock. (pages 23.22, 23.23)

Ambulance Calls

1. In this case, you have a young woman who suffered unspecified deceleration injuries serious enough to render her unconscious. The damage to the car—a caved-in dashboard and smashed windshield—also hints at significant head and chest injury. (pages 23.14, 23.15)

a. The major threats to this woman's airway are the following:

(1) Her tongue, which is liable to fall back against her posterior pharynx

(2) Blood or broken teeth in her mouth

(3) Vomitus

(4) Possible injury to the airway (eg, ruptured larynx)

b. In assessing the adequacy of her *breathing,* you must

(1) LOOK for:

(a) Signs of respiratory embarrassment (nasal flaring, intercostal or supraclavicular retractions)

(b) Tracheal deviation

(c) Obvious bruises or open wounds of the chest

(d) Paradoxical movement of any part of the chest

(2) LISTEN for:

(a) Sucking chest wound

(b) Inequality of breath sounds

(c) Dullness or hyperresonance to percussion

(3) FEEL for:

(a) Tracheal deviation

(b) Subcutaneous emphysema

(c) Instability of the rib cage

c. What needs to be done immediately to ensure adequate breathing is as follows:

(1) Suction out the mouth as needed.

(2) Administer 100% supplemental oxygen.

d. To evaluate and manage the *circulation* during the initial assessment, you must do the following:

(1) Identify and control significant external bleeding.

(2) Check the pulse (quality, rate, regularity, presence of paradoxus).

(3) Note the skin condition (color, moisture, temperature).

(4) Check capillary refill.

(5) Assess neck veins for distention.

2. a. The patient who has a shotgun wound to the chest in a "friendly" encounter has an open pneumothorax (answer C), indeed a quite significant one (a 2-inch hole would be hard not to notice!). The wound inflicted by a shotgun at close range is essentially a blast injury, and so you would expect in addition a considerable amount of damage to the lung tissue beneath, probably with disruption of major blood vessels as well. (pages 23.9, 23.18, 23.19)

b. The steps in managing this patient are the following:

(1) Make certain that the "friend" with the shotgun has left the scene or has been "neutralized" by police.

(2) Seal the open chest wound with an occlusive dressing as quickly as possible. Tape the dressing on three sides only, so that air can escape from it during exhalation.

(3) Administer 100% supplemental oxygen, preferably by nonrebreathing mask. Try to avoid giving oxygen under positive pressure.

(4) Start transport.

(5) Start an IV en route, with lactated Ringer's solution.

3. The elderly woman struck by a car has very well localized pain over the fifth right rib as well as diminished breath sounds and hyperresonance on that side of the chest. (pages 23.8, 23.9, 23.18, 23.19–23.22)

a. This woman probably has a **rib fracture** together with a simple pneumothorax on the right.

b. The principal danger associated with rib fracture is the development of atelectasis because of the patient's reluctance to breathe deeply. Atelectasis, in turn, predisposes the patient to develop pneumonia.

c. The treatment necessary in the field is as follows:

(1) Administer 100% supplemental oxygen by nonrebreathing mask.

(2) Encourage the patient to take periodic deep breaths; have her splint the fractured rib against a pillow each time she does so.

(3) Given the mechanisms of injury (MOI), it would be a good idea as well to immobilize the spine.

d. (1) When the patient becomes suddenly "shocky," while at the same time she shows signs of increased venous pressure (neck veins distended), she has probably developed a tension pneumothorax.

(2) If you are more than 2 to 3 minutes from the hospital when that happens, stop the vehicle and decompress the chest with a needle.

4. All that the initial assessment has revealed to you about the man ejected from his convertible is that he has a partially obstructed airway, is bleeding, and is in shock and therefore is critically injured. In fact, that is all you need to know to start appropriate treatment. Although the following steps of treatment are listed in sequence, you shall, in practice, have to accomplish the first few steps almost simultaneously.

a. Open the airway by jaw thrust. As soon as the equipment to do so is available, suction out the mouth and pharynx.

b. With the hand that is maintaining jaw thrust, seal off the bleeding wound of the neck. Apply a pressure dressing as soon as possible. Then, apply a pressure dressing to the scalp wound.

c. Administer 100% supplemental oxygen as soon as it is available.

d. Immobilize the spine.

e. Start transport.

f. Start at least one large-bore IV en route. Run it wide open.

g. Monitor cardiac rhythm. (pages 23.16, 23.17)

5. You are treating a passenger in a car that was struck from the right side by a truck running a red light. The right-hand front door of the car is rammed in, deforming the passenger compartment of the car. The patient, a middle-aged woman, is conscious and in considerable distress. Her skin is cold and moist. Her neck veins are distended. Her chest moves only minimally on respiration, and you have difficulty hearing breath sounds on the right. You can't really assess the percussion note because of all the noise at the scene. The woman's pulse is 120 beats/min and weak, and her respirations are 36 breaths/min and shallow. (pages 23.9–23.10, 23.19–23.22)

The clues to this patient's tension pneumothorax are the signs of shock in the face of distended neck veins and decreased breath sounds on one side.

a. Steps to take at the scene:

(1) Administer supplemental oxygen.

(2) Decompress the chest with a cannula in the second right intercostal space, midclavicular line.

(3) Immobilize the patient on a long backboard.

(4) Communicate with medical control or receiving hospital.

    b. Steps to be taken en route:

        (1) Perform a detailed physical exam.

        (2) Start a large-bore IV with fluids.

        (3) Recheck vital and neurologic signs every 5 minutes.

6. Asessment (pages 23.14–23.16)

    a. Mental status (AVPU)

    b. Airway while providing manual stabilization

        (1) Check for obstructions

    c. Breathing

        (1) Look for abnormal respirations

        (2) Palpate chest (evidence of instability, crepitus, subcutaneous emphysema)

        (3) Look for jugular vein distention

        (4) Auscultate lung sounds (note absent or decreased breath sounds)

        (5) Observe for signs and symptoms of hypoxia

        (6) Check for signs of hypocarbia

    d. Circulation

        (1) Examine for external bleeding

        (2) Obtain a complete set of vital signs and oxygen saturation

        (3) Look and feel skin

    e. Disability

        (1) Check extremities for pulses

    f. Focused history and physical exam (depending on the severity of the patient)

        (1) SAMPLE history

    g. Detailed exam with head-to-toe assessment

    Management (pages 23.19–23.22)

    a. Ensure the airway is maintained.

    b. Provide oxygen (consider the need for ventilatory assistance and endotracheal intubation).

    c. Consider the need for a needle decompression.

    d. Control any external bleeding.

    e. Take frequent vital signs.

    f. Attach patient to pulse oximeter and capnography if intubated.

    g. Monitor ECG.

    h. Complete cervical spine immobilization before transport.

7. In working out the answers to this question, you may have noticed that the mechanisms and signs of various chest injuries may be very similar to one another. If it is hard to distinguish such injuries in the relative calm and quiet of your study, consider how difficult it is at midnight in a ditch by the side of the interstate highway in the pouring rain—which is where you will inevitably be making such determinations.

    a. D. This patient's *distended neck veins* tell you that something is increasing pressure on the venae cavae. The two most likely possibilities are air in the pleural space or blood in the pericardium. Because the breath sounds are equal, the best bet is cardiac tamponade, and the apparent pulsus paradoxus supports that diagnosis. Under ideal conditions, you might also be able to appreciate that the heart sounds are muffled, but conditions in the field are seldom ideal, and even evaluating breath sounds is usually quite challenging (pages 23.22, 23.23).

        (1) Provide oxygen.

        (2) Start transport.

        (3) Monitor cardiac rhythm.

        (4) Start an IV with lactated Ringer's or normal saline en route.

    b. E. This is the classic picture of traumatic asphyxia, the so-called bloated frog appearance, and it bespeaks massive, often fatal chest injury. Steps of management (page 23.25):

        (1) Provide cervical spine precautions.

(2) Establish an airway. Don't take time at the scene for endotracheal intubation unless absolutely necessary.

(3) Administer 100% supplemental oxygen.

(4) Start transport.

(5) Start at least one IV en route.

c. C. If a patient has three ribs broken in two places, it's a good bet he's got a **flail chest.** You may not actually be able to see the paradoxical movement of the chest, especially if the patient is conscious and splinting the injured part of the chest (which he will do automatically, to reduce the pain that breathing causes him). But the nature of the injury tells you that there probably *is* a flail, and the asymmetry of chest movements supports the hypothesis. Steps of management (pages 23.17, 23.18):

(1) Administer 100% supplemental oxygen by nonrebreathing mask. Be prepared to intubate and provide positive pressure ventilations.

(2) Splint the flail segment by having the patient hold a pillow against it or by taping the unstable segment to the adjacent stable segment.

(3) Encourage the patient to take deep breaths. If he is unable to do so, assist ventilations *gently* with a bag-mask device. *Be alert for pneumothorax.*

(4) Start transport.

(5) Monitor cardiac rhythm.

(6) Start an IV lifeline en route, at a keep-open rate.

d. A. Here again, distended neck veins point to a process that is increasing intrathoracic pressure or otherwise preventing venous return to the heart. The decrease in breath sounds on the right side tells you that the problem is in the right chest, and the hyperresonance argues for a tension pneumothorax there. Steps of management (pages 23.19–23.22):

(1) Administer 100% supplemental oxygen by nonrebreathing mask.

    a. Obtain orders from medical control as required by protocols

    b. Identify the second right intercostal space in the midclavicular line.

    c. Prep the point you have identified (with povidone-iodine).

    d. Use a 14-gauge Intracath or whatever other 14-gauge needle is at hand to pop through into the pleural space and vent the pneumothorax. Secure the catheter or needle in place. Use a flutter valve if possible.

(2) Immobilize the spine.

(3) Start transport.

(4) Start an IV en route.

e. B. Like the patients with cardiac tamponade and tension pneumothorax, this patient with massive hemothorax is showing signs of shock (cold, sweaty skin; rapid, weak pulse). But in contrast to the others, his venous pressure is low (neck veins *not* distended), which makes one suspect hypovolemia. The decreased breath sounds in the left chest indicate that something is going on there, and the dullness to percussion suggests that fluid (blood) has taken the place of air in that side of the chest. It all adds up to massive bleeding within the chest. (Given the location of the stab wound, it is not unreasonable to consider the possibility of myocardial trauma and pericardial tamponade as well.) Steps of management (page 23.22):

(1) Administer 100% supplemental oxygen.

(2) Start transport.

(3) Start two large-bore IVs en route.

True/False

1. T (page 23.8)   **6.** T (page 23.12)

2. F (page 23.9)   **7.** F (page 23.13)

3. F (page 23.10)   **8.** F (page 23.19)

4. T (page 23.11)   **9.** T (page 23.20)

5. F (page 23.12)   **10.** T (page 23.23)

Short Answer

What you need to remember to answer this question correctly is that *any injury below the nipples is an abdominal injury as well as a chest injury.* The bullet apparently took a straight line through the right upper quadrant (RUQ), and it could be expected to have hit the liver, kidney, and perhaps part of the lung. (page 23.12)

Word Find

```
P B S E T R N M A Y X X A H E
B E U U I R U E N O A Z E O L
R N R B G N A E E R R M M A C
O I S I R A Z C O L O T S N I
N P I E C L H H H T P T A T V
C S T F H A T P H E O S V E A
H S F I X O R O O M A N A R L
I Y D T M S R D A S I N C I C
P E Z U G A H C I L E O K O L
O O E N X S H A R U E L P R I
N N U J Q F E O X Z M Q G L V
P L M E D I A S T I N U M Y E
M G A R H P A I D H E A R T R
A K Z D O P O O H O H N D F Y
A N E V X C E B S C A P U L A
```

1. The thoracic cavity lies within a bony, protective cylinder. The **ribs** encircle the whole thorax, articulating with the thoracic **spine** posteriorly and the **sternum anteriorly**. Also forming part of the bony protection on each side of the chest is the strong shoulder blade, or **scapula**, posteriorly and the collar bone, or **clavicle**, anteriorly. The inferior boundary of the thoracic cavity is formed by the **diaphragm**.

2. The **lungs** nearly fill the thoracic cavity. Each of them is covered with a smooth, slippery membrane called the visceral **pleura**; a similar membrane, the parietal pleura, lines the inner wall of the thoracic cavity. Ordinarily there is no space between those two membranes. Injury to the chest, however, may permit air to enter between the two membranes, creating a **pneumothorax**; blood can also accumulate in the space between the two membranes, a situation called **hemothorax**.

3. Some of the most important organs of the body are located in a region in the center of the thoracic cavity called the **mediastinum**. The structures located there include the **heart**, **aorta**, **vena cava**, **trachea**, **bronchi**, and **esophagus**.

4. When two or more ribs are broken in two or more places, a condition called flail chest may develop. Tamponade occurs when the **pericardium** becomes filled with blood, preventing the heart from contracting normally.

5. Because of the way the diaphragm is shaped, several abdominal organs actually lie partially or almost wholly within the chest, for example, the **spleen**, the **liver**, and the **stomach**. Those organs are thus liable to be injured whenever there is serious thoracic trauma.

Skill Drills

1. *Needle Decompression (Thoracentesis) of a Tension Pneumothorax* (page 23.21)

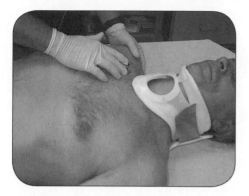

Step 1: Assess the patient.

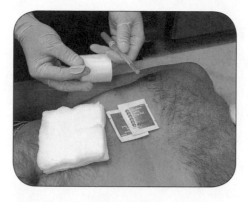

Step 2: Prepare and assemble all necessary equipment. Obtain orders from medical control

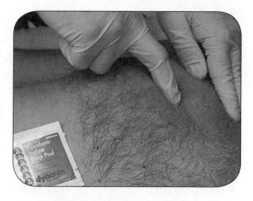

Step 3: Locate the appropriate site between the second and third rib.

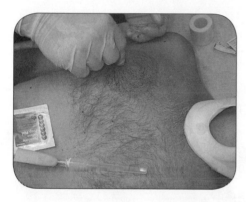

Step 4: Cleanse the appropriate area using aseptic technique.

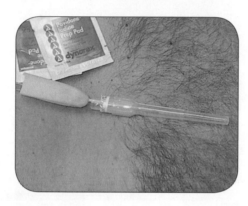

Step 5: Make a one-way valve or flutter valve.

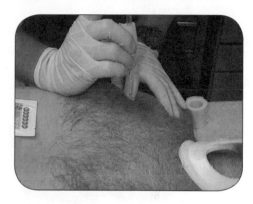

Step 6: Insert the needle at a 90° angle.

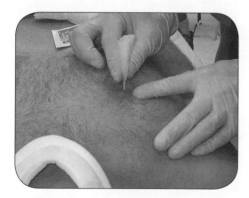

Step 7: Remove the needle and listen for release of air. Properly dispose of the needle in the sharps container.

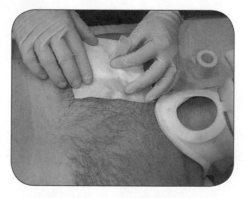

Step 8: Secure the catheter in place. Monitor the patient closely for recurrence of the tension pneumothorax.

Chapter 24: Abdomen Injuries

Matching

1. C (page 24.6)
2. B (page 24.11)
3. B (page 24.11)
4. D (page 24.11)
5. D (page 24.11)
6. F (page 24.11)
7. G (page 24.14)
8. B (page 24.11)
9. A (page 24.10)
10. B (page 24.10)

Multiple Choice

1. D (page 24.13)
2. D (page 24.14)
3. C (page 24.16)
4. C (page 24.6)
5. E (page 24.9)
6. C (page 24.15)
7. D (page 24.5)
8. D (page 24.4)
9. A (page 24.14)
10. D (page 24.13)

Labeling

1. Organs in the peritoneum (page 24.5)

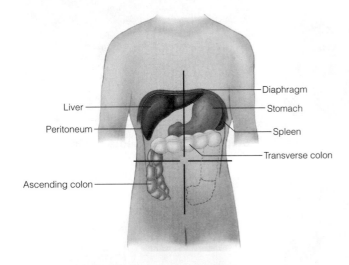

2. Organs in the retroperitoneal space (page 24.5)

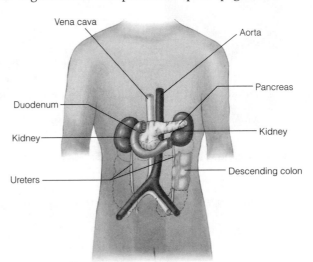

3. Organs in the pelvis (page 24.5)

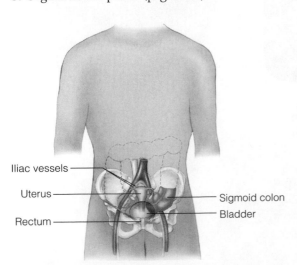

Fill-in-the-Blank

1. PASG (page 24.17)

2. Grey Turner's sign (page 24.12)

3. Cullen's sign (page 24.12)

4. Pancreas, kidneys (page 24.11)

5. Liver (page 24.5)

6. Hollow (page 24.5)

Identify

1. a. Chief complaint: Patient denies any complaint. EMS was called by police for possible stab wound.

    b. Vital signs: Pulse is 120 beats/min and regular; skin is ashen, cool, and diaphoretic; oxygen saturation is 90%; blood pressure 86/60 mm Hg; and sinus tachycardia on the ECG

    c. Pertinent negatives: He denies chest pain or other injuries.

2. a. Chief complaint: Evisceration, abdominal trauma

    b. Vital signs: Pulse is 100 beats/min and irregular; skin is pale, warm, and dry; oxygen saturation is 97% on room air; blood pressure 160/90 mm Hg

    c. Pertinent negatives: He is currently denying chest pain.

Ambulance Calls

1. The evaluation of a patient who has abdominal trauma must be systematic, keeping the entire patient in mind and prioritizing injuries accordingly. (page 24.12)

    a. The mechanisms of injury, including damage to the vehicle and type of seat belt worn (if any) if the patient is the victim of a motor vehicle crash.

    b. The patient's complaints referable to the abdomen, specifically complaints of nausea, vomiting, hematemesis, or abdominal pain.

    c. External signs of abdominal injury, such as abrasions, contusion, seat belt marks, lacerations, or evisceration.

    d. Tenderness or rigidity to palpation.

2. The case of evisceration described in this question is based on an actual case (see Majernik TG, et al. Intestinal evisceration resulting from a motor vehicle accident. *Ann Emerg Med.* 1984;13:633). List the injuries:

    a. Bruise over the right lower ribs

    b. Small bowel evisceration

    c. Avulsion in the right side of the abdomen

    d. Fractured right elbow

The published case report does not record what care was given at the scene, but the care that *should* have been given at the scene is based on the fact that this patient is in shock. The priorities should be the following:

    a. Administer 100% oxygen.

    b. Anticipate vomiting, and have suction at hand.

    c. Assist ventilations with a bag-valve mask.

    d. Cover the eviscerated bowel with sterile dressing; use an occlusive dressing over the wet sterile dressings or with sterile universal dressings that have been soaked in sterile saline. Cover the dressings, in turn, with a towel, to minimize heat loss across the wound.

    e. Immobilize the spine, taking care not to place any straps across the eviscerated bowel. Include the right arm within the straps, to hold the fractured elbow immobile.

    f. Start transport.

    g. Start two large-bore IVs en route, and run in lactated Ringer's as rapidly as possible.

3. The principles of managing an impaled object in the abdomen are fundamentally the same as for an impaled object anywhere else: *leave the impaled object in place.* (page 24.14)

    a. Administer oxygen.

    b. Stabilize the impaled object in place. Buttress it on all sides with universal dressings or with triangular bandages formed into "doughnut" rings. Then, tape the buttress material securely so that the knife cannot move in any direction.

    c. Start transport.

    d. Start an IV en route.

True/False

1. F (page 24.10)   **5.** T (page 24.3)

2. F (page 24.10)   **6.** T (page 24.14)

3. T (page 24.12)   **7.** F (page 24.16)

4. F (page 24.14)   **8.** T (page 24.17)

Fill-in-the-Table

1. The hollow and solid organs of the abdomen are as follows: (pages 24.10, 24.11)

Hollow Organs	Solid Organs
1. Stomach	**1.** Liver
2. Small intestine	**2.** Spleen
3. Pancreas	**3.** Kidneys
4. Large intestine	**4.** Adrenal glands
5. Gallbladder	
6. Ureters	
7. Urinary bladder	

Short Answer

1. a. kidneys (page 24.8)   **c.** bladder (page 24.6)

   b. liver (page 24.10)   **d.** liver (page 24.5)

Crossword Puzzle

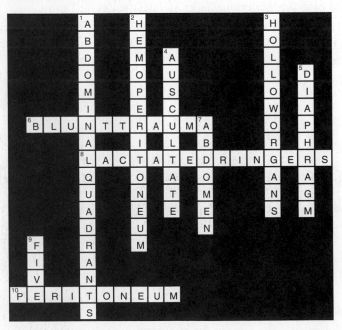

Secret Message

a. Abdominal cavity

b. Liver

c. Umbilicus

d. Mechanism of injury

e. Blast injuries

   Secret Message Answer: BLUNT TRAUMA

Chapter 25: Musculoskeletal Injuries

Matching

1. H (page 25.13)	**5.** D (page 25.30)
2. A (page 25.13)	**6.** E (page 25.37)
3. B (page 25.30)	**7.** G (page 25.38)
4. F (page 25.35)	**8.** C (page 25.13)

Multiple Choice

1. B (page 25.3)	**6.** D (page 25.17)
2. D (page 25.3)	**7.** B (page 25.19)
3. B (page 25.7)	**8.** D (page 25.23)
4. A (page 25.14)	**9.** A (page 25.28)
5. D (page 25.16)	**10.** B (page 25.31)

Labeling

1. Bones in the Foot and Ankle (page 25.6)

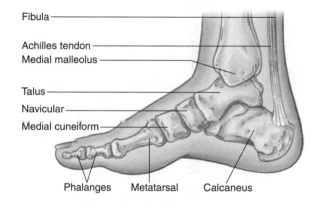

2. Types of Fractures (page 25.15)

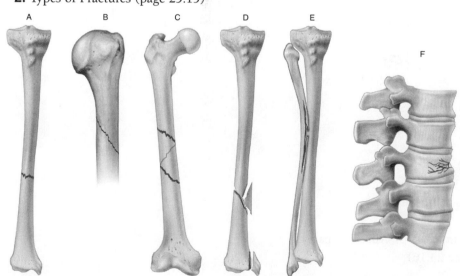

A. Transverse fracture of the tibia
B. Oblique fracture of the humerus
C. Spiral fracture of the femur
D. Comminuted fracture of the tibia
E. Greenstick fracture of the fibula
F. Compression fracture of a vertbral body

3. Three Types of Muscles (page 25.9)

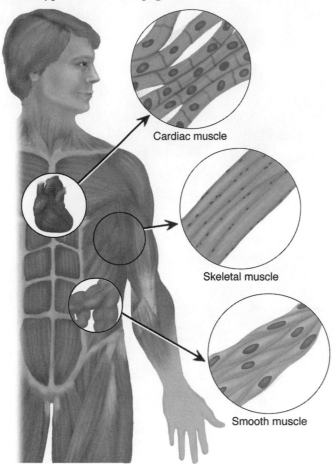

Cardiac muscle

Skeletal muscle

Smooth muscle

Fill-in-the-Blank

1. a. atrophy (page 25.10)

   b. arthritis (page 25.17)

   c. articulations (page 25.6)

   d. axilla (page 25.39)

   e. clavicle (page 25.4)

   f. diaphysis (page 25.7)

   g. patella (page 25.5)

   h. plantar (page 25.12)

   i. pectoral girdle (page 25.4)

2. The signs and symptoms of fracture are usually not terribly subtle:

   a. Unnatural shape: DEFORMITY (page 25.15)

   b. Reduced length: SHORTENING (page 25.15)

   c. Fracture of the small finger: BOXER'S FRACTURE (page 25.30)

   d. Black-and-blue mark: ECCHYMOSIS (referenced throughout)

   e. Grating: CREPITUS (page 25.16)

   f. Devastating consequence of musculoskeletal injuries: DISABILITY (page 25.27)

   g. Protecting from movement: GUARDING (page 25.16)

   h. Hurts to touch it: POINT TENDERNESS (25.19)

   i. Patient may report this: HEARD A SNAP (page 25.33)

   j. Strange moves: UNNATURAL POSITION (page 25.15)

k. Clavicle: COLLAR BONE (page 25.4)

l. Seen in open fracture: EXPOSED BONE ENDS (page 25.16)

Identify

1. a. Chief complaint: Right ankle pain; severe wrist pain. He denies LOC, head or neck pain. The patient denies any respiratory distress and denies any current chest discomfort. He denies any medical condition that may have caused him to fall. He adamantly states that he simply slipped on ice and fell.

b. Vital signs: His baseline vital signs reveal a pulse of 116 beats/min and irregular, respirations of 16 breaths/min nonlabored, oxygen saturation on room air at 98%, blood pressure of 150/90 mm Hg. ECG is rapid atrial fibrillation. PEARRL. Normal capillary refill <2 seconds. Skin color is normal, warm and dry.

c. Pertinent negatives: After questioning the patient you realize that he has a previous medical history of angina, atrial fibrillation, and hypertension. He also takes one aspirin a day and an antihypertensive drug.

2. a. Chief complaint: She tripped on the curb in the parking lot and fell to the ground. Luckily, she wasn't trampled by the hordes of bargain shoppers as the doors opened. She did catch herself with her two outstretched arms. Besides her injured pride she complains of bilateral wrist injuries and is found in extreme pain. As you approach the patient she is sitting in a chair with ice packs already applied and mall security providing first aid. You notice that both her wrists appear bruised and deformed.

b. Vital signs: Her initial vital signs indicate a patient that is conscious and alert. Her skin is slightly ashen and diaphoretic, and she has positive distal motor and neurologic sensations in both hands. She denies other injuries. Her capillary refill is >2 seconds, and she has bilateral radial pulses that appear to be equal. Her blood pressure is obtainable only by palpation at 86. Her oxygen saturation is 96% on ambient air. She denies taking any medications or allergies.

c. Pertinent negatives: The patient denies LOC, head or neck pain. The patient denies any respiratory distress and denies any current chest discomfort. She denies any medical condition that may have caused her to fall.

3. a. Chief complaint: A farm mishap where a tractor rolled on top of and is pinning a 64-year-old man. The patient is unresponsive with airway compromise.

b. Vital signs: Patient is unresponsive with a GCS <8. He has delayed capillary refill and sinus tachycardia of 128 beats/min. His blood pressure is 64 by palpation.

c. Pertinent negatives: There are no pertinent negatives indicated

Ambulance Calls

1. The presence of some injuries may also give clues to the possible presence of other injuries that share the same mechanism of injury (MOI).

a. A young man jumped from a second-story window to escape a fire. He complains of severe pain in the left heel, which is quite black and blue. His calcaneal fracture mandates that you check for fracture of the other calcaneus as well as fracture of the lumbar vertebrae, especially around L1–L2. (page 25.13)

b. A 50-year-old woman was the front-seat passenger in a car that was hit head-on by an oncoming vehicle. Her right knee is bruised and swollen. This is the classic dashboard injury. The same forces that smashed up the knee may well have acted anywhere along the femur to cause a femoral fracture or to ram the femur backward, producing fracture or dislocation of the hip. (page 25.12)

c. A 60-year-old man fell sideways onto his outstretched hand. There is ecchymosis and tenderness at the base of his thumb. In this case of probable schaphoid fracture, the forces are transmitted from the hand, along the radius and ulna, through the elbow, and up the humerus into the shoulder, so look for injuries anywhere along that axis, specifically fracture of the distal radius/ulna, fracture/dislocation of the elbow, fracture of the shaft of the humerus, fracture/dislocation of the shoulder, or fracture of the clavicle. (page 25.13)

d. A construction worker has been extricated from under a pile of concrete blocks that fell on top of him, pinning him prone, when part of a building collapsed. He has bruising over the left shoulder blade, and he cannot move the shoulder on that side. The obvious fracture is the fracture of the scapula, which is a tip-off to the powerful forces involved in the injury. Thus, you need to start looking for rib fractures, vertebral fractures, and damage to underlying soft tissues (pulmonary contusion, renal injury). (page 25.13)

2. It's all well and good to memorize the signs and symptoms of musculoskeletal injuries, but what counts is whether you can recognize the injuries when you see them and whether you then take the appropriate action.

a. Starting with the boy who fell off his skateboard: (page 25.30)

(1) The most likely field diagnosis is a fractured elbow. If you want to be more exact, you could specify that it's a supracondylar fracture of the humerus, but probably it won't be possible (or necessary) in the field to know exactly what is broken and what isn't. The fact that the elbow is involved in a fracture is reason enough to feel a sense of urgency.

(2) Yes, there is a special danger in this case, the danger of the patient developing Volkmann's ischemic contracture as a result of the blood supply to his forearm being jeopardized. He's already showing signs of a compromised blood supply (his hand is cool and pale), and the broken end of the humerus is probably pinching his radial nerve as well (he has a sensory loss in the distribution of the radial nerve). Those are *danger signals!*

(3) If this boy is to retain the use of his right hand, urgent measures must be taken to restore the blood supply to the area. Those measures are best taken by an expert—an orthopedic surgeon—in the hospital; so, if you are close to the hospital, splint the elbow as you found it, and hit the road—notifying the hospital of your ETA so that they can summon an "orthopod" (ie, orthopedic surgeon) to be standing by in the ED. If you are any distance from the hospital, however, contact medical command for orders; you may be instructed to apply traction along the axis of the humerus and straighten the elbow slightly, until the patient's hand "pinks up."

b. The boy's mother tripped over his skateboard in her haste to assist him (there's a lesson in that!). She's done something to her wrist. (page 25.30)

(1) The most likely field diagnosis is a Colles' fracture, that is, a fracture of the distal radius and ulna. The "dinner-fork deformity" is classic for the Colles' fracture, as is the way the woman walked over to you, holding the injured wrist in her other hand and using her body as a splint.

(2) No, there is not ordinarily any special danger in a Colles' fracture, although you must, as always, check the circulation and neurologic function distal to the injury, just to be certain.

(3) A padded aluminum ladder splint, bent into a right angle at the elbow and supported in a sling is probably the most comfortable splint for this woman. But you may also use an air splint (provided it comes up over the elbow) or a padded board splint. In either of those two cases, transport the woman supine, with her splinted arm supported on a pillow, to elevate the injured part.

c. Here is another classic dashboard injury. (page 25.37)

(1) The most likely diagnosis is posterior dislocation of the hip. That is what one would expect given the mechanisms of injury (MOI) (deceleration forces, femur driven backward), and the patient has characteristic signs: The affected hip is flexed, adducted, and internally rotated, and the leg appears shorter than the leg on the uninjured side.

(2) Yes, there is a particular danger associated with posterior hip dislocation. Two dangers, in fact. The most feared complication is avascular necrosis of the head of the femur, which leads to total destruction of the hip joint. There is also danger of damage to the sciatic nerve and consequent foot drop.

(3) The most important treatment for a dislocated hip is early reduction of the dislocation. If you are within 20 minutes or so of the hospital, the best thing to do is immobilize the patient on a long backboard, generously padded with pillows, and transport immediately. If you are at a considerable distance from the hospital, contact medical control. If you are given instructions to do so, try once to reduce the dislocation.

d. The other patient from the same crash was the driver, found unconscious.

(1) The most likely *orthopedic* field diagnosis in this case is a fractured pelvis. But this patient has some other very serious, even life-threatening injuries as well. Loss of consciousness in a patient with trauma means head injury until proved otherwise, and head injury in multitrauma means spinal cord injury until proved otherwise.

(2) Yes, indeed there is a particular danger in this case. There are several particular dangers. For starters, the patient is unconscious, so his airway is in jeopardy. He also seems to be in shock, perhaps from blood loss related to his pelvic fracture, but perhaps from blood loss elsewhere as well.

(3) After the scene size-up, conduct an initial assessment on this patient. The steps in the IA involve a general impression and your "MS-ABC Priority Plan" searching for and managing life threats.

General Impression: unconscious male trauma patient

MS: "U" unresponsive to pain

(a) Open his airway (chin lift or jaw thrust); insert an oropharyngeal airway to help keep it open.

(b) Determine whether he is breathing adequately; if not, assist his breathing with a bag-mask device. In any event, give supplementary oxygen.

(c) Assess the circulation (pulse, capillary refill in children), and control external bleeding.

Priority: high

Given the patient's condition, you're not going to have time to do a lot more in the field except the following:

(a) Manage the ABCs.

(b) Secure the patient to the backboard.

(c) Then, start transport.

(d) En route, get a set of vital signs, if you haven't done so already.

(e) Start at least one and preferably two large-bore IVs, and run a 500-mL fluid challenge.

(f) Complete the detailed physical exam as best you can.

(g) Keep the patient warm.

e. Apparently, it's only when you get back to base that your partner mentions how much his ankle is hurting. (page 25.34)

(1) The most likely diagnosis is a sprained ankle, although you can't be 100% sure without an X-ray.

(2) No, there is no particular danger associated with a sprained ankle.

(3) The treatment is to immobilize the ankle (eg, air splint, pillow splint), apply a cold pack, elevate the ankle, and transport your partner to the ED to be checked over.

f. The high school quarterback who ended up under a pile of 225-pound linemen was subject to significant crushing forces. (page 25.35)

(1) The most likely diagnosis is posterior sternoclavicular dislocation.

(2) Yes, there is a particular danger in this case, and that is damage to critical underlying structures. In fact, there is already evidence that such damage has occurred, for the boy says he is "choking"—an indication of possible tracheal damage.

(3) The most important aspect of this boy's treatment will be expeditious transport to the hospital. Administer supplementary oxygen en route. If he is comfortable lying down, keep him supine, with his left arm abducted and a pillow or rolled towel under his left shoulder; that position may take the pressure off the trachea or whatever structures are being compressed by the proximal end of the clavicle.

g. The pedestrian suffered a direct blow to the shin. (page 25.33)

(1) The most likely diagnosis is an open fracture of the tibia, probably a transverse fracture.

(2) Yes, there is a particular danger associated with tibial fractures, and that is the development of a compartment syndrome. Indeed, the patient's paresthesias suggest that there may already be pressure on the sensory nerves supplying the foot.

(3) To treat the patient in the field, apply manual traction to straighten out the angulation and splint the limb (padded board splint, long-leg air splint). Keep the patient supine so that you can elevate the injured leg. Apply cold packs. Transport the patient without delay, and notify the receiving hospital to have an orthopod standing by.

h. In today's less than tranquil society, gunshot wounds are frequent sources of musculoskeletal trauma. (page 25.33)

(1) The most likely diagnosis in this case is a fractured femur. The location of the wound and the shortening of the injured leg are the tip-offs.

(2) **Yes,** there is a particular danger in this case. Aside from the danger of **shock** that attends every femoral fracture, there is apparently some compromise to distal circulation (the dorsalis pedis pulse is weak). There may also be a danger to *you* if the person who did the shooting is still wandering around with a loaded gun—did you bother to check on that before you ran over to attend the patient?

(3) This is another case that involves setting priorities:

(a) Administer supplemental oxygen.

(b) Cover the open wound(s) with sterile dressings.

(c) Immobilize the injured leg in a traction splint.

(d) Start transport.

(e) Start a large-bore IV en route to the hospital.

(f) Keep rechecking the dorsalis pedis pulse. Document all your findings.

(4) The purposes of splinting in general are as follows:

(a) To relieve pain

(b) To prevent further injury

(c) To help control bleeding

i. The skier who ended up at the bottom of a pileup doubtless suffered a hyperextension injury of the leg. (page 25.37)

(1) The most likely diagnosis is dislocation of the knee (it may also be fractured).

(2) Yes, there is a particular danger associated with that diagnosis, the danger of damage to the popliteal artery and consequent ischemic damage to the lower leg.

(3) The treatment under these circumstances—where you are on the ski slopes, at some distance from a hospital—is to try once to reduce the dislocation, before muscle spasm makes it impossible to do so. Use a traction splint if you have one available. Otherwise, apply manual traction in the long axis of the leg. Then, get the patient to the hospital as quickly as possible, and notify the hospital in advance of your impending arrival.

3. a. As you shall see in the next chapter, when dealing with a severely injured patient, knowing what to do is not enough. One has to know what to do *first* and what to do *next* and what to do after that. If you remember the alphabet, you'll be in good shape.

> **16**   Start an IV.
>
> **9**   Take the vital signs.
>
> **5**   Cut away the trouser leg. (You will want to control the bleeding in the leg if it is excessive, which is part of step C.)
>
> **3**   Determine whether he is breathing (he is) (step B).
>
> **14**   Secure patient to backboard.
>
> **12**   Apply the PASG/MAST [if your protocols allow], while holding the right leg in traction.
>
> **7**   Put manual pressure on the bleeding site (part of step C, Circulation).
>
> **2**   Open the airway (chin lift) (step A).
>
> **15**   Start transport.
>
> **10**   Move the patient to a backboard.
>
> **5**   Check for a carotid pulse (pulse is present) (first part of step C, Circulation).
>
> **11, 13**   Check for a dorsalis pedis pulse on the right. (You need to do this both before and after you have applied the splint, which in this case is the PASG/MAST [if your protocols allow].)
>
> **1**   Do AVPU check (the "mental status" in MS-ABC Priority Plan).
>
> **4**   Check for open or tension pneumothorax (part of checking the adequacy of breathing, step B).
>
> **8**   Pressure dressing over open wound of leg. (In practice, you'll do this whenever the dressing material becomes available.)

In actual practice, you will be carrying out some of the preceding steps very nearly simultaneously. While holding the airway open and observing the movements of the chest, for instance, you will also have a finger on the carotid pulse. But it is useful to consider the actions separately to review priorities.

b. Yes, at least one step has been omitted. The patient was not given supplemental oxygen!

4. An open fracture of the tibia is a serious injury with serious potential complications (such as compartment syndrome), but it does *not* pose an immediate threat to life; nor are there any signs so far of other injuries that do jeopardize the patient's life. (page 25.33)

a. Steps to be taken in the field:

(1) Rapid trauma assessment.

(2) Cover the wound on the leg with a sterile dressing.

(3) Straighten and splint the fractured leg.

(4) Start a large-bore IV (or could be done en route).

b. Steps to be taken en route:

(1) Communicate with medical control or receiving hospital.

(2) Recheck pulse and sensation distal to the fracture every 5 minutes.

(3) Start a large-bore IV (if not done yet).

5. A spinal cord injury is a tragic injury, but ordinarily it does *not* pose an immediate threat to life unless there is a transection high in the cervical spine that paralyzes all muscles of breathing. This patient has a traumatic paraplegia, but no evidence of spinal shock or any other life-threatening condition.

a. Steps to be taken at the scene:

(1) Manually stabilize the head/neck and apply a cervical collar.

(2) Initial assessment.

(3) Immobilize the patient on a long backboard.

b. Steps to be taken en route:

(1) Communicate with medical command or receiving hospital.

(2) Start an IV with normal saline.

(3) Conduct an ongoing assessment, rechecking vital and neurologic signs every 5 minutes.

True/False

1. T (page 25.24)
2. T (page 25.25)
3. T (page 25.24)
4. F (page 25.27)

5. T (page 25.25)
6. T (page 25.23)
7. T (page 25.26)

Fill-in-the-Table

The bones that belong in the various joints are as follows. (pages 25.4, 25.5)

Joint	Bones That Make Up the Joint
Shoulder	Scapula, humerus
Elbow	Humerus, ulna
Wrist	Radius, ulna, carpals
Hip	Ilium, ischium, pubis, femur
Knee	Femur, tibia
Ankle	Tibia, fibula, tarsals

Short Answer

1. The compartment syndrome may be heralded by any or several of the **six Ps**, which are symptoms and signs of an ischemic limb (page 25.28):
   a. Pain is the earliest and most reliable sign.
   b. Pallor.
   c. Pulselessness.
   d. Paresthesias.
   e. Paresis or paralysis.
   f. Puffiness.

2. In examining the patient injured on the ski slope, it's a good idea to start by eliciting his **chief complaint**. Although his deformed right knee may be the most obvious injury to *you,* there may be other injuries that are bothering the *patient* more. If you don't ask, you may not find out. In conducting the physical assessment, pay particular attention to the following (page 25.28):
   a. The position in which the extremities are found (as always, compare the injured to the uninjured limb).
   b. The circulatory status of the injured limb. Check the following:
      (1) Skin condition
      (2) Capillary refill
      (3) Distal pulses (anterior tibial and dorsalis pedis)
   c. The neurologic status of the injured limb. Check the following:
      (1) Sensation to pinprick over the heel and dorsum of the foot
      (2) Motor function: ability to plantar flex and dorsiflex the foot

3. Equipment to grab and take with you when you rush to the side of a severely injured patient should include the following:
   a. Long backboard with at least three straps
   b. Cervical collar and head immobilizer (eg, blanket roll)
   c. Portable oxygen and suction
   d. Oropharyngeal or nasopharyngeal airways
   e. Pocket mask or bagmask device
   f. Wound kit
   g. Stethoscope, blood pressure cuff, and flashlight

Word Find

Musculoskeletal injuries are usually not nearly as difficult to find as the words in this grid.

```
L A S R A T A T E M F P T D T
T L A L S R F N L M X X R T A
I E C I U O I E A N B O B R S
B E N B E I R T B A I H C S A
I T S O M T A E L U I X H U L
A A Q O N C A A M S L M A L I
T P R W A A H B C U S A N O I
M C K R Z P R H U K H B T E E
A P P E N D I C U L A R E L S
A A N L U U I L E M U T R L T
L Z U L M C L P D L G M L A E
A L U P A C S J Q P O U D M R
C L A V I C L E R A D I U S N
E N I P S P U B I S G L E J U
W I N W A L V G H M I I I S M
```

1. The part of the skeleton made up of the upper and lower extremities is called the **appendicular** skeleton. The rest of the skeleton, the part made up of the **skull**, **spine**, **sternum**, and **ribs**, is called the **axial** skeleton. (pages 25.3, 25.4)

2. The highest point of the shoulder is called the **acromion**. (page 25.39)

3. The pelvis is made up of three bones, the **ilium**, **ischium**, and **pubis**. The three come together laterally to form the depression, called the **acetabulum**, in which the head of the thigh bone fits. (page 25.5)

4. (page 25.39) Here are the "translations" into medical terminology:

   a. Shoulder blade: **scapula**

   b. Collar bone: **clavicle**

   c. Funny bone: **ulna**

   d. The funny part of the funny bone: **olecranon**

   e. The bone that articulates with the funny bone and whose name sounds funny: **humerus**

   f. Knee cap: **patella**

   g. Shin bone: **tibia**

   h. Finger bone: **phalanx**

   i. "Hip bone": greater **trochanter**

5. The bone that runs along the thumb side of the forearm is called the **radius**. It articulates at the wrist with the carpal bones, which in turn articulate with the **metacarpal** bones of the hand. (page 25.5)

6. The **fibula**, the smaller bone of the lower leg, forms the lateral **malleolus** in its distal articulation with the **tarsal** bones. Those in turn articulate with the **metatarsal** bones of the foot. (page 25.6)

Fill-in-the-Table

1.

Potential Blood Loss from Fracture Sites	
Fracture Site	**Potential Blood Loss (mL)**
Pelvis	1,500-3,000
Femur	1,000-1,500
Humerus	250-500
Tibia or fibula	250-500
Ankle	250-500
Elbow	250-500
Radius or ulna	150-250

(page 25.19)

Problem Solving

(page 25.19)

1. 1,000 mL
2. 4,500 mL
3. 1,000 mL

Section 4 Case Study: Answers and Summary

1. What immediate care is required for this patient?

This patient has multiple significant mechanisms of injury. Each one must be addressed based on severity (ie, what will kill the patient first). Continue to have the firefighter maintain manual stabilization of the patient's head while you and your partner perform the following interventions:

- **Control external hemorrhage**
  - All external bleeding must be stopped immediately. Your partner can accomplish this while you tend to the patient's airway.
    - The stab wound to the left anterior chest should be covered with an occlusive dressing. Any open wound to the chest could indicate underlying pulmonary injury and an open pneumothorax (sucking chest wound).
- **100% supplemental oxygen**
  - Although increased, this patient's respiratory effort is adequate (good tidal volume); therefore, 100% supplemental oxygen via a nonrebreathing mask should be applied.
    - Monitor this patient's respiratory effort carefully and be prepared to initiate positive-pressure ventilatory support if his breathing becomes inadequate (eg, reduced tidal volume, profoundly labored).

Teamwork between you and your partner is critical to providing effective patient care. Had the firefighters not been present to assist with spinal immobilization (meaning that your partner would have to), your first priority would have been to control the external bleeding. Only after the external bleeding is controlled would you apply oxygen. You must treat injuries in the order of what is going to kill the patient *first*. Severe external bleeding can cause death within a few seconds if not immediately controlled. Delaying oxygen therapy for the 1 or 2 minutes that it takes to control the severe bleeding will not kill the patient.

2. What does jugular venous distention in this patient suggest?

The stab wound to the left side of the chest and jugular venous distention should make you suspicious of a *pericardial tamponade*. The presence of bilaterally equal breath sounds rules out a tension pneumothorax, another potential cause of jugular venous distention.

The heart is encased in a fibrous, inelastic membrane called the pericardium. The pericardial space, which is actually a potential space that normally contains 20 to 30 mL of lubricating fluid, exists between the pericardium and the heart. Blood can enter the pericardial space if small myocardial blood vessels (eg, coronary arteries) are torn or if direct penetration of the myocardium occurs. As a result, a condition called hemopericardium occurs. As more blood enters the pericardial space, a pericardial tamponade can develop **(Figure 4-1)**.

Pericardial tamponade is most commonly associated with stab wounds to the chest. Larger penetrating injuries, such as gunshot wounds, often create a large enough hole in the pericardium for blood to exit the pericardial space and are typically associated with exsanguination into the thoracic cavity rather than pericardial tamponade.

Because the tough, fibrous pericardium does not stretch, accumulating blood puts pressure on the heart, affecting both the systolic and diastolic phases of the cardiac cycle. Pressure on the heart impairs venous return to the heart (preload) and limits right ventricular filling. As venous pressure increases, the jugular veins become distended.

3. What additional signs may accompany jugular venous distention in a patient with penetrating chest trauma?

In the adult patient, the pericardial space can hold 200 to 300 mL of blood before signs of a pericardial tamponade become evident; however, smaller volumes of blood can still significantly reduce cardiac output. Progression of a pericardial tamponade depends on how fast blood is filling the pericardial space.

As previously discussed, pericardial tamponade causes an increase in venous pressure and jugular venous distention. In addition, right ventricular expansion (and filling) is impaired, which compromises output through the pulmonary arteries and subsequent venous return to the left side of the heart. This causes a *decreased cardiac output and systemic hypotension*. A *reflex tachycardia* attempts to (but cannot) compensate for the low cardiac output state.

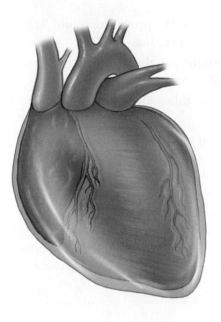 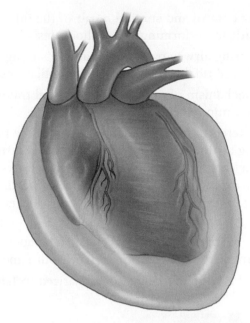

■ **Figure 4-1** Pericardial tamponade occurs when blood or other fluids accumulate in the pericardial sac. As bleeding into the pericardium continues, the myocardium is compressed, which impairs venous return and cardiac output.

Because myocardial contractility is compromised, the patient's systolic blood pressure decreases. Additionally, decreased ability of the myocardium to fully relax causes an increase in the diastolic blood pressure. This results in a *narrowed pulse pressure* (the difference between the systolic and diastolic blood pressure).

Pulsus paradoxus, which is characterized by a drop in systolic blood pressure of greater than 10 mm Hg during inspiration, may also occur and is caused when the expanding lungs literally stop the heart in animation by putting additional pressure on the already compressed myocardium. Pulsus paradoxus can be determined clinically by noting a diminished or even disappearing radial pulse upon inspiration.

Increasing amounts of blood in the pericardium may also cause *muffled or distant heart sounds*; however, this is often difficult to hear, especially in a loud environment such as the back of a moving ambulance.

Beck's triad, a classic finding in pericardial tamponade, is characterized by three clinical signs: (1) jugular venous distention, (2) muffled heart sounds, and (3) a narrowing pulse pressure. However, all three of these clinical signs may not be present, especially if the patient is hypovolemic from other injuries (eg, pelvic fracture), which is possible in this patient because of his pelvic pain. The physical findings of a pericardial tamponade are summarized in **Table 4-1**.

Table 4-1   Physical Findings of a Pericardial Tamponade
Tachycardia and hypotension
Bilaterally equal breath sounds
Midline trachea
Beck's triad
• Jugular venous distention
• Muffled or distant heart sounds
• Narrowing pulse pressure

4. What specific treatment is required to treat this patient's condition?

Patients with pericardial tamponade require rapid transport to a trauma center with continuous monitoring of airway, breathing, and circulation en route. As with any critical trauma patient, unnecessary delays must not occur in the field.

Treatment for patients with pericardial tamponade includes removing blood from the pericardium by a procedure called *pericardiocentesis*. This procedure, however, is almost exclusively performed in the emergency department and is only a temporizing intervention until bleeding control and surgical repair of the injury can occur in the operating room. Refer to locally established protocols in regards to performing pericardiocentesis in the prehospital setting.

Prehospital management begins by ensuring airway patency and administering 100% supplemental oxygen. If the patient's respiratory effort is inadequate (eg, reduced tidal volume), assisted ventilations with 100% oxygen will be necessary.

Perform spinal immobilization if the mechanism of injury suggests spinal trauma. Because this patient was pushed out of a moving vehicle, he will clearly require immobilization.

Crystalloid IV fluids should be administered to increase venous return to the right atrium (preload). By increasing pre-load, the full and vigorously contracting atrium will force blood into the ventricles, thus stretching its walls. Stretching of the ventricular wall enhances contractility and the force with which it ejects blood out to the body. Increased cardiac contractility due to stretching of the myocardial wall is called the *Frank-Starling mechanism*; which, by administering IV fluids, will be enhanced, and can maintain cardiac output until a pericardiocentesis can be performed.

Continuous cardiac monitoring is essential in the management of a patient with pericardial tamponade. Decreased cardiac output and hypoperfusion can result in life-threatening dysrhythmias. Pericardial tamponade is also associated with pulseless electrical activity (PEA), a condition in which a cardiac rhythm is present on the cardiac monitor but a palpable pulse is not present.

Management for the patient with a pericardial tamponade is summarized in **Table 4-2**.

Table 4-2   Management for a Pericardial Tamponade
Ensure airway patency • Immobilize the spine if the mechanism of injury suggests spinal trauma.
Administer 100% supplemental oxygen • Assist ventilations with 100% oxygen if the patient is breathing inadequately.
Establish two large-bore IV lines • Infuse isotonic crystalloids to increase preload and maintain cardiac output.
Continuous cardiac monitoring • Be alert for cardiac dysrhythmias or cardiac arrest (PEA).
Rapid transport to a trauma center • Notify the receiving facility early. • Reassess the patient frequently while en route.

Summary

Pericardial tamponade is a condition in which blood accumulates in the pericardium and causes hemodynamic compromise. It is most often the result of penetrating trauma, specifically stab wounds to the chest. A small tear in a myocardial blood vessel or direct penetrating trauma to the myocardium causes blood to seep into the myocardium, which puts pressure on the heart and impairs its performance. The progression of a pericardial tamponade depends on the rate at which blood is accumulating within the pericardium.

Patients with pericardial tamponade typically present with signs of shock (eg, tachycardia, hypotension, diaphoresis) as well as jugular venous distention, muffled heart sounds, and a narrowing pulse pressure (Beck's triad). If the patient is severely hypovolemic from other injuries, however, jugular venous distention may not be present.

Complications associated with pericardial tamponade include cardiac dysrhythmias, such as ventricular fibrillation or ventricular tachycardia, or cardiac arrest with PEA.

A careful, systematic assessment of the patient is required to identify the signs of pericardial tamponade and initiate the most appropriate treatment. Prehospital management consists of ensuring a patent airway, administering 100% oxygen (or ventilatory support if needed), immobilizing the spine if the mechanism of injury suggests spinal trauma, infusing IV crystalloids to increase venous return, and rapidly transporting the patient to a trauma center. Cardiac monitoring en route is essential in being able to identify and treat life-threatening cardiac dysrhythmias.

A pericardiocentesis is required to remove blood from the pericardium, thus improving cardiac output. However, this is almost exclusively performed in the emergency department by a physician and is only a temporizing intervention until the injury can be repaired surgically.

Section 5: Medical

Chapter 26: Respiratory Emergencies

Matching

1. F (page 26.6)
2. J (page 26.8)
3. C (page 26.10)
4. H (page 26.17)
5. A (page 26.29)

6. E (page 26.33)
7. B (page 26.38)
8. I (page 26.6)
9. G (page 26.8)
10. D (page 26.8)

Multiple Choice

1. B (page 26.7)
2. C (page 26.35)
3. D (page 26.43)
4. C (page 26.11)
5. A (page 26.14)

6. C (page 26.22)
7. C (page 26.23)
8. B (page 26.25)
9. D (page 26.28)
10. A (page 26.27)

Labeling

1. The Upper Airway (page 26.6)

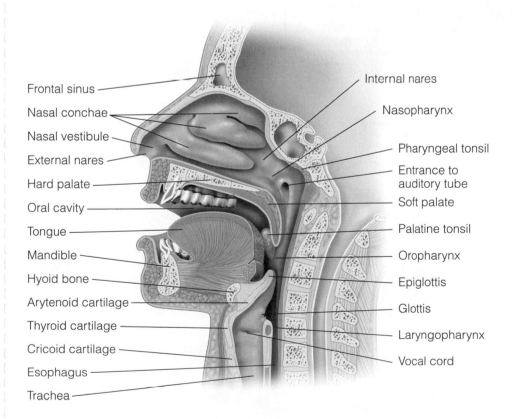

Frontal sinus
Nasal conchae
Nasal vestibule
External nares
Hard palate
Oral cavity
Tongue
Mandible
Hyoid bone
Arytenoid cartilage
Thyroid cartilage
Cricoid cartilage
Esophagus
Trachea

Internal nares
Nasopharynx
Pharyngeal tonsil
Entrance to auditory tube
Soft palate
Palatine tonsil
Oropharynx
Epiglottis
Glottis
Laryngopharynx
Vocal cord

2. The Larynx (page 26.7)

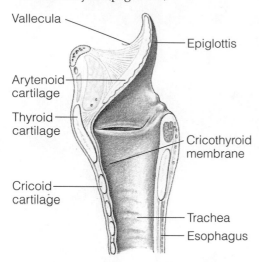

3. Respiratory Patterns (page 26.13)

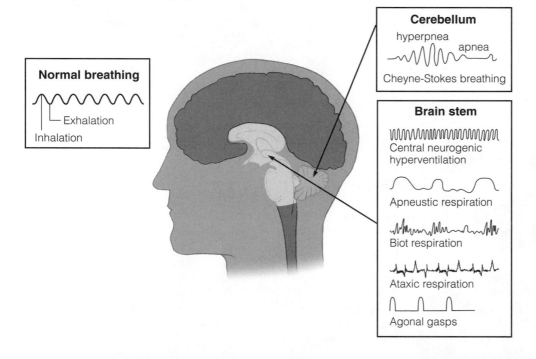

Fill-in-the-Blank

1. Atelectasis (page 26.10)
2. Cilia (page 26.8)
3. Polycythemia (page 26.10)
4. Flail chest (page 26.12)
5. Orthopnea (page 26.15), cyanosis (page 26.17)
6. Paroxysmal nocturnal dyspnea (page 26.18)
7. Tactile fremitus (page 26.20)
8. three, two (page 26.21)
9. End-tidal (page 26.24)
10. Nasogastric tube (page 26.26)

Identify

1. Chief complaint: Unresponsive, not breathing

2. Vital signs: Heart rate 46 beats/min, oxygen saturation is 54%

3. Pertinent negatives: No chest rise and fall

Tommy was **unconscious** and **not breathing.** He had **no chest rise and fall** upon trying to ventilate him. He did have a faint brachial pulse, which identified that compressions were not need yet because his airway had not been blocked for very long. Oxygen saturation was 54%, heart rate (HR) was 46 beats/min and no spontaneous respirations. Blood pressure was unattainable. After the airway is opened, Tommy quickly returns to normal with 100% supplemental oxygen.

Ambulance Calls

1. a. Although it is *possible* for a 22-year-old to suffer a heart attack, it is not very likely; so, when you are confronted with a patient of that age complaining of chest pain, you need to think about other possibilities—such as a pulmonary embolism, a spontaneous pneumothorax, or, as this case turns out to be, hyperventilation syndrome. The tip-offs are the paresthesias around the mouth, the carpopedal spasm, and, incidentally, the increased respiratory rate. That last is significant because, strangely enough, often tachypnea and hyperpnea are *not* the most prominent features of hyperventilation syndrome and, as in this case, other signs or symptoms may predominate.

b. The *steps in management* are

  (1) Calm and reassure the patient.

  (2) Help her to take conscious control of her breathing by telling her to breathe as you slowly count (about one number every 5 seconds).

  (3) (If the acute episode *doesn't* pass, the patient needs to be evaluated in the emergency department.)

c. This woman's arterial PCO_2 is probably lower than normal because her minute ventilation is increased; that is, she is blowing off more carbon dioxide than usual. (pages 26.37, 26.38)

2. The 985,500 cigarettes (give or take a few) that Mr. Koff has smoked over the past 45 years seem to be catching up with him. You can do the arithmetic yourself: 3 packs/day × 20 cigarettes/pack × 365 days/year × 45 years. (pages 26.16, 26.17)

a. Now you find him in respiratory distress. *Signs of respiratory distress* include the following:

  (1) Nasal flaring

  (2) Tracheal tugging

  (3) Retraction of intercostal muscles

  (4) Use of accessory muscles in the neck to assist breathing

  (5) Paradoxical respiratory movement with sucking in of the epigastrium on inhalation (normally the belly bulges *out* on inhalation)

b. What needs to be done *immediately* on encountering a patient in this condition is to administer supplemental oxygen before you ask any more questions or proceed any further with your examination. It is also a good idea to attach the patient to a cardiac monitor at this stage because a hypoxic patient is a patient who is very likely to develop serious, possibly life-threatening cardiac arrhythmias—and you'd like to have some warning that they are coming!

c. In *taking the history,* the following are the pieces of information you would like to know (page 26.18):

Regarding the dyspnea, the OPQRST questions are in order:

  (1) O: Onset—when it did start?

  (2) P: We already have a general idea of what provoked the symptoms (probably it was being in the recumbent position for several hours); but it would be useful to know what palliates them. Is there a position in which the patient is more comfortable? Has he taken anything to try to relieve his symptoms? If so, did it help?

  (3) Q: What is the quality of the dyspnea? Is it the same as his usual shortness of breath or qualitatively different?

  (4) R: Radiates—does pain go anywhere else?

  (5) S: How severe is the dyspnea? Ask the patient to rate it against his usual dyspnea, in terms of ability to do specific things (eg, walk up a flight of stairs) on a 1 to 10 scale, with 1 being nothing, and 10 being the worst.

  (6) T: What was the timing of this particular attack? When specifically did it come on? What symptom came first, and then what came next?

  (7) Take a SAMPLE history.

3. In conducting the *physical assessment*, you are looking for some very specific signs. (pages 26.16–26.20)

Part of the Body	What I Am Looking for in Particular
General appearance	Position; level of consciousness (to indicate cerebral oxygenation); degree of distress; skin—sweating cyanosis
Vital signs	Tachycardia; abnormal respiratory rate, depth, or pattern; noisy breathing
Head	Cyanosis of mucous membranes; nasal flaring
Neck	Tracheal tugging or deviation; use of neck muscles to breathe; distended neck veins
Chest	Barred chest; abnormal or unequal breath sounds; inadequate air exchange
Abdomen	Paradoxical respiratory movement; painful, palpable liver in right upper quadrant
Extremities	Cigarette stains; clubbing of the fingers; pedal edema

4. a. 2. This patient is most likely suffering from an acute decompensation of chronic obstructive pulmonary disease (COPD). (page 26.30)

b. The *steps of management* should include the following:

- Administer supplemental *oxygen!* (You should have done that already.)
- Keep the patient sitting up (he probably won't allow you to do otherwise).
- Start an IV fluids at TKO rate.
- Monitor cardiac rhythm.

If you chose to withhold oxygen from this patient, or even to give it in a stingy fashion, you flunk—because the patient may die. Go back and reread the section in your textbook on COPD. *No, oxygen should not be withheld from this patient,* nor should it be given in very low flows. *The treatment of choice for COPD in decompensation is oxygen, oxygen, oxygen.* That is the only drug that can save the patient's life.

The doctor has ordered for the patient as well. You shall see in a moment whether that was a judicious choice, but meanwhile it gives you an opportunity to review the pharmacology of albuterol. (page 26.31)

5. a. The 56-year-old man with the sudden onset of dyspnea and pleuritic chest pain has most probably suffered a pulmonary embolism (answer 1), to which his chronic heart disease predisposed him.

b. Prehospital *management* of the case includes the following steps:

(1) Administer 100% supplemental oxygen.

(2) Start an IV large bore with fluid to keep a vein open.

(3) Monitor cardiac rhythm.

(4) Transport without delay. (page 26.36)

6. a. The *first* thing you should do for the firefighter overcome by smoke is give him oxygen (even in the old days, long before there were paramedics, firefighters knew the importance of "getting the good gas in and the bad gas out").

b. Among the things you would like to find out in *taking the history* of this exposure are (page 26.18):

(1) Did the firefighter lose consciousness during the exposure? If so, for how long?

(2) Was he in a closed space with toxic fumes?

(3) What was burning? That is important information for the emergency department (ED) staff.

(4) Does the firefighter have any significant underlying medical problems? A period of hypoxia during the fire, for example, could have much more serious implications for a patient with underlying heart disease than one with normal coronary arteries.

c. Warning *signs* that should alert you to the possibility *of respiratory tract injury* after a toxic inhalation include the following:

(1) Facial burns

(2) Singed eyebrows or nasal hairs

(3) Blisters in the mouth

(4) Sooty sputum

(5) Brassy cough

(6) Hoarseness

(7) Stridor

d. In particular, if you hear *stridor,* you should be alerted to the possibility that the airway is about to close off altogether. Stridor, therefore, is a signal to get moving as fast as possible to the hospital. (page 26.39)

True/False

1. T (page 26.6)	**11.** F (page 26.30)
2. F (page 26.8)	**12.** T (page 26.30)
3. F (page 26.10)	**13.** F (page 26.31)
4. T (page 26.14)	**14.** T (page 26.32)
5. F (page 26.15)	**15.** T (page 26.34)
6. F (page 26.17)	**16.** T (page 26.42)
7. T (page 26.18)	**17.** F (page 26.42)
8. T (page 26.19)	**18.** F (page 26.43)
9. F (page 26.20)	**19.** T (page 26.44)
10. T (page 26.23)	**20.** F (page 26.44)

Short Answer

1. a. Four things that can cause a pulmonary embolism are the following (page 26.36):

    (1) Fat embolism from a broken bone

    (2) Amniotic fluid leakage

    (3) Air embolism from trauma or IV

    (4) Blood clot caused by heart rhythms or lifestyle

  b. Diagnosis of a pulmonary embolism is cyanosis that does not resolve with the administration of supplemental oxygen. A good history, finding out about such events as a recent surgery or broken bone, also helps with the diagnosis. Cardiac history and your patient's current heart rhythm also help. The patient may have a history of deep vein thrombus. Also, the patient may present with an acute pain centered in the chest that doesn't radiate. Lungs sounds are generally good with maybe a small area of diminished sounds. (page 26.36)

2. There are no contraindications to oxygen in the prehospital setting (page 26.39)!

3. Not everything that wheezes is an acute asthmatic attack. Other causes of wheezing include the following (page 26.22):

  a. Left heart failure

  b. Smoke inhalation or inhalation of toxic fumes

  c. Chronic bronchitis

  d. Foreign body obstruction of a major airway (eg, the patient who has a peanut lodged in a bronchus or a tumor compressing a bronchus)

4. Signs that should alert you to the seriousness of an asthmatic attack in a child include the following (page 26.28):

  a. Sleepiness

  b. Pulsus paradoxus

  c. Cyanosis

  d. Hyperinflation of the chest

  e. A silent chest

Crossword Puzzles

```
 A     B R O N C H O S P A S M
 E           E       M       L     H
 R           M     C M       A     E
 C R O U P   C O   A   O     R     P
 A   S       R  P A R E N C H Y M A
 R   O       I   T   I   I   N
 P   L     T A C H Y P N E A       X
 O         O   O   S   A
 P N E U M O N I T I S   S M O O T H
 E         D     S     H
 D E A D S P A C E   D I U R E T I C S
 A         A       N           L
 L       T U R B I N A T E S   U
 S       T           P         B
 P       I           A         B
 A N T I C H O L I N E R G I C S   I
 S       A           E         N
 M       G           R         G
       G R E E N F I E L D
```

Problem Solving

1. **a.** 200 mL
   b. 700 − 200 = 500
   500 − 150 = 350 mL

2. **a.** 120 mL
   b. 600 − 120 = 480 mL
   480 − 150 = 330 mL

(page 26.8)

Fill-in-the-Table

1.

Breathing Patterns	
Pattern	**Signs and Symptoms**
Agonal	Irregular gasps that are few and far between. Usually represent stray neurologic impulses in the dying patient. It is not unusual for patients who are pulseless to have an occasional agonal gasp.
Apneustic	When the pneumotaxic center in the brain is damaged, the apneustic center causes a prolonged inspiratory hold (fish breathing). This ominous sign indicates severe brain injury.
Ataxic	Completely irregular respirations that indicate severe brain injury or brain-stem herniation.
Biot respirations	Respirations with an irregular pattern, rate, and depth with intermittent patterns of apnea. Indicative of severe brain injury or brain-stem herniation.
Bradypnea	Unusually slow respirations.
Central neurogenic hyperventilation	Tachypneic hyperpnea. Rapid and deep respirations caused by increased intracranial pressure or direct brain injury. Drives carbon dioxide levels down and pH levels up, resulting in respiratory alkalosis.
Cheyne-Stokes respirations	Crescendo-decrescendo breathing with a period of apnea between each cycle. It is not considered ominous unless grossly exaggerated or in the context of a patient who has brain trauma.
Cough	Forced exhalation against a closed glottis; an airway-clearing maneuver. Also seen when foreign substances irritate the airways. Controlled by the cough center in the brain. Antitussive medications work on the cough center to reduce this sometimes-annoying physiologic response.
Eupnea	Normal breathing.
Hiccup	Spasmodic contraction of the diaphragm causing short exhalations with a characteristic sound. Sometimes seen in cases of diaphragmatic (or phrenic nerve) irritation from acute myocardial infarction, ulcer disease, or endotracheal intubation.
Hyperpnea	Unusually deep breathing. Seen in various neurologic or chemical disorders. Certain drugs may stimulate this type of breathing in patients who have overdosed. It does not reflect respiratory rate—only respiratory depth.
Hypopnea	Unusually shallow respirations.
Kussmaul respirations	The same pattern as central neurogenic hyperventilation, but caused by the body's response to metabolic acidosis; the body is trying to rid itself of blood acetone via the lungs. Kussmaul respirations are seen in patients who have diabetic ketoacidosis, and are accompanied by a fruity (acetone) breath odor. The mouth and lips are usually cracked and dry.
Sighing	Periodically taking a very deep breath (about twice the normal volume). Sighing forces open alveoli that close in the course of day-to-day events.
Tachypnea	Unusually rapid breathing. This term does not reflect depth of respiration, nor does it mean that the patient is hyperventilating (lowering the carbon dioxide level by breathing too fast and too deep). In fact, patients who breathe very rapidly frequently move only small volumes of air and are *hypo*ventilating (much like a panting dog).
Yawning	Yawning seems to be beneficial in the same manner that sighing is. It also appears to be contagious!

(page 26.14)

Section 5: Medical

Chapter 27: Cardiovascular Emergencies

Part 1: Cardiac Function

Matching

1. D (page 27.40)	**6.** A (page 27.33)
2. J (page 27.38)	**7.** I (page 27.31)
3. G (page 27.36)	**8.** F (page 27.25)
4. E (page 27.36)	**9.** H (page 27.23)
5. B (page 27.34)	**10.** C (page 27.21)

Multiple Choice

1. B (page 27.7)	**6.** A (page 27.25)
2. B (page 27.7)	**7.** D (page 27.27)
3. D (page 27.14)	**8.** C (page 27.25)
4. B (page 27.16)	**9.** A (page 27.30)
5. C (page 27.21)	**10.** B (page 27.31)

Labeling

1. Coronary arteries (page 27.8)

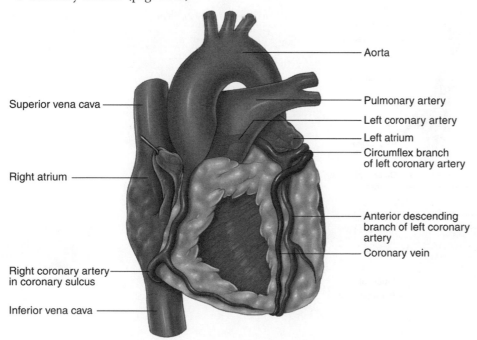

Aorta

Superior vena cava

Pulmonary artery

Left coronary artery

Left atrium

Circumflex branch
of left coronary artery

Right atrium

Anterior descending
branch of left coronary
artery

Coronary vein

Right coronary artery
in coronary sulcus

Inferior vena cava

2. Structures of a blood vessel (page 27.11)

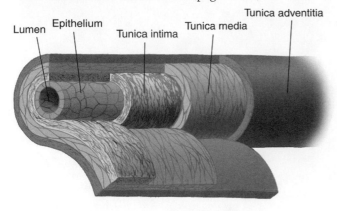

Lumen   Epithelium   Tunica intima   Tunica media   Tunica adventitia

3. The major arteries and veins (page 27.12)

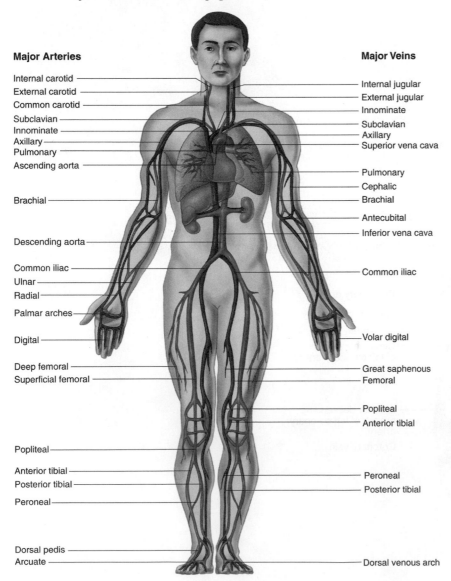

Major Arteries

Internal carotid
External carotid
Common carotid
Subclavian
Innominate
Axillary
Pulmonary
Ascending aorta
Brachial
Descending aorta
Common iliac
Ulnar
Radial
Palmar arches
Digital
Deep femoral
Superficial femoral
Popliteal
Anterior tibial
Posterior tibial
Peroneal
Dorsal pedis
Arcuate

Major Veins

Internal jugular
External jugular
Innominate
Subclavian
Axillary
Superior vena cava
Pulmonary
Cephalic
Brachial
Antecubital
Inferior vena cava
Common iliac
Volar digital
Great saphenous
Femoral
Popliteal
Anterior tibial
Peroneal
Posterior tibial
Dorsal venous arch

Fill-in-the-Blank

   1. Collateral circulation (page 27.7)
   2. Aortic (page 27.8)
   3. Diastole, systole (page 27.9)
   4. Pulmonary circulation (page 27.10)
   5. Arteriole, aorta (page 27.11)
   6. Stroke volume (page 27.13)
   7. Gatekeeper (page 27.14)
   8. Depolarize (page 27.14)
   9. Absolute refractory period (page 27.16)
  10. T wave (page 27.16)

True/False

   1. T (page 27.41)   **6.** T (page 27.34)
   2. F (page 27.39)   **7.** F (page 27.33)
   3. F (page 27.37)   **8.** F (page 27.30)
   4. T (page 27.36)   **9.** T (page 27.29)
   5. T (page 27.36)   **10.** T (page 27.28)

Crossword Puzzle

Fill-in-the-Table

1. (page 27.15)

Role of Electrolytes in Cardiac Function	
Electrolyte	**Role in Cardiac Function**
Sodium (Na^+)	Flows into the cell to initiate depolarization

Potassium (K^+)	Flows out of the cell to initiate repolarization
	    *Hypo*kalemia → increased myocardial irritability
	    *Hyper*kalemia → decreased automaticity/conduction

Calcium (Ca^{++})	Has a major role in the depolarization of pacemaker cells (maintains depolarization) and in myocardial contractility (involved in contraction of heart muscle tissue)
	    *Hypo*calcemia → decreased contractility and increased myocardial irritability
	    *Hyper*calcemia → increased contractility

Magnesium (Mg^{++})	Stabilizes the cell membrane; acts in concert with potassium, and opposes the actions of calcium
	    *Hypo*magnesemia → decreased conduction
	    *Hyper*magnesemia → increased myocardial irritability

2. (page 27.16)

Components of the ECG	
ECG Representation	**Cardiac Event**
P wave	Depolarization of the atria
P-R interval	Depolarization of the atria and delay at the AV junction
QRS complex	Depolarization of the ventricles
ST segment	Period between ventricular depolarization and beginning of repolarization
T wave	Repolarization of the ventricles
R-R interval	Time between two ventricular depolarizations

Part 2: Heart Rhythms and the ECG

Matching

1. G (page 27.43)

2. C (page 27.43)

3. I   (page 27.44)

4. D (page 27.45)

5. B (page 27.47)

6. F (page 27.48)

7. E (page 27.51)

8. A (page 27.54)

9. J   (page 27.56)

10. H (page 27.61)

Multiple Choice

1. B (page 27.61)	**6.** C (page 27.78)
2. D (page 27.65)	**7.** D (page 27.80)
3. C (page 27.69)	**8.** A (page 27.83)
4. A (page 27.72)	**9.** B (page 27.86)
5. B (page 27.75)	**10.** A (page 27.43)

Fill-in-the-Blank

1. Sinus arrest (page 27.49)

2. Supraventricular tachycardia (page 27.50)

3. Accelerated junctional rhythm (page 27.53)

4. Third-degree heart block (page 27.55)

5. Ventricular fibrillation (page 27.58)

6. Bigeminy, trigeminy (page 27.58)

7. Asystole (page 27.59)

8. Delta wave (page 27.61)

9. Unifocal, multifocal (page 27.58)

10. Sinus bradycardia (page 27.47)

True/False

1. T (page 27.42)	**6.** F (page 27.52)
2. F (page 27.44)	**7.** T (page 27.54)
3. F (page 27.46)	**8.** F (page 27.56)
4. T (page 27.47)	**9.** T (page 27.57)
5. F (page 27.50)	**10.** F (page 27.60)

Short Answer

1. Shave body hair to prevent movement and facilitate skin contact. Wipe chest area with an alcohol swab to remove oil and dead tissue. Wait for alcohol to dry before application. Always attach electrodes to the cable before applying them to the chest area. Confirm the proper placement of all electrodes. (page 27.42)

2. The P wave is the depolarization of the sinoatrial (SA) node. P-R interval occurs while the impulse is delayed at the atrioventricular (AV) node. This delay allows the ventricles to fill fully. QRS complex is the depolarization of both the ventricles. The T wave represents the repolarization of both ventricles. (pages 27.43–27.45)

3. A 12-lead echocardiogram (ECG) "looks" at the heart as a whole. It gives views of the heart different from the standard 3 leads. It helps in localizing the site of injury in the heart. (page 27.65)

4. Always start with scene safety and body substance isolation (BSI) procedures. Check for responsiveness, open the airway and assess breathing, and if the patient is not breathing, give 2 breaths. Check pulse and start compressions if needed. Ready your defibrillator and check the patient's rhythm. After the rhythm is established, follow advanced cardiac life support (ACLS) and/or your local protocol. (pages 27.73, 27.74)

5. You and the medical director should practice different scenarios in preparation for having to deliver any bad news. You should role-play and discuss the correct way to break the news of the death of the patient to the family. You must feel comfortable and develop strategies in advance for dealing with these situations. (pages 27.77, 27.78)

Word Find

```
C C N P B Q N W V S L M X H Q P H I A
F O P O Q R W F C R H S Y D R T Y D T
K N M A I X A I H T Q P R E E N P I R
E L X P P S T D Y L O B C D B A O O I
Z J A R L E R H Y V M O O C U L K V A
E R O C R E R E O C R C P J L U A E L
E P Q U O L T L V D A C E Y H G L N L
K I I C A F E E I O S R R E U A E T A
I D W N P M I A H L I F D O Z O M R N
P N O W I S L T P E X D Q I B C I I O
S G U A A L O Q L O A N R V A I A C I
A V S N E V A W P U S R I A L T A U T
E J O A P O V Y M E M M T T C N V L C
S D D A I M H T Y H R R A B R A I N U
E S T A C H Y C A R D I A H L A W R U
N O I T A L L I R B I F E D C O T Q J
U N I F O C A L U U P F V P R N C E O
K G W B Y V R A Z A J N B R I G Y K S
K D N Z L P N X B T L N J O G Q P S N
```

1. Arrhythmia (page 27.41)
2. P wave (page 27.43)
3. Synch (page 27.45)
4. Tachycardia (page 27.47)
5. Bradycardia (page 27.47)
6. Atrial (page 27.50)
7. Multifocal (page 27.51)
8. SA node (page 27.52)
9. Junctional (page 27.52)
10. Unifocal (page 27.58)
11. Idioventricular (page 27.56)
12. Agonal rhythm (page 27.59)
13. Spike (page 27.60)
14. Hypokalemia (page 27.61, 27.62)
15. Complete heart block (page 27.64)
16. Precordial leads (page 27.65)
17. Code (page 27.72)
18. Hypovolemia (page 27.75)
19. Cardioversion (page 27.78)
20. Defibrillation (page 27.80)
21. Nitrates (page 27.84)
22. Diuretics (page 27.86)
23. Anticoagulant (page 27.87)

Part 3: Putting It All Together

Matching

1. I (page 27.86)
2. B (page 27.86)
3. E (page 27.86)
4. F (page 27.86)
5. A (page 27.86)
6. C (page 27.86)
7. H (page 27.86)
8. D (page 27.87)
9. J (page 27.87)
10. G (page 27.87)

Labeling

1. Electrical conduction system (page 27.14)

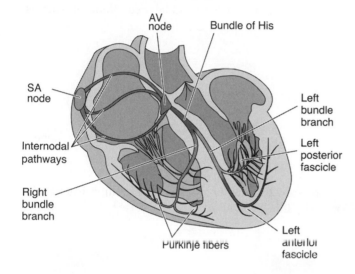

2. Schematic representation of a 12-lead ECG (page 27.70)

I	aVR	V₁	V₄
LCA		LCA	LCA
Lateral wall LV		Septum LV	Anterior wall LV
II	**aVL**	**V₂**	**V₅**
RCA	LCA	LCA	LCA
Inferior wall LV	Lateral wall LV	Septum LV	Lateral wall LV
III	**aVF**	**V₃**	**V₆**
RCA	RCA	LCA	LCA
Inferior wall LV	Inferior wall LV	Anterior wall LV	Lateral wall LV

Ambulance Calls

1. **a.** Chief complaint: Severe chest pain

   Vital signs: Skin pale and cool, pulse is 82 beats/min and thready. Respirations are 32 breaths/min and shallow. Blood pressure is 90/62 mm Hg, and oxygen saturation is 91% on room air.

   b. (1) Apply high-flow supplemental oxygen.

   (2) Listen to lung sounds.

   (3) Apply heart monitor.

   (4) Start an intravenous (IV) medication line.

   He is not a candidate for nitroglycerin at this point, but having the patient chew 325 mg of aspirin would be appropriate. (page 27.53)

    c. (1) Yes

      (2) About 135 beats/min

      (3) Hidden in QRS, some are seen as inverted after QRS

      (4) Not present

      (5) Not present

      (6) 0.12 seconds

      (7) Present and upright

      (8) Junctional tachycardia (page 27.53)

  d. Without a 12-lead ECG, you cannot confirm an acute myocardial infarction (AMI). However, the patient has chest pain, and so AMI and chest pain protocols should be followed.

  e. Treatment should consist of ACLS guidelines. Nitrates would not be good for this patient because of the low blood pressure.

2. a. Chief complaint: Severe dyspnea

    Vital signs: Cyanotic, pulse of 102 beats/min and irregular. Respirations are 60 breaths/min and labored. Blood pressure is 170/94 mm Hg. Lungs have crackles, and oxygen saturation is 86%.

  b. (1) Provide high-flow supplemental oxygen.

      (2) Monitor the ECG.

      (3) Obtain a 12-lead ECG if possible.

      (4) Start an IV. Keep the patient sitting up. (page 27.37)

  c. Right-sided heart failure (page 27.36)

  d. Provide oxygen to help bring up saturations. Follow ACLS guideline for pulmonary edema, and drop the patient's blood pressure with a nitrate after an IV has been started. (page 27.37)

3. a. Chief complaint: Syncope/low heart rate

    Vital signs: Pulse is regular and heart rate is 44 beats/min. Respirations are 22 breaths/min. Oxygen saturation is 94%. Chest pain is not measurable, skin is cool, and blood pressure is 82/40 mm Hg. Lungs are clear. (page 27.48)

  b. (1) Decreased cerebral perfusion

      (2) Arrhythmias

      (3) Increased vagal tones

      (4) Heart lesions (page 27.24)

        More reasons for syncope are stated in Chapter 28.

  c. (1) Provide high-flow oxygen.

      (2) Start an IV. Atropine 0.5 mg can be used to speed up the heart rate. An epinephrine drip or a bolus of epinephrine can also be used. Consult your protocols. (page 27.48)

  d. Transcutaneous pacing (TCP) (page 27.48)

4. a. Chief complaint: Feeling poorly

    Vital signs: Pulse is 76 beats/min and irregular, blood pressure is 110/74 mm Hg. Oxygen saturation is 97%. Lungs are clear, and the skin is cool.

  b. (1) No (irregular)

      (2) 76 beats/min (approx.)

      (3) Absent

      (4) Not present

      (5) n/a (P waves not present)

      (6) None

      (7) QRS complex is normal.

      (8) Atrial fibrillation

      (9) Treatment is supportive, and monitor the patient. Do not convert A Fib in the field unless absolutely necessary. (page 27.52)

5. a. Accelerated idioventricular rhythm (page 27.56)

  b. Sinus arrhythmia (page 27.49)

  c. Atrial flutter (page 27.51)

d. Second-degree heart block, Mobitz type II (page 27.55)

e. Polymorphic ventricular tachycardia (page 27.57)

f. Third-degree heart block (page 27.55)

g. Accelerated junctional rhythm (page 27.53)

h. Junctional rhythm (page 27.52)

i. Idioventricular rhythm (page 27.56)

j. Sinus arrest (page 27.49)

k. Multifocal atrial tachycardia (page 27.51)

l. Second-degree heart block, Mobitz type I (page 27.55)

m. Monomorphic ventricular tachycardia (page 27.57)

n. First-degree heart block (page 27.54)

o. Wandering atrial pacemaker (page 27.50)

p. Supraventricular tachycardia (page 27.50)

q. Sinus bradycardia (page 27.48)

r. Ventricular fibrillation (page 27.59)

6. a. Premature junctional complexes (page 27.54)

b. Premature ventricular complex (page 27.57)

c. Premature atrial complex (page 27.50)

Crossword Puzzle

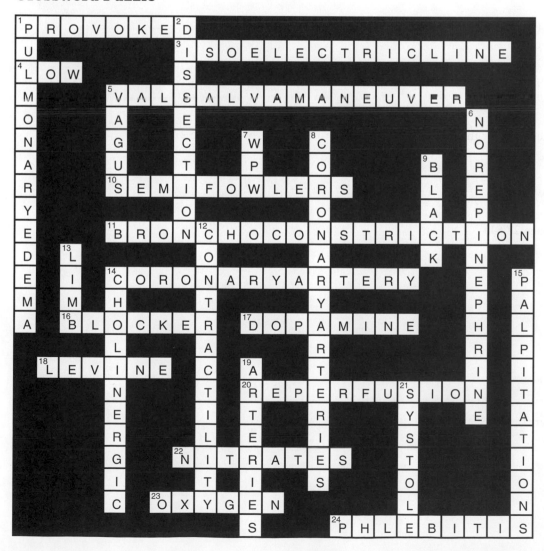

Problem Solving

1. 75 mL/min × 72 mL = 5,400 mL/min (page 27.13)

2. 100 beats/min × 90 mL = 9,000 mL/min (page 27.13)

3. **a.** L (page 27.34)

   b. R (page 27.36)

   c. R (page 27.36)

   d. L (page 27.35)

   e. R (page 27.36)

   f. R (page 27.36)

   g. L (page 27.34)

4. MAP = DBP + $\frac{1}{3}$ (SBP – DBP) (page 27.40)

   a. 109 (approx.)

   b. 156 (approx.)

   c. 107 (approx.)

5. 0.04 seconds (page 27.43)

6. 5 (page 27.43)

7. **a.** Altered level of consciousness (LOC) and mental status

   b. Chest pain

   c. Hypotension

   d. Other signs of shock

   e. Heart rate above 150 beats/min (page 27.81)

8. Adenosine (page 27.81)

9. Amiodarone (page 27.81)

10. Begin transcutaneous pacing (TCP) (if the patient is conscious, consider analgesic if that can be accomplished rapidly) (page 27.79)

11. **a.** Epinephrine 1 mg (page 27.76)

    b. Vasopressin 40 units (as a replacement for the first or second epinephrine, but not both) (page 27.76)

    c. Atropine 1 mg (page 27.76)

    d. Atropine 0.5 mg (page 27.79)

    e. Epinephrine 2–10 µg/min (page 27.79)

    f. Adenosine 6 mg (page 27.81)

    g. Amiodarone 150 mg/10 min (page 27.81)

12. Hypovolemia

    Hypoxia

    Hydrogen ion (acidosis)

    Hypo/hyperkalemia

    Hypoglycemia

    Hypothermia

    Toxins

    Tamponade, cardiac

    Tension pneumothorax

    Thrombosis (coronary or pulmonary)

    Trauma (hypovolemia) (page 27.81)

Chapter 28: Neurologic Emergencies

Matching

(page 28.28)

1. B
2. B
3. A
4. A
5. B

6. B
7. B
8. B
9. A
10. A

Multiple Choice

1. D (page 28.5)
2. C (page 28.6)
3. A (page 28.8)
4. B (page 28.13)
5. C (page 28.14)

6. C (page 28.18)
7. A (page 28.20)
8. D (page 28.23)
9. D (page 28.33)
10. B (page 28.35)

Labeling

1. Parts of the Brain (page 28.6)

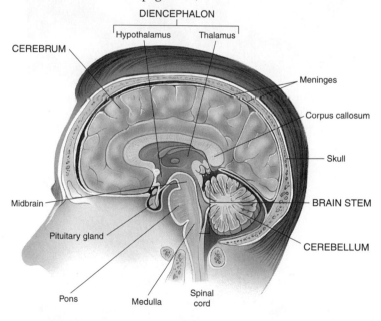

2. Parts of a Neuron (page 28.8)

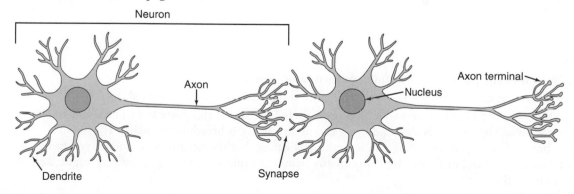

3. Pupil Responses (page 28.19)

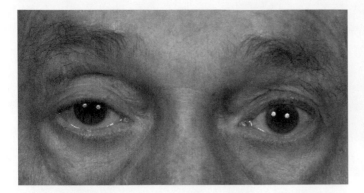

A. Normal

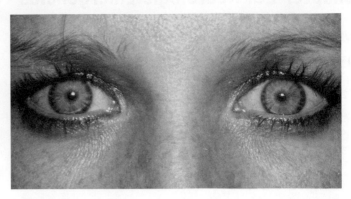

B. Constricted (pin point)

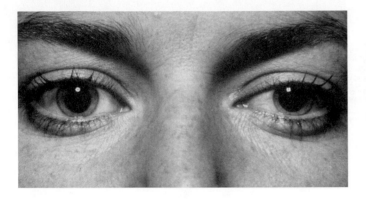

C. Dilated

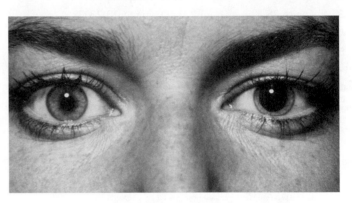

D. Unequal

Fill-in-the-Blank

1. Pons (page 28.6)

2. Neurotransmitters (page 28.7)

3. Endotoxin (page 28.10)

4. Brain, blood, cerebrospinal fluid (page 28.12)

5. Decrease, increase (page 28.15)

6. 15, 3 (page 28.17)

7. Expressive aphasia (page 28.18)

8. Glucose, 60–120 (page 28.20)

9. Ischemic, hemorrhagic (page 28.24)

10. Febrile, generalized (grand mal), petite mal (page 28.29)

Identify

1. Chief complaint: General weakness, visual disturbance

2. Vital signs: blood pressure is 128/76 mm Hg, pulse is 84 beats/min, oxygen saturation is 98%

3. Pertinent negatives: No pain, vital signs in normal ranges, no facial droop, no trauma, temperature is normal.

Wow, what a tricky patient! Vital signs are all pretty normal, blood pressure is 128/76 mm Hg, pulse is 84 beats/min and regular, and oxygen saturation is 98%. The patient is alert and has a patent airway. He is breathing regularly. His blood glucose level is 112 mg/dL. What the vital signs are telling you is nothing is wrong, but the negatives are telling you more. The patient has no signs of trauma, infection, or illness. He is not in any pain. His symptoms and signs are very vague, and supportive care and transport are all that are required.

Ambulance Calls

1. The next seizure case you have to deal with is a lot more serious; it is a case of *status epilepticus.*

   a. When you get around to doing a rapid medical assessment, you will want to be particularly alert for the following (page 28.31):

      (1) Irregularities in the pulse

      (2) The combination of bradycardia and hypotension, which would suggest increasing intracranial pressure as a cause of the seizures

      (3) Evidence of head trauma as either cause or result of the seizures

      (4) Inequality of the pupils, again suggesting rising intracranial pressure

      (5) Breath odors (alcohol, ketones, poisons)

      (6) Gingival hypertrophy, suggesting long-term phenytoin use

      (7) Stiff neck, suggesting the patient has bled into the cerebrospinal fluid (CSF)

      (8) Injuries, especially posterior dislocation of the shoulder

      (9) Medical identification tag

      (10) Medication bottles in pockets

   b. The steps in *treating* a patient in status epilepticus are (page 28.31):

      (1) Protect the patient from injury.

      (2) Ensure an open airway, which will mean whipping in an endotracheal tube the first chance you get. After the tube is in, insert an oropharyngeal airway as well, to prevent the patient from biting down on the endotracheal tube, and secure them both in place. (Patients having seizures have been known to bite an endotracheal tube in half!)

      (3) Administer supplemental oxygen. Remember: Deaths from seizures are hypoxic deaths.

      (4) Start an IV with a large-bore catheter and secure it *very* well.

   c. The medication most commonly used in the field for status epilepticus is diazepam (Valium) (page 28.31).

      (1) The *contraindications* to giving diazepam are in patients who are pregnant and those who have already taken other sedative drugs or alcohol.

      (2) The correct *dosage* is 5.0 mg slowly IV given *after* you have measured a baseline blood pressure. Then, wait a few minutes, and recheck the blood pressure. You may repeat diazepam every 10 to 15 minutes with 5.0 mg (total dosage should not exceed 30 mg). You may also use lorazepam 0.05 mg/kg (maximum dose at one time is 4 mg). Repeat the lorazepam in 10 to 15 minutes with a maximum dose of 8 mg in a 12-hour period. (page 28.31)

      (3) The possible *side effects* of intravenous diazepam include hypotension and even respiratory or cardiac arrest (those more serious complications are more likely to occur in elderly patients). (You may need to refer to the pharmacology chapter for more details on the drug.)

2. For once the person calling 9-1-1 got it right: The woman with a "possible stroke" has almost certainly had a stroke.

   a. She is most likely right-handed. You know that the stroke involves the left side of her brain because the right side of her body is paralyzed. You suspect that the left side of her brain is the dominant side because the stroke has robbed her of speech. Most right-handed people are "left-dominant," that is, the left side of the brain is the dominant side in terms of speech and several other functions. (page 28.19)

   b. The steps in *treating* this woman are as follows (page 28.19):

      (1) Protect her airway because she cannot (she has no gag reflex). Suction secretions as needed, and keep her in the stable side position.

      (2) Administer supplemental oxygen by nasal cannula.

      (3) Monitor cardiac rhythm, and be prepared to deal with arrhythmias.

      (4) Start an IV with a microdrip infusion set, and hang normal saline at a keep-open rate.

      (5) Protect the paralyzed extremities. The patient should be lying on her nonparalyzed (left) side so that she can feel if she is putting too much pressure on an arm or leg.

      (6) Maintain a running conversation with the patient, and provide honest reassurance.

3. Here you have a patient in coma of unknown cause.

   a. The easiest way to remember the possible causes of coma is through the mnemonic AEIOU-TIPS (page 28.29):

      (1) A Alcohol/acidosis

      (2) E Epilepsy/electrolyte imbalance/endocrine

      (3) I Insulin (hypoglycemia)

(4) O Overdose/poisoning

(5) U Uremia

(6) T Trauma/temperature abnormalities

(7) I Infection

(8) P Psychogenic

(9) S Stroke/space-occupying lesion

b. (1) Establish an airway (hold off intubation, though, until you can assess the results of dextrose and naloxone).

(2) Administer supplemental oxygen.

(3) Establish an IV in a large vein.

(4) Give thiamine, 100 mg slowly IV.

(5) Give 50% dextrose, 50 mL slowly IV, preferably after checking the blood glucose level.

(6) If the patient does not wake in response to dextrose and there is reason to suspect narcotic overdose (eg, pinpoint pupils), give naloxone, 0.8 mg slowly IV; if there is no response after 2 to 3 minutes, repeat the dose.

(7) If there is no response to two doses of naloxone, intubate the trachea.

(8) Monitor cardiac rhythm.

Other steps include: Keep a flow sheet of neurologic and vital signs; protect the patient's eyes: tape them shut; and transport the patient to the hospital (page 28.29).

True/False

1. T (page 28.5)

2. F (page 28.6)

3. F (page 28.7)

4. T (page 28.9)

5. T (page 28.11)

6. F (page 28.12)

7. T (pages 28.14, 28.15)

8. T (page 28.17)

9. F (page 28.18)

10. F (page 28.22)

11. T (page 28.22)

12. F (page 28.23)

13. F (page 28.27)

14. T (page 28.28)

15. F (page 28.30)

Short Answer

1. Vocabulary:

a. Hemiparesis: weakness of one half (side) of the body (hemi- + -paresis) (page 28.18)

b. Neuropathy: disease of nerves (neuro- + -pathy) (page 28.37)

2. a. Seizure disorders

b. Diabetes

c. Atrial fib/blood clots

Word Find

```
X P N J S U T M A F I K D R T N D N
S T R S E T I R D N E D W I Z Y D E
Y U Z M I O M A I A B S C E S S V U
N E O X Z X Y D F T D Q I T Y T R R
C X J V U Y E C I A A R O I S A P O
O O T Y R G L H B X R N H G L G M T
P T M W E E I G A I I E L U A M M R
E O E S N N B N A M U C P P U E A A
H X N M I G C I I C I R V L S D N N
A I I H P I H Y P O T H A L A M U S
X N N U B E L A S E H D E A R U L M
P S G M S R R E R V P B Z T B I L I
N K I T L E T A R B E R E C E D A T
G L T S S O K M T R X N O I R D V T
A M I I O G A O E U Z F I T E E Z E
K O S H H T L C R W R M L S C B A R
L W J S O U P W N T R E M O R S H N
A I O Y O S N A T D S E S P A N Y S
```

1. Nervous (page 28.5)
2. Medulla (page 28.6)
3. Reticular (page 28.6)
4. Hypothalamus (page 28.7)
5. Cerebellum (page 28.7)
6. Synapses (page 28.7)
7. Limbic (page 28.7)
8. Neurotransmitter (page 28.7)
9. Dendrites (page 28.8)
10. Myelin (page 28.9)
11. Spina bifida (page 28.10)
12. Exotoxins (page 28.10)
13. Meningitis (page 28.13)
14. Decerebrate (page 28.14)
15. Coma (page 28.16)
16. Ptosis (page 28.17)
17. Nystagmus (page 28.18)
18. Hemiparesis (page 28.18)
19. Ataxia (page 28.19)
20. Tremors (page 28.20)
21. Oxygen, glucose, temperature (page 28.21)
22. Strokes (page 28.24)
23. Seizures (page 28.29)
24. Postictal (page 28.30)
25. Syncope (page 28.31)
26. Abscess (page 28.33)
27. Dystonia (page 28.34)
28. Cerebral palsy (page 28.36)

Fill-in-the-Table

1. (page 28.17)

Glasgow Coma Scale		
	Adult	**Pediatric Patient (< 5 y)**
Eye opening	4. Spontaneous	4. Spontaneous
	3. Voice	3. To shout/voice
	2. Pain stimulation	2. Pain stimulation
	1. None	1. None
Verbal	5. Oriented	5. Cry, smile, coo, words correct for age
	4. Disoriented	4. Cries, inappropriate words for age
	3. Inappropriate words	3. Inappropriate scream or cry
	2. Incomprehensible	2. Grunts
	1. None	1. None
Motor	6. Obeys	6. Spontaneous
	5. Localizes pain	5. Localizes pain
	4. Withdraws from pain	4. Withdraws from pain
	3. Decorticate	3. Decorticate
	2. Decerebrate	2. Decerebrate
	1. None	1. None

2. (page 28.29)

A. Abscess, AIDS, alcohol

B. Birth defect, brain infections, brain trauma

D. Diabetes mellitus

F. Fever

I. Idiopathic, inappropriate medication dosage

O. Organic brain syndromes

R. Recreational drugs

S. Stroke, systemic infection

T. Tumor, transient ischemic attack (TIA)

U. Uremia

Problem Solving

Cincinnati Prehospital Stroke Scale (page 28.27)

1. Smile is not equal

2. Uses sentence, "You can't teach an old dog new tricks"

3. Closes her eyes and right arm drifts down

Los Angeles Prehospital Stroke Screen (page 28.27)

1. Age is greater than 45.

2. Smile is unequal.

3. Blood glucose is normal.

4. Her grip strength is not equal.

5. Right arm drift.

6. Patient is not bedridden.

7. Symptom onset is less than 24 hours.

8. No history of seizures or epilepsy.

Chapter 29: Endocrine Emergencies

Matching

1. E (page 29.19)	**8.** N (page 29.7)
2. B (page 29.8)	**9.** K (page 29.9)
3. D (page 29.8)	**10.** M (page 29.7)
4. G (page 29.13)	**11.** I (page 29.6)
5. F (page 29.5)	**12.** H (page 29.18)
6. A (page 29.5)	**13.** L (page 29.6)
7. C (page 29.14)	**14.** J (page 29.9)

Multiple Choice

1. D (page 29.4)	**9.** C (page 29.11)
2. C (page 29.4)	**10.** A (page 29.13)
3. B (page 29.5)	**11.** D (page 29.14)
4. A (page 29.5)	**12.** A (page 29.16)
5. B (page 29.6)	**13.** D (page 29.17)
6. B (page 29.7)	**14.** A (page 29.18)
7. B (page 29.8)	**15.** D (page 29.19)
8. B (page 29.11)	

Labeling

1. The body's response to stress (page 29.6)

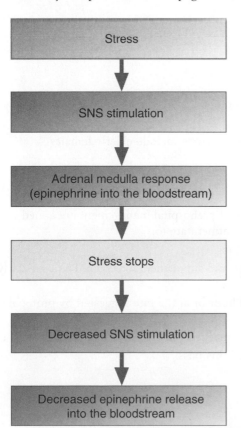

Stress

↓

SNS stimulation

↓

Adrenal medulla response
(epinephrine into the bloodstream)

↓

Stress stops

↓

Decreased SNS stimulation

↓

Decreased epinephrine release
into the bloodstream

2. The adrenal cortex and the adrenal medula (page 29.8)

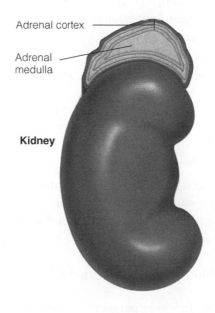

Adrenal gland

Adrenal cortex

Adrenal
medulla

Kidney

Fill-in-the-Blank

1. Myxedema coma (page 29.18)
2. Thyroid-stimulating hormone (page 29.17)
3. Salt; potassium (page 29.16)
4. Rehydration, electrolyte (page 29.14)
5. Head injury, seizures, traumatic (page 29.12)
6. Seizure,thirst (page 29.11)
7. Type 1, type 2, medical management (page 29.10)
8. Islets of Langerhans, glucagons, insulin (page 29.8)
9. Master gland, endocrine (page 29.5)
10. Feedback systems, negative feedback (page 29.4)

Identify

1. **a.** Chief complaint: Altered level of consciousness
   b. Vital signs: Respirations are shallow and the patient is diaphoretic. Her pulse is 118 beats/min, and her blood pressure is 104/88 mm Hg.
   c. Pertinent negatives: Her blood glucose is 48 mg/dL.
   d. Nature of the endocrine disorder: Type 1 diabetes.
   This patient is likely suffering from hypoglycemia. Hypoglycemia in the insulin-dependent diabetic is often the result of having taken too much insulin, too little food, or both. Her vital signs include a mental status of being unresponsive, a tachycardia of 118 beats/min, and a blood pressure of 104/88 mm Hg. Her skin indicates diaphoresis as well as blood glucose of 48 mg/dL. (page 29.11)

2. **a.** Chief complaint: Shortness of breath
   b. Vital signs: Rapid breathing. He is tachycardic with a blood pressure of 108/82 mm Hg.
   c. Pertinent negatives: Fruity, acetone breath. He has poor skin turgor and skin tenting is present.
   d. Nature of the endocrine disorder: Diabetic patient
   This patient is likely suffering from diabetic ketoacidosis. His vitals include tachycardia, an elevated blood glucose level, and blood pressure of 108/82 mm Hg. Oxygen saturation is 95%. (page 29.14)

3. **a.** Chief complaint: Altered mental status
   b. Vital signs: Bradycardic and hypotensive
   c. Pertinent negatives: Can't get a pulse oximeter reading, acting confused and psychotic
   d. Nature of the endocrine disorder: Myxedema coma
   This patient is most likely suffering from myxedema coma. The hallmarks of myxedema coma include elderly females, behavioral/mental status changes, and hypothermia. (page 29.18)

Ambulance Calls

1. The patient is showing characteristic signs of diabetic ketoacidosis (DKA). The steps of prehospital management are aimed primarily at stabilizing vital functions and restoring fluid. The goals of prehospital treatment are to:
   a. begin rehydration and to correct the patient's electrolyte and acid–base abnormalities.
   b. Follow the procedure for any comatose patient with regard to airway maintenance and supplemental oxygen. Be particularly alert for vomiting and have suction ready.
   c. Start an intravenous (IV) and infuse up to 1 L of normal saline over the first half hour or at the rate suggested by protocol or online Medical Control.
   d. Monitor cardiac rhythm. Changes in serum potassium caused by DKA can lead to marked myocardial instability. (page 29.14)

2. A young salesman has had a grand mal seizure while waiting for an appointment with his boss.
   a. The causes of seizures include: (*Students should provide six of the following*)
      (1) Stroke
      (2) Head trauma
      (3) Brain tumor
      (4) Hypoxemia

(5) Hypoglycemia

(6) Toxins, **drugs, or withdrawal** from drugs or alcohol

(7) Meningitis

(8) Idiopathic epilepsy

(9) In a pregnant woman, **eclampsia**

Note that this list is very nearly identical to the list of causes of coma. So, if you can't remember the causes of seizures, just go through the AEIOU-TIPS roster. (page 29.12)

b. The steps in treating this patient are:

(1) Management of the ABCs.

(2) Remember that a patient whose gag reflex is absent can't protect his or her own airway from aspiration and should be intubated at the earliest opportunity.

(3) If breathing is abnormally slow or shallow, assist breathing with bag-mask ventilation.

(4) Administer oxygen whether the patient is breathing spontaneously or being ventilated.

(5) If the patient has altered mental status, establish an IV with 0.9% normal saline or a saline lock.

(6) Make an immediate determination of the blood glucose level and initiate treatment if the reading is less than 60 mg/dL. Give 25 g of D50; this dose will reverse most cases of hypoglycemia.

(7) If you have any other reason to suspect a narcotics overdose (pinpoint pupils, needle tracks on the arms, depressed respirations), then consider administration of naloxone (Narcan).

(8) Monitor the cardiac rhythm of every comatose patient.

(9) Transport the comatose patient supine if he or she is intubated.

(10) Transport the patient in the stable side position (unless injuries preclude that position).

(11) If the patient must be supine (e.g., because of suspected spine injury) and can't be intubated, keep the mouth and pharynx suctioned free of secretions, vomit, and blood.(page 29.12)

c. Almost magically, just moments after you've given the glucose, the patient becomes fully alert and also apparently restored to his "sweet" disposition—prima facie evidence that the source of his problem was undoubtedly **hypoglycemia.** (The patient's remark about how he shouldn't have skipped breakfast suggests that he had come to the same conclusion.) (page 29.20)

d. The *advice* to give this patient is

(1) Get yourself a **medical identification tag that states you are a diabetic and wear it at all times.**

(2) Pay attention to **early warning signs of hypoglycemia,** and do something about them before the attack progresses.

(3) Always **carry a candy bar** or other source of sugar with you, to eat when you feel hypoglycemic symptoms.

3. a. Probable underlying illness(es): Hypoglycemia (page 29.21)

b. Probable underlying illness(es): diabetes

c. The patient has an insulin pump. The possibilities include a malfunctioning pump, the patient didn't load the insulin into the pump, and regardless of the pump the patient disregarded proper dietary control causing a hypoglycemic emergency. (page 29.11)

d. Don't let a known diagnosis of diabetes prevent you from considering other causes of coma. Diabetics are not immune to head injury, stroke, seizures, meningitis, and other traumatic injuries or conditions. Keep an open mind and assess the patient thoroughly. (page 29.12)

True/False

1. T (page 29.20)
2. F (page 29.19)
3. T (page 29.18)
4. T (page 29.17)
5. F (page 29.16)
6. T (page 29.13)
7. F (page 29.12)
8. T (page 29.11)

9. T (page 29.11)
10. F (page 29.10)
11. T (page 29.9)
12. T (page 29.8)
13. F (page 29.8)
14. T (page 29.6)
15. F (page 29.4)

Short Answer

1. Vocabulary:

   a. Hypoglycemia: Hypoglycemia in the insulin-dependent diabetic is often the result of having taken too much insulin, too little food, or both. Unlike other tissues, which can usually metabolize fat or protein in addition to sugar, the tissues of the central nervous system (including the brain) depend entirely on glucose as their source of energy. If the level of glucose in the blood drops dramatically, the brain is literally starved. (page 29.11)

   b. Diabetic ketoacidosis (DKA): A life-threatening condition, DKA occurs when certain acids accumulate in the body because insulin is not available. Patients who suffer from this condition tend to be young—teenagers and young adults. In DKA, the deficiency of insulin prevents cells from taking up the extra sugar. (page 29.13)

   c. Thyrotoxicosis: A toxic condition caused by excessive levels of circulating thyroid hormone. Although hyperthyroidism can cause thyrotoxicosis in some patients, the two conditions are not identical. Thyrotoxicosis may also be caused by goiters, autoimmune disease (Grave's disease—the most common cause of hyperthyroidism), and thyroid cancer. Grave's disease, which has an incidence of 1.4 cases per 1,000 persons, has a chronic course with remissions and relapses. If left untreated, it may be fatal. (page 29.19)

   d. Insulin: Hormone produced by the pancreas that's vital to the control of the body's metabolism and blood glucose level. Insulin causes sugar, fatty acids, and amino acids to be taken up and metabolized by cells. (page 29.23)

   e. Cushing's syndrome: A condition caused by an excess of cortisol production by the adrenal glands or by excessive use of cortisol or other similar steroid (glucocorticoid) hormones. (page 29.23)

2. Treatment:

   a. Myxedema coma: Administer supplemental oxygen therapy to correct hypoxia. Intubation and ventilation are indicated for patients with diminished respiratory drive or those who are unable to protect their airway; these measures help prevent respiratory failure. Monitor the patient's cardiac status. Hypotension may respond to crystalloid therapy, and vasopressive agents may be necessary (dopamine). Administer 25 to 50 g of D50 if glucose levels are less than 60 mg/dL. Treat hypothermia with passive rewarming methods because aggressive rewarming may lead to vasodilation and hypotension. Hemodynamically unstable patients with profound hypothermia, however, require active rewarming. Avoid sedatives, narcotics, and anesthetics because of the delayed metabolism. (page 29.18)

   b. Adrenal insufficiency: The treatment for adrenal insufficiency is based on the clinical presentation and findings, and is geared toward maintaining the airway, breathing, and circulation until arrival at the emergency department. Other goals of prehospital treatment are to begin rehydration of the patient and to correct the electrolyte and acid–base abnormalities. Follow the procedure for a patient with altered mental status or comatose patient with regard to airway maintenance and supplemental oxygen. Be alert for vomiting and have suction ready. Start an IV and infuse up to 1 L of 0.9% normal saline. If the patient is hypotensive, administer a normal saline bolus at 20 mL/kg. Remember, a patient in adrenal insufficiency may be severely dehydrated, often to the point of shock, and needs volume. Check the patient's glucose level. Administer 25 to 50 g of D50 to correct the hypoglycemia. D_5NS is the preferred IV fluid, but a second IV administering D_5W can be used to maintain the patient's blood glucose level. Monitor cardiac rhythm because changes in serum electrolytes can lead to marked myocardial instability. (page 29.16)

   c. Hyperosmolar nonketotic coma: The treatment of hyperosmolar nonketotic coma/hyperosmolar hyperglycemic nonketotic coma (HONK/HHNC) in the prehospital setting follows the pathway for dehydration and altered mental status. Airway management is the top priority. The comatose patient is often unable to maintain and protect his or her airway. For this reason, endotracheal intubation may be indicated and should be completed as early as possible. Cervical spine immobilization should be used for all unresponsive patients found down, unless witnesses can validate that no fall occurred. Large-bore IV access should be gained as soon as possible, but do not delay transfer while initiating the IV. If necessary, obtain IV access during the transport to the emergency department. Also obtain a blood glucose level as soon as possible. After you have initiated the IV, a bolus of 500 mL 0.9% normal saline is appropriate for nearly all adults who are clinically dehydrated. In patients with a history of congestive heart failure and/or renal insufficiency, a 250-mL bolus may be a more appropriate starting point. Fluid deficits in HONK/HHNC patients may amount to 10 L or more. These patients may receive 1 to 2 L in the first hour. If the glucose level is less than 60 to 80 mg/dL, then (depending on your local protocols) administer 25 g of D50 as soon as possible. (page 29.15)

Crossword Puzzle

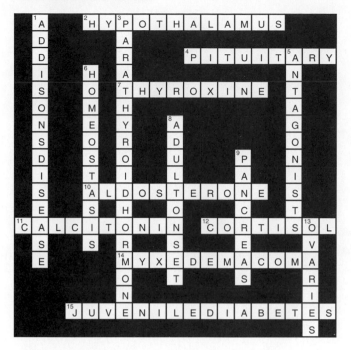

Fill-in-the-Table

1. (page 29.8)

Hormones of the Adrenal Glands	
Cortisol	Increases metabolic rate, using fat and protein for energy
Aldosterone	Reabsorbs sodium and water from the urine, and excretes excess potassium
Epinephrine/norepinephrine	Stimulates sympathetic nervous system receptors

2. (page 29.9)

Hormones of the Gonads	
Male	
Testosterone	Main sex hormone in males Responsible for secondary sex characteristics: voice deepening, growth of facial hair, muscle development, pubic hair, growth spurts
Female	
Estrogen	Responsible for secondary sex characteristics: breast growth, fat accumulation at hips and thighs, pubic hair, growth spurts Involved in pregnancy Regulation of menstrual cycle
Progesterone	Involved in pregnancy Regulation of menstrual cycle Prevents maturation of additional egg during ovulation

3. (page 29.14)

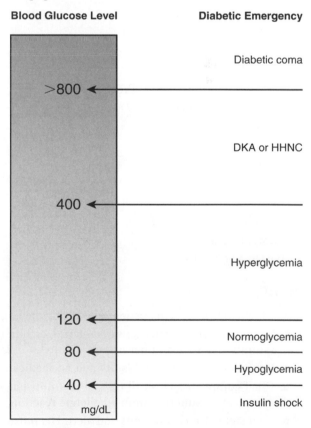

Blood Glucose Level	Diabetic Emergency
>800	Diabetic coma
	DKA or HHNC
400	
	Hyperglycemia
120	Normoglycemia
80	Hypoglycemia
40	Insulin shock
mg/dL	

Chapter 30: Allergic Reactions

Matching

1. D (page 30.4)
2. C (page 30.4)
3. B (page 30.3)
4. A (page 30.3)
5. C (page 30.4)
6. A (page 30.3)
7. D (page 30.4)
8. C (page 30.4)
9. A (page 30.4)
10. D (page 30.4)

Multiple Choice

1. D (page 30.10)
2. D (page 30.12)
3. B (page 30.13)
4. D (page 30.13)
5. D (page 30.13)
6. D (page 30.13)
7. C (page 30.16)
8. A (page 30.3)
9. C (page 30.5)
10. C (page 30.5)

Labeling

(page 30.6)

1. Antigen is introduced into the body
2. Mast cells
3. Bronchospasm, vasoconstriction
4. Decreased cardiac output, decreased coronary flow
5. Vasodilation, leakiness
6. Pruritis, urticaria, edema

Fill-in-the-Blank

1. Acquired immunity (page 30.7)
2. Natural immunity (page 30.7)
3. Antigen (page 30.3)
4. Mast (page 30.6)
5. Histamine (page 30.6)
6. Noisy upper airway (page 30.10)
7. Life-threatening (page 30.12)
8. Epinephrine (page 30.13)
9. Glucagon (page 30.13)
10. Oxygen (page 30.13)

Identify

1. a. Chief complaint: This patient is probably having a localized reaction at the sting site.
   b. Vital signs: She is conscious and alert. Her skin color is normal, warm, and dry. Capillary refill is normal. Her oxygen saturation is 99% and her blood pressure is 112/68 mm Hg. PEARRL.
   c. Pertinent negatives: No history and no medications.
2. a. Chief complaint: This call isn't all that unusual, especially given the recent concerns about Lyme disease. This patient doesn't appear to be suffering from an allergic reaction.
   b. Vital signs: He is conscious and alert. His pulse is 110 beats/min and regular. Blood pressure is 142/84 mm Hg, PEARRL, skin warm/moist.
   c. Pertinent negatives: No previous medical history, no allergies and no known drug allergies.

3. a. Chief complaint: This call seems as though it's a true medical emergency. Many schools and classrooms are "peanut free." The patient presents as being in noticeable distress with a well-documented allergy history. In fact, many restaurants and bakeries have signs posted regarding their ingredients and the use of products that may cause allergic reaction.

   b. Vital signs: Pulse of 124 beats/min, oxygen saturation of 90%, blood pressure is 90/62 mm Hg. Pertinent negatives: None.

   c. Pertinent negatives: None indicated.

4. a. Chief complaint: It's not uncommon to respond to a reported allergic reaction only to find the patient in minor distress. What's not really clear is the time the patient had dinner. If several hours have gone by, it is less likely that the cause is an allergic reaction. A number of ailments can cause GI upset included bacterial and viral infections.

   b. Vital signs: Her vitals signs are: pulse of 124 beats/min, oxygen saturation of 90%, blood pressure is 112/62 mm Hg.

   c. Pertinent negatives: None.

5. a. Chief complaint: Once again, this is a true life-threatening emergency. It's hard to predict how babies and small children may present after receiving routine inoculations. The vast majority of small patients suffer only from minor systemic complications, such as pain and fever. But, occasionally you may encounter a child who has had serious side effects. Remember to aggressively maintain ABCs, contact medical control immediately, and follow Pediatric Advanced Life Support as well as local protocols.

   b. Vital signs: Apical pulse of 190 beats/min. Delayed capillary refill, mottled skin.

   c. Pertinent negatives: None.

Ambulance Calls

1. This 52-year-old man who was stung by a bee is also suffering an anaphylactic reaction, but because of his age, you have to be a little more careful in giving epinephrine.

   a. The treatment is as follows:

   (1) Ensure that his airway stays patent.

   (2) Administer high-flow oxygen.

   (3) Monitor the ECG throughout (keep the beep tone on).

   (4) Start a large-bore IV.

   (5) Give epinephrine as follows: First, dilute 0.1 mg (0.1 mL) of 1:1,000 epinephrine in 10 mL of normal saline and inject it over 10 minutes. If the patient is not getting better by then, start an infusion at 1 μg per minute.

   (6) Remove the stinger from the patient's skin, taking care not to squeeze it. If the site is on an extremity, put a constricting band (venous tourniquet) proximal to the sting site.

   (7) Consult medical command regarding any other pharmacotherapy.

   (8) Transport without delay.

   b. Epinephrine, if given in excessive dosage, may cause the following:

   (1) extreme hypertension.

   (2) angina.

   (3) cardiac arrhythmias and consequent palpitations. (page 30.12)

2. If you want to stay out of trouble on your night off, stay out of restaurants! The lady at the next table is suffering an anaphylactic reaction, apparently to something she ate. The sensation of a lump in the throat along with her squeaky voice indicates that she is in a lot of trouble. The steps in management are as follows:

   a. Administer albuterol by a metered-dose inhaler to try to buy some time for the airway (but have your cricothyrotomy kit at hand just in case).

   b. Administer supplemental oxygen by nasal cannula.

   c. Start transport.

   d. Start an IV with a large-bore cannula.

   e. Give diphenhydramine, 50 mg IM.

   f. If you are a long way from the hospital, give hydrocortisone, 500 mg IV over 5 minutes. (page 30.12)

3. a. Patient A is showing classic signs of choking, and a shot of epinephrine will not help him a bit (except during resuscitation from the cardiac arrest he will surely suffer if you failed to diagnose his choking and act immediately).

   b. Patient B is simply experiencing a very common untoward side effect of erythromycin, about which he *should* have been warned by the doctor who prescribed the drug.

   c. Patient C *is* suffering an anaphylactic reaction.

4. Use the following steps to manage patient C:

  a. Ensure that his airway stays open. It is already in jeopardy, judging from his hoarse voice. If you are unable to whip an endotracheal tube in, administer 4 to 10 sprays of 1:1,000 racemic epinephrine, and get moving at once to the hospital, administering oxygen throughout.

  b. Monitor the ECG; cardiac dysrhythmias are likely.

  c. Start at least one large-bore IV and run it wide open.

  d. Unfortunately, in this particular case, you probably cannot use a constricting band to isolate the injection site because what the patient in all probability got was two shots of penicillin, one in each buttock, so there's no place to put the venous tourniquet!

  e. You *can,* however, give epinephrine, 0.1 mg/kg of a 1:10,000 solution (about 5–10 mL) *slowly* IV. (page 30.12)

5. The *contraindications* to diphenhydramine are the following:

  a. Asthma or chronic obstructive pulmonary disease

  b. Glaucoma

  c. Prostate problems

  d. Ulcer disease

  e. Pregnancy (page M.8)

6. The *dosage* in this case would be 25 to 50 mg *slowly* IV. (page M.8)

7. Possible *side effects* of diphenhydramine include the following:

  a. Drowsiness

  b. Blurring of vision

  c. Dry mouth

  d. Wheezing

  e. Difficulty in urinating

Before you finish with this case, be sure to have a word with your medical director—so that he or she can have a word with the people at the Public Health Clinic. They need to be reminded that it just won't do to give a patient a parenteral antibiotic (or any other drug) and whip him out the door! Patients should remain under observation for at *least* 30 minutes after any parenteral medication. (page M.8)

True/False

1. F (page 30.14)   **6.** T (page 30.4)

2. T (page 30.14)   **7.** T (page 30.5)

3. F (page 30.13)   **8.** F (page 30.5)

4. F (page 30.12)   **9.** T (page 30.7)

5. F (page 30.12)   **10.** F (page 30.12)

Short Answer

1. Effects produced by mast-cell mediators include the following:

  a. Systemic vasodilatation

  b. Pulmonary vasoconstriction

  c. Increased capillary permeability

  d. Bronchoconstriction

  e. Decreased coronary blood flow

  f. Decreased strength and contractility of the heart

  g. Increased tendency for arrhythmias (page 30.8)

2. Agents commonly responsible for anaphylactic reactions fall into three general categories: drugs, foods, and insect venoms.
Students should provide four of the following:

DRUGS	Penicillin
	Blood products
	Horse serum products
	Vaccines
	Biologic extracts
FOODS	Nuts
	Seafood
	Egg whites
	Fruits
INSECT VENOMS	Hymenoptera
	Fire ants

(page 30.4)

Word Find

1. Unlike the words in the box, the signs and symptoms of anaphylaxis are rarely obscure.

```
P M M D B U K N N E E U U J G
B D P W E C R I H H D Y P H W
L Z M A O Y K T C L I E L T F
O G B H P O A I C F Y M W Q
A N S C A I D R A C Y H C A T
T I W F I A C S Z Q A D S R W
I H M K E T O S E Y R R K M H
N S Z H P S D E T T G I I J E
G U P Y T Y A N I G N A V A E
A L E M S Y A E H R R A I D Z
E F F P A M H S T R I D O R E
S I N Q I R A R I C O U G H S
U E H X U P C A R Y Q P G T F
A F T N F Q N O K A E B N W Y
N T I G H T C H E S T W F Q D
```

SIGNS AND SYMPTOMS (page 30.10)

Cardiovascular
a. Angina
b. Arrhythmia
c. Shock
d. Tachycardia

Respiratory
e. Hoarseness
f. Stridor
g. Cough
h. Wheezes
i. Dyspnea
j. Tight chest

Gastrointestinal
k. Cramps
l. Bloating
m. Nausea
n. Diarrhea

Skin
o. Warm
p. Edema
q. Flushing
r. Urticaria

Central Nervous
s. Headache

Secret Message

This secret message should not have been a big surprise.

a. Antibody

b. Antigen

c. Allergen

d. Anaphylaxis

e. Histamine

f. Wasp

g. Itch

h. Drip

i. Widow

j. Tort

k. To

l. gtt

Secret Message: A PATIENT WITH STRIDOR IS A PATIENT IN DANGER. DON'T ALLOW HIM TO ASPHYXIATE.

Fill-in the Table

Antigen	Examples
Drugs	Antibiotics, colloids, enzymes, vaccines
Insect stings	Bees, yellow jackets, hornets, wasps, fire ants
Foods	Peanuts, fish, shellfish, egg, soy, milk
Latex	Gloves and other medical materials
Animals	Long-haired animals, horse serum, gamma globins

(page 30.4)

Problem Solving

1. 0.3 to 0.5 mL from a 1 mg/1 mL ampule

2. 1:10,000 epi, 0.1 mg per 10 mL, 3 to 5 mL

3. 30 gtt/minute

4. Benadryl (diphenhydramine), 50 mg (page 30.12)

Chapter 31: Gastrointestinal Emergencies

Matching

1. F (page 31.15)
2. G (page 31.19)
3. J (page 31.19)
4. K (page 31.21)
5. C (page 31.11)
6. L (page 31.16)
7. H (page 31.27)
8. N (page 31.27)
9. M (page 31.27)
10. O (page 31.27)
11. B (page 31.27)
12. A (page 31.16)
13. E (page 31.18)
14. J (page 31.23)
15. D (page 31.24)

Multiple Choice

1. A (page 31.11)
2. C (page 31.8)
3. B (page 31.12)
4. C (page 31.21)
5. A (page 31.17)
6. D (page 31.11)
7. C (page 31.23)
8. A (page 31.25)
9. D (page 31.12)
10. B (page 31.13)

Labeling

1. Abdominal Organs (page 31.5)

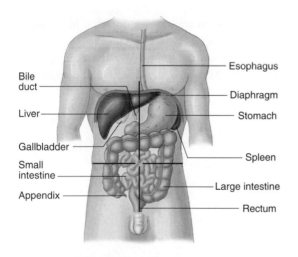

2. The Stomach (page 31.6)

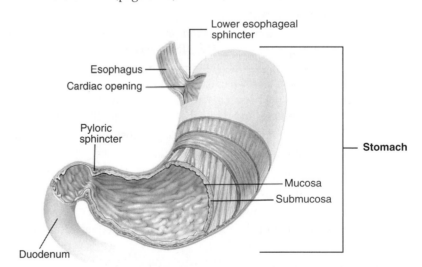

Fill-in-the-Blank

1. Hepatitis, longer (page 31.25)
2. Alcohol, smoking, mucosal (page 31.4)
3. Portal, venous, absorbed (page 31.6)
4. Duodenum, jejunum, ileum (page 31.7)
5. Immunocompromised, food-borne (page 31.9)
6. *Helicobacter pylori,* nonsteroidal (page 31.11)
7. Cholecystitis, gallbladder, duodenum (page 31.11)
8. Diverticulitis (page 31.12)
9. Ulcerative colitis, hereditary (page 31.13)
10. Hemorrhage, catecholamines, epinephrine (page 31.15)

Identify

1. **a.** Chief complaint: Gastrointestinal (GI) bleed, hypovolemic shock, and near syncope
   b. Vital signs: Skin is diaphoretic, ashen, cool; blood pressure is 88 mm Hg by palpation; heart rate is 118 beats/min; oxygen saturation is 89%
   c. Pertinent negatives: None indicated for this call
2. **a.** Chief complaint: Per law enforcement, "man down"; per the patient, abdominal pain
   b. Vital signs: CTC: jaundiced, cool, dry; delayed capillary refill; sinus tachycardia; oxygen saturation is 94%; blood pressure is 142/86 mm Hg; blood glucose level is 110 mg/dL
   c. Pertinent negatives: Patient denies any injuries or falls
3. **a.** Chief complaint: Severe abdominal pain
   b. Vital signs: ECG, sinus rhythm, equal bilateral radial pulses, normal capillary refill. Pulse is 92, strong and regular, oxygen saturation is 98%, skin color is normal, and skin is warm and diaphoretic.
   c. Pertinent negatives: No recent injury or trauma

Ambulance Calls

1. **a.** The patient in this ambulance call has a classical presentation of appendicitis. (page 31.20)
   b. (1) Oxygen
   (2) IV access
   (3) Volume resuscitation as necessary
   (4) Dopamine for septicemia if indicated
   (5) Pain management
   (6) Nausea management (page 31.24)
   c. *Diphenhydramine:* It can cause drowsiness and a decline in blood pressure.
   Hydroxyzine: Be cautious when administering this medication to patients who have taken any medication that has central nervous system (CNS) depressive effects because it acts synergistically to increase the CNS depression.
   Promethazine: Be cautious when administering this medication to patients who have taken any medication that has CNS depressive effects because it acts synergistically to increase the CNS depression. Because this medication is formulated with phenol, promethazine has a pH between 4 and 5.5, and so it produces a marked burning sensation during injection. Administer it very slowly (over 10 to 15 minutes), and dilute the drug in 10 to 20 mL of normal saline if it will be administered by the IV route. (page 31.23)
2. **a.** Aggressive management of ABCs, including positioning to facilitate drainage and suctioning
   b. Rapid but safe immediate transport
   c. Fluid resuscitation
   d. Pharmacologic management of nausea and vomiting (page 31.23)
3. **a.** Body substance isolation (BSI)
   b. Effective positioning of the patient will ensure adequate drainage of material out of the mouth
   c. Oxygen
   d. Listen to lung sounds.
   e. Administer hypotonic solution.
   f. Consider pain management.
   g. Consider medications that may be administered for management of nausea. (page 31.22)

True/False

1. T (page 31.23)
2. F (page 31.21)
3. T (page 31.21)
4. T (page 31.20)
5. F (page 31.18)
6. F (page 31.17)
7. T (page 31.16)
8. T (page 31.16)
9. T (page 31.15)
10. F (page 31.15)

Short Answer

1. **a.** Borborygmi: A bowel sound characterized by increased activity within the bowel. (page 31.16)
   b. Cholecystitis: Inflammation of the gallbladder. (page 31.20)
   c. Scaphoid: A concave shape of the abdomen. This can be caused by evisceration. (page 31.16)
   d. Mallory Weiss syndrome: The junction between the esophagus and the stomach tears. (page 31.11)
2. **a.** Somatic (page 31.17)
   b. Appendicitis (page 31.20)
   c. Irritation or injury to tissue, causing activation of peripheral nerve tracts (page 31.17)
3. **a.** Somatic (page 31.17)
   b. Usually occurs after an initial visceral, parietal, nerve tracts causing "pain" in distant locations. (page 31.17)

Word Find

```
G G N G Z L V H I D T S D B U
A E M V I Y C E L G N B I O I
L V O V Y A R O E K P L M I C
L Q E M M E G H U O E C U B M
B R M O C B X H M D V T N J N
L S T L R E C T U M G U U N P
A S A I G F P C O L Q Z J S E
D E K E O M T X M U P D E D F
D M E B R F H P P L J J J Q U
E C K L X C M U U O V H F V N
R W O W E X N V T J B J N F F
Z Q E L O N R A L B H U E V J
S B K U O Z P F P E D I K O I
Y H 7 T P N S U T Y A C D C D
M U N E D O U D J Z X V C N I
```

GASTROINTESTINAL SYSTEM

1. Bile duct (page 31.5)
2. Colon (page 31.24)
3. Duodenum (page 31.6)
4. Gallbladder (page 31.6)
5. Ileum (page 31.7)
6. Jejunum (page 31.7)
7. Liver (page 31.7)
8. Pancreas (page 31.12)
9. Rectum (page 31.20)
10. Stomach (page 31.20)

Fill-in-the-Table

1. The patient's symptoms and signs can tell you a lot.

Finding	What the Finding Tells Me
Coffee-ground vomitus	The patient is bleeding into his stomach, and the blood has been there for some time.
Severe bradycardia	This may be a cardiac and not an abdominal problem.
Melena	The patient is bleeding somewhere in the gastrointestinal tract.
Tenting of the skin	The patient is severely dehydrated.
Patient very still	The patient probably has peritonitis.
Pulsatile abdominal mass	Likely abdominal aortic aneurysm.
Rigid abdomen	Almost certainly peritonitis.

Chapter 32: Renal and Urologic Emergencies

Matching

1. D (page 32.8)
2. A (page 32.10)
3. C (page 32.7)
4. E (page 32.7)
5. B (page 32.8)

6. H (page 32.8)
7. J (page 32.8)
8. F (page 32.8)
9. G (page 32.8)
10. I (page 32.8)

Multiple Choice

1. C (page 32.3)
2. B (page. 32.3)
3. B (page 32.4)
4. D (page 32.4)
5. A (page 32.7)

6. B (page 32.7)
7. C (page 32.8)
8. A (page 32.10)
9. B (page 32.11)
10. A (page 32.17)

Labeling

1. The Urinary System (page 32.3)

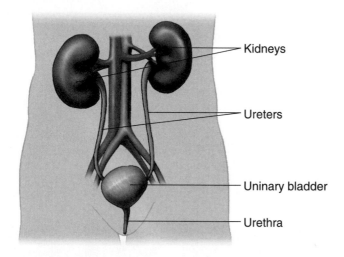

2. The Glomerulus of the Kidneys (page 32.5)

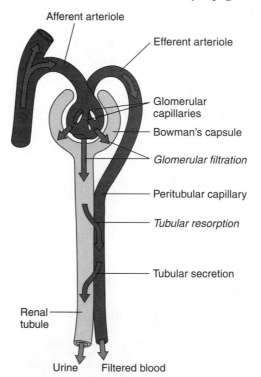

3. Male Reproductive System (page 32.14)

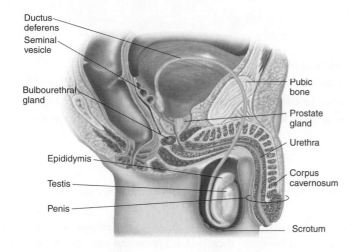

Ductus deferens
Seminal vesicle
Bulbourethral gland
Epididymis
Testis
Penis
Pubic bone
Prostate gland
Urethra
Corpus cavernosum
Scrotum

4. Female Reproductive System (page 32.13)

SIDE VIEW

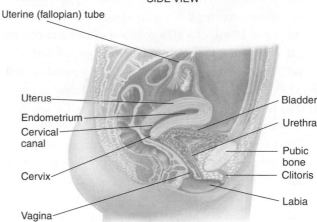

Uterine (fallopian) tube
Uterus
Endometrium
Cervical canal
Cervix
Vagina
Bladder
Urethra
Pubic bone
Clitoris
Labia

Fill-in-the-Blank

1. Comfort support (page 32.17)
2. Cortex, medulla, pelvis (page 32.4)
3. Antidiuretic hormone (page 32.6)
4. Hemodialysis (page 32.9)
5. Disequilibrium syndrome (page 32.11)
6. Priapism (page 32.13)
7. Visceral (page 32.15)
8. Cardiac (page 32.16)
9. Pain relief (page 32.17)
10. Lower (page 32.7)

Identify

1. Chief complaint: Kidney stone, abdominal pain
2. Vital signs: Alert, oxygen saturation is 98%, respirations are 18 breaths/min, lungs are clear. Pulse is 96 beats/min, sinus tachycardia, blood pressure is 148/94 mm Hg. Blood glucose is 96 mg/dL, skin is warm and dry, with a temp of 98.6°F. The pain is 10/10.
3. Pertinent history: History of salty food and drink with no water consumption.

Ambulance Calls

1. The first patient with abdominal pain you had to deal with is a 42-year-old man.
   a. Poorly localized, crampy pain associated with other autonomic symptoms such as nausea is called visceral pain. (page 32.15)
   b. Visceral pain usually comes about because of obstruction of a hollow organ that causes distention and stretching of the organ wall.
   c. Visceral pain is characteristic of conditions such as bowel obstruction, urethral stone, or a stone in the bile duct.
2. E. The patient is in obvious pain and is probably bleeding internally as a result of the trauma to the kidneys. Remember that kidneys are solid organs that filter the blood and they hold a lot of blood. Rapid assessment of this patient with IV support should be established quickly, and then he should be transported to the regional trauma center. (page 32.11)
3. With more and more patients being maintained on chronic renal dialysis, paramedics will find themselves dealing more often with the problems to which dialysis patients are prone.
   a. (1) The patient who feels too weak to move and has peaked T waves on his ECG is most likely suffering from hyperkalemia. (page 32.16)

(2) The steps to take are as follows:

  (a) Continue to monitor his cardiac rhythm carefully.

  (b) Give atropine, 0.5 mg rapidly IV.

  (c) Give 10 mL of a 10% solution of calcium chloride IV.

  (d) Make sure the calcium chloride has infused. Then give 50 mEq of sodium bicarbonate IV.

  (e) Transport without delay, and be prepared to deal with a cardiac arrest en route. (page 32.17)

b. (1) The patient with paroxysmal nocturnal dyspnea has classic signs of **congestive heart failure** (CHF).

  (2) The treatment is very nearly the same as for any other patient with CHF except that some of the medications usually given in CHF will probably be useless. (page 32.17)

  (a) Keep the patient sitting up with legs dangling.

  (b) Administer supplemental oxygen with positive pressure.

  (c) You can try giving sublingual nitroglycerin, but it is not likely to work. Don't bother trying diuretics such as furosemide (Lasix)—for certain those will not work.

  (d) Transport without delay, and notify the receiving facility that the patient will require emergency dialysis, which is the treatment of choice for his CHF. If the receiving hospital does not have the means to carry out an emergency dialysis, ED physicians may have to perform a phlebotomy of about a unit of blood as a temporizing measure until the patient can reach a dialysis unit.

c. (1) The patient with a postdialysis headache and signs of increased intracranial pressure is *probably* suffering from disequilibrium syndrome as a consequence of the dialysis, but at that point you cannot rule out a subdural hematoma.

  (2) You have to assume the worst and treat him for a possible subdural (page 32.17):

  (a) Ensure an open airway; be alert for vomiting and be prepared to suction.

  (b) Administer supplemental oxygen.

  (c) **Monitor** cardiac rhythm.

  (d) **Transport** without delay.

True/False

1. T (page 32.18)   **6.** F (page 32.6)

2. F (page 32.16)   **7.** T (page 32.6)

3. F (page 32.3)   **8.** T (page 32.6)

4. T (page 32.4)   **9.** F (page 32.7)

5. F (page 32.5)   **10.** T (page 32.8)

Short Answer

1. a. Oliguria: very small urine output

  b. Perinephric: around the kidney

  c. Hepatomegaly: enlargement of the liver

  d. Anasarca: Generalized massive edema affecting all parts of the body

  e. Excessive urination: polyuria

  f. Tumor of the liver: hepatoma

  g. Looking at (inside) the bladder: cystoscopy

  h. Urine (products) in the blood: uremia

2. We scarcely ever think very much about our kidneys and how much they do for us. It is only when the kidneys are *not* working that we can begin to appreciate all the things they do when they *are* functioning. And when they aren't working, a whole lot of other things start going wrong as well. Thus, patients with chronic renal failure are much more prone to the following conditions (page 32.9):

  a. Congestive heart failure

  b. Malignant hypertension

  c. Acute myocardial infarction

  d. Cardiac arrhythmias

e. Cardiac tamponade
f. Subdural hematoma
g. Septicemia
h. Bleeding disorders

Crossword Puzzle

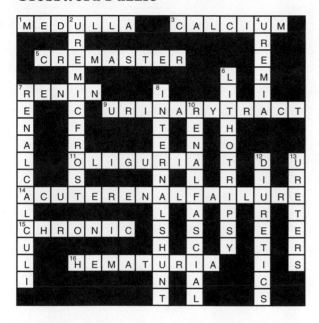

Fill-in-the-Table

1. (page 32.8)

Signs and Symptoms of Acute Renal Failure	
Prerenal acute renal failure	Hypotension Tachycardia Dizziness Thirst
Intrarenal acute renal failure	Flank pain Joint pain Oliguria Hypertension Headache Confusion Seizure
Postrenal acute renal failure	Pain in lower flank, abdomen, groin, and genitalia Oliguria Distended bladder Hematuria Peripheral edema

Chapter 33: Toxicology: Substance Abuse and Poisoning

Matching

1. J	(page 33.19)	**9.** D	(page 33.33)
2. N	(page 33.33)	**10.** M	(page 33.9)
3. A	(page 33.23)	**11.** C	(page 33.26)
4. I	(page 33.31	**12.** H	(page 33.30)
5. O	(page 33.9)	**13.** F	(page 33.14)
6. L	(page 33.11)	**14.** E	(page 33.28)
7. B	(page 33.29)	**15.** K	(page 33.9)
8. G	(page 33.34)		

Multiple Choice

1. C	(page 33.4)	**9.** C	(page 33.15)
2. D	(page 33.6)	**10.** D	(page 33.20)
3. A	(page 33.9)	**11.** D	(page 33.20)
4. D	(page 33.10)	**12.** D	(page 33.22)
5. D	(page 33.11)	**13.** A	(page 33.29)
6. A	(page 33.11)	**14.** C	(page 33.31)
7. B	(page 33.5)	**15.** C	(page 33.36)
8. B	(page 33.9)		

Fill-in-the-Blank

1. Poison; drug (page 33.4)

2. Toxicologic emergencies; intentional; unintentional (page 33.4)

3. Ingestion; inhalation; injection; absorption (page 33.5)

4. Toxidromes; clinical umbrella (page 33.7)

5. Malnutrition; injury (page 33.9)

6. Respiratory depression; gag reflex (page 33.10)

7. Heroin; lucid (page 33.19)

8. Hypotension; rhythm disturbances; breathing (page 33.20)

9. Poisoning; oxygen; hemoglobin (page 33.21)

10. Water-soluble, alkalis, alkalis (page 33.24)

11. Sildenafil (Viagra); nitrites; hypotension (page 33.24)

12. Inhalant; hearing; function; equilibrium; death (page 33.27)

13. Gastric irritation; pain; toxicity; death (page 33.28)

14. Tricyclic antidepressants; tachycardia; depression; seizures (page 33.29)

15. Monoamine oxidase; hyperkalemia; acidosis (page 33.29)

Identify

1. a. Sedative and hypnotic

   b. *Students should provide two of the following:*

     (1) Phenobarbital

     (2) Diazepam

     (3) Thiopental (page 33.8)

2. a. stimulant

   b. *Students should provide two of the following:*

     (1) Amphetamine

     (2) Methamphetamine

     (3) Cocaine

     (4) Diet aids

     (5) Nasal decongestants (page 33.8)

3. The odor of alcohol (ETOH) along with nausea and vomiting may indicate ingestion and poisoning as a result of alcohol. (page 33.8)

4. A seizing patient could be consistent with amphetamines, camphor, cocaine, strychnine, arsenic, carbon monoxide (CO), or petroleum poisoning. Depressed respirations could be indicative of narcotic, alcohol, propoxyphene, CO, or barbiturate poisoning. The type of poisoning common to both symptoms might lead you to be suspicious of a narcotic overdose. CO doesn't seem likely because family members are able to give you some information and there is no indication that they're suffering any of the same symptoms. (page 33.8)

Ambulance Calls

1. a. Questions to ask the patient's neighbors include the following:

     (1) When was the patient last seen?

     (2) Do you have any idea of what happened to him?

     (3) Is he known to suffer any chronic illnesses (eg, diabetes, epilepsy)?

     (4) Has he been injured recently?

     (5) Did he complain of any symptoms when last seen?

     (6) Is he a known abuser of drugs or alcohol?

   b. Besides the neighbors, the **scene itself** may provide valuable information about what may have caused the patient's coma. Check out:

     (1) The bathroom and bedroom for medicine bottles or drug paraphernalia

     (2) The kitchen for insulin in the refrigerator or other medications on the counter

     (3) The living room and the kitchen trash for empty liquor bottles.

   c. The patient's physical findings can also help narrow down the possible causes of his coma:

Finding	Possible Diagnostic Significance
Cold, dry skin	Overdose of alcohol or sedative drugs
Pulse = 110 beats/min, thready	Hypovolemia, hypoglycemia, overdose of barbiturates
Blood pressure = 90/60 mm Hg	Hypovolemia
Respirations = 12 breaths/min and shallow	Overdose with sedative drugs
Pupils dilated and do not react to light	Cerebral anoxia, barbiturate overdose, certain eye drops
Breath smells of alcohol (ETOH)	Patient ingested alcohol
Left arm is cold and blue	Patient has been lying for a long time on his left arm

   d. The patient is best described as comatose, answer C.

   e. The steps in managing this patient are as follows:

     (1) Open the airway by manual methods, and insert an oral airway. If the patient accepts the oral airway, be prepared to intubate.

     (2) Administer supplemental oxygen by bag-mask device.

     (3) Check blood glucose. Administer dextrose 50% IV if hypoglycemic.

     (4) Consider administering naloxone (Narcan) per local protocol and/or Medical Control.

     (5) Intubate.

     (6) Monitor cardiac rhythm.

     (7) Frequently recheck vitals and neurological function, and note any trends.

(8) Splint the patient's left arm in a position of function.

(9) Transport. (page 33.8)

2. When Junior, or anyone else for that matter, swallows something he shouldn't have swallowed, it's important to obtain details of the ingestion.

   a. What was swallowed? (Bring the container to the hospital with the patient if possible.)

   b. When was it swallowed?

   c. How much was swallowed? (Check to see how much is left in the container if there's any uncertainty—that will give you an upper limit, anyway, of the amount that could have been ingested.)

   d. What else was swallowed? Did Junior perhaps sample some washing powder as an hors d'oeuvre, or maybe a bit of furniture polish as a chaser?

   e. Did he vomit? (page 33.11)

3. When a person is found unconscious and there is reason to suspect a toxic cause, the physical assessment should focus not only on the evaluation of the level of consciousness but also on parameters that might provide clues to a specific toxic agent. *Students should provide four of the following:*

   a. Unusual odors on the breath

   b. A precise assessment of the level of consciousness, charted on a patient care report (PCR)

   c. The condition of the skin (CTC: color, temperature, condition)

   d. The respirations, for signs of respiratory depression or metabolic acidosis

   e. Abnormalities of the pulse and blood pressure

   f. Abnormalities of the pupils (very dilated or very constricted) (page 33.8)

4. When the teenager swallows his father's antihypertensive medications:

   a. Activated charcoal is given to absorb poisonous compounds to its surface and thereby effectively remove them from the body.

   b. There are poisonings in which activated charcoal is *not* effective. *Students should provide three of the following:*

   (1) Methanol ingestion

   (2) Acid or alkali ingestion

   (3) Organophosphate poisoning

   (4) Cyanide poisoning

   c. Follow local protocol and medical control regarding dosing of activated charcoal.

   d. The *steps in treatment* for this teenager:

   (1) Give activated charcoal as early as possible if indicated by local protocol and Medical Control.

   (2) Maintain ABCs and administer high-flow supplemental oxygen.

   (3) Initiate IV access.

   (4) **Monitor** cardiac rhythm and vital signs frequently.

   (5) **Transport** the patient to the hospital.(page 33.20)

5. The gentleman who swallowed crystalline Drano ingested a very strong alkali that will continue burning holes in everything it touches until it is removed from the body.

   a. The objective of prehospital treatment is primarily to *dilute* the alkali:

   (1) Maintain ABCs and administer high-flow supplemental oxygen.

   (2) Initiate IV access.

   (3) Monitor cardiac rhythm and vital signs frequently.

   (4) Transport the patient to the hospital. (page 33.24)

6. Down by the railway, some of the community's homeless population have congregated to console themselves with whatever they can find to drink. Sometimes, the substances chosen as cheap substitutes for ethanol can have disastrous consequences when ingested.

   a. The first patient is showing classic signs of ethylene glycol toxicity. The pleasant taste of the substance, the gastrointestinal symptoms some hours later, and the severe respiratory distress about 24 hours later are all characteristic.

   b. The steps of management are as follows:

   (1) Administer supplemental oxygen, as for any patient whose lungs are full of fluid. (page 33.25)

    (2) Follow local protocol and medical control regarding the administration of activated charcoal. (page 33.26)

    (3) Start an IV.

    (4) Contact medical control for consideration of sodium bicarbonate IV. (page 33.26)

    (5) Transport the patient to the hospital.

  c. The second patient, who appears drunk, is most likely suffering from methyl alcohol poisoning.

  d. The care plan for a patient with suspected methanol poisoning is the same as for ethylene glycol poisoning, with the exception of possibly getting an order from medical control to administer 10 mL of 10% calcium gluconate via slow IV push.

    (1) Administer supplemental oxygen, as for any patient whose lungs are full of fluid. (page 33.26)

    (2) Follow local protocol and medical control regarding the administration of activated charcoal. (page 33. 26)

    (3) Start an IV.

    (4) Contact medical control for consideration of sodium bicarbonate IV. (page 33.26)

    (5) Transport the patient to the hospital.

    (6) Get an order from medical control to administer 10 mL of 10% calcium gluconate via slow IV push.

7. a. The woman who swallowed silver polish most probably swallowed cyanide, as evidenced by the smell of almonds on her breath, flushing of the skin, and tachycardia and hypotension. (page 33.8)

  b. The drug that can buy some time is amyl nitrite, which in effect pulls cyanide away from the cellular enzymes it is poisoning. (Cyanide antidote kits also contain 25% sodium thiosulfate, for added effect.) (page 33.22)

  c. Amyl nitrite is given by breaking a vial into a gauze pad and having the patient inhale through the handkerchief for 20 seconds, immediately followed by the inhalation of 100% supplemental oxygen for about 40 seconds. (page 33.23)

  d. The *side effects* of amyl nitrite include hypotension. In anticipation of the hypotensive effects, keep the patient recumbent during amyl nitrite administration. (page 33.23)

  e. The steps of management, then, for this victim of cyanide poisoning are as follows:

    (1) Maintain a patent airway; if her level of consciousness continues to deteriorate, maintaining the airway may require endotracheal intubation.

    (2) Give 100% supplemental oxygen by tight-fitting nonrebreathing mask.

    (3) Administer amyl nitrite as just described.

    (4) Start an IV and give enough fluid to maintain the blood pressure. (page 33.23)

    (5) Monitor cardiac rhythm.

    (6) Notify the receiving hospital to ready a sodium thiosulfate infusion.

    (7) Transport the patient without delay; amyl nitrite is only a temporizing measure, and you cannot keep it up for very long.

8. There's something called too much of a good thing, and too much insulation of a cabin heated by a wood stove is definitely in the too-much-of-a-good-thing category!

  a. In the case in question, *everyone* inside the cabin is showing signs of carbon monoxide poisoning.

  b. The steps to take are as follows:

    (1) Bundle up in warm clothes and open all the windows of the cabin.

    (2) Get everyone outdoors as quickly as possible.

    (3) Call for an ambulance. Don't trust yourself or anyone else under the influence of carbon monoxide to drive.

    (4) As soon as the ambulance arrives, give 100% supplemental oxygen by a nonrebreathing face mask to all exposed victims, but give priority to the baby, who is clearly the most severely affected.

    (5) Keep everyone at rest to minimize metabolic demand for oxygen.

    (6) Monitor the baby's cardiac rhythm.

    (7) Ask medical command to start inquiries regarding the nearest hyperbaric facility. (page 33.21)

9. a. The patient stricken with a "possible heart attack" while sitting out on the lawn is in fact the victim of his next-door neighbor's insecticide spray. Although you must take very seriously the possibility of acute myocardial infarction in any middle-aged man who complains of weakness, nausea, and a tight feeling in his chest, the hypersalivation combined with constricted pupils and severe bradycardia all point to organophosphate poisoning. And, indeed, your partner returns from his discussion with Mr. Dimbledirt carrying the offending bottle of parathion.

  b. The drug used to treat organophosphate poisoning is the parasympathetic blocking agent atropine sulfate.

  c. Massive doses of atropine are often required to counteract the effects of organophosphates. Paramedics administer 1 mg IV. Thereafter, atropine is administered 1 mg IV every 3–5 minutes until the patient is atropinized.

d. (1) Treatment for organophosphate poisoning starts with decontamination and removal of all contaminated clothing *before* initiating care or loading the patient into the ambulance. Contaminated clothing should be placed in plastic bags and disposed of as hazardous materials. Ideally, the patient should be scrubbed with soap and water. After that, patient care includes the following measures:

  (2) Establish and maintain the airway. Consider an advanced airway as needed.

  (3) Suction as needed.

  (4) Give high-flow supplemental oxygen.

  (5) Establish vascular access.

  (6) Administer 1.0 mg atropine IV push, and repeat the dose every 3 to 5 minutes until symptom reversal (that is, atropinization) occurs.

  (7) Administer 1 to 2 g of pralidoxime (2-PAM) infused with normal saline over 5 to 10 minutes.

  (8) Apply the ECG monitor, pulse oximeter, and capnometer.

  (9) Immediately transport to the appropriate facility. (pages 33.20–33.21)

10. The boy who suffered a seizure after inhaling typewriter correction fluid should be treated as any other postictal patient:

  a. Protect his airway by positioning him on his side; suction secretions as needed.

  b. Administer supplemental oxygen by nasal cannula.

  c. Monitor cardiac rhythm; arrhythmias and "sudden sniffing death" are not unheard of after inhalation of typewriter correction fluid.

  d. Start an IV.

  e. Transport without delay. (page 33.27)

True/False

1. T (page 33.5)

2. F (page 33.6)

3. T (page 33.10)

4. T (page 33.7)

5. F (page 33.9)

6 T (page 33.10)

7 T (page 33.10)

8. F (page 33.11)

9. T (page 33.13)

10. T (page 33.30)

11. T (page 33.24)

12. T (page 33.28)

13. T (page 33.29)

14. F (page 33.31)

15. F (page 33.37)

Short Answer

1. The patient whom you are tempted to write off as "just another drunk" is in fact much more vulnerable to a host of injuries and medical problems than the more sober John Q. Citizen. The conditions to which alcoholics are particularly susceptible include the following:

  a. Subdural hematoma

  b. Gastrointestinal bleeding

  c. Pancreatitis

  d. Hypoglycemia

  e. Pneumonia

  f. Burns

  g. Hypothermia

  h. Seizures

  i. Arrhythmias

  j. Cancer (page 33.10)

Word Find

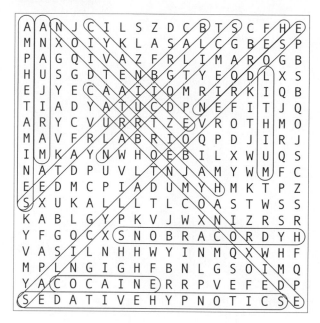

1. Cocaine; heroin (page 33.7)
2. Marijuana (page 33.15)
3. Amphetamines (page 33.42)
4. Barbiturates (page 33.17)
5. Sedative-hypnotics (page 33.42)
6. Cyanide (page 33.22)
7. Narcotics (page 33.19)
8. Carbon monoxide (page 33.21)
9. Hydrocarbons (page 33.26)
10. Lithium (page 33.30)
11. Habituation (page 33.9)
12. Salicylate overdose (page 33.31)

Fill-in-the-Table

1. You don't have to look very far to find commonly ingested poisons. Just check your own home. (page 33.5–33.6)

Type of Poison	Examples
Strong acid	**Toilet bowl cleaner, battery acid, bleach disinfectant**
Strong alkali	**Drain buildup remover (Drano), Clinitest tabs, chlorine bleach, dishwasher detergent**
Volatile hydrocarbon	**Naphtha, kerosene**
Toxic plant	**Lantana, dieffenbachia, caladium, castor bean**

2.

Signs and Symptoms of Acetaminophen Toxicity		
Stage	Timeframe	Signs and Symptoms
I	< 24 h	Nausea, vomiting, loss of appetite, pallor, malaise
II	24–72 h	Right upper quadrant abdominal pain; abdomen tender to palpation
III	72–96 h	Metabolic acidosis, renal failure, coagulopathies, recurring GI symptoms
IV	4–14 d (or longer)	Recovery slowly begins, or liver failure progresses and the patient dies

(page 33.31)

Chapter 34: Hematologic Emergencies

Matching

1. E (page 34.15)
2. J (page 34.15)
3. H (page 34.15)
4. A (page 34.15)
5. I (page 34.15)
6. B (page 34.15)
7. G (page 34.15)
8. C (page 34.15)
9. D (page 34.15)
10. F (page 34.15)

Multiple Choice

1. D (page 34.9)
2. D (page 34.10)
3. D (page 34.12)
4. A (page 34.5)
5. C (page 34.5)
6. C (page 34.6)
7. C (page 34.7)
8. A (page 34.8)
9. B (page 34.13)
10. D (page 34.3)

Labeling

1. Components of the Blood System (page 34.5)

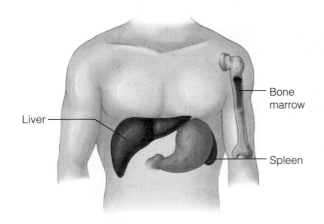

Bone marrow

Liver

Spleen

2. Normal RBCs and Sickle Cells (page 34.9)

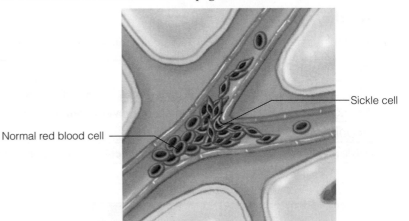

Sickle cell

Normal red blood cell

Fill-in-the-Blank

1. Life (page 34.3)
2. Hematopoietic (page 34.3)
3. Red blood cells, white blood cells, platelets, and plasma (page 34.3)
4. Stem cells (page 34.4)
5. RBC count, hemoglobin level, and hematocrit (page 34.4)
6. Platelets (page 34.4)
7. Von Willebrand (page 34.8)
8. Sickle cell disease (page 34.9)
9. Fatigue, headaches, dyspnea (page 34.10)
10. Pain (page 34.11)

Identify

1. **a.** Chief complaint: Extreme weakness, fatigue, and dyspnea.
   b. Vital signs: Pulse is 86 beats/min, slightly irregular, and difficult to palpate; blood pressure is 92/P. Skin is pale, warm, and dry. Pupils are equal and reactive to light. Oxygen saturation is 91% on ambient air.
   c. Pertinent negatives: Denies chest pain or shortness of breath.
2. **a.** Chief complaint: Altered mental status and possible syncope.
   b. Vital signs: His radial pulses are equal bilaterally and regular at 86 beats/min. Skin is jaundiced, but cool and dry. PEARRL. Oxygen saturation is 98% on a nonrebreathing face mask.
   c. Pertinent negatives: Not sure if he lost consciousness.
3. **a.** Chief complaint: acute sickle cell crisis, pain.
   b. Vital signs: Vital signs are pulse of 112 beats/min regular, skin is warm/moist, pulse oximetry of 91%, blood pressure 148/96 mm Hg. PEARRL.
   c. Pertinent negatives: None.

Ambulance Calls

1. **a.** The patient who develops back pain, diaphoresis, cyanosis, and so forth during a blood transfusion is showing signs of a hemolytic reaction to the blood transfusion. (answer 2)
   b. To deal with this situation, you need to do the following:
   (1) *Stop the transfusion!* Disconnect the blood bag and save it for testing.
   (2) Keep the IV line open with D_5W (if signs of shock develop, switch to normal saline or Ringer's).
   (3) Draw a blood sample (red-top tube) from a site other than the IV line.
   (4) Notify the physician and request orders.
2. **a.** Hemophilia is a bleeding disorder in which clotting does not occur or occurs insufficiently (von Willebrand disease). (page 34.8)
   b. Take care of the ABCs, and be alert for signs of acute blood loss (pallor, weak pulse, and hypotension). Note any bleeding of unknown origin, such as nosebleeds, bloody sputum, and blood in the urine or stool (melena). Patients who complain of respiratory problems should receive high-flow oxygen. Note ECG findings, and treat symptomatic arrhythmias as appropriate. IV therapy may be necessary in cases of unstable hypotension. Some patients will have significant pain, so analgesics may be appropriate. This disease is a form of hemophilia.

True/False

1. F (page 34.3)
2. F (page 34.4)
3. T (page 34.5)
4. F (page 34.5)
5. T (page 34.8)
6. F (page 34.8)
7. T (page 34.9)
8. T (page 34.9)
9. F (page 34.10)
10. T (page 34.10)

Short Answer

1. Blood disorders present differently from other typical injuries and diseases encountered by paramedics. Please provide some of the common findings as they relate to the following organs and systems: (page 34.10)
   a. Skin
   Uncontrolled bleeding
   Chronic bruising
   Itching
   Pallor
   Jaundice
   b. Gastrointestinal tract
   Bloody nose
   Bleeding or infected gums
   Melena
   Liver failure

    c. Cardiovascular system

      Dyspnea

      Tachycardia

      Chest pain

      Hemoptysis

2. Assessment and treatment of patients with blood disorders may differ slightly from assessment and treatment of patients with more typical diseases encountered by paramedics. Please describe how the treatment and assessment of the following diseases differ.

    a. Leukemia (page 34.10)

      i. Depends on stage.

      ii. Patient complains of fatigue, headaches, or dyspnea.

      iii. Fever, bone pain, and diaphoresis may be present.

      iv. Vital signs may indicate shock.

      v. Treatment includes ABCs, IV access, and pain medications.

    b. Hemophilia (page 34.8)

      i. Acute and chronic bleeding may occur at any time.

      ii. Spontaneous intracranial bleeding may be common.

      iii. Be supportive of patients and families.

      iv. Treatment includes ABCs, IV access, treat all bleeding as potentially life threatening.

    c. Polycythemia (page 34.8)

      i. Characterized by an overabundance of red blood cells.

      ii. Can be caused by a rare disorder or congestive heart failure.

      iii. Can lead to strokes, TIAs, headaches, and abdominal pain.

      iv. Found more frequently in adults older than 50 years.

      v. Clinical treatment includes phlebotomy.

      vi. Provide and support ABCs.

3. Provide definitions for the following terms:

    a. Leukopenia: reduction in the number of WBCs

    b. Polycythemia: overproduction of RBCs, WBCs, and platelets

    c. ABO system: antigen classification system used to classify blood

    d. Reticuloendothelial system: primarily used to defend against infection

    e. Pruritus: unspecified itching

    f. Hematocrit: the percentage of RBCs in total blood volume

    g. Melena: blood in the stool

Word Find

```
R O B Y S O Q Y E B X T E R W S A S H
L E L O I N H F A Z H H S Y L I I T E
E X D M N T E S T R C T A L I S M E M
G H Z R M E O G O L I Z E E K A E M A
R O T Q O P M M I R D C S Y N T C E T
A C A X H S B A C T D K I X C S U C O
J G U I E O I O R O N A D D A O E L P
K T L C C F T D O R M A L A U E L L O
V S B Y Q A S L C S O B L N M E S I
I U T D M O B W A I O W E Y X O R I E
L E U E H E Z L T K T C W I H D V T
S I H E T S P L E E N Y E C Z A P A I
W M V I U N I V E R S A L D O N O R C
C H H E M O G L O B I N K O E R O G M
L W Q Z R N P O F Q J W C V M J M L J
A I M E H T Y C Y L O P I C R E D Z P
S A M O H P M Y L N T S S B P R H X R
E R Z R W T G G C R I C U D I Z S X U
R O N M D T T T S A A V A S G P S Y T
```

1. Plasma (page 34.3)
2. Hematopoietic (page 34.3)
3. Stem cells (page 34.4)
4. Hematocrit (page 34.4)
5. Hemoglobin (page 34.4)
6. White blood cells (page 34.3)
7. Thrombocytes (page 34.3)
8. Basophils (page 34.4)
9. Spleen (page 34.5)
10. Bone marrow (page 34.5)
11. Liver (page 34.5)
12. Universal donor (page 34.6)
13. Antigens (page 34.15)
14. Homeostasis (page 34.6)
15. Hemolytic disorder (page 34.6)
16. Sickle cell disease (page 34.9)
17. Leukemia (page 34.7)
18. Polycythemia (page 34.8)

Fill-in-the-Table

Blood Types			
Blood Type	ABO Antigens	ABO Antibodies	Acceptable Blood Donor Types
A	A	Anti-B	A, O
B	B	Anti-A	B, O
AB	A, B	None	A, B, AB, O
O	None	Anti-A Anti-B	O

(page 34.6)

Chapter 35: Environmental Emergencies

Matching

(page 35.15)

1. HL
2. HP
3. HL
4. HL
5. HP
6. HP

7. HL
8. HP
9. HL
10. HL
11. HP

Multiple Choice

1. D (page 35.9)
2. C (page 35.5)
3. B (page 35.6)
4. A (page 35.8)
5. D (page 35.10)

6. A (page 35.15)
7. B (page 35.16)
8. B (page 35.23)
9. C (page 35.26)
10. D (page 35.14)

Labeling

1.

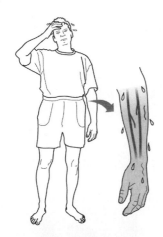

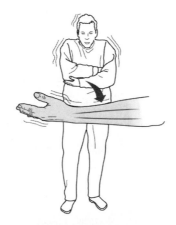

Hot Environment

- Hypothalamus stimulated
- Blood vessels dilate, maximizing heat loss from skin
- Body sweats, causing evaporation and cooling

Body temperature *decreases*

Cold Environment

- Hypothalamus stimulated
- Blood vessels constrict, minimizing heat loss from skin
- Muscles shiver, generating heat

Body temperature *increases*

(page 35.5)

Fill-in-the-Blank

1. **a.** For the human body to maintain a nearly constant core temperature, it must balance heat loss with heat production.

Sources of Body Heat

(1) Basal metabolism

(2) Exercise

(3) Absorption of heat

(4) Evaporation of sweat

Ways of Shedding Heat

(1) Radiation

(2) Convection

(3) Conduction

b. The body's mechanisms for dissipating excess heat have certain limitations. First, all of the mechanisms depend on peripheral vasodilatation to shunt blood from the core to the body surface. Furthermore, three of the body's cooling mechanisms require a temperature gradient between the body and the outside to be effective. None of these three mechanisms—radiation, convection, or conduction—can work if the outside is not at least a few degrees cooler than the body core. Finally, one of the body's cooling mechanisms is dependent on the ambient humidity. When the humidity is high, that mechanism—namely, evaporation of sweat—is ineffective in lowering the core temperature.

c. A hatless hiker standing still on a mountaintop on a windless day loses heat from his head by radiation. A breeze picks up. Now the hiker loses heat by convection as well.

d. A white-water enthusiast who capsizes his canoe in a swift-running stream loses body heat by conduction.

e. A soldier on maneuvers in the desert in ambient temperatures of more than 37.7°C (100°F) can shed heat only by evaporation of sweat. (pages 35.6, 35.7)

Identify

1. a. Chief complaint: Fell through ice.

   b. Vital signs: Patient is shivering. ECG rhythm is regular with Osborn waves.

   c. Pertinent natives: None. (page 35.16)

   d. *Students should provide three of the following:*

   (1) Time in water

   (2) Patient temperature

   (3) Neurologic assessment

   (4) Amount of alcohol ingested and when

   (5) Any drugs taken

   (6) Blood glucose

   e. B. (Conduction) This is the transfer of heat from a hotter object to a cooler object by direct physical contact. (page 35.6)

   f. 500 mL (page 35.17)

Ambulance Calls

1. a. The patient probably had a heat syncope episode that occurs in people who may be under heat stress and who experience peripheral vasodilatation that possibly may be exacerbated by dehydration. One group in which this seems prevalent is those attending mass outdoor gatherings. An additional contributing factor may be alcohol intake (beer). Some other factors that should be considered but that might not yet be identified are medical conditions such as diabetes, drug intake, and amount of physical exertion done by the patient. (pages 35.7, 35.9)

   b. Maintain the airway and provide oxygen, place in a cool environment in the supine position, and provide fluid replacement either orally or by IV. (page 35.9)

   c. If the patient does not quickly respond in the supine position, suspect heat exhaustion or heat stroke. (pages 35.9, 35.10)

2. a. The fullback who is acting "crazy" after practicing on a hot, humid afternoon is most probably suffering from exertional heat stroke. You were fortunate to be able to record a temperature and obtain conclusive evidence. In many cases, the patient is too combative to allow you to measure the temperature, and you can only suspect the diagnosis on the basis of his symptoms and signs alone. (page 35.10)

   b. The steps in managing exertional heat stroke in this patient are as follows:

   (1) Move him to a cooler environment, preferably your air-conditioned ambulance with the fans blowing.

   (2) Strip off his clothing and football gear.

   (3) Apply ice packs to his flanks while massaging his neck and torso. Spray the patient with tepid water, and keep a **fan** blowing in his direction.

   (4) Start an IV bolus 200 cc of fluids.

   (5) Monitor temperature and cardiac rhythm.

   (6) Be prepared for seizures.

   (7) Transport without delay. (page 35.11)

3. a. The running back writhing in pain is most likely suffering from heat cramps. (page 35.8)

b. The steps in treating him are as follows:

(1) Tell the coach to stop massaging the boy's legs!

(2) Move the boy to a cooler environment.

(3) If he is not nauseated, give him salt-containing fluids to drink (at least a quart). If the patient is too nauseated to take the fluids by mouth, insert an IV and infuse normal saline rapidly (consult Medical Control for the IV rate).

(4) Do not allow the boy to return to practice that day. He should go home and rest in a cool place. Instruct him to seek medical attention if he develops headaches, dizziness, nausea, or severe fatigue. (page 35.8)

4. a. The quarterback may indeed be coming down with mononucleosis, but it could be fatal to miss a case of heat exhaustion. (page 35.9)

b. You should treat him in the field as follows:

(1) Move the boy to a cooler environment.

(2) Remove most of his clothing, down to his undershorts, and sponge him with cool water.

(3) Start an IV and run it wide open.

(4) Monitor cardiac rhythm and vital signs.

(5) Transport to the hospital. (page 35.9)

c. By now, one would think Coach would have reached the conclusion that football practice in the searing heat is not healthy for a teenager. But you should in any case suggest to him that if he *must* conduct practice during the "dog days" of August, he should schedule the heavy exertion for the early morning and late afternoon hours.

5. a. The baby at the supermarket is suffering from classic heat stroke. The inside of an automobile that is parked in the sun in 37.7°C (100°F) temperatures can very quickly reach a temperature of around 82°C (180°F)—not high enough to bake a cake, perhaps, but certainly high enough to bake a baby. This infant is in severe danger and may die. (page 35.10)

b. Treatment is extremely urgent:

(1) Open the airway. Intubate as soon as you have a chance.

(2) Administer supplemental oxygen.

(3) Strip off all the baby's clothing.

(4) Spray and fan the baby continuously until you reach the hospital.

(5) If you are able to do so, start an IV en route to the hospital with 5% dextrose in half normal saline, and run it at about 150 mL per hour.

(6) Monitor rectal temperature.

(7) Transport without delay. (page 35.11)

6. It only happens to paramedics—a ski vacation turns into a search-and-rescue mission.

a. The first skier has deep frostbite. You don't really have the means to rewarm his leg in the field, nor can you ensure that it won't simply freeze again during transport to the ski lodge. (page 35.14)

b. The management therefore is as follows:

(1) Move him to a sheltered place, such as that cabin behind the trees, until the snowmobile comes.

(2) Give him some calories, preferably a candy bar or some other carbohydrate source. Give him a hot, sweet drink if you're carrying a thermos.

(3) Leave the frostbitten extremity frozen. Don't attempt any rewarming in the field.

(4) Pad the frostbitten leg to prevent it from being bruised during transport.

(5) Protect the rest of the patient's body from the cold with insulating blankets.

c. The second skier has a more superficial frostbite. (page 35.13)

d. The management therefore is as follows:

(1) Move him to a sheltered place, such as that cabin behind the trees, until the snowmobile comes.

(2) Give him some calories, preferably a candy bar or some other carbohydrate source. Give him a hot, sweet drink if you're carrying a thermos.

(3) Try to warm the frostbitten foot with your hands (or by putting it in *your* armpit!).

(4) Splint the frostbitten leg to prevent it from being bruised during transport.

(5) Protect the rest of the patient's body from the cold with insulating blankets.

e. The third lost skier is suffering from severe hypothermia. Only his very occasional breathing tips you off that he's not (yet) in cardiac arrest. (pages 35.17, 35.18)

f. In managing him:

(1) As long as his airway is not obstructed, it's best not to touch him at all until the ambulance arrives. Send someone down to the road to intercept the ambulance, help carry equipment, and guide the paramedics to the patient.

(2) Move the patient *very* gently onto the stretcher, and carry the stretcher *very* gently to the ambulance.

(3) Maintain the airway manually until the patient has been well ventilated with 100% oxygen by bag-mask device for at least 3 minutes. Then, intubate the trachea rapidly and smoothly.

(4) Apply monitoring electrodes, and check the cardiac rhythm. If asystole should occur, start cardiopulmonary resuscitation (CPR), but give basic life support (BLS) only. If you see *ventricular fibrillation (VF) on the monitor, give one shock, resume CPR immediately for a 2-minute cycle, and then attempt to deliver another shock. Continue until three shocks have been given. If VF persists, put the defibrillator away and just continue basic life support all the way to the hospital. It is important that CPR be uninterrupted with quality compressions at a rate of 100 per minute. Medical Control can be contacted to determine if additional shock should be provided.*

(5) If the patient's clothing is wet, *gently* cut away wet clothing and replace it with dry blankets.

(6) Notify the receiving hospital of the nature of the case and your estimated time of arrival (ETA).

(7) Keep the ambulance interior around 15.5°C (60°F).

(8) Instruct the driver to make it a smooth ride to the hospital.

7. The speedboat driver who is *plunged* into cold lake water is a likely candidate for hypothermia by the process of conduction. Heat loss is 25% faster in water than in air and can occur after relatively short exposure because of the rapidity with which water conducts heat away from the body. In managing such a case, you should observe these guidelines:

a. Try to prevent the victim from exerting himself. Toss him a rope and pull him to shore, or send one of the other boats over to haul him aboard and bring him ashore. But in any case, discourage him from thrashing about in the water.

b. As soon as you have the victim ashore, carry him to a sheltered place, preferably the inside of your ambulance, and cut away his wet clothes. Be sure to keep him absolutely still.

c. Monitor his cardiac rhythm.

d. Cover him with insulating materials, and cover those with blankets.

e. Wrap chemical hot packs in towels, and place them in his armpits and near the groin.

f. Give him a hot, caffeine-free, sugary drink.

g. Keep him recumbent.

h. Transport him to the hospital. (pages 35.6, 35.17)

8. The "vagrant" in the bus station represents a classic example of the kind of case that is too often misdiagnosed.

a. Any patient found in the circumstances described must be suspected to be suffering from one of the following:

(1) Hypothermia

(2) Hypoglycemia

(3) Stroke

or all of the above until proved otherwise. (pages 35.16, 35.17)

b. In view of those possibilities, the steps in management are as follows:

(1) Administer warmed, humidified oxygen (if available).

(2) Complete the rapid medical assessment. Obtain vital signs, and check for injuries with particular attention to the head.

(3) Start an IV (using warmed IV fluid).

(4) Give 50% dextrose, 50 mL IV.

(5) Monitor cardiac rhythm.

(6) Cover the patient with warm blankets.

(7) Transport to the hospital. (page 35.17)

9. a. Ask if the headache is throbbing and worse over the temporal or occipital areas and if it is exacerbated by a valsalva maneuver. If the answer to any of these questions is yes, there is a likelihood the patient has acute mountain sickness. (page 35.27)

b. (1) Dyspnea at rest

(2) Cough

(3) Chest tightness

(4) Two of the following suggests high-altitude pulmonary edema: central cyanosis, rales or wheezing in at least one lung field, tachypnea, or tachycardia. (page 35.27)

c. (1) Give supplemental oxygen (4–6 L/min) until the condition improves.

(2) Descend as soon as possible, with minimal exertion.

(3) A portable ventilator can be used, if available, provided descent is not possible or no oxygen is accessible. If you can't descend, give your friend nifedipine and add dexamethasone if neurologic deterioration occurs. (page 35.28)

10. a. The diver ascended from his dive without exhaling constantly to vent air from the lungs or he held his breath during the ascent. The result is that he probably has sustained pulmonary overpressurized syndrome (POPS), also known as "burnt lungs," which has probably caused arterial gas embolism (AGE). (page 35.23)

b. (1) Ensure an adequate airway, intubate if a basic life support (BLS) airway is not effective (fill the cuff with saline if the patient is to be placed in a hyperbaric chamber).

(2) Administer 100% supplemental oxygen.

(3) Transport in the supine position (use ground transport if cabin pressure is an issue).

(4) Establish an IV en route.

(5) Place on and ECG monitor.

(6) Have medication ready for seizures and dopamine for hypotension, and follow protocol for direct referral to a hyperbaric chamber facility. (page 35.25)

c. Decompression sickness (page 35.24)

True/False

There are a lot of folk remedies for frostbite. Some of them are downright dangerous. Do you know the truth about frostbite?

1. F (page 35.13)   **6.** T (page 35.12)
2. T (pages 35.13, 35.14)   **7.** T (page 35.9)
3. T (page 35.14)   **8.** F (page 35.10)
4. F (page 35.13)   **9.** F (page 35.11)
5. F (page 35.13)   **10.** T (page 35.6)

Short Answer

1. Heat is a form of cardiovascular stress because the body responds to heat by vasodilatation. Increasing the diameter of the blood vessels increases their volume so that the heart must increase its output to prevent a fall in blood pressure. The heart increases output by increasing both its rate and stroke volume, which inevitably means an increase in cardiac work. (page 35.6)

2. A person's risk of suffering significant heat illness in response to heat stress can be increased by the following factors. Students should provide five of the following:

a. Exertion or anything else that increases endogenous heat production (e.g., fever, hyperthyroidism)

b. High humidity

c. Obesity

d. Diabetes

e. Alcoholism

f. Dehydration

g. Cardiovascular or cerebrovascular disease

h. Heavy or occlusive clothing

i. Drugs such as diuretics and some tranquilizers (page 35.7)

3. a. The dog days of summer also put *you* at risk of heat illness, especially if you have to carry heat-stricken, 300-pound patients down four flights of stairs. So, take some precautions to protect yourself on very hot days. *Students should provide five of the following:*

(1) Wear light-colored, loose-fitting clothing. If your service does not have an appropriate summer uniform, ask your union to demand one!

(2) Stay in cool places whenever you can.

(3) Park the ambulance in the shade.

(4) Increase your fluid intake. Carry cold drinks with you in the vehicle, and partake frequently.

(5) Wear a cool, damp towel around your neck.

(6) Put a fan on the dashboard of the ambulance.

(7) Seek medical attention at the first symptom of heat illness. (page 35.11)

b. Of course, to seek attention at the first symptom of heat illness, you have to know what the symptoms *are*!

(1) Headache

(2) Fatigue or lack of energy

(3) Dizziness

(4) Nausea or vomiting (page 35.11)

4. Let's hear it for all the moms out there! They've been right all along.

a. "Don't go out without a hat and scarf; it's freezing out there."

Mother was right because most heat loss from the body occurs from the head and neck. By trapping some of that heat within insulating layers, a hat and scarf can reduce convective heat loss from above the shoulders. (page 35.6)

b. "Stop rolling around in the snow. You'll get a death of a chill."

Mother was right because snow conducts heat away from the body faster than air does. And when the snow melts and your clothes get wet, cooling by conduction is even faster. (page 35.6)

c. "Get out of those wet clothes this minute."

Mother was right because wearing wet clothing promotes heat loss by conduction while the clothes remain wet and by evaporation as the clothes dry. (page 35.6)

d. "Those skates are much too tight. Your toes will fall off."

Mother was right because anything that interferes with the circulation to the extremities predisposes them to frostbite. (page 35.13)

e. "Make sure you wear your windbreaker. It's blowing a gale out there."

Mother was right because exposure to the wind increases heat loss by convection. (page 35.6)

f. "Eat. Eat. You have to have something to keep going in this weather."

Mother was right because metabolic heat production requires fuel, so you need to maintain your caloric intake, especially in the form of carbohydrates, before anticipated exposure to cold temperatures. (page 35.5)

5. It's important to follow Mother's advice because, by itself, the body does not have a lot of ways to defend itself against the cold. The three ways it can do so are as follows:

a. By peripheral vasoconstriction, to shunt blood away from the body shell to the body core

b. By shivering, to increase heat production by skeletal muscle

c. By increasing the basal metabolic rate, to increase overall metabolic heat production (page 35.7)

6. Some people are more likely to suffer cold injury than others are.

a. Factors that predispose a person to *frostbite* include the following:

(1) Tight clothing, especially tight shoes or gloves

(2) Smoking

(3) Hunger, fatigue, or dehydration

(4) Hypothermia (generalized cooling) (page 35.12)

b. Many factors predispose a person to suffer hypothermia. *Students should provide four of the following:*

(1) Old age

(2) Infancy

(3) Alcoholism

(4) Chronic illness

(5) Poor planning for outdoor activity; unpreparedness (page 35.15)

7. Even our nursery rhyme companions were in danger of cold exposure:

a. When the three little kittens lost their mittens, they became most vulnerable to frostbite of the paws. (page 35.12)

b. Sitting on an ice-cold tuffet, Miss Muffet was losing heat by conduction from her bottom to the tuffet and by radiation, mostly from her head and neck, to the surrounding atmosphere. If there was any breeze, she was losing heat by convection as well. (page 35.6)

c. Jack Sprat has a greater risk of hypothermia than his wife does because he has less natural insulation. (page 35.15)

d. Little Jack Horner had the right idea eating his Christmas pie before going out into the cold because he knew that one needs calories to increase internal heat production in cold weather. (page 35.5)

e. When the wind blows, the cradle rocks, and baby loses heat by convection. (page 35.6)

Word Find

1. Afterdrop (page 35.11)	**10.** Drowning (page 35.20)	**19.** Narcosis (page 35.23)
2. Altitude (page 35.27)	**11.** Environmental (page 35.4)	**20.** Orthostatic (page 35.9)
3. Ataxia (page 35.31)	**12.** Frostnip (page 35.31)	**21.** Osborn (page 35.16)
4. Blackout (page 35.32)	**13.** Gangrene (page 35.14)	**22.** Radiation (page 35.6)
5. Cerebral (page 35.32)	**14.** Homeostasis (page 35.5)	**23.** Saturation (page 35.22)
6. Classic (page 35.10)	**15.** Hyperthermia (page 35.11)	**24.** Thermolysis (page 35.6)
7. Core (page 35.31)	**16.** Hyponatremia (page 35.9)	**25.** Wind chill (page 35.6)
8. Cramps (page 35.8)	**17.** Lassitude (page 35.32)	
9. Decompression (page 35.25)	**18.** Metabolic (page 35.5)	

Fill-in-the-Table

1. The slang expression "Cool it!" means to take it easy, to simmer down. And that is precisely what happens to the major systems of the body when cooled: They all slow down. (page 35.16)

Body System	Effects of Hypothermia
Central nervous system	**Apathy, lethargy** **Impaired reasoning** **Dysarthria** **Ataxic gait, uncoordinated movements**
Cardiovascular system	**Contracted intravascular space** **Increased blood viscosity with sludging in the capillaries** **Edema** **Bradycardia, arrhythmias, susceptibility to ventricular fibrillation**
Respiratory system	**Slowing of respiratory rate** **Increased tracheobronchial secretions** **Decreased cough and gag reflexes**
Muscular system	**Weakness and stiffness**
Metabolic system	**Hypoglycemia** **Ketoacidosis** **Slowed hepatic drug metabolism**

Chapter 36: Infectious and Communicable Diseases

Matching

1. E (page 36.6)
2. H (page 36.7)
3. C (page 36.6)
4. A (page 36.6)
5. D (page 36.6)

6. F (page 36.24)
7. G (page 36.24)
8. B (page 36.28)
9. I (page 36.4)
10. J (page 36.20)

Multiple Choice

1. D (page 36.4)
2. D (page 36.6)
3. B (page 36.6)
4. D (page 36.7)
5. D (page 36.8)

6. A (page 36.10)
7. C (page 36.11)
8. A (page 36.12)
9. C (page 36.14)
10. D (page 36.18)

Fill-in-the-Blank

1. Standard precautions (page 36.8)
2. Handwashing (page 36.8)
3. Postexposure follow-up (page 36.10)
4. Life-threatening conditions (page 36.12)
5. Epstein-Barr, oral (page 36.16)
6. Immunocompromised (page 36.18)
7. Sexually transmitted diseases (page 36.16)
8. Viral hepatitis (page 36.19)
9. Patient, patient, unwashed (page 36.24)
10. Mammals, birds (page 36.25)

Identify

1. a. Chief complaint: Flu-like symptoms that include fever, chills, dry cough.
   b. Vital signs: Respiratory rate of 20 breaths/min. Oxygen saturation on ambient air 95%, pulse 106 beats/min and regular, blood pressure of 128/68 mm Hg, skin warm and dry. Victim is conscious and alert.
   c. Pertinent negatives: He denies medication, allergies to medication, international travel, other previous medical history.
2. a. Chief complaint: Infestation of lice; patient is contaminated.
   b. Vital signs: Pulse of 88 beats/min and irregular, blood pressure 98/72 mm Hg, oxygen saturation 88%. He is tachypneic, and there is obvious skin tenting and delayed capillary refill.
   c. Pertinent negatives: He just put on the "new clothing" this morning and rarely "needs" to take any pills.
3. a. Chief complaint: ALS interfacility transport.
   b. Vital signs: Blood pressure as noted on the noninvasive monitor is 98/54 mm Hg with a heart rate of 62 beats/min.
   c. Pertinent negatives: Patient is "stable" for transport.

Ambulance Calls

1. a. The college student with fever, headache, stiff neck, vomiting, and an altered state of consciousness is showing typical signs of meningitis, perhaps meningococcal.
   b. The paramedic can minimize the risk of catching meningitis from a patient by wearing a mask and washing hands after the call. (page 36.14)
2. a. The 54-year-old man with hemoptysis, night sweats, and weight loss most probably has tuberculosis.

   b. The paramedic can minimize the risk of contracting the infection by wearing a mask and washing hands after the call. It is also a good idea to check, about 2 months later, for evidence of new TB infection by having a tuberculin test. (page 36.14)

3. a. The intravenous drug user with yellow eyes, dark urine, anorexia, and distaste for cigarettes has classic symptoms of viral hepatitis, most likely type B in view of his intravenous drug use.

   b. To minimize the risk of contracting hepatitis from a patient, the paramedic should employ universal precautions, including barrier protection (mask, gown, gloves) and extreme caution with needles and IV equipment. And, oh yes, wash your hands after the call. (page 36.19)

4. a. The 8-year-old with fever, sore throat, and swelling around the angles of the jaw most likely has mumps.

   b. The paramedic's best protection against mumps is immunization, either by mumps vaccine or by having had the illness as a child. The paramedic who is not immunized should wear a mask. And whether immune or not, wash your hands after the call. (page 36.13)

5. a. The young lady with fever, conjunctivitis, and spots has measles.

   b. If *you* haven't had measles, or immunization against measles, you can try wearing a mask, but in all likelihood you will soon have measles, too—just wait about 10 days. Be sure to wash your hands after the call though, to minimize the risks to the next patients you treat. (page 36.12)

6. a. (1) Wear PPE

   (2) Leather gloves

   (3) Face/eye protection

   (4) Turn-out gear (page 36.8)

   b. Completely restock the vehicle and replace any used items. Clean/cold sterilize any reusable patient contact equipment, and clean all exposed surfaces with disinfectant. (page 36.26)

   c. Assuming that appropriate PPE was used during and after the call, there is nothing that really needs to be completed. A soiled uniform/gear should be changed and laundered at work. If there was an exposure, your designated infection control officer should be contacted. Disinfect the vehicle and its equipment. Commercially available antiviral and antibacterial cleansers should be used or use a 10% bleach and water mixture. (pages 36.8, 36.26)

True/False

1. F (page 36.21)   **6.** T (page 36.20)

2. T (page 36.20)   **7.** F (page 36.21)

3. T (page 36.21)   **8.** F (page 36.21)

4. F (page 36.21)   **9.** T (page 36.17)

5. F (page 36.21)   **10.** F (page 36.16)

Short Answer

1. a. What illnesses did you have as a child or up to this point?

   b. What did your personal immunization survey turn up? Are you completely covered, or do you have some deficits to make up?

   c. If your last tetanus booster was more than 10 years ago, or if you never had an immunization against hepatitis B, make sure you remedy those and any other immunization deficits *before* you take your first call. And be sure to wash your hands.

2. There's no need to be panicky about AIDS or any other communicable disease if you know something about it.

   a. There are only three ways in which AIDS can be transmitted from one person to another:

   (1) Sexual contact

   (2) Through contaminated blood or blood products (eg, being stuck by a needle used on an HIV-positive person)

   (3) From mother to fetus

   b. Things one can do to minimize the risk of acquiring HIV from a patient are categorized under the heading of "standard precautions". *Students should provide three of the following:*

   (1) Wear latex gloves for any contact with a patient's blood or body fluids.

   (2) Use additional barrier protection (eg, mask, eye wear) for any procedures that may involve the splashing of blood or body fluids.

   (3) Wash your hands after every patient contact!

   (4) Handle needles and other sharp instruments with extreme caution. Do not recap needles. Dispose of them safely. (page 36.20)

Crossword Puzzle

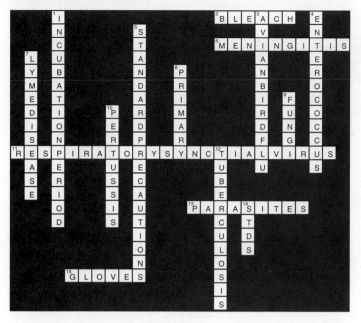

Secret Message

1. Lady Macbeth probably would not have made a very good paramedic because there were certain fundamental deficiencies in her character. But one thing she *did* have going for her: She washed her hands frequently!

    a. Fomite

    b. Virus

    c. Tuberculin

    d. Icterus

    e. Orchitis

    f. Dysuria

    g. Rash

    h. Night sweats

    i. Cough

    j. Fatigue

    k. Nausea

    l. Cyanosis

    m. Gag

    n. Dilate

    o. Banana

    p. DOT

    q. Tea

    Secret Message: THE BEST SAFEGUARD AGAINST CATCHING OR TRANSMITTING A CONTAGIOUS DISEASE IS TO WASH YOUR HANDS AFTER EVERY CALL.

Fill-in the Table

1.

Recommended Personal Protective Equipment for Prevention of Transmission of HIV and Hepatitis B Virus in the Prehospital Setting				
Task or Activity	**Disposable Gloves**	**Gown**	**Mask**	**Protective Eyewear**
Bleeding control with spurting blood	Yes	Yes	Yes	Yes
Bleeding control with minimal bleeding	Yes	No	No	No
Emergency childbirth	Yes	Yes	Yes, if splashing is likely	Yes, if splashing is likely
Blood drawing	Not required by CDC, but recommended for EMS	No	No	No
Starting an intravenous line	Yes	No	No	No
Endotracheal intubation, laryngeal mask airway, Combitube use	Yes	No	No, unless splashing is likely*	No, unless splashing is likely*
Oral/nasal suctioning, manually cleaning airway	Yes	No	No, unless splashing is likely*	No, unless splashing is likely*
Handling and cleaning instruments with microbial contamination	Yes	No, unless soiling is likely	No	No
Measuring blood pressure	No	No	No	No
Measuring temperature	No	No	No	No
Giving an injection	Not required by CDC, but recommended for EMS	No	No	No

*Splashing is often likely, so use PPE accordingly.

Adapted from: Centers for Disease Control and Prevention.

(page 36.8)

2.

Disease	Mode(s) of Transmission	Protective Measures
AIDS	Sexual contact; injection of contaminated blood products; from mother to fetus	Gloves, mask, extreme caution with needles and sharp objects, handwashing
Hepatitis type A	Fecal-oral, from ingesting contaminated water, shellfish, etc.	Handwashing
Hepatitis type B	Sexual contact; injection of contaminated blood products	Immunization Gloves, mask, extreme caution with needles and sharp objects, handwashing
Meningitis	Droplet spread	Mask Handwashing
Mumps	Saliva, droplet spread	Immunization, mask Handwashing
Syphilis	Sexual contact, infected saliva, semen, vaginal discharge	Gloves Handwashing
Tuberculosis	Droplet spread	Mask Handwashing

(pages 36.12–36.21)

Chapter 37: Behavioral Emergencies

Matching

1. (page 37.4)

1. P		**6.** O	
2. P		**7.** O	
3. O		**8.** B	
4. B		**9.** O	
5. P		**10.** P	

2. (page 37.6)

1. F		**7.** D	
2. B		**8.** C	
3. E		**9.** D	
4. A		**10.** B	
5. H		**11.** E	
6. G		**12.** H	

Multiple Choice

1. A (page 37.4)	**6.** D (page 37.24)
2. D (page 37.6)	**7.** A (page 37.26)
3. C (page 37.8)	**8.** D (page 37.4)
4. D (page 37.10)	**9.** B (page 37.5)
5. A (page 37.15)	**10.** A (page 37.5)

Fill-in-the-Blank

1. Biological, psychosocial, sociocultural (page 37.4)

2. Clearly, confused, delusional, frequent (page 37.8)

3. Fear, dread (page 37.14)

4. Stress, nightmares (page 37.14)

5. Amitril, Elavil (page 37.16)

6. Hypertensive crisis (page 37.16)

7. Suicide (page 37.16)

Identify

1. Fluoxetine (Prozac) and Valium (page 37.16)

2. Phenelzine (Nardil) and buprion (Wellbutrin) (page 37.16)

3. Aripiprazole (Abilify) (page 37.21)

Ambulance Calls

1. The shortest answer to this question is that the paramedic did just about everything wrong! Furthermore, he or she was inexcusably rude.

a. The paramedic never identified himself (assume it was a male paramedic).

b. The paramedic used a demeaning term to address the patient ("dearie") instead of asking her name and addressing her with respect as Miss, Ms., or Mrs. So-and-so.

c. The paramedic stood in front of the patient, towering over her and also blocking her escape—a very threatening stance. He should have crouched down, so that he was at the same level as the patient, and positioned himself somewhat to the side, so that she wasn't trapped in the corner.

d. The paramedic passed judgment on the patient's feelings ("Big girls don't cry"). Furthermore, he belittled the patient's problem without even waiting to find out what the problem was! ("You're making a mountain out of a molehill.")

e. The paramedic gave inappropriate and premature reassurance, telling the patient in essence that everything will be all right by tomorrow without even knowing what's wrong today.

f. The paramedic tried to forestall the patient's expressions of feeling, urging her to stop crying.

g. The paramedic never gave the patient a chance to talk.

h. The paramedic then turned his back on the patient and asked if someone else could tell him what was going on, implying that the patient's version of things was of no importance.

i. Needless to say, the paramedic in this story was an imposter. No *real* paramedic would ever behave like that. (pages 37.9–37.12)

2. The fact that Mr. Crosby has admitted you to his apartment, even reluctantly, is a hopeful sign.

   a. You might start the interview something like this: "Your neighbors have been worried about you; that's why they called us. They thought there might be some kind of problem here. Is there any way we can help?" If the patient then says something to the effect that there's nothing anyone can do to help, you might comment on his statement: "You seem really discouraged." The object is to indicate that you are a "sympathetic ear," prepared to listen to his troubles. (page 37.9)

   b. The *symptoms of depression* that this patient is showing include the following:

   (1) A sense of worthlessness

   (2) Decreased appetite

   (3) No apparent interest in anything

   (4) Lack of energy (page 37.15)

   c. Other symptoms and signs of depression include

   (1) Sleep disturbances

   (2) Difficulty concentrating

   (3) Psychomotor abnormalities (retardation or agitation)

   (4) Suicidal thoughts (page 37.15)

   d. The *risk factors for suicide* in this patient's history include

   (1) Male, over 55 years old

   (2) Widower

   (3) Socially isolated

   (4) Depressed

   (5) Possible alcohol problem (empty bottles lying around) (page 37.16)

   e. Other risk factors for suicide include the following. *Students should provide four of the following:*

   (1) A previous suicide attempt

   (2) A family history of suicide

   (3) Suicidal thoughts, particularly when there are concrete plans

   (4) Clear warning of intent to commit suicide

   (5) Recent loss of a significant person

   (6) Recent job loss or financial setback (page 37.16)

   f. Among the questions to ask in evaluating this patient's suicide risk are the following:

   (1) Have you ever felt that life wasn't worth living?

   (2) Have you thought about harming yourself?

   (3) How would you go about it—have you made any plans? (page 37.17)

3. The young woman with a "possible heart attack" is unlikely to be suffering a heart attack (although it's not completely out of the question).

   a. Her problem is most likely a panic attack. (page 37.14)

   b. The symptoms and signs that suggest that diagnosis include the following:

   (1) Dyspnea

   (2) Chest tightness

   (3) Feeling faint

   (4) Her feelings of unreality and impending death

   (5) Tachycardia

   (6) Sweating

   (7) Trembling (page 37.14)

   c. Yes, there certainly are other possibilities that must be taken into account.

   (1) Highest on the list is pulmonary embolism.

   (2) One also has to consider the possibility of a cardiac arrhythmia.

   (3) A reaction to a drug

   (4) An anaphylactic reaction

   (5) An acute myocardial infarction, which is seen much more frequently among young people these days because of the widespread use of cocaine

   d. To manage this patient, therefore:

     (1) Separate her from all the panicky bystanders. Move her into a private office, or move everyone out of *her office*.

     (2) Sit down to talk with her.

     (3) Administer supplementary oxygen. Until you know that you are *not* dealing with a pulmonary embolism or cardiac event, you need to cover all bases.

     (4) Apply monitoring electrodes, and check the rhythm on the scope.

     (5) Assuming that there are no abnormal findings, reassure the patient that you cannot find any indication of serious illness and that the chances are she is suffering a panic attack. Tell her that to make absolutely sure, she needs to be checked out in the hospital. If it does turn out that she is having a panic attack, there are effective treatments for that condition. (page 37.14)

4. The police officer who summoned you to the bar was on the right track, even if "psycho case" is not a very specific diagnosis.

   a. The patient is probably in the manic phase of a bipolar disorder. (page 37.18)

   b. The evidence to suggest that diagnosis includes the following:

     (1) His pressure of speech

     (2) His grandiose ideas (big business deals, big spender)

     (3) His apparently euphoric mood that is, nonetheless, very brittle; his good cheer easily turns to a less pleasant affect when he is challenged by the bartender or the police officer

     (4) His hyperactivity, pacing up and down (page 37.18)

   c. In managing this patient, you will have to try to persuade him to go voluntarily to the hospital. If he will not be persuaded, and probably he will not, coercion will be necessary. Consult your medical director first. (page 37.18)

5. The strangely dressed man found wandering down the middle of the street is a good example of disorganized behavior. Because walking in traffic is not a healthy form of activity, the patient must be assumed to be unable to care for himself and probably needs institutional care. From the description, it does not sound as if you will be able to obtain a useful history. You should simply tell the patient gently but firmly that you are going to take him to the hospital for care. He will probably go along without much fuss if you are nonthreatening about it. (page 37.13)

6. The karate expert is seriously ill and probably dangerous.

   a. He is showing signs of psychosis (answer 2)—hallucinations, persecutory delusions, loosening of associations. (page 37.21)

   b. Yes, there are indications that he might become violent.

   c. Indications. *Students should provide four of the following:*

     (1) His body language—sitting there like a coiled spring, gripping the armrests of the chair

     (2) The fact that he is easily startled

     (3) His avoidance of eye contact

     (4) The fact that he views the paramedics as adversaries (he thinks you're the FBI!)

     (5) His hearing voices that tell him to put up a fight

   d. In managing this situation:

     (1) Observe your surroundings. Keep yourself between the patient and the door to his room. Make note of any potential weapons.

     (2) Maintain a safe distance, at least two arm lengths (which will keep you out of range of his foot).

     (3) Identify yourself again as a paramedic.

     (4) Acknowledge the patient's behavior ("You seem very worried.") and state your willingness to help. Don't sound too friendly.

     (5) Encourage the patient to talk about what's bothering him.

     (6) Define your expectations of his behavior.

     (7) If talking to the patient isn't working, back off and get help.

     (8) Explain to the patient's mother that it will be necessary to take the young man to the hospital against his will (she may be required to sign his commitment papers). Call for police backup, and consult medical command.

     (9) *When you have sufficient manpower,* apply restraints as quickly and efficiently as you can. Once the patient is restrained, don't remove the restraints.

     (10) Maintain verbal contact with the patient throughout transport. (page 37.22)

True/False

  1. T (page 37.11)   **4.** F (page 37.13)

  2. F (page 37.13)   **5.** T (page 37.12)

  3. F (page 37.19)   **6.** T (page 37.25)

Short Answer

1. The paramedic needs to develop a "nose for danger" and to be able to predict which situations present a high risk for violence.

   a. Any place where alcohol is being consumed

   b. Crowd incidents

   c. Scenes of violent injury

   b. Diagnostic groups (page 37.24)

2. a. Patients intoxicated with drugs or alcohol

   b. Patients withdrawing from drugs or alcohol

   c. Psychotic patients

   d. Patients with delirium (page 37.24)

Secret Messages

1. Your thought for the day applies to all of the paramedic's work in the field, not just the care of "mental" patients. Every patient who has a functioning brain in his or her head is a "mental" patient.

   a. Hallucination   i. Echolalia

   b. Delusion   j. Anxiety

   c. Perseveration   k. Restlessness

   d. Phobia   l. Flat

   e. Ambivalence   m. Thought

   f. Stereotyped   n. STD

   g. Confusion   o. Envy

   h. Fugue state

Secret Message: THE EVALUATION OF EVERY PATIENT SHOULD INCLUDE AN ASSESSMENT OF HIS PSYCHOLOGICAL STATUS. OBSERVE AND LISTEN TO THE PATIENT CAREFULLY.

Fill-in-the-Table

Selected Disease States That May Produce Psychotic Symptoms	
Disease State	**Psychotic Symptoms**
Toxic and deficiency states	Drug-induced psychoses, especially from: • Digitalis • Steroids • Disulfiram • Amphetamines • LSD, PCP, and other psychedelics Nutrition disorders: • Alcohol abuse • Vitamin deficiencies Poisoning with bromide or other heavy metals Kidney failure Liver failure
Infections	Syphilis Parasites Viral encephalitis (eg, after measles) Brain abscess
Neurologic disease	Seizure disorders (especially temporal lobe seizures) Primary and metastatic tumors of the brain Dementia Cerebrovascular accident Closed-head injury
Cardiovascular disorders	Low cardiac output (eg, in heart failure)
Endocrine disorders	Thyroid hyperfunction (thyrotoxicosis) Adrenal hyperfunction (Cushing's syndrome)
Metabolic disorders	Electrolyte imbalances (eg, after severe diarrhea) Hypoglycemia Diabetic ketoacidosis

Skill Drill

Restraining a Patient (page 37.27)

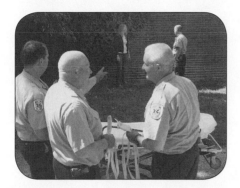

Step 1: If possible, corner the patient in a safe area.

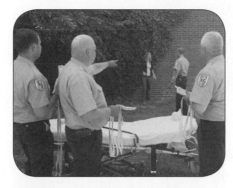

Step 2: Assemble 4 or 5 rescuers and have the stetcher or carrying device and soft restraints nearby. Designate a leader.

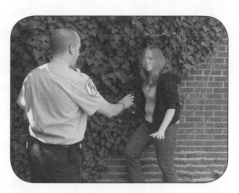

Step 3: Assign positions to each team member: four extremities and the head.

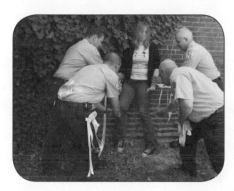

Step 4: On the direction of the team leader, move together toward the patient.

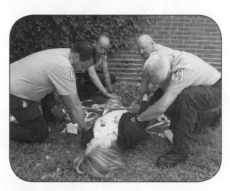

Step 5: Each team member should grasp the assigned body part and carefully, with the least amount of force, bring the patient to the ground.

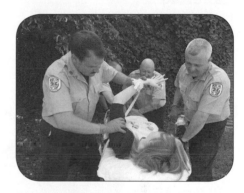

Step 6: Carefully place the patient on the stretcher or carrying device in a face-up position.

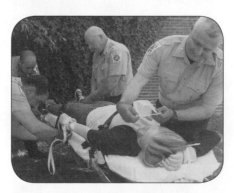

Step 7: Tie the patient with soft restraints at each wrist and ankle as well as the chest and pelvis sheets. If the patient is spitting, place an oxygen mask or surgical mask on his or her face.

Chapter 38: Gynecologic Emergencies

Matching

1. H (page 38.4)
2. C (page 38.4)
3. E (page 38.5)
4. J (page 38.5)
5. A (page 38.6)
6. G (page 38.14)
7. D (page 38.14)
8. F (page 38.15)
9. I (page 38.19)
10. B (page 38.15)

Multiple Choice

1. C (page 38.5)
2. D (page 38.5)
3. B (page 38.8)
4. B (page 38.10)
5. B (page 38.18)
6. A (page 38.15)
7. C (page 38.16)
8. D (page 38.19)
9. B (page 38.20)
10. C (page 38.22)

Labeling

1. Anatomy of the Female Reproductive System (page 38.4)

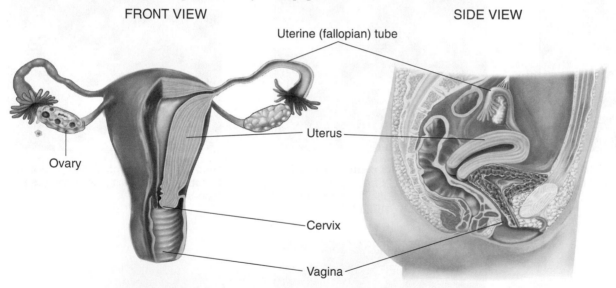

FRONT VIEW

SIDE VIEW

Uterine (fallopian) tube

Ovary

Uterus

Cervix

Vagina

2. Reproductive Systerm with an Ectopic Pregnancy (page 38.9)

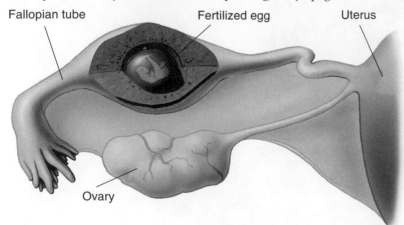

Fallopian tube

Fertilized egg

Uterus

Ovary

Fill-in-the-Blank

1. Vagina (page 38.4)
2. Imperforate hymen (page 38.4)
3. Amenorrhea (page 38.6)
4. Menopause (page 38.5)
5. Endometriosis (page 38.7)
6. Toxic shock syndrome (page 38.9)
7. Scene safety (page 38.11)
8. Modesty (page 38.12)
9. Cullen's, Grey-Turner's (page 38.16)
10. Ketamine hydrochloride (page 38.21)

Identify

1. Chief complaint: Severe abdominal pain.
2. Vital signs: Patient is alert, 10/10 scale for pain, pulse is 120 beats/min, blood pressure is 140/92 mm Hg, sinus tachycardia, oxygen saturation is 99%, respirations are 20 breaths/min, the temperature is 102°F, pupils are PEARRL, and lungs are clear.
3. Pertinent negatives: No illness, no trauma, and no sexual activity yet.

   What is wrong? She has a ruptured ovarian cyst. The lack of sexual activity takes out the possibility of ectopic pregnancy. She is running a fever with no other signs of illness. The rebound tenderness, abdominal distention, and vomiting tell you that this patient is very ill, and because of her vitals, she appears to be in septic shock. Rapid transport is indicated for her.

Ambulance Calls

1. **a.** The 25-year-old woman with fever and abdominal pain that began not long after her menstrual period is most likely suffering from pelvic inflammatory disease (answer E).

   b. (1) The prehospital management is gentle transport.

   (2) In view of the woman's tachycardia, fever, and history of vomiting, she is probably dehydrated, so it is a good idea as well to start an IV with crystalloid and run in fluids en route to the hospital. (page 38.18)

2. **a.** The 24-year-old woman who thinks she has appendicitis more likely has an embryo developing in her right fallopian tube, that is, an ectopic pregnancy (answer D). Crampy, unilateral abdominal pain followed by spotting and signs of early shock are good enough evidence to start treatment.

   b. Treatment is as follows:

   (1) Administer supplemental oxygen.

   (2) Keep the patient recumbent.

   (3) Start a large-bore IV and run it wide open.

   (4) Allow nothing by mouth.

   (5) Keep the patient warm.

   (6) Monitor cardiac rhythm and vital signs.

   (7) Notify the receiving hospital.

   (8) Transport without delay. (page 38.19)

True/False

1. F (page 38.20)		**6.** T (page 38.4)
2. F (page 38.20)		**7.** F (page 38.6)
3. T (page 38.20)		**8.** F (page 38.7)
4. F (page 38.20)		**9.** F (page 38.14)
5. T (page 38.20)		**10.** T (page 38.15)

Short Answer

1. In evaluating a woman of childbearing age whose chief complaint is abdominal pain, you are going to want to know more about the pain, about associated symptoms, and about her obstetric and gynecologic history. (pages 38.13–38.18)

    a. Among the questions you should ask in taking the history, therefore, are the following (students will list ten):

    (1) What provoked the pain? Does anything make it better or worse?

    (2) What is the pain like? Sharp? Dull? Crampy?

    (3) Where is the pain? Does it radiate anywhere else?

    (4) How severe is the pain? Compared to prior experience or on 1 to 10 scale.

    (5) When did the pain start? What is the temporal relationship between the pain and other symptoms?

    (6) What other symptoms has the patient noticed? Has she had vaginal bleeding? Has she felt **dizzy or faint**?

    (7) When was her last normal menstrual period?

    (8) Has she noticed any breast tenderness, urinary frequency, or nausea in the mornings?

    (9) What, if any, type of contraception does the woman use?

    (10) Has she had any vaginal discharge?

    (11) How many previous pregnancies has she had? How many deliveries?

    (12) What gynecologic problems has she had in the past?

    (13) Does she have any serious underlying illnesses?

    b. On physical examination, what you want to look for in particular are the following:

    (1) Signs of hypovolemia, such as anxiety, restlessness, cold and clammy skin, tachycardia, and postural changes in vital signs

    (2) Signs of peritoneal irritation, such as abdominal rigidity or pain on movement

2. Risk factors for ectopic pregnancy include the following (students will list two):

    a. Previous pelvic inflammatory disease

    b. Previous ectopic pregnancy

    c. Using an IUD for contraception

    d. Previous pelvic surgery (page 38.19)

3. The classic triad of findings in ectopic pregnancy are

    a. Abdominal pain

    b. Amenorrhea

    c. Vaginal bleeding (page 38.19)

Crossword Puzzle

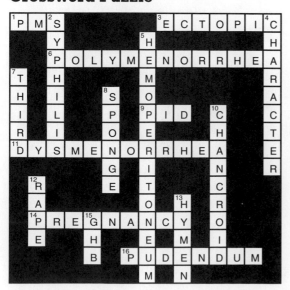

Fill-in-the-Table

1. (page 38.18)

Estimating Blood Volume Loss				
Grade of Hemorrhage/ Blood Loss	**Heart Rate**	**Respiratory Rate**	**Blood Pressure**	**Central Nervous System**
First/< 15%	Minor tachycardia	No change	No change	No change
Second/15%–30%	Tachycardia	Tachypnea	Decreased pulse pressure	Anxiety or combativeness
Third/30%–40%	Marked tachycardia	Marked tachypnea	Systolic hypotension	Altered mental status
Fourth/> 40%	Marked tachycardia	Marked tachypnea	Severe systolic hypotension	Comatose/unresponsive

Source: Adapted from United States Department of Defense. *Emergency War Surgery Nato Handbook.* 2004:Table 7-1. Available at: http://www.bordeninstitute .army.mil/emrgncywarsurg/Chp7Shock&Resuscitation.pdf. Accessed May 18, 2006.

Chapter 39: Obstetrics

Matching

(page 39.16)   (pages 39.14–39.16)

1. C   **6.** D
2. A   **7.** A
3. D   **8.** F
4. E   **9.** C
5. B   **10.** E
                              11. B

Multiple Choice

1. B (page 39.13)   **6.** D (page 39.29)
2. D (page 39.14)   **7.** A (page 39.32)
3. A (page 39.16)   **8.** D (page 39.4)
4. C (page 39.21)   **9.** C (page 39.6)
5. B (page 39.26)   **10.** A (page 39.7)

Labeling

1. Structures of the pregnant uterus. (page 39.5)

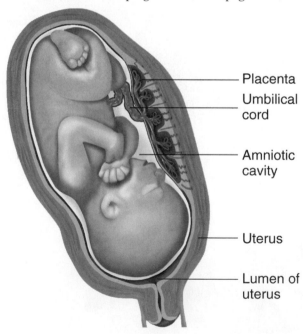

Placenta

Umbilical cord

Amniotic cavity

Uterus

Lumen of uterus

(page 39.5)

2. Causes of hemorrhage. (page 39.14)

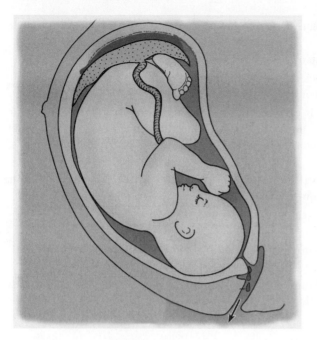

A. Placenta previa

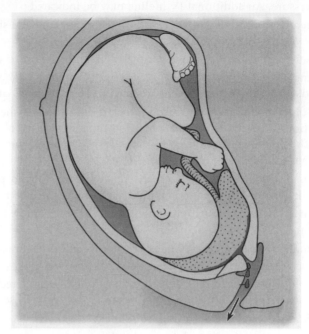

B. Abruptio placenta

Fill-in-the-Blank

1. endometrium (page 39.4)

2. umbilical cord (page 39.5)

3. increases (page 39.7)

4. Preeclampsia (page 39.9)

5. spontaneous abortion (page 39.12)

6. Placenta previa (page 39.14)

7. Multigravida (page 39.16)

8. second stage (page 39.21)

9. transverse (page 39.28)

10. magnesium sulfate (page 39.31)

Identify

1. Chief complaint: "I am bleeding from my vagina"

2. Vital signs: Pulse is 110 beats/min and thready, respirations are 24 breaths/min, blood pressure is 100/70 mm Hg, and the patient is pale and diaphoretic.

3. Pertinent findings: Patient is 35 years old, in her third trimester, multiparity with previous cesarean sections. The blood is bright red, she is painless, thirsty, and says she is weak. The vital signs and physical exam reveal signs of shock. (pages 39.15–39.16)

Ambulance Calls

1. a. The 22-year-old who has passed blood and tissue through the vagina and is showing signs of hemorrhagic shock is most likely having an incomplete abortion (answer C). The passage of tissue indicates some sort of abortion, and the fact that she is continuing to bleed suggests that there is still tissue in the uterus. (page 39.13)

b. She should be treated for shock because her vital signs indicate that she is already in shock:

(1) Keep the woman recumbent, lying on her left side.

(2) Administer 100% supplemental oxygen via nonrebreathing mask at 15 L/min.

(3) Provide rapid transport to a definitive care facility, notifying the facility of the patient's condition en route.

    (4) Start an intravenous (IV) lifeline of normal saline with a large-bore IV catheter. Infuse at a rate necessary to maintain blood pressure. An additional IV lifeline may be indicated.

    (5) Establish an echocardiogram (ECG) and obtain baseline vital signs. Do not attempt to examine the woman internally or pack the vagina with trauma pads.

    (6) Use loosely placed trauma pads over the vagina in an effort to staunch bleeding.

    If bleeding is severe, and significant signs and symptoms of shock are present, pharmacologic management may be indicated. *Tocolytics* are drugs that are used to delay preterm labor. (page 39.15)

2. a. The 32-year-old woman has good reason to be "feeling poorly": she is carrying a dead fetus in her uterus; that is, she has a **missed abortion** (answer D). Her history is typical: a threatened abortion earlier in the pregnancy that seemed to get better, but failure of the pregnancy to develop normally. By 6 months, her uterine fundus should be palpable above the umbilicus, just barely above the pelvic brim. (page 39.13)

   b. The prehospital management of missed abortion is simply to **transport** the patient to the hospital while providing emotional support. At the hospital, surgical evacuation of the uterus will be required. (page 39.13)

3. a. The primigravida with painless vaginal bleeding is experiencing a **threatened abortion** (answer A). The absence of contractions indicates that the abortion is not yet inevitable. (page 39.12)

   b. The prehospital treatment of threatened abortion is simply to **transport**, while providing emotional support to the patient. (page 39.13)

4. a. The 16-year-old who went to the backstreet abortionist has suffered one of the most common results: **septic abortion** (answer E). By the time you reach the scene, the girl already has signs of septic shock, and she may die. (page 39.13)

   b. The prehospital management is to **treat for shock:**

    (1) Keep the woman recumbent, lying on her left side.

    (2) Administer 100% supplemental oxygen via nonrebreathing mask at 15 L/min.

    (3) Provide rapid transport to a definitive care facility, notifying the facility of the patient's condition en route.

    (4) Start an IV lifeline of normal saline with a large-bore IV catheter. Infuse at a rate necessary to maintain blood pressure. An additional IV lifeline may be indicated.

    (5) Establish an ECG and obtain baseline vital signs. Do not attempt to examine the woman internally or pack the vagina with trauma pads.

    (6) Use loosely placed trauma pads over the vagina in an effort to staunch bleeding. (page 39.13)

5. a. The 26-year-old veteran of three previous miscarriages is probably correct; she seems to be having yet another, that is, an **inevitable abortion** (answer B). The severe cramping and uterine contractions that accompany her vaginal bleeding bode ill for the continuation of the pregnancy. (page 39.13)

   b. The prehospital treatment of inevitable abortion is expectant treatment for shock:

    (1) Keep the woman recumbent, lying on her left side.

    (2) Administer 100% supplemental oxygen via nonrebreathing mask at 15 L/min.

    (3) Provide rapid transport to a definitive care facility, notifying the facility of the patient's condition en route.

    (4) Start an IV lifeline of normal saline with a large-bore IV catheter. Infuse at a rate necessary to maintain blood pressure. An additional IV lifeline may be indicated.

    (5) Establish an ECG and obtain baseline vital signs. Do not attempt to examine the woman internally or pack the vagina with trauma pads. (page 39.15)

6. This case concerns a 36-year-old grand multipara with third-trimester bleeding.

   a. Three possible causes of third-trimester bleeding are:

    (1) Abruptio placenta

    (2) Placenta previa

    (3) Uterine rupture (page 39.14)

   b. In this particular case, the most likely diagnosis is **placenta previa.** (page 39.14)

   c. Among the characteristic features of placenta previa manifested by this patient are the following:

    (1) *Painless* vaginal bleeding. (There is severe pain with placental abruption or uterine rupture.)

    (2) *Bright red* blood. (In abruption, bleeding is dark.)

    (3) The *fetus remains viable.*

    (4) The *abdomen* is *soft and nontender.* (page 39.15)

   d. The steps in prehospital management are (page 39.15):

     (1) Keep the woman recumbent, lying on her left side.

     (2) Administer 100% supplemental oxygen via nonrebreathing mask at 15 L/min.

     (3) Provide rapid transport to a definitive care facility, notifying the facility of the patient's condition en route.

     (4) Start an IV lifeline of normal saline with a large-bore IV catheter. Infuse at a rate necessary to maintain blood pressure. An additional IV lifeline may be indicated.

     (5) Establish an ECG and obtain baseline vital signs. Do not attempt to examine the woman internally or pack the vagina with trauma pads.

     (6) Use loosely placed trauma pads over the vagina in an effort to staunch bleeding.

        If bleeding is severe, and significant signs and symptoms of shock are present, pharmacologic management may be indicated. *Tocolytics* are drugs that are used to delay preterm labor. In cases of abruptio placenta and placenta previa, magnesium sulfate may be ordered by Medical Control (4 to 6 g bolus over a 20-minute period, followed by a 2 to 4 g/hr titrated drip). Oxytocin may be ordered in cases of uterine rupture, with an ordered dose of 20 to 40 units (1,000 mL at 100 mL/hour) to encourage uterine contractions.

7. a. The woman with the fainting spells is most probably suffering from supine hypotensive syndrome (answer E) because her pulse and blood pressure improved very quickly after she turned to her side and took the weight of her uterus off her inferior vena cava. Nonetheless, you can't take a chance on missing a concealed hemorrhage. In fact, women whose volume status is already marginal are most vulnerable to the supine hypotensive syndrome. So, you will have to treat the patient as someone who might develop hemorrhagic shock. (page 39.30)

   b. The prehospital management, then, is as follows:

     (1) Administer supplemental **oxygen**.

     (2) Keep the patient in the recumbent position with the bulk of her uterus to the side to avoid vena cava syndrome.

     (3) Start an **IV with saline**.

     (4) **Transport** to the hospital as soon as possible.

     (5) Obtain an ECG. (page 39.30)

8. a. The woman who fell in a downtown department store has a chief complaint unrelated to her pregnancy—a twisted ankle. But, in fact, a careful examination reveals a very serious problem that is related to her pregnancy, preeclampsia (answer B), as manifested by edema and hypertension. (page 39.9)

   b. The initial prehospital treatment, therefore, is as follows:

     (1) **Splint** the injured ankle.

     (2) **Transport** the woman in the semi-Fowler's position (as long as this does not cause any dizziness).

     (3) Start an IV en route so that it will be there if you need it. Pain meds should be discussed with Medical Control before being administered. (pages 39.19–39.20)

   c. And, indeed, you did need that IV—when the woman proceeded to have a grand mal seizure and develop full-blown eclampsia. The steps to take at that point are:

     (1) **Protect the patient from injury** during the tonic-clonic phase of the seizure.

     (2) Ensure an adequate **airway**.

     (3) Administer supplemental **oxygen**.

     (4) Contact **Medical Control** for orders. You may be asked to give **Magnesium sulfate** 10%, 2 to 4 gm IV.

     (5) Notify the receiving hospital. If the woman's seizures cannot be controlled, it may be necessary to take her straight to the operating room for an emergency cesarean section. (page 39.31)

9. When *two* pregnant women are involved in a motor vehicle crash, it's quadruple trouble!

   a. Some of the changes during pregnancy that make a woman more vulnerable to injury or that affect her response to injury include the following (students will list five):

     (1) **Elevation of the diaphragm**, which effectively pushes the abdominal contents into the chest so that abdominal organs are more apt to be injured after a blow to the chest.

     (2) **Forward, upward displacement of the bladder**, rendering it more vulnerable to injury.

     (3) The **uterus** becomes more susceptible to injury as it enlarges and occupies more space in the abdomen.

     (4) **Increase in vascular volume** by as much as 50% so that the pregnant woman can lose a lot of blood (and the fetus can be in big trouble) before she shows signs of shock.

     (5) **Relative tachycardia and hypotension** make it difficult to interpret the pregnant woman's vital signs after injury.

(6) **Redistribution of blood flow** to the pelvic area means that a pregnant woman will bleed much more profusely from injuries such as pelvic fracture.

(7) Delayed gastric emptying during pregnancy makes a pregnant woman more likely to vomit and aspirate after injury. (pages 39.6–39.9)

b. You find the *driver* of the car conscious, but with evidence of steering wheel trauma to the abdomen and indications of impending shock (thirst, tachycardia, slight hypotension). She must, therefore, be **treated for shock** and regarded as a **load-and-go** emergency:

(1) Manually **stabilize the cervical spine.**

(2) Remove the woman from the vehicle on a **long backboard**, with the usual spinal precautions.

(3) In the ambulance, keep the **backboard tilted 30° to the left side.**

(4) Ensure an adequate **airway**; be prepared for vomiting.

(5) Administer supplemental **oxygen.**

(6) Start **transport**, and notify the receiving hospital.

(7) En route, **start at least one large-bore IV**, and run in normal saline to maintain a normal blood pressure.

(8) Obtain an ECG.

c. The pregnant *passenger* does not seem to be seriously injured, although her complaints of neck pain ("whiplash") should prompt appropriate measures to stabilize the cervical spine. In any case, however, you **cannot conclude that there is no injury to the fetus.** Only careful evaluation in the hospital, and observation over several hours, can establish that fact. (page 39.20)

10. Deciding whether you have time to transport a woman in active labor to the hospital is a judgment call, and there is room for debate in some of these situations. As a general rule, you will have a lot more time with nulliparas. Multiparas can progress very rapidly through labor, and so the margin for error is smaller. (pages 39.21–39.22)

a. D A 20-year-old woman in her first pregnancy. She says her water broke about 6 hours ago. Now her contractions are about 2 minutes apart, and she feels a need to move her bowels. You are 20 minutes from the hospital.

The urge to move the bowels indicates that the fetal head is already in the birth canal and delivery is imminent. The delivery may be complicated by fetal infection because the amniotic sac ruptured several hours ago.

b. D A 32-year-old multipara (gravida 10, para 8) who has been in labor about 5 hours. Her contractions are 3 minutes apart. She says she thinks the baby's coming. You are 10 minutes from the hospital.

As a general rule, when a woman who has had eight babies tells you that the baby is coming, she knows what she's talking about! *Complications* seen more commonly in grand multips include uterine rupture and postpartum hemorrhage.

c. T A 25-year-old nullipara (gravida 1, para 0) who has been in labor for 9 hours. Her contractions are 4 to 5 minutes apart. You are 20 minutes from the hospital.

In *this* case, you should have plenty of time. The woman is a beginner, and her contractions are still quite widely spaced.

d. D A 30-year-old gravida 4, para 3, who has been in labor for 6 hours. She had two of her three children by cesarean section. Her contractions are 2 minutes apart, and she is crowning. You are 5 minutes from the hospital.

No doubts here: the woman is crowning! If she's had two previous cesarean sections, she is at increased risk for uterine rupture during labor.

e. T A 28-year-old gravida 1, para 0, whose contractions started 24 hours ago. They do not come at regular intervals, and they have not gotten much more intense since they started. You are 25 minutes from the hospital.

This woman may not even be in labor at all. Her contractions sound suspiciously like Braxton Hicks contractions. If you sit around waiting for her to deliver, you might spend several weeks at the scene!

f. D A 24-year-old gravida 3, para 2, who announces, as you enter her apartment, "Hurry, the twins are coming any minute!" She says she has been in labor "quite a while," and you time her contractions as coming less than 2 minutes apart. You are 20 minutes from the hospital.

With the contractions coming at only 2-minute intervals in a multip, you can't afford to take a chance. The potential complications more likely in a twin birth include cord prolapse, breech presentation, and postpartum hemorrhage. The babies are also likely to be small and therefore to require the kind of special care given to premature babies.

11. Science has not yet established the precise mechanism that stimulates a woman to go into labor, but any experienced emergency medical technician basic (EMT-B) or paramedic can attest to the fact that one thing that can stimulate labor is shopping! That is why paramedics frequently find themselves delivering babies in department stores.

a. When the baby's face is found to be covered by the intact amniotic sac, you should **tear open the amniotic sac,** either with your fingers or a forceps, and carefully peel it away from the baby's face. Then, **suction the baby's nostrils and mouth** with a bulb aspirator. (page 39.25)

b. When the umbilical cord is found *tightly* wound around the baby's neck, the only thing you can do is **put two clamps on the cord, 2 inches apart, and cut the cord between the clamps.**(page 39.25)

c. The steps to take from that point on are as follows:

   (1) Guide the baby's head downward to **allow delivery of the upper shoulder.**

   (2) Guide the baby's head upward to **allow delivery of the lower shoulder.**

   (3) Wipe the baby's mouth and nose free of blood and mucus, and **suction out the mouth and nostrils again.**

   (4) **Tell the mother** and all the salespersons in the lingerie department if it's a boy or a girl.

   (5) **Dry the baby, cover it with a blanket, and put it on the mother's abdomen.**

   (6) **Record the time** of birth and the **Apgar score** while you await the delivery of the placenta.

   (7) When the placenta separates, instruct the mother to bear down.

   (8) *After the placenta has delivered,* **massage the uterus, and put the baby to the mother's breast.**

   (9) Clean up, put a sanitary pad between the mother's legs, bid farewell to the women in the lingerie department, and **transport.** (pages 39.22–39.26)

12. a. What you are dealing with at the ski lodge is a **breech presentation.** That smooth presenting part with a crack down the middle is a buttocks, not a head! (page 39.27)

  b. Management is as follows:

   (1) *Position the mother* with her buttocks at the edge of the bed or stretcher and her legs flexed.

   (2) Allow the buttocks and trunk of the baby to deliver spontaneously. *Do not pull on the baby.*

   (3) Once the baby's legs are clear, *support the baby's body* on the palm of your hand and volar surface of your arm.

   (4) Then, lower the baby slightly so that it very nearly hangs by its own weight downward; that will help the head pass through the pelvic outlet. You can tell when the head is in the vaginal canal because you'll be able to see the baby's hairline at the nape of its neck just below the mother's symphysis pubis.

   (5) *When you can see the baby's hairline,* grasp the baby by the ankles and lift it upward in the direction of the mother's abdomen. The head should then deliver without difficulty.

   (6) If the baby's head does not deliver in 3 minutes, the baby is in danger of suffocation, and immediate action is indicated. Suffocation may occur when the baby's umbilical cord is compressed by its head against the birth canal, which cuts off the baby's supply of oxygenated blood from the placenta, and the baby's face is pressed against the vaginal wall, which prevents it from breathing on its own. Place your gloved hand in the vagina, with your palm toward the baby's face. Form a V with your fingers on either side of the baby's nose, and push the vaginal wall away from the baby's face until the head is delivered.

   (7) Do not attempt to pull the baby out forcibly or allow an explosive delivery. If the head does not deliver in 3 minutes of establishing the airway, provide rapid transport to the hospital, with the mother's buttocks elevated on pillows. If at all possible, try to maintain the baby's airway throughout transport in the manner described. En route, alert the hospital so that they can have the appropriate personnel on hand when the mother arrives. (page 39.27)

13. Prolapsed umbilical cord occurs in only about 1 of every 300 deliveries, but it is more likely with a premature birth like this one. What you have to do is as follows:

   (1) Position the mother supine with her hips elevated as much as possible on pillows.

   (2) Administer 100% supplemental oxygen via nonrebreathing mask.

   (3) Instruct the mother to pant with each contraction, which will prevent her from bearing down.

   (4) If you are trained and authorized to do so, catheterize the mother's bladder; instill 500 mL of saline into the bladder through the catheter; then, clamp the catheter shut. The full bladder helps keep the presenting part off the cord.

   (5) With two fingers of a gloved hand, gently *push the baby* (not the cord) back up into the vagina until the presenting part is no longer pressing on the cord.

   (6) While you maintain pressure on the presenting part, have your partner cover the exposed portion of the cord with dressings moistened in normal saline.

   (7) Somehow, you're going to have to try to maintain that position, with a gloved hand pushing the presenting part away from the cord, throughout *urgent transport* to the hospital. (page 39.28)

14. a. The *special* measures required in delivering twins, as opposed to a single birth, are simply to

   (1) Wait for the second birth after the first is complete. Meanwhile, keep the first baby warm on the mother's abdomen, covered with a blanket.

   (2) Treat both babies as you would preemies, paying scrupulous attention to their warmth, prevention of bleeding, and protection from contamination. (page 39.29)

   b. The mother's *risk factor for postpartum hemorrhage* was the very fact of her twin pregnancy because the placenta covers a larger area in a twin pregnancy, and the uterine muscles become overstretched so that they contract less efficiently. (page 39.29)

   c. Other risk factors for postpartum hemorrhage include (*students will list three of the following*):

   (1) Prolonged labor

   (2) Retained products of conception

   (3) Grand multiparity

   (4) Multiple pregnancy

   (5) Placenta previa

   (6) A full bladder (page 39.29)

   d. The steps that should be taken to manage postpartum hemorrhage in the field are as follows:

   (1) Continue uterine massage.

   (2) Put either or both babies to the breast to start nursing.

   (3) Contact Medical Control to consider administration of oxytocin.

   (4) Begin transport, and notify the receiving hospital.

   (5) Start another IV with a large-bore catheter to infuse crystalloid rapidly.

   (6) Manage external bleeding from perinatal tears with a sanitary napkin and direct pressure. (page 39.30)

True/False

1. F (page 39.21)   **5.** F (page 39.26)

2. T (page 39.19)   **6.** F (page 39.26)

3. F (page 39.22)   **7.** T (page 39.27)

4. T (page 39.24)

Short Answer

1. The functions of the placenta include (students will list four):

   a. Respiratory gas exchange

   b. Transport of nutrients

   c. Excretion of wastes

   d. Transfer of heat

   e. Hormone production

   f. Formation of a barrier (page 39.5)

2. Any four of the following:

   a. Prolonged labor or delivery of multiple babies

   b. Retained products of conception

   c. Grand multiparity

   d. Multiple pregnancy

   e. Placenta previa

   f. A full bladder (page 39.29)

Word Find

```
O F G P U O N G L V Y U G D R
Y S B Y U G N P E A G Y V R W
S Y X H B I L R U M O U C O C
E B U T N A I P O L L A F C P
S F B W C U B Y N V S C X L R
S D O E Z C T Z A C A K I A E
L R N M U V O E I X J K V C P
C T Y L N O I T R O B A R I A
A E A P S B O P D U X L E L R
F M O V D I V A R G S E C I T
E B V I N V A G I N A D O B U
T R Z M P R I M I P A R A M M
U Y A O V U L A T E D Z R U R
S O D H W D O U N T X N K R E
K E D O S U T K K F F H B H T
```

On around the 14th day of the cycle, women **ovulate**, that is, a Graafian follicle located in the left or right ovary ruptures and releases an egg, or **ovum**. If a sperm should happen along just about the time when the egg is released, fertilization may take place, usually in the **fallopian tube**, where the fertilized egg remains for about 3 days before entering the **uterus** and implanting in the endometrium. Between the third and eighth week of development, the fertilized egg is called an **embryo**. Thereafter, it is called a **fetus** until delivery. After delivery, it is officially a **baby**.

Specialized structures develop during pregnancy to support the developing baby. The baby is enclosed in a fluid-filled **amniotic sac**. It is nourished by a large, vascular organ of pregnancy called the **placenta**, which attaches to the baby via the **umbilical cord**.

At about 40 weeks after conception, the baby reaches maturity, or **term**, and is ready to make its debut in the world. (When a baby is expelled early, before the 20th to 28th week of gestation, the woman is said to have had a miscarriage, or **abortion**.) At that point, the woman goes into labor, the process by which the baby is expelled from the womb, and the pregnant, or **gravid**, womb begins contracting. As it does so, the **cervix** progressively effaces and dilates until the womb becomes continuous with the birth canal, or **vagina**. The period of uterine contractions are of shorter duration in a **primipara**, a woman who has already had a delivery in the past, than it is in a nullipara. Delivery is imminent when the presenting part becomes visible, that is, when **crowning** occurs. At that point, it is important to control the rate at which the baby emerges; otherwise, there may be injury to the mother's external genitalia (**vulva**) or to the skin between the anus and the opening of the birth canal, an area called the perineum. All events occurring before delivery are called antepartum, or **prepartum**, while those occurring after delivery are called postpartum.

Fill-in-the-Table

1. The Stages of Labor: Nullipara versus Multipara (page 39.21)

The Stages of Labor: Nullipara Versus Multipara		
Stage of Labor	**Nullipara**	**Multipara**
First stage	8 to 12 hours	6 to 8 hours
Second stage	1 to 2 hours	30 minutes
Third stage	5 to 60 minutes	5 to 60 minutes

Section 5 Case Study: Answers and Summary

1. What initial management is indicated for this patient?

■ 100% oxygen via nonrebreathing mask

- This patient's respirations are adequate (normal rate and depth); therefore, she is not in need of positive pressure ventilator this time.
- Patients with any alteration in mental status should be assumed to be suffering from cerebral hypoxia, and should receive 100% supplemental oxygen as soon as possible.

2. What is your interpretation of this cardiac rhythm?

The characteristics of this cardiac rhythm (**Figure 5-1**) are consistent with *first-degree atrioventricular (AV) block*. The rhythm is regular, has a rate of approximately 65 beats/min, and has monomorphic P waves, all of which are consistently followed by narrow QRS complexes, and a PR interval greater than 0.20 seconds (0.31 seconds, to be exact).

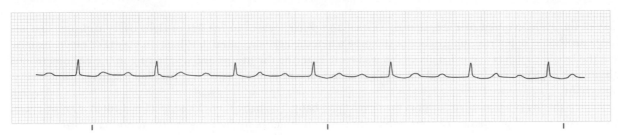

■ **Figure 5-1** Your patient's cardiac rhythm.

First-degree AV block is typically a benign cardiac rhythm. It is characterized by a prolongation of the PR interval (>0.20 seconds), which represents an abnormal delay at the AV junction. The normal PR interval ranges from 0.12 to 0.20 seconds.

Treatment for first-degree AV block is typically not required unless accompanied by symptomatic bradycardia. It is doubtful that this cardiac rhythm is related to this patient's signs and symptoms.

3. What is your field impression of this patient?

The first thing to note is the patient's extremely elevated blood pressure of 210/170 mm Hg, which is clearly indicative of a hypertensive emergency. Furthermore, the following assessment findings support a field impression of *acute hypertensive encephalopathy:*

- Disorientation
- Severe headache
- Nausea
- Diplopia (double vision) and photophobia (light sensitivity)

Hypertensive encephalopathy is a life-threatening complication of severe hypertension, in which the diastolic blood pressure is 140 mm Hg or greater. If the condition is left untreated, it can result in irreversible damage to the heart, kidneys, or brain within a matter of a few hours.

Signs and symptoms of acute hypertensive encephalopathy include severe headache, nausea and vomiting, visual disturbances, and confusion. In severe cases, paralysis, coma, and seizures may occur.

Although conditions such as intracranial hemorrhage and pheochromocytoma (an adrenal tumor that produces epinephrine) can cause hypertensive encephalopathy, it is most commonly the result of noncompliance with antihypertensive medications in a patient with an established history of hypertension.

4. Are the patient's vital signs and SAMPLE history consistent with your field impression?

The patient's diastolic blood pressure (≥140 mm Hg) is consistent with a hypertensive crisis. Her respiratory and pulse rates are within normal limits; however, her pulse is bounding, which is common when the blood pressure is excessively elevated.

Any time a patient tells you that he or she is having the worst headache of their life, you should be concerned. That information alone will usually ensure that a computed tomographic (CT) scan of the head is performed at the hospital.

The patient's history of hypertension clearly predisposes her to hypertensive crisis, and her antihypertensive medications reinforce her history.

- Prazosin (Minipress) is a selective alpha-adrenergic blocker used to treat hypertension. Prazosin dilates arterioles and veins, thereby decreasing total peripheral vascular resistance and decreasing diastolic blood pressure more so than systolic blood pressure. Unlike beta-blocking drugs, prazosin does not cause a decrease in heart rate or cardiac output, since it does not have an effect on the heart (selective beta).

- Chlorothiazide (Diuril) is a thiazide diuretic drug commonly prescribed in combination with alpha- or beta-blocking drugs in the treatment of hypertension. Thiazides promote diuresis by decreasing the rate at which sodium and chloride are reabsorbed in the distal renal tubules in the kidney. This effect promotes the excretion of additional water from the body. Thiazides also have an antihypertensive effect, which is attributed to direct dilation of the arterioles as well as a reduction in the total fluid volume of the body.

5. What specific treatment is required for this patient's condition?

The goal in treating a hypertensive emergency involves a *rapid, yet controlled* lowering of the patient's blood pressure. If the blood pressure is lowered too fast, infarction of the heart, brain, or kidneys can occur.

In most circumstances, pharmacological therapy for hypertensive encephalopathy is initiated in controlled setting of a hospital; however, if transport to the hospital is lengthy, or in severe cases (eg, when the patient is unconscious), medical control may order one of the following medications:

- **Labetalol (Trandate, Normodyne)**
  - 20 mg via slow IV push administered over 2 minutes
  - May repeat at 40 to 80 mg every 10 minutes until the desired effect is achieved or a total dose of 300 mg has been administered
- **Nitroglycerin (Nitro-Bid, Tridil, Isordil, NTG)**
  - Start the IV infusion at 10 µg/min and titrate to the desired effect. Do not exceed 20 mcg/min.
  - Must predilute in D_5W, place in a glass bottle, and use an infusion pump
- **Nitroprusside sodium (Nipride)**
  - Mix 50 or 100 mg in 250 mL of D_5W *only*.
  - Start the IV infusion at 0.10 µg/kg/min and titrate upward until the desired effect is achieved. The maximum dose is 5 µg/kg/min.
  - Place opaque material around IV bottle, use an infusion pump, and carefully monitor the patient's blood pressure

Nitroglycerin would be the most common pharmacological agent used for acute hypertensive emergencies in the field, as Labetalol and Nipride are not commonly carried on the ambulance.

Placing the patient in a comfortable position and dimming the lights in the ambulance may afford the patient some relief from her headache. The patient must be transported to the hospital immediately, while monitoring airway, breathing, and circulation en route.

6. Is further treatment required for this patient?

Although the patient is less confused and disoriented, she is still dangerously hypertensive and complaining of a severe headache. At the discretion of medical control, additional medication dosing may be required. Depending on the medication that you are administering, this may involve titrating the infusion upwards (eg, Nipride, NTG), or administering another bolus dose (eg, Labetalol).

Further treatment for this patient should be supportive, which involves continuous monitoring of her airway, breathing, and circulation, and making her as comfortable as possible.

7. Are there any special considerations for this patient?

This patient is at risk for acute hemorrhagic stroke because of her significant hypertension; therefore, you must continually monitor her signs and symptoms that would indicate stroke.

Signs of acute hemorrhagic stroke include a sudden loss of consciousness and signs of increased intracranial pressure, such as bradycardia, posturing, and irregular respirations that are either fast or slow. If signs of a hemorrhagic stroke become evident, nitroglycerin would be contraindicated and should be stopped if it is being administered. Nitroglycerin would exacerbate intracranial bleeding due to its vasodilatory effects. Preparations for endotracheal intubation should be made for definitive airway control in the event that intubation becomes necessary.

Summary

Hypertensive emergencies can pose a unique challenge for the paramedic, usually because the medications used to treat them are not available for field use (eg, Nipride, Labetalol), or protocols will not allow for the emergent lowering of the blood pressure in the prehospital setting.

The priorities of care are to identify the hypertensive emergency, take measures to support airway, breathing, and circulation, and immediately transport the patient to the hospital where the blood pressure can be rapidly lowered in a controlled environment. If the patient is unconscious or otherwise unable to protect their own airway, intubation should be performed.

In a conscious patient, dimming the lights in the ambulance and allowing the patient to assume a comfortable position may provide relief from the severe headache that classically accompanies a hypertensive emergency.

Hypertensive encephalopathy, if left untreated, can result in irreversible damage to the heart, kidneys, and brain. Damage to these organs may be so severe that they are no longer able to support life.

Section 6: Special Considerations

Chapter 40: Neonatology

Matching

1. H (page 40.30)	**8.** E (page 40.10)
2. N (page 40.26)	**9.** C (page 40.31)
3. I (page 40.7)	**10.** G (page 40.30)
4. A (page 40.19)	**11.** M (page 40.9)
5. K (page 40.20)	**12.** J (page 40.21)
6. B (page 40.6)	**13.** L (page 40.11)
7. D (page 40.10)	**14.** F (page 40.16)

Multiple Choice

1. D (page 40.7)	**6.** A (page 40.18)
2. A (page 40.7)	**7.** D (page 40.10)
3. C (page 40.9)	**8.** C (page 40.19)
4. C (page 40.10)	**9.** A (page 40.20)
5. D (page 40.19)	**10.** D (page 40.21)

Labeling

1.

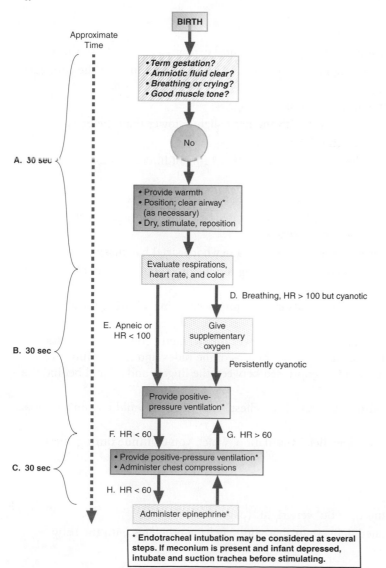

(page 40.15)

Fill-in-the-Blank

1. Transition, pulmonary, oxygen (page 40.7)
2. 37, 38, 42 (page 40.7)
3. Umbilical cord, blood supply, pressure (page 40.8)
4. Cyanotic, vigorous, thermoregulation (page 40.9)
5. Pneumothorax, compressions, palpable (page 40.10)
6. Rarely, obstruction, choanal atresia (page 40.10)
7. Decompression, orogastric, diaphragmatic (page 40.14)
8. Seizure, newborn (page 40.21)
9. Infections, temperature, hypoglycemia, metabolic (page 40.23)
10. Hypoglycemia, apnea, feeding, lethargy, seizures (page 40.24)
11. Mucus, blood, uncommon (page 40.24)
12. Antiemetics, resuscitation, fontanelle (page 40.25)
13. Dehydrated, obtunded, compressions (page 40.26)
14. Community hospital, equipment, regional center (page 40.27)
15. Viral infection (page 40.25)

Identify

1. **a.** If the umbilical cord comes out ahead of the baby, the blood supply through the umbilical cord may be cut off. In this case:
   (1) Relieving pressure on the cord (by gently moving the presenting part of the body off the cord and pushing the cord back) can be lifesaving.
   (2) When the baby's head is delivered, suction the mouth and nose with a bulb syringe.
   (3) After the infant is delivered, keep the baby at the level of the mother, with the head slightly lower than the body.
   (4) Clamp the umbilical cord in two places, and then cut between the clamps.
   (5) Your initial rapid assessment of the newborn may be done simultaneously with any treatment interventions.
   (6) Note the time of delivery, and monitor the ABCs.
   (7) In particular, assess respiratory rate, respiratory effort, pulse rate, color, and capillary refill. (page 40.8)

2. **a.** If the baby is apneic (ie, has a 20-second or longer respiratory pause) or has a pulse rate less than 100 beats/min after 30 seconds of drying and stimulation and supplemental free-flow (blow-by) oxygen:
   (1) Begin positive-pressure ventilation (PPV) by bag-mask device, being sure to use a newborn-sized bag mask.
   (2) You should use caution when squeezing the bag to avoid inadvertently delivering too much volume, potentially resulting in a pneumothorax. (page 40.15)

   b. Chest compressions are indicated if the pulse rate remains less than 60 beats/min despite positioning, clearing the airway, drying and stimulation, and 30 seconds of effective PPV:
   (1) With the thumb (two-rescuer) technique, two thumbs are placed side by side over the sternum between the nipples, and the hands encircle the torso. With the two-finger (one-rescuer) technique, the tips of the index and middle fingers are placed over the sternum between the nipples and the sternum is compressed between the fingers and a hand behind the baby's back.
   (2) The depth of compression is one third of the anteroposterior diameter of the chest. Your fingers should remain in contact with the chest at all times.
   (3) In neonates, the chest compressions occur in synchrony with artificial ventilation, which you continue during chest compressions.

Ambulance Calls

1. If you were expecting problems in delivering this 38-year-old multip, you were right. (page 40.6)
   a. Yes, there are several indications that this may be a complicated delivery or that you may have problems with the baby afterward:
   (1) Maternal age greater than 35 years
   (2) No prenatal care
   (3) Prolonged labor

   (4) Meconium staining of the amniotic fluid

   (5) Probable postterm baby (It's hard to know how much to trust the mother's estimate of the gestational age.) (page 40.6)

b. Students should provide four of the following. Other risk factors for obstetric and neonatal complications include:

   (1) Maternal diabetes

   (2) Maternal drug or alcohol abuse

   (3) Antepartum hemorrhage

   (4) Twin pregnancy

   (5) Abnormal presentation

   (6) Prolapsed umbilical cord

   (7) Fetal distress

c. When the baby's head delivers and is found to be covered with meconium:

   (1) Clean the mouth and nostrils with sterile gauze.

   (2) Use a bulb aspirator to suction the mouth and nostrils.

d. Once the baby is fully delivered:

   (1) Quickly dry off the baby.

   (2) Clamp and cut the cord.

   (3) Hand off the baby to your partner to intubate and suction as needed.

   (4) If the baby does not breathe spontaneously, give several breaths with bag-mask device and oxygen.

   (5) Finish drying the baby, and cover with warm blankets.

2. *Return of the Spider Monster* is not recommended viewing for an impressionable woman in the third trimester of pregnancy. Look what can happen!

a. When you find yourself holding a newborn premature infant that had the temerity to be born before you could even open your obstetrics (OB) kit, take the following steps:

   (1) Suction the mouth and nostrils with a bulb syringe.

   (2) Quickly dry the baby with whatever you have available.

   (3) As soon as possible, wrap the baby in something warm.

   (4) When your partner brings the OB kit, clamp and cut the cord. (page 40.8)

b. Hypothermia is an increased risk for morbidity and mortality. However, if the newborn appears otherwise healthy, it is appropriate to clamp and cut the cord. It may also be necessary to cut and clamp the cord to resuscitate in the prehospital setting. (pages 40.29, 40.23)

c. The things you can do to try to prevent the baby from becoming hypothermic are the following:

   (1) Dry the baby thoroughly.

   (2) Place cap on the baby's head.

   (3) Cover the baby with a warm blanket.

   (5) Keep the baby on the mother's body.

   (6) In the ambulance, turn on the heaters full blast until the ambient temperature increases to around 35°C (95°F), even if it's summer! (page 40.23)

d. Besides keeping the baby warm, you need to do the following:

   (1) Take particular care to maintain a patent airway.

   (2) Administer supplemental oxygen into a tent or by blow-by.

   (3) Wear a surgical mask and gown to protect the baby from infection.

3. You think this case is exaggerated? You don't believe that teenage girls give birth on the toilet? In fact, this scenario is based on an actual case managed by real paramedics.

a. Immediately upon rescuing the infant from the toilet, you must do the following:

   (1) Dry off the baby, preferably with warm towels, and cover with a warm blanket.

   (2) Suction the mouth and nostrils.

   (3) Stimulate the baby to breathe.

   (4) Clamp and cut the umbilical cord.

   (5) Administer supplemental oxygen.

b. The indications for starting artificial ventilation are as follows:

   (1) Apnea

   (2) A heart rate less than 100 beats/min

   (3) Persisting central cyanosis despite 100% supplemental oxygen

c. After a minute of artificial ventilation, you find the heart rate to be 84 beats/min. You should continue artificial ventilation only.

d. When you check again, however, the pulse rate has dropped below 60 beats/min, so at that point you should start external chest compressions at 120 per minute.

e. The indications for epinephrine are

   (1) Asystole

   (2) A heart rate persistently below 80 beats/min despite adequate artificial ventilation with 100% supplemental oxygen and high-quality external chest compressions

f. The recommended concentration for newborns is 1:10,000. The recommended dose is 0.1 to 0.3 mL/kg of 1:10,000.

True/False

1. T (page 40.13)   **6.** F (page 40.29)

2. F (page 40.19)   **7.** F (page 40.17)

3. T (page 40.8)   **8.** F (page 40.26)

4. T (page 40.29)   **9.** T (page 40.25)

5. T (page 40.23)   **10.** T (page 40.19)

Short Answer

1. Catheterization of the Umbilical Vein. (page 40.16)

a. Clean the cord with alcohol or another antiseptic. Place a sterile tie firmly, but not too tightly, around the base of the cord to control bleeding. Place a sterile drape over the site. Maintain sterile technique as much as possible.

b. Prefill a sterile 3.5F to 5F umbilical vein line catheter (a comparable-size sterile feeding tube can be used in an emergency) with normal saline using a 3-mL syringe.

c. Cut the cord with a scalpel below the clamp placed on the cord at birth about 1 to 2 cm from the skin (between the clamp and the cord tie).

d. The umbilical vein is a large, thin-walled vessel usually found at the 12 o'clock position, as compared to the two thick-walled umbilical arteries usually found at 4 and 8 o'clock . Insert the catheter into this vein for a distance of 2 to 4 cm (less in preterm infants) until blood can be aspirated. If the catheter is advanced into the liver, the infusion of hypertonic solutions may lead to irreversible damage. If the catheter is advanced into the heart, arrhythmias may develop.

e. Flush the catheter with 0.5 mL of normal saline and tape it in place.

2. Intubate a Neonate. (page 40.13)

a. Be sure the newborn is preoxygenated by bag-mask ventilation with 100% supplemental oxygen prior to making an intubation attempt.

b. Suction the oropharynx to remove any secretions.

c. Place the laryngoscope blade in the oropharynx, and then visualize the vocal cords. Place the endotracheal (ET) tube between the vocal cords until the black line on the tube is at the level of the cords.

Word Find

```
Y Q F O J S N P I N I F F D N W S
T R E V E Q L L S I S O D I C A H
M I E T F O R A M E N O V A L E U
R U E T W J E C V V M B M X F E N
P J I R R T R E T L D C M L M A T
L R O N A A N N Y A R Y U Y D G X
A C E N O A L T L C U T E R U S C
Y E O M C C H A G I A Z N A U N E
M E N A A X E N C L D T I V Y R K
N I V P D T B M V I N K R O Y I R
F A A S A X U L V B L C E I O J M
B H H O H U X R C M I I P W A K I
L E R P U E W E E U K O B G L G C
O T G B P T Z N Q S C I X M W S F
A D V N G X D W K C V F K I U P R
V Q C J Z N K C O H S Z N M L Z G
S U S O I R E T R A S U T C U D B
```

1. Oxygenated blood from the **placenta** (page 40.7) enters the fetus in the **umbilical vein** (Figure 40.1). It flows through the liver into the inferior **vena cava** (Figure 40.1). Leaving that vessel, a large proportion of the oxygenated blood flows directly across the **atria** through a hole called the **foramen ovale** (Figure 40.1), thereby bypassing the lungs. When blood goes from the right side of the heart to the left side of the heart without picking up oxygen in the lungs, it is called a **shunt** (Figure 40.1). Another direct connection, the **ductus arteriosus** (Figure 40.1), links the fetal pulmonary artery to the **aorta** (Figure 40.1). Both of these connections close very soon after birth. After circulating through the fetus, blood enters an **umbilical artery** (Figure 40.1) to return to the placenta.

2. The newborn, or **neonate** (page 40.6), is very vulnerable to hypothermia. It is important to try to prevent hypothermia from occurring in the newborn because hypothermia may lead to **acidosis** (page 40.18), which in turn may lead to **shock** (page 40.10). A baby born before the 38th week of pregnancy or weighing less than 2.5 kg is considered to be **premature** (page 40.20) and is at higher risk of hypothermia.

3. When fetal stool, called **meconium** (page 40.30), is expelled into the amniotic fluid, it may find its way into the fetal airway before birth and then be aspirated deep into the airway when the baby takes its first breath. The result may be a complete failure to breathe at all, called **apnea** (page 40.19).

4. The womb: **uterus** (page 40.7)

5. The organ where eggs reside: **ovary**

6. The region between the vagina and the anus: **perineum** (page 40.29)

Fill-in-the-Table

1.

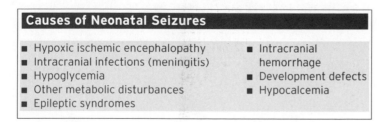

Causes of Neonatal Seizures	
■ Hypoxic ischemic encephalopathy	■ Intracranial hemorrhage
■ Intracranial infections (meningitis)	
■ Hypoglycemia	■ Development defects
■ Other metabolic disturbances	■ Hypocalcemia
■ Epileptic syndromes	

(page 40.21)

Problem Solving

1. The Apgar score is: 4

2. The Apgar score is: 13 (page 40.10)

Skill Drill

1. *Intubation of a Neonate* (page 40.14)

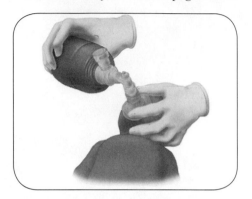

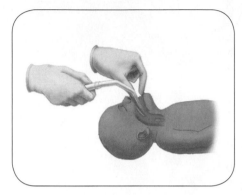

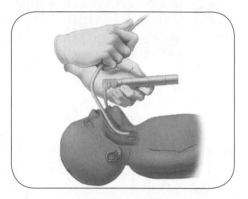

Step 1: Preoxygenate the infant by bag-mask ventilation with 100% supplemental oxygen.

Step 2: Suction the oropharynx. Provide bag-mask ventilation if bradycardia results.

Step 3: Place the laryngoscope blade in the oropharynx. Visualize the vocal cords. Place the endotracheal (ET) tube between the vocal cords until the black line on the ET tube is at the level of the cords.

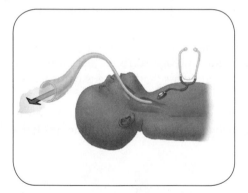

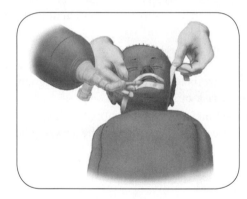

Step 4: Confirm placement. Observe chest rise, auscultate laterally and high on the chest, note the absence of significant air sounds over the stomach, and note mist in the ET tube.

Step 5: Tape the ET tube in place. Monitor the newborn closely for complications.

Chapter 41: Pediatrics

Matching

1. E	(page 41.8)	**9.** E (page 41.7)
2. A	(page 41.7)	**10.** A, B, C, D, E (page 41.47)
3. D	(page 41.7)	**11.** D (page 41.7)
4. B	(page 41.7)	**12.** B (page 41.7)
5. A, B	(page 41.7)	**13.** A (page 41.7)
6. D, E	(page 41.7)	**14.** E (page 41.7)
7. A	(page 41.6)	**15.** D (page 41.7)
8. A, B, C, D, E (page 41.15)		

Multiple Choice

1. C (page 41.48)	**6.** D (page 41.10)
2. C (page 41.49)	**7.** A (page 41.52)
3. D (page 41.50)	**8.** D (page 41.55
4. D (page 41.8)	**9.** C (page 41.58)
5. B (page 41.9)	**10.** C (page 41.22)

Labeling

1.

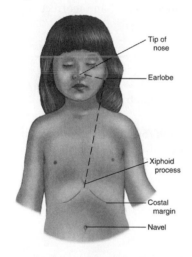

Tip of nose

Earlobe

Xiphoid process

Costal margin

Navel

(page 41.30)

Fill-in-the-Blank

1. Tolerated, oropharyngeal (page 41.22)

2. Blow-by technique (page 41.24)

3. Always, ventilation, airway management (page 41.24)

4. Teeth, aspiration, bradycardia, placement (page 41.26)

5. Parasympathetic, bradycardia, cardiac, pulse oximeter (page 41.27)

6. Hypovolemic, distributive, cardiogenic. (page 41.31)

7. Hypovolemic, tachypnea, pale, mottled, cyanotic (page 41.32)

8. Sunken eyes, mucous membranes, turgor, delayed (page 41.32)

9. Compartment syndrome, injury, infection (page 41.33)

10. Uncommon, congenital, rhythm (page 41.34)

Identify

1. a. Chief complaint: Respiratory distress (probably the croup)

b. Vital signs: Normal capillary refill, oxygen saturation of 95%, conscious alert, audible stridor

c. Pertinent negatives: Age-appropriate behavior, recognizes her mother

2. a. Chief complaint: Infant unrestrained and ejected during fatal motor vehicle crash

b. Vital signs: Age-appropriate LOC, skin color normal, skin is warm and dry. Normal capillary refill. Oxygen saturation of 96%. Pulse rate of 150 beats/min.

c. Pertinent negatives: No obvious external bleeding; assessment is unremarkable

3. a. Chief complaint: Seizure, probably a febrile seizure.

b. Vital signs: Skin ashen, warm, and dry. A rectal temperature of 100.3°F. Patient responds to pain. Her oxygen saturation is 98%. Pupils are sluggish but equal. Patient has equal bilateral breath sounds. The remainder of exam is unremarkable.

c. Pertinent negatives: The patient's mother denies any other medications, history, or allergies to medications. She further denies any recent injury or trauma to the child.

Ambulance Calls

1.The scene of a collision where a child has been injured is probably the most stressful environment that a paramedic will enter.

a. (1) Fracture of the left femur

(2) Ruptured spleen

(3) Injury to the right side of the head

b. Perhaps hardest to deal with at a collision scene like the one described are the feelings and behaviors of the child's parents.

(1) Obviously, there is no "correct" answer to the question of how you feel when assaulted by an angry parent. If you're normal, however, you'll probably feel angry.

(2) What you do with your feelings is another matter, and there is a correct way to handle the situation and an incorrect way. The correct way is as follows:

(a) Mentally count to 10 before you reply to the angry father.

(b) Stay calm.

(c) Don't raise your voice.

(d) Try to enlist the father's help in caring for the child; give him something constructive to do, such as fetching the backboard from the ambulance or folding triangular bandages into cravats. (page 41.8)

c. The child's vital signs (pulse = 120 beats/min, respirations = 24 breaths/min, and blood pressure = 90/60 mm Hg) are normal for his age (answer 3). The slight tachycardia is easily explained by the pain and excitement of the situation.

2. When 2-year-old Tammy starts barking in the middle of the night, it's a great attention-getter.

a. The vital signs are abnormal for her age. There is tachycardia and tachypnea.

b. The most likely diagnosis is croup.

c. The steps of prehospital management are as follows:

(1) Give humidified supplemental oxygen while you set up a nebulizer.

(2) Nebulized epinephrine is available in two formulations: racemic epinephrine and L-epinephrine. The dose for racemic epinephrine (2.25%) is 0.5 mL mixed in 3 mL of normal saline. The dose for L-epinephrine is 0.25 to 0.5 mg/kg of the 1:1,000 solution (maximum, 5 mg per dose); this form can be diluted with normal saline to bring the volume to 3 mL. (page 41.19)

(3) Place the child in a position of comfort.

(4) **Notify** the receiving hospital of the case.

(5) **Transport** without delay.

3. Diffuse wheezing and respiratory distress in a child under a year of age are the tip-offs in this case.

a. The vital signs are abnormal. The baby has tachycardia, tachypnea, and a slight elevation in blood pressure. (page 41.21)

b. The most likely diagnosis is bronchiolitis.

c. The steps of prehospital management are as follows:

(1) Give humidified oxygen.

(2) Assist ventilations gently with a bag-mask ventilator.

(3) Consult medical command as to whether to give a trial of bronchodilators.

(4) Keep the intubation kit handy in case of apnea.

(5) Monitor cardiac rhythm.

(6) Transport without delay. (page 41.21)

4. a. When little Bobby develops severe respiratory distress and signs of airway obstruction over a very short time, and he does not have a high fever, the most likely diagnosis is foreign body obstruction of the airway, that is, choking.

b. The steps of managing a choking child are as follows:

(1) Kneel on one knee behind the child, and circle his or her body by placing both arms around the child's chest. Prepare to give abdominal thrusts by placing your fist just above the patient's umbilicus and well below the xiphoid process. Place your other hand over that fist.

(2) Give the child rapid, distinct abdominal thrusts in an upward direction. Be careful to avoid applying force to the lower ribcage or sternum.

(3) Repeat this standing technique until the child expels the foreign body or becomes unresponsive.

(4) If the child becomes unresponsive, place him or her supine on a firm, flat surface and inspect the airway using the head tilt–chin lift. If you can see the foreign body, try to remove it. Do not perform blind finger sweeps.

(5) Attempt rescue breathing. If the first attempt fails, reposition the head and try again.

(6) If the airway remains obstructed, begin cardiopulmonary resuscitation (CPR) with chest compressions at the 30:2 compression/ventilation ratio and prepare for immediate transport. If you manage to clear the airway obstruction in an unresponsive child (older than 1 year), but he or she remains apneic and pulseless, begin CPR and attach the automated external defibrillator (AED) as soon as possible, using appropriately sized AED pads. If you are unable to relieve the obstruction after several attempts, transport immediately.

(7) If the child loses consciousness, start CPR. Initiate transportation. Consider **direct laryngoscopy** to remove the foreign body under direct vision. (page 41.18)

c. Compress the chest about one third to one half its total depth. Push hard and fast (100 compressions/min), and allow full chest recoil.

d. Check the femoral pulse in infants and young children and the carotid pulse in older children and adolescents. (page 41.12)

e. Place the heel of your hand over the middle of the sternum (between the nipples). Avoid compression over the lower tip of the sternum, which is called the xiphoid process. (page 41.2)

f. The defibrillation dosage for a 12-kg child is 24 joules (2 joules/kg).

g. Anything that can be administered IV can be administered through an intraosseous line (such as isotonic fluids, medications). (page 41.33)

5. A sudden, severe sore throat along with a high fever should start some warning lights blinking in your brain.

a. The vital signs are abnormal. The child has both tachycardia and tachypnea, not to mention his very **high fever.**

b. The most likely diagnosis is epiglottitis.

c. The steps in prehospital management are as follows:

(1) Approach the child very gently so as not to disturb him.

(2) Give humidified supplemental oxygen.

(3) Place the child in a position of comfort.

(4) Notify the receiving hospital to have the appropriate specialists standing by.

(5) Transport without delay. (page 41.20)

d. The special *danger* threatening this child is complete airway obstruction from epiglottal swelling, which may occur literally within minutes.

6. The little boy having an asthmatic attack during nature study is already in bad shape by the time you arrive on the scene.

a. Five signs that suggest he is in bad shape are his

(1) Drowsiness (a sign of carbon dioxide retention)

(2) Pulsus paradoxus of 40 mmHg

(3) Cyanosis, indicating hypoxemia

(4) Hyperinflated chest, indicating obstruction to exhalation

(5) Silent chest, indicating that practically no air is moving in and out (page 41.20)

b. The steps in managing this case are as follows:

(1) Give humidified supplemental oxygen by mask while preparing the nebulizer.

(2) Start an IV.

(3) Give a nebulized bronchodilator, such as albuterol, 0.5 mL in 3 mL of normal saline, with oxygen as the carrier gas.

(4) Monitor cardiac rhythm.

(5) Ask your dispatcher to notify the child's parents and request that they meet you in the emergency department.

(6) Transport the child in a position of comfort.

7. Most calls you receive for asthmatic attacks will be for patients already known to have asthma. Such patients will not call for help unless there is something different about this particular attack.

a. Questions to ask in taking the history of a child having an acute asthmatic attack include the following:

(1) How long has the attack been going on?

(2) What medications has the child already taken? When? In what dosage?

(3) How much fluid has the child managed to take?

(4) Does the child have any allergies?

(5) Has the child had any hospitalizations for asthma? If so, when? (page 41.20)

b. It's easier to remember medications to give in an acute asthmatic attack if you know what you are giving them *for.* When giving albuterol, you need to know:

(1) The *contraindication* in children: diabetes

(2) The possible *adverse side effects:* palpitations, tremors, nervousness, dizziness, nausea

(3) Metered dose inhaler (MDI) with a spacer-mask device. Unit doses of 2.5 mg of albuterol premixed with 3 mL of normal saline are often used for nebulization and represent an acceptable starting dose for most young children. (page 41.21)

8. There is no easy answer to the question of how to respond in a case of sudden infant death syndrome (SIDS). Each case will be a little different, and your response should be guided by local protocols and personal judgment. You need to make a quick appraisal to decide whether the mother already realizes that the baby is dead. If not, it might be worth starting CPR, so that she can feel, afterward, that everything possible was done. If you do start CPR, do it right; go through all the steps as you would for a baby you expected to survive. If, on the other hand, you feel that the mother already knows that her baby is dead, it may be better to take the more difficult option, and that is to confirm her worst fears. Should you do so, you must be prepared to spend time with the mother and to deal with her grief.

As this case illustrates, when you do confront a case of crib death, you will have to make an instant decision on the spot regarding how to proceed. If you haven't prepared yourself ahead of time for such decisions, it could be one of the longest instants of your experience. (page 41.46)

9. Seizures in children are a lot like seizures in adults, but they tend to be considerably more upsetting to all concerned.

a. Seizures in children result from the following causes. *Students should provide five of the following:*

(1) Head trauma

(2) Meningitis

(3) Fever

(4) Hypoglycemia

(5) Hypoxia

(6) Failure of a known epileptic to take prescribed medications

(7) Abuse of drugs (yes, in children) (page 41.42)

b. There are specific questions to ask in taking the history of a child who has had a seizure. *Students should provide five of the following:*

(1) Is this the child's first seizure?

(2) How many seizures has the child had today?

(3) Has the child had a fever? Stiff neck? Headache?

(4) Might the child have ingested a toxic product?

(5) Is there a family history of seizures?

(6) If the child is known to have seizures, did he take his medication today?

(7) What did the seizure look like? (page 41.43)

c. In performing the physical assessment of a child who has had a seizure, look in particular for the following signs. *Students should provide five of the following:*

   (1) Changes in the state of consciousness

   (2) Skin temperature and moisture (febrile seizure?)

   (3) Evidence of head trauma

   (4) Equality and reactivity of the pupils

   (5) Stiff neck

   (6) Signs of injury sustained during the seizure (eg, dislocation of the shoulder) (page 41.43)

d. From all of the information you obtain about this child, you conclude that he probably had a febrile seizure. The prehospital treatment is as follows:

   (1) Maintain the airway.

   (2) Transport him to the hospital. (page 41.43)

10. The 14-year-old, unlike the previous patient, is in status epilepticus.

a. The steps in treatment are as follows:

   (1) Treatment at the scene will be limited to supportive care if the seizure has stopped by the time of your arrival.

   (2) Status epilepticus requires more extensive intervention. For a child with ongoing seizure activity, open the airway using the chin-lift or jaw-thrust maneuver. Very proximal airway obstruction is common during a seizure or postictal state because the tongue and jaw fall backward as a result of the decreased muscle tone associated with altered mental status.

   (3) If the airway is not maintainable with positioning, consider inserting a nasopharyngeal airway.

   (4) Suction for secretions or vomitus, and consider the lateral decubitus position in case of ongoing vomiting. Do not attempt to intubate during an active seizure because endotracheal intubation in this setting is associated with serious complications and is rarely successful. You are better off using BLS airway management, stopping the seizure, and then considering the child's need for ALS airway support.

   (5) Provide 100% supplemental oxygen to the patient, and start bag-mask ventilation as indicated for hypoventilation. Consider placing a nasogastric (NG) tube to decompress the stomach if the patient requires assisted ventilation.

   (6) Assess the child for IV sites. Measure the serum glucose level, and treat any documented hypoglycemia.

   (7) Consider your options for anticonvulsant administration. (page 41.43)

b. The *contraindications* to giving diazepam are pregnancy, respiratory depression, hypotension, and previous ingestion of alcohol or sedative drugs.

c. The possible *side effects* include apnea, hypotension, and even cardiac arrest. (page 41.44)

11. Whenever you are called to deal with injury in an infant or very young child, you must always keep the possibility of child abuse in the back of your mind.

a. What's fishy about this particular story is the claim that the 10-month-old "stepped on a cigarette." At the age of 10 months, most babies are just beginning to stand up (holding on) and are not yet walking, so it's hard to imagine how a 10-month-old would manage to step on a cigarette.

b. Clues to child abuse include the following:

   (1) Parental behavior: vague, evasive, hostile

   (2) Discrepancies in the history

   (3) Delay in seeking care

   (4) A child who looks generally neglected (dirty, unkempt)

   (5) A child who does not turn to his parents for comfort

   (6) A child who does not cry

   (7) The presence of multiple bruises of multiple vintages

   (8) Injuries in and around the mouth

   (9) Suspicious burns (as in the present case; or scald burns without splash marks)

   (10) Fractures in an infant less than a year old

c. The steps in caring for this particular child are as follows:

   (1) Put a sterile dressing on the burn.

   (2) Transport the child to the hospital.

   (3) Notify the physician in private of your suspicions.

(4) Fill out whatever legal forms are required.

(5) Document everything on your PCR.

d. What if the parent refuses to permit you to transport the child? Your service should have a policy established in advance to deal with such situations. Here are some suggestions:

(1) Try to persuade the parent to change his or her mind. Do so in a calm, professional manner.

(2) Call for law enforcement.

(3) Document the entire call, including a list of whom you notified, on your PCR.

Remember, the abused child may be in life-threatening danger. If you fail to report a suspected case of child abuse, the next call to the same address may be for a dead child. (page 41.47, 41.48)

12. The baby who fell from the balcony has sustained a serious head injury. (Did you notice the signs of increasing intracranial pressure?) The prehospital treatment is as follows:

a. Maintain an open airway (use an oropharyngeal airway if the baby becomes unconscious). Anticipate vomiting, and have suction at hand.

b. Administer supplemental oxygen.

c. Immobilize the spine with a baby backboard or a pediatric backboard with folded towels to elevate the baby's back slightly.

d. Start transport.

e. Ventilate the baby with a bag-mask device.

f. Notify the receiving hospital. (page 41.51)

13. You have two injured children in this collision.

a. The first child has an *abdominal injury* and early *shock*. He is therefore in the load-and-go category. His prehospital treatment is as follows:

(1) Maintain an open airway. Anticipate vomiting, and keep suction at hand.

(2) Administer oxygen.

(3) Immobilize the child on a backboard

(4) Start transport.

(5) Notify the receiving hospital.

(6) Start an IV en route to the hospital.

(7) Splint the broken arm. (page 41.52)

b. The second child has a *tension pneumothorax* (the clues were his extreme respiratory distress, tracheal deviation, and a point of maximal impulse (PMI) shifted to the left). He is also in the load-and-go category, but only after critical interventions, including decompression of the pneumothorax, have been carried out.

(1) Ensure a patent airway.

(2) Administer supplemental oxygen.

(3) Decompress the pneumothorax by inserting a 14-gauge angiocath into the fourth right intercostal space in the midclavicular line.

(4) Immobilize the child on a backboard.

(5) Start transport.

(6) Notify the receiving hospital.

(7) Monitor cardiac rhythm (myocardial contusion is likely).

(8) Start an IV lifeline en route to the hospital. (page 41.52)

14. a. The infant removed from the smoky house fire should be intubated because he was unconscious in a smoky environment and therefore at high risk for respiratory complications.

b. Other factors that put a pediatric fire victim at high risk for airway obstruction and that are therefore indications for immediate intubation include the following. *Students should provide five of the following:*

(1) Stridor

(2) Wheezing

(3) Signs of respiratory distress

(4) Facial burns

(5) Singed eyebrows

(6) Red, edematous mouth

(7) Carbonaceous sputum (page 41.55)

15. a. Abdominal thrusts (Heimlich maneuver) are recommended to relieve a severe airway obstruction in a conscious child. Have little Johnny's mom call 9-1-1. Hopefully, you can dislodge the peanuts and uneventfully return to the football game. But what if you can't?

  b. Follow these steps to remove a foreign body obstruction from a conscious child who is in a standing position:

   (1) Kneel on one knee behind the child, and circle his or her body by placing both arms around the child's chest. Prepare to give abdominal thrusts by placing your fist just above the patient's umbilicus and well below the xiphoid process. Place your other hand over that fist.

   (2) Give the child rapid, distinct abdominal thrusts in an upward direction. Be careful to avoid applying force to the lower ribcage or sternum.

   (3) Repeat this standing technique until the child expels the foreign body or becomes unresponsive.

   (4) If the child becomes unresponsive, place him or her supine on a firm, flat surface and inspect the airway using the head tilt–chin lift. If you can see the foreign body, try to remove it. Do not perform blind finger sweeps.

   (5) Attempt rescue breathing. If the first attempt fails, reposition the head and try again.

   (6) If the airway remains obstructed, begin CPR with chest compressions at the 30:2 compression-to-ventilation ratio and prepare for immediate transport. If you manage to clear the airway obstruction in an unresponsive child (older than 1 year), but he or she remains apneic and pulseless, begin CPR. (page 41.18)

True/False

1. F (page 41.13)   **9.** F (page 41.26)

2. F (page 41.40   **10.** T (page 41.26)

3. T (page 41.6)   **11.** T (page 41.26)

4. T (page 41.9)   **12.** F (page 41.6)

5. T (page 41.49)   **13.** T (page 41.55)

6. F (page 41.50)   **14.** F (page 41.52)

7. F (page 41.22)   **15.** T (page 41.37)

8. F (page 41.31)

Short Answer

1. Signs of hypovolemia and shock in infants and children include the following. *Students should provide six of the following:*

  a. Apathy and listlessness

  b. Cold, pale, mottled skin

  c. Prolonged capillary refill (longer than 2 seconds)

  d. Collapsed veins

  e. Increasing abdominal girth

  f. Tachycardia and tachypnea

  g. Scanty urine output (page 41.32)

2. Load-and-go situations in children include the following. *Students should provide ten of the following:*

  a. Fall from a height of more than 2 times the height of child

  b. Child involved in an collision with fatalities

  c. Child ejected from a car in a motor vehicle crash

  d. Child who was struck by a car while walking or biking

  e. Child in whom you are unable to secure an airway

  f. Respiratory arrest

  g. Open pneumothorax

  h. Tension pneumothorax

  i. Cardiac arrest

  j. Shock

  k. Uncontrollable bleeding

  l. Coma or deteriorating level of consciousness

  m. Signs of increasing intracranial pressure (page 41.52)

Word Find

```
O K Q F T M R S P J R N G B V I I Q W B J W K Z I D K Y
D E Z H G K N Y M S G V R W S Y Y L B W P H L I Q E A G
I E M A F I E X H G B W Z U X C H Z B O F O R C A E B M
E Z Z O F V U H U L Z I C H Q I O R D X V F Z L I U I H
N H U F R H Q M Y R N J J B L Q T O Z A D E C E P F P X
P S I E D D I H B P Z P Q G W S F X A G Z T K M G P D P
T N E V E G N I N E T A E R H T E F I L T N E R A P P A
G G O P P I H Y N L Y A N J U Y S J K J Y Z H T J U H L
H E B W D U C X S L M U M O H V Y N N T X P D C C L N M
P H G U Q S E Q T Y M E L B S K O V I M Z C J M K X E R
A V I P N W T P U T B P A A I L V D R N O T H X Y H B R
Q L C H U C Y E T O O A H C G N I L T T O M D Y E K Z Y
Q Z V A D P B T B M G V B W R G W A W S J L C T P F V U
R M S F L J W E X P Z D T N I O V J C T L T K R H N J Y
E Z W F D W O C B K R O I R E P C G J M T H X E C E X S
C M H Y Q S L H K J H B L M U K D Y M O V N A G A J G Y
U U T R K A B I D L L A N E O N A T A L P E R I O D U D
T Y I Z L S B A Y C H D X G X A N H U N M U T R F T S P
N W O Q R O C L I C P V X G U Z R Y S U O K R L P L Q R
U E P R O B Q L U R K P V X Y V O F B X S Y T R L K U
Y W N J R R M N O G N L G C X B Q Q D K G W I Q G N G E
G X D V T J C R A E J L E H N W O J Q I K J Z S I C Q D
O E F H S Z C K G K I F K P E M L D Y K R E Q L H E J Z
V X U X U B R T E N J L U R F D G D S L J T Z U C L Q H
Q V B U L A Z S P X P G B Q I S B R N M W C S R N U B J
L Z X V M A V B U D O D E S C C C Q B X P S P M O R F Y
A P C U O A X N X L M B M G P O Z K U O P V R N H E B K
I A V H G L D X B E N D L H R P P G Y Q D E S W R G Q H
```

1. Shaken baby syndrome (page 41.48)
2. Croup (page 41.9)
3. Nuchal rigidity (page 41.41)
4. Sniffing (page 41.10)
5. Mottling (page 41.10)
6. Stridor (page 41.12)
7. Blow-by technique (page 41.24)
8. Petechial (page 41.41)
9. Rhonchi (page 41.16)
10. Acrocyanosis (page 41.11)
11. Neonatal period (page 41.6)
12. Apparent life-threatening event (page 41.47)

Fill-in-the-Table

1. Even in a non-load-and-go situation, you must be able to perform the physical exam of the injured child quickly. To do so, you must know precisely what you are looking for at each step.

Body Area	What I Am Looking for in Particular
Head	Bulging or sunken **fontanelles** in infants **Battle's sign, raccoon's eyes,** blood or clear **fluid draining from the nose or ears** Unequal pupils
Neck	**Tenderness; tracheal deviation**
Chest	Location of the **point of maximal impulse (PMI)** Bruises, instability Inequality of breath sounds
Abdomen	**Bruises, seat belt marks** Distention, tenderness, rigidity
Extremities	**Deformity, bruises** Peripheral pulses **Movement** and **sensation**

2.

Normal Respiratory Rate by Age	
Age	**Respiratory Rate (breaths/min)**
Infant	25–50
Toddler	20–30
Preschool-age child	20–25
School-age child	15–20
Adolescent	12–16

(page 41.12)

3.

Normal Pulse Rates for Age	
Age	**Pulse Rate (beats/min)**
Infant	100–160
Toddler	90–150
Preschool-age child	80–140
School-age child	70–120
Adolescent	60–100

(page 41.12)

4.

Normal Blood Pressure for Age	
Age	**Minimal Systolic Blood Pressure (mm Hg)**
Infant	> 70
Toddler	> 80
Preschool-age child	> 80
School-age child	> 80
Adolescent	> 90

(page 41.13)

Problem Solving

1. Minimal systolic blood pressure = 80 + (2 × Age in years)

a. 92 mm Hg

b. 100 mm Hg

c. 90 to 92 mm Hg (page 41.13)

2. a. 5.5 mm

b. 6.25 mm (page 41.29)

Skill Drills

1. a. The initial energy setting is 2 J/kg or 36 joules. (page 41.40)

b. Subsequent defibrillations should occur at 4 J/kg or 72 joules. (page 41.40)

2. a. Epinephrine should be given by the subcutaneous (SQ) or intramuscular (IM) route at a dose of 0.01 mg/kg of the 1:1,000 solution, to a maximum dose of 0.3 mg. This patient should be given 0.01 mg/kg or the maximum dose of 0.3 mg of 1:1,000 solution. (page 41.19)

b. Diphenhydramine (dose: 1 to 2 mg/kg IV to a maximum of 50 mg), or 27 to 50 mg IV (page 41.19)

c. Bronchodilators may be delivered by nebulizer or metered-dose inhaler (MDI) with a spacer-mask device. Unit doses of 2.5 mg of albuterol premixed with 3 mL of normal saline are often used for nebulization and represent an acceptable starting dose for most young children. (page 41.21)

3. *One-Rescuer Bag-Mask Ventilation for a Child* (page 41.25)

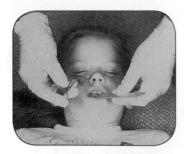 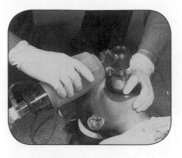 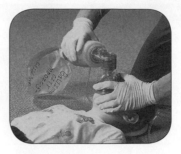 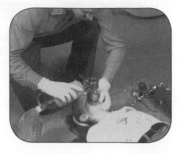

Step 1: Open the **airway**, and **insert** the appropriate airway adjunct.

Step 2: Hold the **mask** on the patient's face with a one-handed **head tilt–chin lift** technique (E-C clamp). Ensure a good **mask-to-face** seal while maintaining the airway.

Step 3: **Ventilate** at a rate of **20 breaths/min** for children. Allow adequate time for exhalation.

Step 4: Assess effectiveness of ventilation by assessing **bilateral** rise and fall of the **chest**.

4. *Performing Chest Compressions on a Child* (page 41.37)

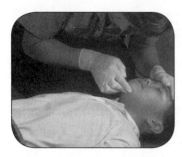 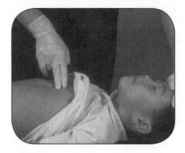 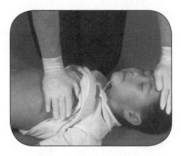 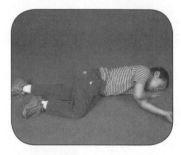

Step 1: Place the child on a firm surface, and use one hand to maintain the head tilt–chin lift.

Step 2: Place the heel of your hand over the middle of the sternum (between the nipples); avoid compression of the xiphoid process.

Step 3: Coordinate compression with ventilation in a 30:2 ratio, pausing for ventilation.

Step 4: Reassess breathing and pulse after 2 minutes and at 2-minute intervals thereafter. If the child resumes effective breathing, place him or her in the recovery position.

Chapter 42: Geriatrics

Matching

1. H (page 42.9)
2. J (page 42.5)
3. E (page 42.13)
4. I (page 42.6)
5. D (page 42.8)
6. A (page 42.16)

7. K (page 42.13)
8. G (page 42.8)
9. F (page 42.9)
10. C (page 42.13)
11. B (page 42.11)

Multiple Choice

1. B (page 42.5)
2. A (page 42.6)
3. C (page 42.6
4. A (page 42.7)
5. D (page 42.8)

6. C (page 42.9)
7. D (page 42.10)
8. D (page 42.11)
9. A (page 42.13)
10. D (page 42.19)

Labeling

1. Lower gastrointestinal (GI) system hemorrhage. (page 42.23)

2. Upper GI system hemorrhage. (page 42.22)

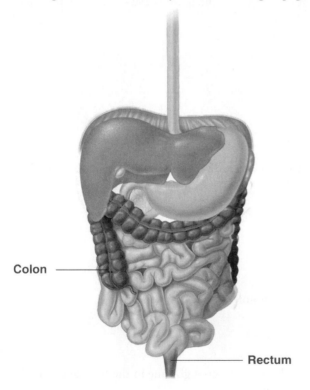

Colon

Rectum

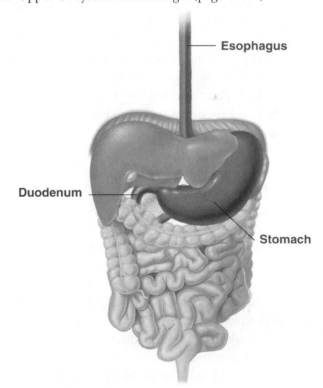

Esophagus

Duodenum

Stomach

Fill-in-the-Blank

1. Elderly, emergency (page 42.5)
2. Just getting old (page 42.6)
3. Hypertrophies (page 42.6)
4. Respiratory, reductions (page 42.7)
5. Nephron units, filtering (page 42.7)

6. Appetite, saliva, dryness (page 42.8)

7. Intervertebral, compression, height (page 42.8)

8. Meniere disease, cycles, months (page 42.9)

9. Wrinkling, resiliency, drier, fragile (page 42.9)

10. Morbidity, mortality, 70 (page 42.10)

Identify

1. a. Chief complaint: Right-sided midthigh pain

   b. Vital signs: Her pulse is 84 beats/min and very irregular. Her oxygen saturation is 88% on room air. Blood pressure is 106/86 mm Hg. The patient's skin turgor is poor, with delayed capillary refill of >2 seconds. Pupils are Equal and Round, Regular in size, and react to Light (PEARRL). An echocardiogram (ECG) shows a sinus rhythm with frequent premature ventricular contractions (PVCs) and short runs of ventricular tachycardia.

   c. Pertinent negatives: She denies chest pain, shortness of breath, dizziness, nausea, or vomiting. She also denies a trip and fall. The area appears to be clear of obstacles, rugs, or other obvious trip hazards.

2. a. Chief complaint: Patient is conscious but not alert to person, place, time, or purpose.

   b. Vital signs: Blood glucose of 66 mg/dL. His pulse rate is 92 beats/min and regular, blood pressure is 160/72 mm Hg. His skin is warm and moist, and he has normal capillary refill and oxygen saturation of 96% on room air.

   c. Pertinent negatives: There is minimally detectable damage to the vehicle as well as the vehicles that were struck.

Ambulance Calls

1. As noted, one way to try to make sure you don't miss any important symptoms is to conduct a review of systems, which should include questions such as the following:

   a. Have you had any pain or discomfort in your chest (cardiovascular system)?

   b. Have you had any palpitations (cardiovascular system)?

   c. Have you been short of breath (cardiovascular/respiratory systems)?

   d. Have you been coughing (respiratory system)?

   e. Have you felt dizzy or fainted (cardiovascular/nervous system)?

   f. Have you had any difficulty speaking (cardiovascular/nervous system)?

   g. Have you had any severe headaches (nervous system)?

   h. Have you noticed any funny sensations in your arms or legs, or have you had any difficulty walking (nervous system)?

   i. Have you had any changes in your appetite or weight (digestive system)?

   j. Has there been any change in your bowel movements (digestive system)?

   k. Have you had any pain or difficulty in urinating (urinary system)? (page 42.20)

2. One of the most frequent geriatric calls is for a patient who has fallen.

   a. Questions to ask in taking the history might include the following:

     (1) How did it happen?

     (2) Did you feel dizzy before you fell, or have any other similar warning symptoms?

     (3) Did you feel anything snap before you fell?

     (4) Are you taking any new medications?

     (5) Where does it hurt?

   b. The past medical history of an elderly patient may be quite extensive, and there isn't enough time in the field to elicit all the details. The things you *need* to know to render appropriate emergency care are:

     (1) Major underlying illnesses (e.g., diabetes, angina)

     (2) Recent hospitalizations (Where? What doctor?)

     (3) Allergies

     (4) Current medications (That means *all* medications—prescribed and over-the-counter varieties. Collect them all in a bag and take them with the patient to the hospital.)

   c. *Students should provide six of the following.* In performing the physical assessment, one should look in particular for:

     (1) The patient's state of **dress** and **grooming**, as an indication of her general ability to care for herself

(2) The level of consciousness (AVPU or Glasgow Coma Scale)

(3) The position in which the patient is found

(4) An elevated blood pressure, which might signal increasing intracranial pressure, or a decreased blood pressure, which might suggest shock

(5) A very slow pulse, suggesting either increasing intracranial pressure or the source of a syncopal episode

(6) An increased respiratory rate, which may signal shock or a variety of other serious conditions

(7) Signs of head injury (e.g., cerebrospinal fluid leak, Battle's sign)

(8) Neck tenderness

(9) Instability or tenderness of the ribs

(10) Deformity in the limbs

(11) The state of the surroundings, another indication of the patient's overall ability to care for herself. (page 42.20)

  d. *Students should provide three of the following.* The elderly are more susceptible than younger people to:

(1) Subdural hematoma (page 42.16)

(2) Compression of the cervical spinal cord (page 42.8)

(3) Rib fracture (page 42.16)

(4) Hip fracture (page 42.16)

3. Factors related to geriatric suicide:

  a. If depression goes unrecognized or untreated, it is associated with a higher suicide rate in the elderly population than in any other age group.

  b. The majority of elder suicides occur in people who have recently been diagnosed with depression.

  c. The majority of suicide victims have seen their primary care physician within the month before the event.

  d. Geriatric patients typically do not make suicidal gestures or attempt to get help.

  e. The rate of completed suicide is disproportionately high in the geriatric population. (page 42.15)

True/False

1. T (page 42.6)   **6.** F (page 42.9)

2. F (page 42.13)   **7.** T (page 42.10)

3. F (page 42.19)   **8.** F (page 42.25)

4. T (page 42.30)   **9.** F (page 42.29)

5. T (page 42.9)   **10.** T (page 42.29)

Short Answer

1. Among the attributes that make caring for the elderly particularly challenging are the following. *Students should provide five of the following:*

  a. Many physiologic functions are diminished. (page 42.6)

  b. Typical symptoms and signs of disease may be absent, altered, or delayed. (page 42.17)

  c. Physical illness often presents as a mental disorder. (page 42.13)

  d. Multiple problems coexist in the same patient, producing multiple symptoms. (page 42.17)

  e. Adverse reactions to drugs occur frequently. (page 42.20)

  f. Psychosocial factors have an increased impact on health. (page 42.5)

2. Among the psychosocial stresses that accompany advancing age are the following:

  a. Retirement from work, with the attendant loss of community status, sense of usefulness, and the structure that a job gives to one's daily life. (page 42.5)

  b. Bereavement, as more and more friends (and often a spouse) die. (page 42.5)

3. A number of changes in the body occur as part of the normal aging process. *Students should provide two changes per organ system.*

  a. CARDIOVASCULAR (page 42.6)

(1) Increase in blood pressure

(2) Decrease in cardiac output

(3) Cardiac hypertrophy

(4) Electric conduction system atrophy

b. RESPIRATORY (page 42.7)

(1) Decreased vital capacity

(2) Increased residual volume

(3) Decreased air flow

(4) Decreased arterial PO2

(5) Decreased cough, gag, and ciliary clearance

c. RENAL (page 42.7)

(1) Decreased renal blood flow

(2) Decreased nephron mass

(3) Impaired thirst mechanism

(4) Decreased ability to maintain salt and fluid balance

d. DIGESTIVE (page 42.8)

(1) Decreased sense of taste

(2) Decreased secretion of saliva and gastric juice

(3) Less efficient hepatic detoxification

e. MUSCULOSKELETAL   (page 42.8)

(1) Decreased bone mass

(2) Decreased muscle mass

f. NERVOUS (page 42.9)

(1) Decreased visual acuity

(2) Loss of high-tone hearing

(3) Impaired proprioception

g. HOMEOSTATIC (page 42.9)

(1) Impaired temperature regulation

(2) Blunted febrile response to infection

(3) Impaired blood glucose control

4. *Students should provide four of the following.* Responses to illness common among the elderly include:

a. Acute confusion or other change in mental status (page 42.9)

b. Weakness (page 42.9)

c. Dizziness (page 42.16)

d. Dyspnea (page 42.21)

e. Fatigue (page 42.22)

5. A number of problems are involved in taking a history from an elderly patient, but most of those obstacles can be overcome with a little patience, tact, and ingenuity.

a. Obstacle: The patient has trouble hearing you.

What you can do about it: Sit facing the patient, in good light, and speak slowly and clearly.

b. Obstacle: Patient may not report important symptoms.

What you can do about it: Conduct a review of systems to screen the major organ systems for serious abnormality.

c. Obstacle: The patient has several chief complaints.

What you can do about it: Ask, "What happened *today*?" or "What is bothering you the most? How is it different from the way it was yesterday?"

d. Obstacle: The patient is too confused to give a history.

What you can do about it: Try to obtain information from the family or other caregivers. (page 42.20)

6. Acute myocardial infarction and congestive heart failure occur commonly in the elderly, but are as likely as not to present with atypical signs and symptoms: (page 42.10)

Condition	Possible Signs and Symptoms in the Elderly
ACUTE MYOCARDIAL, INFARCTION	Confusion, weakness, dyspnea, stroke, syncope, incontinence
CONGESTIVE HEART FAILURE	Fatigue

7. Conditions that may present as delirium in the elderly include the following. *Students should provide five of the following:*

   a. Acute myocardial infarction

   b. Congestive heart failure

   c. Pneumonia

   d. Dehydration

   e. Electrolyte abnormalities (e.g., hyponatremia)

   f. Drug toxicity (page 42.24)

8. Among the drugs used in prehospital care, those most likely to cause problems in the elderly include the following:

   a. Lidocaine (page 42.5)

   b. Furosemide (page 42.27)

   c. Morphine (page 42.27

Crossword Puzzle

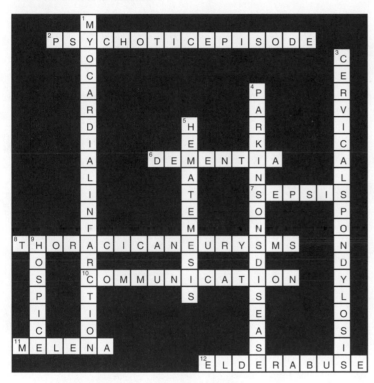

Fill-in-the-Table

1.

Causes of Falls in the Elderly	
Cause	**Clues to Suggest This Cause**
Extrinsic (accidental)	Obvious environmental hazard at the scene, such as poor lighting, scatter rugs, uneven sidewalk, ice or other slippery surface
Intrinsic drop attacks	Sudden fall; patient found on the ground somewhat confused, often temporarily paralyzed and unable to get up; no premonitory symptoms
Postural hypotension	Fall when getting up from a recumbent or sitting position (Check medications the patient is taking, and ask about occult blood loss, such as presence of black stools. Measure blood pressure in recumbent and sitting positions.)
Dizziness or syncope	Marked bradycardia or tachyarrhythmias
Stroke	Other characteristic signs of stroke, such as hemiparesis, hemiplegia, or aphasia
Fracture	Patient felt something snap before falling.

(page 42.16)

Chapter 43: Abuse, Neglect, and Assault

Matching

(page 43.9)

1. C

2. B

3. A

4. D

5. B

(page 43.7)

1. A

2. A

3. B

4 A

5. B

Multiple Choice

1. C (page 43.3)

2. D (page 43.4)

3. A (page 43.5)

4. D (page 43.6)

5. C (page 43.7)

6. B (page 43.9)

7. A (page 43.11)

8. D (page 43.7)

9. D (page 43.5)

10. C (page 43.8)

Fill-in-the-Blank

1.

A: Affect

B: Bruises of varying stages

U: Unusual injury patterns

S: Suspicious circumstances

E: Environmental clues (page 43.5)

2. Mandated (page 43.6)

3. Active (page 43.7)

4. Polypharmacy (page 43.13)

5. Sexual assault, rape (page 43.11)

6. Physical, emotional, economic; sexual (page 43.9)

7. Understaffed, poor training (page 43.7)

8. Objective, subjective (page 43.11)

9. Stocking, doughnut (page 43.5)

10. 85 (page 43.4)

Identify

1. Chief Complaint: Stomach hurts

2. Vital Signs: Pulse of 130 beats/min and thready, blood pressure is 70/40 mm Hg, and the respirations are 36 breaths/min.

3. Significance of the Findings: Abdominal bruising and rigidity

Ambulance Calls

1. a. Injury to top of the head.

b. Multiple bruises in various stages of healing.

c. Location of bruises: back and buttocks.

d. Burn marks on hands.

e. Child has little affect (sitting on couch, no talking or eye contact). (page 43.5)

2. a. Active Neglect

    (1) No companionship

    (2) Not getting her medicine

    (3) No assistance with transportation

  b. Passive Neglect

    (1) Ignored and isolated (page 43.7)

3. Physical: Kicking and hitting

  Emotional: Calls her names and makes negative comments

  Economic: Undercut attempt to get a job

  Sexual: Forces sex (page 43.9)

True/False

1. T (page 43.3)	**9.** T (page 43.7)
2. F (page 43.4)	**10.** T (page 43.13)
3. F (page 43.4)	**11.** F (page 43.9)
4. T (page 43.5)	**12.** T (page 43.9)
5. T (page 43.5)	**13.** F (page 43.5)
6. T (page 43.5)	**14.** F (page 43.5)
7. F (page 43.6)	**15.** T (page 43.11)
8. F (page 43.7)	

Short Answer

1. a. Repeated calls to the family residence

  b. Multiple bruises in various stages of healing

  c. Bruises in the area of the body that is not expected, such as buttocks, back, face, or upper legs

  d. Bite or burn marks

  e. Stocking/glove burns or doughnut burns that indicate the child has been immersed in hot water

  f. Multiple fractures or fractures in various stages of healing

  g. Scalp wounds with signs or symptoms of hematoma and concussion

  h. Child does not become agitated when a parent leaves the room or does not look to the parent for reassurance (pages 43.5, 43.6)

Word Find

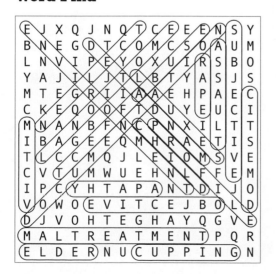

1. Neglect (page 43.13)
2. Abuse (page 43.13)
3. Maltreatment (page 43.4)
4. Environmental (page 43.5)
5. Affect (page 43.5)
6. Apathy (page 43.5)
7. Cupping (page 43.13)
8. Mandated (page 43.13)
9. Domestic (page 43.8)
10. Elder (page 43.6)
11. Child (page 43.3)
12. Profile (page 43.7)
13. Emotional (page 43.9)
14. Sexual (page 43.13)
15. Rape (page 43.13)
16. Assault (page)
17. Victim (page 43.11)
18. Document (page 43.11)
19. Objective (page 43.10)
20. Subjective (page 43.11)

Fill-in-the-Table

Mnemonic	What the Letter Represents
C	Consistency of the injury with the child's developmental age
H	History consistent with injuries
I	Inappropriate parental concerns
L	Lack of supervision
D	Delay in seeking care
A	Affect
B	Bruises of varying stages
U	Unusual injury patterns
S	Suspicious circumstances
E	Environmental clues

(page 43.5)

Chapter 44: Patients With Special Needs

Matching

1. I   (page 44.11)
2. G   (page 44.4)
3. A   (page 44.9)
4. L   (page 44.15)
5. H   (page 44.4)
6. B   (page 44.8)
7. K   (page 44.10)
8. F   (page 44.6)
9. E   (page 44.8)
10. D   (page 44.12)
11. J   (page 44.14)
12. C   (page 44.14)

Multiple Choice

1. D   (page 44.6)
2. D   (page 44.7)
3. D   (page 44.8)
4. C   (page 44.8)
5. C   (page 44.9)
6. D   (page 44.10)
7. D   (page 44.16)
8. D   (page 44.17)
9. D   (page 44.18)
10. D   (page 44.8)

Labeling

1. American Sign Language for terms related to illness and injury (page 44.5)

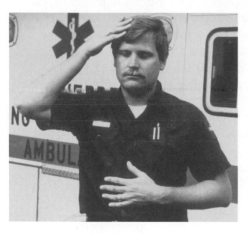

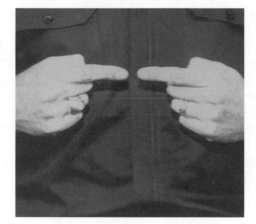

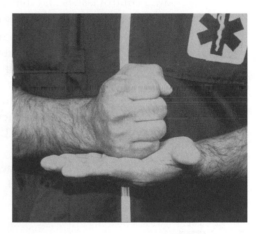

sick   hurt   help

Fill-in-the-Blank

1. Conductive, sensorineural (page 44.4)
2. Impaired, lipreading (page 44.5)
3. Psychological, injury, hearing (page 44.6)
4. Disorders, hoarseness, harshness, resonance (page 44.7)
5. Vulnerable, accident, hearing, smell (page 44.7)
6. Pickwickian, hypoxemia, hypercapnia, polycythemia (page 44.9)
7. Down syndrome (page 44.10)
8. Patient, tone, expressions, language (page 44.11)
9. Exaggerated, visual, seizures, retardation (page 44.13)
10. Birth defect, pregnancy, column, develop (page 44.15)

Identify

1. **a.** Chief complaint: Terminally ill patient
   b. History of present illness: Irregular breathing, apnea, unconscious
   c. Other medical history: Do Not Resuscitate Order (DNR)
2. **a.** Chief complaint: Seizures
   b. History of present illness: Seizures that haven't responded to rectal diazepam
   c. Other medical history: Down syndrome, multiple medications, seizures
3. **a.** Chief complaint: Fever
   b. History of present illness: Cloudy urine, has a Foley catheter
   c. Other medical history: Quadriplegic, tracheotomy, colostomy, feeding tube, can't verbalize his complaints and concerns, uses a writing board

Ambulance Calls

1. **a.** It's best to ask the patient how to move her in the safest and most comfortable manner. She may have a special lift or assist devices that will make the transfer easier for both the crew and patient. It's important to try to protect her dignity and privacy. Calling emergency medical services (EMS) can sometimes be embarrassing, especially when her deformity is revealed. It's often better to work as a team. If more assistance is required, it should be requested. The goal is to provide safe movement for the patient and crew.
   b. The patient may have some level of paralysis; especially in her lower trunk and extremities (if present). The patient may have bowel control issues and may have a Foley catheter. Some patients have shunts placed in their brain to relieve excess cerebrospinal fluid. If the patient has suffered other injuries, she might not even know. (page 44.15)
2. **a.** As with any patient who's had a seizure, your concern is to maintain adequate ABCs. Based on the initial assessment, it's obvious that this patient probably needs aggressive airway and breathing support. This should be accomplished by opening the airway with a head tilt–chin left. Suctioning is also important, as well as high-flow oxygen. If the patient needs ventilatory assistance, using a bag-mask device would be indicated. It would also be appropriate to transport the patient away from the crowd and concert to avoid an embarrassing episode when she regains consciousness. The patient's mom is probably well versed in her medical history and care. It's important to include the mother in any treatment decisions and have her assist as appropriate. If the patient doesn't recover in a reasonable period of time, transport to an appropriate hospital is required.
   b. Patient may present with a round head with a flat occiput; an enlarged, protruding tongue; wide-set eyes; and folded skin on either side of the nose. (page 44.10)

True/False

1. T (page 44.4)	**6.** T (page 44.10)
2. F (page 44.5)	**7.** F (page 44.11)
3. T (page 44.6)	**8.** T (page 44.13)
4. T (page 44.7)	**9.** F (page 44.14)
5. F (page 44.8)	**10.** T (page 44.15)

Short Answer

1. **a.** Oftentimes, it most beneficial to focus on the prevailing health condition of the patient and the need to seek treatment. A frank discussion regarding the risk/benefit of refusing treatment can often convince a patient to seek treatment. Properly documenting a patient's refusal, including exam finding, chief complaint, and risks of refusal, will usually convince a patient to be transported, especially when you ask the patient to sign this document.
   b. This is something that you need to reference and investigate in your response area. Each location has its own specific rules, regulations, laws, and customs. Discuss your concern with your medical director and develop a preplan to handle these cases.

c. You should research the location of free clinics and health care resources in your community for those patients who may benefit from an alternative in a nonemergency situation. Each state has its own rules and regulations. However, it is important to note that no patient should be refused transport to an emergency care facility based on his or her ability to pay.

d. Federal laws allow patients to be seen and evaluated regardless of their ability to pay. (page 44.18)

2. Many of the patients a paramedic encounters have a hearing impairment. Sometimes this impairment is readily noticeable. (page 44.5)

a. What clues would indicate to you that your patient has a hearing impairment?

(1) Presence of hearing aids

(2) Poor word pronunciation

(3) Failure to respond to your questions

b. How would you go about communicating with someone that has a hearing impairment?

(1) Face the patient; position yourself about 18 inches directly in front of the patient.

(2) Ask the patient how he or she would like to communicate with you, such as by using American Sign Language.

(3) Use written communication.

(4) Speak slowly.

(5) Use a low-pitched voice.

(6) Try the "reverse stethoscope" technique.

(7) Have only one person interview the patient to avoid confusion.

(8) Make sure the patient is using his or her hearing aid and that it's turned on.

3. a. Request and plan for extra help.

b. Plan the safest and easiest exit route.

c. Avoid lifting the patient by one limb.

d. Use a team approach to coordinate and preplan each move.

e. Use specialized equipment if available.

f. Notify the receiving hospital.

g. Be respectful of the patient's dignity. (page 44.8)

4. a. What are some of the causes of visual impairments?

(1) Congenital defects

(2) Disease

(3) Injury

(4) Infection

(5) Degeneration of the eyeball, optic nerve, or nerve pathways

b. What can paramedics do to alleviate some of the fears felt by patients with visual impairments?

(1) Make yourself known when entering the room and introduce yourself and others.

(2) Tell the patient what is happening.

(3) Identify noises.

(4) Describe the situation and surroundings.

(page 44.7)

Word Find

1. Aphasia (page 44.6)
2. Arthritis (page 44.12)
3. Cerebral palsy (page 44.12)
4. Conductive deafness (page 44.4)
5. Cystic fibrosis (page 44.13)
6. Developmental disability (page 44.10)
7. Down syndrome (page 44.10)
8. Emotional/mental impairment (page 44.11)
9. Hemiplegia (page 44.8)
10. Mental illness (page 44.9)
11. Multiple sclerosis (page 44.13)
12. Muscular dystrophy (page 44.14)
13. Myasthenia gravis (page 44.15)
14. Obesity (page 44.8)
15. Osteoarthritis (page 44.12)
16. Quadriplegia (page 44.8)
17. Poliomyelitis (page 44.14)
18. Paraplegia (page 44.8)
19. Sensorineural deafness (page 44.4)
20. Spina bifida (page 44.15)
21. Terminal illness (page 44.16)

Fill-in-the-Table

Special Need	Associated Patient Care Need
Speech impairments	Talk to patients as adults. Patience is important. Ask the patient how he or she prefers to communicate. (page 44.7)
Visual impairments	Introduce yourself; use visual aids if helpful; identify noises, the situation, and surroundings. (page 44.7)
Paralysis	Patients may rely on a ventilator and other specialized equipment, and they may have feeding tubes, Foley catheters, and colostomies. Be aware of potential complications. (page 44.8)
Obesity	Put the patient at ease. Communicate your plan to help. Request extra assistance for moving and transport. (page 44.8)
Developmental disabilities	Treatment should be based on the complaint, unless the illness is related to the mental disability. (page 44.10)
Pathologic challenges	Formulate your treatment plan with special consideration of these patients. Pathologies may include cancer, arthritis, cerebral palsy, muscular dystrophy, polio, previous head injury, and myasthenia gravis. (page 44.12)

Chapter 45: Acute Interventions for the Chronic Care Patient

Matching

1. C (page 45.27)
2. I (page 45.11)
3. A (page 45.30)
4. J (page 45.20)
5. D (page 45.9)

6. E (page 45.23)
7. F (page 45.11)
8. G (page 45.11)
9. B (page 45.11)
10. H (page 45.20)

Multiple Choice

1. A (page 45.4)
2. C (page 45.5)
3. A (page 45.30)
4. D (page 45.6)
6. C (page 45.9)
7. D (page 45.11)
8. D (page 45.15)

9. C (page 45.14)
10. D (page 45.15)
11. C (page 45.20)
12. D (page 45.23)
13. A (page 45.25)
14. D (page 45.28)
15. C (page 45.14)

Fill-in-the-Blank

1. Chemotherapy, cytotoxic, cytotoxic (page 45.27)
2. Home setting, nursing home (page 45.26)
3. Postpartum depression, depression (page 45.25)
4. Serous exudate, purulent exudate (page 45.23)
5. Colostomy (page 45.20)
6. Vascular access devices, attempt (page 45.16)
7. Ventilators, breathing, intrapulmonary pressure (page 45.11)
8. Oxygen concentrators (page 45.09)
9. Pre-event phase, postevent (page 45.05)
10. Neurologic, apnea monitor (page 45.26)
11. Stressor, sympathetic, tachycardia (page 45.27)
12. Ureterostomy, suprapubic, urinary bladder (page 45.20)

Identify

1. a. Chief Complaint: Blocked catheter, possible urinary tract infection
   b. Vital Signs: Loss of consciousness (LOC), not alert; oxygen saturation is 92%; blood pressure 124/78 mm Hg; sinus tachycardia; PEARRL (Pupils Equal And Round, Regular in size, react to Light)
   c. PertinentNegatives: None indicated
2. a. Chief Complaint: Interfacility transport
   b. Vital Signs: Blood pressure 90/60 mm Hg, pulse 120 beats/min, oxygen saturation is 89%, skin turgor is poor; patient's skin is ashen, warm, and dry
   c. Pertinent Negatives: This patient is being treated for long-term rehabilitation of a severe motor vehicle crash–related head injury. She is tachycardic, hypotensive, and has a very low oxygen reading for someone who is intubated and is purportedly stable and appropriate for transport by ambulance. The paramedics would be correct to contact medical control and question whether she is an appropriate candidate for interfacility transport.
3. a. Chief Complaint: An unconscious, unresponsive patient
   b. Vital Signs: None detected
   c. Pertinent Negatives: A Do Not Resuscitate (DNR) order

Ambulance Calls

1. a. Wash your hands and apply a mask, goggles, and clean nonlatex gloves.

   b. Open supplies may be used.

   c. Remove the inner cannula.

   d. Attach the catheter to negative pressure. Check the suction and clear the catheter by drawing up a small amount of saline.

   e. Have the patient take a deep breath or preoxygenate him or her.

   f. Insert the catheter into the trachea without suction. Apply intermittent suction while removing the catheter. Repeat as necessary. Keep the patient well oxygenated during the procedure.

   g. Clean the inner cannula with the tracheostomy brush, rinse, replace, and lock into place. Omit this step for a one-piece tracheostomy.

   h. Remove your gloves and wash your hands.

   i. Document the procedure and assessment on your patient care report (PCR). (page 45.12)

2. To draw blood from a central venous catheter:

   a. Wash your hands and apply a mask, goggles, and nonlatex gloves.

   b. Draw the flush solution (usually normal saline but may be a heparin solution) into a syringe.

   c. Set up the supplies, including the port access kit.

   d. Swab the port with an appropriate cleansing solution (eg, Betadine) or clamp the catheter and remove the cap.

   e. Attach an empty syringe or Vacutainer adapter to the hub or port.

   f. Release the clamp (if clamped), and aspirate 5 mL of blood.

   g. Reclamp the catheter if necessary and discard the aspirated blood.

   h. Attach a new syringe or adapter.

   i. Obtain the blood samples.

   j. Reclamp the catheter if necessary and attach the syringe with the flush solution.

   k. Release the clamp and flush the line.

   l. Reclamp and recap the line.

   m. Identify the tubes of blood by writing the date and time drawn and the paramedic's name on the side of the tube.

   n. Document the procedure and assessment on the PCR.

   o. Dispose of contaminated equipment. (page 45.15)

3. a. Describe several of the factors involved in your scene size-up.

   (1) Pets that live in homes with chronically ill persons may be agitated.

   (2) Families may keep a variety of weapons.

   (3) Caregiver stress, exhaustion, and pressure may cause some family members to react negatively to you.

   (4) The house may have been renovated to accommodate large equipment that may make entrances unsafe.

   (5) Perform a quick assessment of the supporting equipment. (page 45.6)

   b. Describe the factors involved in the focused history and physical exam for the chronic care patient.

   (1) In a trauma patient, stabilize the patient's cervical spine, perform a rapid physical exam, provide comfort, and assess for other injuries.

   (2) In a medical patient, gather a SAMPLE history, perform an assessment of the chief complaint, and take the patient's vital signs before you develop the plan of care.

   (3) After you have obtained the history, you may complete a physical exam. Treatment is based on both history and exam.

   c. Describe the factors involved in your patient's detailed physical exam.

   (1) Most calls to the chronic home care setting are medical in nature.

   (2) The chief complaint may give you a clue about the mechanism of injury or cause of the illness.

   (3) The level of detail required for a physical exam in the home care setting is similar to any other physical exam.

   (4) The need for a comprehensive examination depends on the acuity of the patient and the risk factors for further injury or illness.

True/False

1. T (page 45.4)
2. F (page 45.4)
3. F (page 45.5)
4. T (page 45.6)
5. F (page 45.6)
6. T (page 45.7)
7. F (page 45.8)
8. T (page 45.9)

9. T (page 45.14)
10. F (page 45.18)
11. F (page 45.20)
12. T (page 45.23)
13. F (page 45.23)
14. T   (page 45.25)
15. F (page 45.28)

Short Answer

1. a. Manage the disease process
   b. Manage chemotherapy side effects
   c. Analgesic medications (page 45.27)
2. a. Active listening, be supportive.
   b. Suggest methods or agencies for securing additional resources.
   c. Offer injury prevention guidance. (page 45.5)
3. a. Medicare
   b. Medicaid
   c. Private insurance
   d. Out of pocket
   e. Local and state-funded programs (page 45.5)
4. a. Hand washing
   b. Waterless gel with at least 60% alcohol content
   c. Gloves
   d. Mask, goggles, gown (page 45.6)
5. a. Inoperative or damaged equipment
   b. Inoperative IVs, tubes, artificial airways, and ventilators (page 45.7)
6. a. Opening
   b. Repositioning
   c. Clearing (page 45.12)
7. a. A sudden onset of chest pain
   b. Shortness of breath
   c. Decreased cardiac output (page 45.16)

Fill-in-the-Table

1.

Serious Complications Associated With Vascular Access Devices	
Complication	**Assessment Findings**
Occlusion	Cannot aspirate blood; infusion doesn't run
Catheter thrombosis	Swelling of arm, neck, or shoulder; pain
Sepsis	Fever, chills, malaise
Catheter migration	Change in length of exposed catheter
Catheter breakage	Leaking or bleeding from catheter
Embolism (air)	Chest pain, shortness of breath, tachycardia, hypotension, decreased level of consciousness
Embolism (PICC/midline catheter)	Inadvertent removal with distal portion of catheter missing

(page 45.7)

Crossword Puzzle

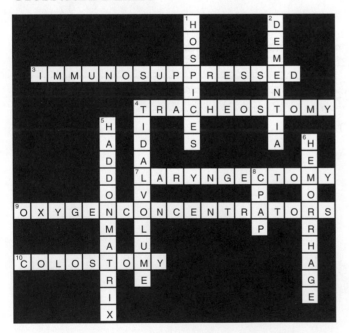

Skill Drills

1. *Replacing an Ostomy Device*

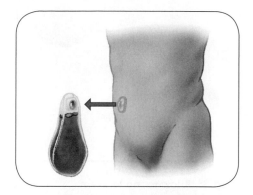

Step 1: Empty/remove the current appliance and dispose of it appropriately.

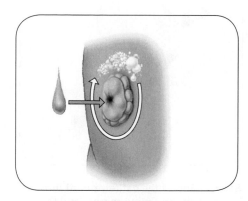

Step 2: Wash the area around the stoma with soap and water. Cleanse the stoma with water.

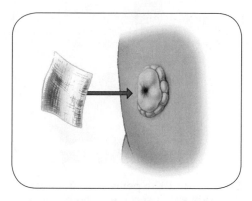

Step 3: Place a clean gauze pad over the stoma.

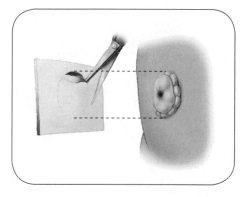

Step 4: Cut the wafer to the correct size using the patient's measurement for tracing.

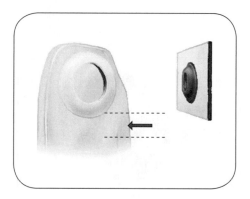

Step 5: Attach the appliance to the wafer.

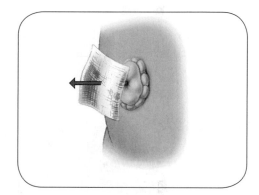

Step 6: Remove the gauze.

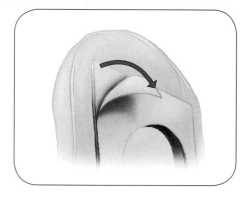

Step 7: Remove the paper backing from the wafer.

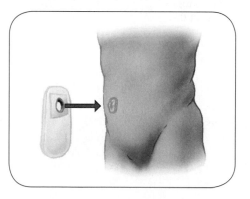

Step 8: Apply the appliance with the stoma centered in the wafer cutout.

2. *Catheterizing an Adult Male Patient*

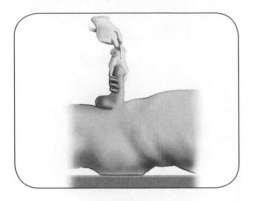 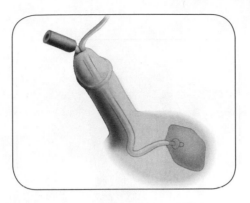 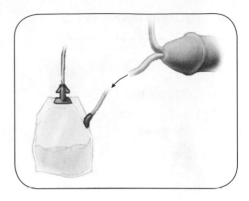

Step 1: Hold the penis at a **90°** angle to the body and insert the catheter.

Step 2: Insert the catheter until the Y between the drainage port and the **balloon** port is at the tip of the penis. For a straight catheter, insert approximately 1 inch more.

Step 3: Allow **urine** to drain.

3. *Catheterizing an Adult Female Patient*

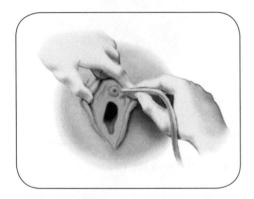 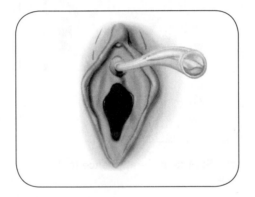 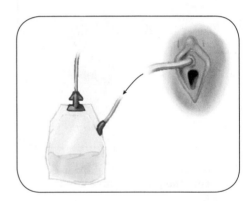

Step 1:   Locate the urinary meatus anterior to the vagina and insert the catheter.

Step 2: When **urine** is evident in the tubing, insert the catheter another 1 to 3 inches.

Step 3: Allow the urine to **drain.**

Section 6 Case Study: Answers and Summary

1. What is your initial treatment for this child?

■ **Minimize the child's anxiety**

Although the child is clearly ill, your findings in the initial assessment do not warrant immediate separation of her from her mother. If possible, continue your assessment of the child while her mother is holding her. This will minimize the child's anxiety and may facilitate a more accurate assessment.

■ **100% supplemental oxygen**
 • Pediatric nonrebreathing mask or blow-by technique

Although the child's respirations are increased, they are unlabored and are producing adequate tidal volume; therefore, ventilatory assistance is not indicated at this point. Administer passive oxygenation in a nonthreatening manner to avoid increasing the child's anxiety. If she becomes more irritable after applying a nonrebreathing mask, have the mother hold oxygen tubing near her nose and mouth.

Continue to monitor the child's respiratory effort and closely observe for signs of inadequate ventilation, such as a shallow depth of breathing (reduced tidal volume) or a decreasing mental status. Be prepared to assist ventilations with a bag-valve-mask device if signs of inadequate breathing are observed.

2. What is your field impression of this child?

This child's clinical presentation is highly suggestive of meningitis. The following signs, symptoms, and historical findings support this field impression:

■ **Fever**

■ **Headache**
 • Young children will often grab the sides of their head or place their hand on their head when they are experiencing a headache. Older children are usually able to tell you that their head hurts.

■ **Irritability**
 • Irritability is a very common sign of meningitis in smaller children. You should be especially suspicious if the child tends to become more irritable when she is picked up (paradoxical irritability); this indicates increased pain as traction is pulled on the inflamed meninges surrounding the spinal cord.

■ **Apparent nuchal rigidity (neck stiffness)**
 • The fact that the child will not move her head suggests that she is experiencing nuchal rigidity—a classic sign of meningitis.
 • Nuchal rigidity may not be a reliable sign in children less than 18 to 24 months of age.

Meningitis, also referred to as spinal meningitis, is an inflammation of the meningeal layers that surround and protect the brain and spinal cord. The infection can be bacterial, viral, or even fungal in origin. In many cases, meningitis is preceded by upper respiratory infection (URI) symptoms. In the prehospital setting, it is not possible to determine the etiologic pathogen causing the disease (eg, bacterial, viral, fungal); therefore, you should assume the disease to be bacterial in origin (the most life-threatening) until proven otherwise.

Bacterial meningitis remains a significant cause of mortality and morbidity in children. According to the Centers for Disease Control and Prevention (CDC), 3% to 6% of cases of meningitis in children are fatal; 20% of the patients who survive experience hearing loss or other long-term sequelae (eg, neurological impairment).

Relative to viral (aseptic) meningitis, which typically does not pose the risk of permanent neurological damage, bacterial meningitis is a potentially life-threatening infection. It is often associated with an altered mental status, seizures, and increased intracranial pressure (ICP). If left untreated, bacterial meningitis can result in severe sepsis, permanent neurological damage, and even death.

Prior to 1990, *Haemophilus influenzae* type b (Hib) was the most common cause of bacterial meningitis; however, because a vaccine for Hib is now administered to children as part of their routine immunizations, the occurrence of *H. influenzae* has

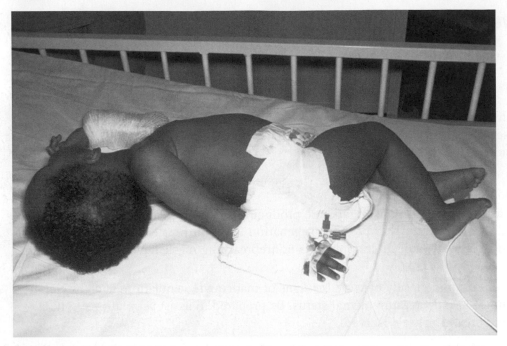

■ **Figure 6-1** Nuchal rigidity is a sign of meningitis, particularly in children older than 18 to 24 months of age.

decreased. According to the CDC, the incidence of Hib-related meningitis between 1980 and 1990 was approximately 40 to 100 per 100,000 children under 5 years of age. Since vaccinations against Hib began, the incidence has decreased to 1.3 per 100,000 children in that same age group. *Neisseria meningitidis* (*N. meningitidis*), also called meningococcal meningitis, and *Streptococcus pneumoniae* (also called pneumococcal meningitis) are currently the leading causes of bacterial meningitis in children greater than one month of age. In neonates (birth to 1 month of age), meningitis is usually caused by *Escherichia coli* (*E. coli*), group B streptococcus, or *Listeria monocytogenes*.

Classic signs and symptoms of bacterial meningitis include high fever, headache, and nuchal rigidity (**Figure 6-1**). In infants, the clinical presentation is commonly that of increased irritability, poor feeding, vomiting, a bulging fontanelle (sign of increased ICP), and inconsolability. Because infants and children less than 18 to 24 months of age often lack adequately developed neck musculature, nuchal rigidity may not manifest; therefore, it is an unreliable sign in this age group. Only in children older than 18 to 24 months of age are headache and nuchal rigidity reliable manifestations of meningitis.

The signs and symptoms of meningitis (**Table 6-1**) can develop over several hours or a few days, and may vary depending on the child's age. For example, infants may present with increased irritability, poor feeding, and difficulty in being consoled; older children are often unable to maintain a comfortable position secondary to muscle stiffness.

In older children, the inability to extend the legs with the hips flexed (Kernig sign) and/or involuntary flexion of the hip, knee, or ankle when the neck is passively flexed (Brudzinski sign) are suggestive of meningeal irritation. However, the absence of these clinical findings does not rule out meningitis.

Bacterial meningitis is a contagious disease. The primary mode of transmission is via the airborne droplet route, such as the exchange of respiratory secretions (eg, coughing, sneezing, kissing). Unlike the common cold or flu, however, the bacteria are not spread via casual contact with an infected person. Nonetheless, the appropriate BSI precautions—gloves and facial protection—must be strictly followed when caring for a patient with suspected meningitis.

Table 6-1   Signs and Symptoms of Bacterial Meningitis
Fever
Headache (in children > 18 to 24 months of age)
Nuchal rigidity (in children > 18 to 24 months of age)
Photophobia (sensitivity to light)
Nausea and vomiting • Projectile vomiting may occur with increased ICP.
Irritability/difficult to console • Paradoxical irritability in infants
Bulging fontanelle (in infants)
Decreased level of consciousness/lethargy
Skin rashes • Petechiae or purpura
Seizures

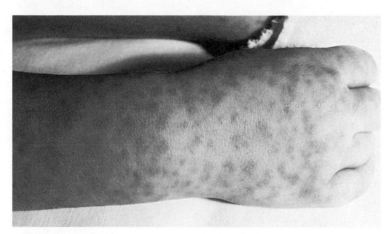

■ **Figure 6-2**   Petechial rash in a child with meningococcal meningitis.
(Courtesy of the Centers for Disease Congrol and Prevention.)

3. What are petechiae and purpura? What do they indicate?

Petechiae are small (< 0.05 cm) circumscribed areas of superficial bleeding into the skin. Initially, they appear as red pinpoint-sized spots and then turn purple or dark blue. A petechial rash (**Figure 6-2**) is not a disease itself, but a manifestation of an underlying problem. The presence of petechiae indicates a low platelet count (thrombocytopenia) and is associated with a severe systemic infection (sepsis).

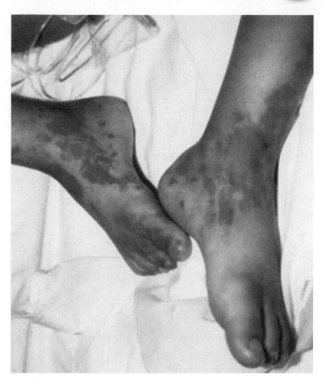

■ **Figure 6-3**   Purpura in a child with meningococcal meningitis.

Approximately 25% of children with meningococcal meningitis develop an erythematous (red) maculopapular rash followed by petechiae or purpura, most commonly located on the extremities. Purpura, also a manifestation of thrombocytopenia, appears as purple circumscribed skin lesions greater than 0.5 cm in size (**Figure 6-3**).

Although petechiae and purpura are classically seen in children with meningococcal meningitis, they can also occur in conjunction with other infectious diseases, viral or bacterial.

4. What treatment will you provide to this child en route to the hospital?

Children with suspected meningitis must be closely monitored for the presence of increased intracranial pressure, seizures, and signs of septic shock. Because infants and small children have relatively immature immune systems, they are particularly vulnerable to sepsis.

If respiratory depression develops (suggestive of increased ICP), assist the child's ventilations with a bag-valve-mask device and 100% oxygen. Endotracheal intubation may be necessary if you are unable to provide effective bag-valve-mask ventilations or your transport time to the hospital will be lengthy.

Provided the child remains hemodynamically stable, allow him or her to remain with the caregiver. Continue oxygen therapy as tolerated and promptly transport the child to the hospital. If signs and symptoms of septic shock (**Table 6-2**) are present, obtain IV or IO access and administer 20-mL/kg boluses of normal saline or lactated Ringer's as needed to maintain adequate perfusion. If the child is hemodynamically stable, consider deferring IV therapy until the child is in the emergency department. Remember, you should avoid any unnecessary procedures; these will likely increase the child's anxiety and could cause acute deterioration of his or her clinical condition.

If the child experiences a seizure, administer a benzodiazepine drug such as diazepam (Valium) or midazolam (Versed). If IV or IO access is not available, diazepam can be given via the rectal route; midazolam can be given intramuscularly if needed. Follow locally established protocols or contact medical control as needed regarding the pediatric doses of these drugs.

Table 6-2 Signs and Symptoms of Septic Shock
Weak, rapid peripheral pulses
Rapid, shallow respirations
Poor muscle tone
Cool, pale extremities
• Unless profound peripheral vasoconstriction is present, the child's skin may remain warm or hot secondary to high fever.
Capillary refill time greater than 2 seconds
• Most reliable in children less than 6 years of age
Decreased level of consciousness
• Failure to recognize parents
• Difficult to arouse
Petechial or purpuric rash
Hypotension (late sign)

If, despite two or three crystalloid fluid boluses, the child remains hypotensive, medical control may order an infusion of one of the following vasoactive drugs, both of which should be titrated as necessary to improve perfusion:

■ **Epinephrine: 0.1 to 1 µg/kg/min**

■ **Dopamine: 2 to 20 µg/kg/min**
  • Usual starting dose is 5 to 10 µg/kg/min.

Definitive treatment for a child with meningitis and septic shock involves the administration of antibiotics—an intervention that cannot be provided in the prehospital setting. Therefore, rapid transport to an appropriate medical facility is essential.

Summary

Meningitis remains a significant cause of mortality and morbidity in children. *Neisseria meningitidis* (*N. meningitidis*), or meningococcal meningitis, and *Streptococcus pneumoniae* (also called pneumococcal meningitis), are the most common causes of bacterial meningitis in children older than 1 month of age. *Haemophilus influenzae* type b (Hib) has been virtually eradicated as a cause of bacterial meningitis in children due to Hib vaccinations that began in the late 1980s. If left untreated, bacterial meningitis may result in septic shock, permanent neurological impairment, or death.

Meningitis should be suspected in any child who presents with fever, headache, and nuchal rigidity; however, headache and nuchal rigidity are most reliably assessed in children older than 18 to 24 months of age. Other signs and symptoms include nausea and vomiting, irritability, photophobia, signs of increased intracranial pressure, seizures, and a petechial or purpuric rash. In infants, common signs include paradoxical irritability, poor feeding, a bulging fontanelle, and inconsolability.

Prehospital care for a child with meningitis begins by taking the appropriate BSI precautions, including gloves and facial protection; bacterial meningitis is a contagious disease that is spread by the airborne droplet route. Obtain and maintain the child's airway and provide supplemental oxygen or assisted ventilation as needed. If signs of hypoperfusion are present, 20-mL/kg IV or IO crystalloid fluid boluses should be given. Vasopressor therapy (eg, epinephrine, dopamine) may be required for fluid-refractory hypoperfusion. If the child is hemodynamically stable, consider deferring IV therapy to avoid causing unnecessary anxiety. Promptly transport the child to an appropriate medical facility, while closely monitoring his or her ABCs en route. Meningitis is diagnosed in the emergency department with a lumbar puncture (spinal tap) and is treated definitively with antibiotic therapy.

Section 7: Operations

Chapter 46: Ambulance Operations

Matching

1. G (pages 46.13–46.15)	**6.** G (pages 46.13–46.15)
2. G (pages 46.13–46.15)	**7.** A (pages 46.13–46.15)
3. A (pages 46.13–46.15)	**8.** A (pages 46.13–46.15)
4. A (pages 46.13–46.15)	**9.** G (pages 46.13–46.15)
5. G (pages 46.13–46.15)	**10.** G (pages 46.13–46.15)

Multiple Choice

1. A (page 46.5)	**6.** C (page 46.13)
2. B (page 46.4)	**7.** C (page 46.14)
3. C (page 46.10)	**8.** A (page 46.14)
4. B (page 46.10)	**9.** C (page 46.15)
5. C (page 46.12)	**10.** D (page 46.8)

Labeling

1. Landing Zone (LZ) (page 46.14)

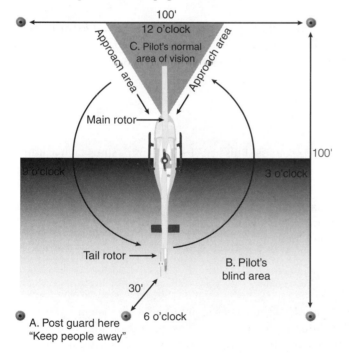

Fill-in-the-Blank

1. There's room for some discussion regarding what things are absolutely essential during the first few minutes with a patient who has been critically injured in a road collision. With experience, you may want to modify your list. In general, you will have to make a trade-off between all the equipment you would like to have immediately at hand and what you can carry comfortably during your first, hurried dash—often over difficult terrain—to the patient.

_____	Long-leg air splint	X	Stethoscope
_____	Drug box	X	Flashlight
X	Portable suction unit	X	Triangular bandages
X	Oxygen cylinder	_____	Chemical cold packs
_____	OB kit	X	Cervical collar
X	Pocket mask	_____	Traction splint
X	Oropharyngeal airways	X	Nonrebreathing mask
_____	Intravenous fluid bags	X	Long backboard/straps
X	Dressing materials	_____	Oral thermometer
X	Large-bore IV cannulas	X	Fire extinguisher
X	Head immobilizer	_____	Bed pan
X	Self-adhering roller bandage	X	Heavy-duty scissors
_____	Selection of board splints	_____	Emesis basin
_____	Wheeled cot stretcher	X	Handheld radio
_____	ECG monitor	_____	Adhesive bandages
_____	Contact lens remover		

Other equipment that might be needed: Depending on the circumstances, you might require some light rescue and extrication equipment. And you may prefer a bag-mask device to a pocket mask. Finally, emergency medical technicians-Basic (EMT-Bs) and paramedics should, in this era of acquired immune deficiency syndrome (AIDS), don plastic or rubber gloves when they have to come in contact with a patient's blood or secretions.

Identify

a. Chief complaint: Deformity to left collarbone, possible internal trauma.

b. Vital signs: Alert, respirations are 22 breaths/min, shallow; decreased left lung sounds. Pulse is 114 beats/min, sinus tachycardia with PVC, blood pressure is 132/84 mm Hg. Pain is 9/10, PEARRL, skin is warm.

c. Pertinent negatives: No loss of consciousness, right lung sound clear.

Walt and Dave did a great job in thinking on their feet. Because of the collar bone a C-collar isn't going to work. The use of the towels and tape is the next best thing. They also went to the regional trauma center. The patient has a few PVCs and decreased lung sounds on the left which, is consistent with the seat belt injuries. They should be watching the left chest for a possible pneumothorax and the pericardial tamponade.

Ambulance Calls

1. a. Cory and Bill should have worked out their differences before arriving on the scene. They should know who is going to act as lead, and both of them should know what equipment to grab before leaving the squad. It is not a good idea to have a lay person digging through your squad looking for your equipment. Their actions on scene were very unprofessional and detrimental to the patient's outcome.

b. There are many questions that could be asked on scene. Here are six that would be beneficial at this scene.

(1) How far did the patient fall?

(2) How did he land?

(3) Has he been unconscious the whole time or has he made any noises or movements since he fell?

(4) Do you know any of his medical history?

(5) What is his name and who will be contacting family?

(6) What made him fall?

c. What kind of transport decision would you make right away? This patient needs to be at a trauma center. Most likely he has a head injury, and because he is unconscious as a result of a fall from a second-story roof he is a definite regional trauma center candidate. If air medical is available and able to get the patient to the trauma center more quickly than by ambulance, they should be called within the first minute of arriving on the scene. Cory and Bill should be thinking of the "platinum 10 minutes" and the "golden hour" when treating this patient. (pages 46.13–46.15)

2. a. Jeff and Larry should know better than to skip checking the squad. You should always recheck after every change in crews. Tires can leak during downtime; people forget to refuel. A turn signal may be working in the morning but quits sometime during the day. Checking the squad also mentally prepares you for the coming shift. It gives you confidence in your equipment because **you** know that it is ready to go, instead of relying on someone else. Everything should be checked once a day. (page 46.7)

b. A visual check should include a quick walk around to ensure that there are no flat tires or fluids dripping from the engine. Many services have a checklist beside the squad so that you can see when the last check was made on the unit and the equipment. The responding crew could have someone in the back check other equipment on the way to the scene. Every department is different, so make sure you understand the checks that are designed for your unit and make sure when your call is over that all supplies are stocked and ready for the next call. (pages 46.6 and 46.7)

True/False

1. F (page 46.5)   **6.** T (page 46.8)

2. T (page 46.5)   **7.** F (page 46.9)

3. T (page 46.5)   **8.** T (page 46.9)

4. F (page 46.6)   **9.** F (page 46.10)

5. F (page 46.7)   **10.** T (page 46.14)

Short Answer

There are many ways to save time without cutting corners in the management of the critically injured, among them are the following:

1. Get rolling at once when dispatched. Don't wait until you have all the details; all you need to get on the road is the *address*—you can find out the rest en route.

2. Know the map, and take the shortest route to the scene.

3. While en route to the scene, assemble the equipment you will need when you get there.

What other ideas did you come up with for saving time? It is always possible to find a more efficient way to do a job.

Secret Message

a. Parking on a roadway at night can be DANGEROUS.

b. A LANDING zone should be 100 feet by 100 feet.

c. System Status Management (SSM) attempts STRATEGIC deployment to minimize response time.

d. As a paramedic, you should always act as an ADVOCATE for your patient.

e. Padded cabinet corners were installed to prevent INJURY to the emergency medical technician (EMT).

f. WHEEL bounce is a vibration synchronous with road speed.

g. Wheel WOBBLE is a common finding at low speeds.

Secret Message: ALWAYS DRIVE WITH DUE REGARD

Fill-in-the-Table

1. (page 46.14)   **2.** (page 46.14)

Advantages of Using an Air Ambulance
■ Specialized skills or equipment is needed
■ Rapid transport is possible
■ Can provide access to remote areas
■ Helicopter hospital helipads are available

Disadvantages of Using an Air Ambulance
■ Weather/environment
■ Altitude limitations
■ Airspeed limitations
■ Aircraft cabin size
■ Terrain
■ Cost
■ Patient's condition

Skill Drills

1. *Loading the Patient* (page 46.11)

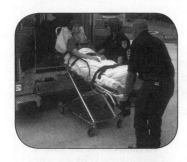

Step 1: Tilt the head of the cot upward, and place it into the patient compartment with the wheels on the floor.

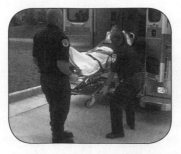

Step 2: The second paramedic on the side of the cot releases the undercarriage lock and lifts the undercarriage.

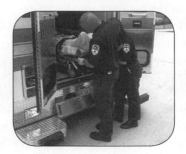

Step 3: Roll the cot into the back of the ambulance.

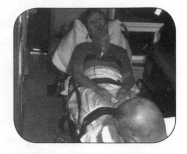

Step 4: Secure the cot to the brackets mounted in the ambulance.

2. *Unloading the Patient* (page 46.12)

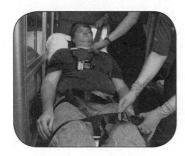

Step 1: Ensure that the patient is secured to the stretcher.

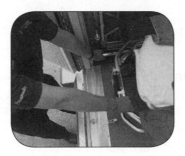

Step 2: Unlock the head and foot locks.

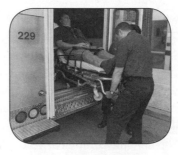

Step 3: Lifting with your legs, carefully roll the stretcher forward until the undercarriage engages.

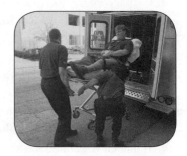

Step 4: With your partner steadying the stretcher from the side, gently bring the stretcher forward out of the ambulance.

Chapter 47: Medical Incident Command

Matching

1. E (page 47.8)	**6.** D (page 47.11)
2. H (page 47.8)	**7.** J (page 47.12)
3. B (page 47.7)	**8.** C (page 47.12)
4. G (page 47.6)	**9.** I (page 47.12)
5. A (page 47.10)	**10.** F (page 47.11)

Multiple Choice

1. B (page 47.4)	**6.** A (page 47.13)
2. B (page 47.5)	**7.** C (page 47.16)
3. C (page 47.9)	**8.** D (page 47.13)
4. C (page 47.10)	**9.** A (page 47.14)
5. D (page 47.12)	**10.** B (page 47.9)

Labeling

1. Diagram of an MCI (page 47.11)

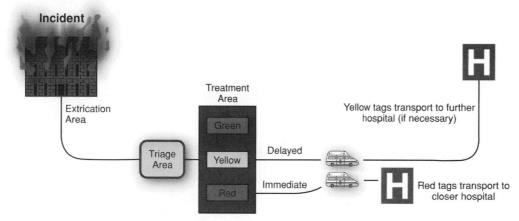

2. The START algorithm (page 47.15)

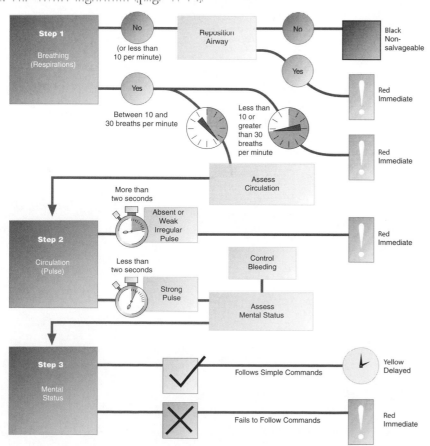

3. The JumpSTART Algorithm (page 47.17)

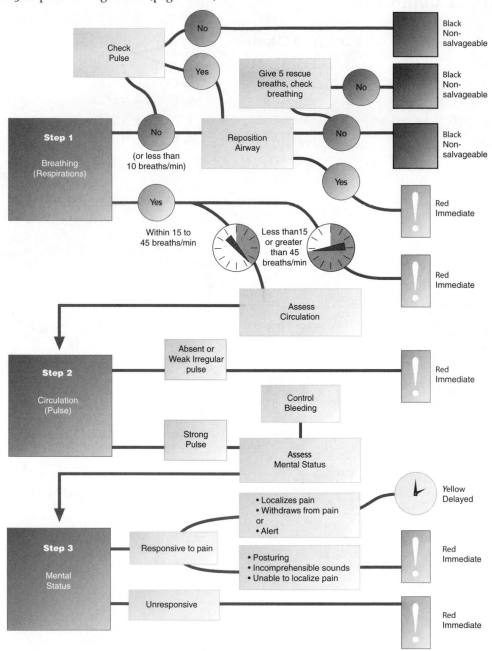

Fill-in-the-Blank

1. Multiple-casualty incident (page 47.4)

2. Closed (page 47.5)

3. Finance (page 47.6)

4. Safety, PIO, liaison (page 47.7- 47.8)

5. Preparedness (page 47.8)

6. Transportation (page 47.11)

7. Primary, secondary (page 47.13)

8. Rapid (page 47.14)

9. Jump (page 47.15)

10. Staging (page 47.11)

Identify

1. Chief complaint: Impaled object in left buttock
2. Vital signs: Respiration is 20 breaths/min, oxygen saturation is 97%, clear lungs, pulse is 98 beats/min, normal sinus rhythm, blood pressure is 136/88 mm Hg, patient is 7/10 on scale for pain, skin is warm and dry.
3. Pertinent negatives: Remained alert during the whole time, not a lot of bleeding, which indicates a tamponade effect inside where the wood is pressing against the veins and arteries.

   Your patient provides a small challenge because of the need to stabilize him to a backboard as a result of the blast knocking him down. However, the impaled object is not letting you lay him. This is where you do the best job possible and move him as little as possible. A scoop stretcher may be a better tool to use to "pick" up the patient.

Ambulance Calls

1. This call may be the most stressful event you ever respond to. Remember to take care of yourself as soon as possible, and debrief. Don't be a "hero"; take your turn in the rehab section. Don't become a victim! Please stay on top of scene safety and don't get lulled into a false sense of security. Stay on your toes!

   a. Everyone's answers may be different because there is no right or wrong answers here. Work as a group to develop a list of the best items to carry.
      (1) Communication radio
      (2) Multi tool
      (3) Gloves
      (4) Pen and paper
      (5) Flashlight
      (6) AM/FM radio
      (7) Trauma bandages
      (8) Pocket face mask
      (9) Leather gloves
      (10) Orange vest (page 47.7)

   b. Once again there will be a lot of different answers. Two heads are always better than one. Tell them help will be coming soon, to stay away from downed powerlines, and not to move patients unless they are in extreme danger. Try to account for everyone in the area. Stay in a group. Do not go back into a destroyed building.

   c. Remember, anything can become a hazard during a disaster. People, animals, burst water and gas mains, downed electric lines, fires, falling debris, sewage, and the weather. Can you think of any others?

2. a. If you have emergency management people that are trained for this, they should take command. If the fire station is unharmed, it would make a great central command post. The nursing home should also have a command post that reports back to central command because of the large volume of people in that area. The fire station can also serve as a rehab center or staging area because a lot of supplies are already there. The fire station will be a logical gathering area for incoming help.

   b. Because the high school has not be touched it would be a logical place to go. It has large open spaces and a large kitchen that could be used to feed people. Churches, community buildings, libraries, and senior citizen centers are all good places to use. Check to see if the local grocery store is able to start bringing food and water to your chosen site.

3. a. Your emergency response team should have a list of these agencies and phone numbers to call for help right away. If your dispatch center is still operating, it may have already alerted these agencies. Red Cross Disaster Services will probably be the first to arrive. You may have church agencies and state and local governmental agencies that will also respond.

True/False

1. F (page 47.11)
2. T (page 47.7)
3. T (page 47.4)
4. T (page 47.5)
5. F (page 46.5)
6. T (page 47.8)
7. F (page 47.8)
8. T (page 47.10)
9. F (page 47.13)
10. T (page 47.14)

Short Answer

1. In the first stage of the START triage system, you will use a strong, commanding voice to shout out to the victims. You need to tell them if they can walk or are uninjured to move to a specific landmark away from the disaster site. In this way, you have just effectively triaged all the walking wounded into one area with out actually looking at each patient. (page 47.14)

2. In the second stage of START, you begin with the first patient you reach. Assess the respiratory status by opening the airway. If the patient is not breathing, tag the person black and move to the next patient. A patient breathing faster than 30 breaths/min should be tagged red. If the breathing rate is less than 30 breaths/min, move on to the assessment of the circulatory system. If the person has no radial pulse, tag him or her red; if not, move again to the neurologic assessment. If the patient is unconscious or unable to follow a simple command, tag him or her red. If the person can follow the command, tag the person yellow and move on to the next patient. (page 47.15)

3. Children and infants may not be able to understand your commands. Children with special needs will be confused and need to be taken to the treatment center as soon as possible. Remember that children go into cardiac arrest because of respiratory arrest, and so the assessment process is a little different for children. (page 47.15)

4. Always take advantage of a debriefing after a large incident. It can really help to manage stress after the initial event. Encourage participation, but do not force people to attend. The quicker you can return to active work after an incident, the better off you will be in the long run. (page 47.16)

Crossword Puzzle

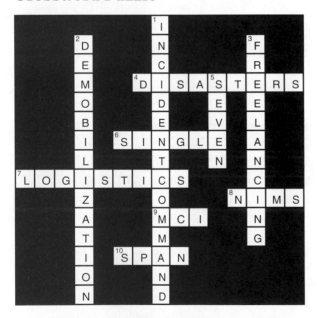

Fill-in-the-Table

1. (page 47.7)

MCI Equipment and Supplies*	
Airway control	PPE (gloves, face shield, HEPA or N95 mask) Oral airways, nasal airways Suction units (manual units) Rigid tip Yankauer and flexible suction catheters LMA, Combitube, ET tubes* Laryngoscope and blades* Tube check, tube restraint, tape, syringes, stylet* End-tidal CO_2 device
Breathing	Pocket mask and one-way valve Bag-mask device(s) (adult and child), spare masks Oxygen delivery devices (nonrebreathing mask, cannula, extension tubing) Oxygen tank, regulator Occlusive dressings Large-bore IV catheter for thoracic decompression*
Circulation	Dressings, bandages, tape Sphygmomanometer, stethoscope Burn dressings, burn sheets, sterile water for irrigation One-handed tourniquets 1,000 mL bags of normal saline, IV start kits, catheters*
Disability	Rigid collars (one size fits all) Head beds, wide tape, backboard straps Flashlights, spare batteries
Exposure	Space blanket to cover patients Scissors
Logistic/Command	Sector vests (triage, treatment, transport, staging, command, rescue) Pads of paper, pencils, pens, markers Triage tags or kits used by your regional system Assessment cards

Note: The items denoted by * could be packaged in an ALS kit.

Chapter 48: Terrorism and Weapons of Mass Destruction

Matching

1. I (page 48.12)
2. C (page 48.8)
3. F (page 48.10)
4. E (page 48.14)
5. G (page 18.14)

6. A (page 48.13)
7. J (page 48.14)
8. B (page 48.19)
9. H (page 48.20)
10. D (page 48.11)

Multiple Choice

1. C (page 48.4)
2. D (page 48.6)
3. A (page 48.8)
4. C (page 48.9)
5. B (page 48.10)

6. A (page 48.11)
7. B (page 48.14)
8. D (page 48.15)
9. C (page 48.16)
10. A (page 48.19)

Labeling

1.

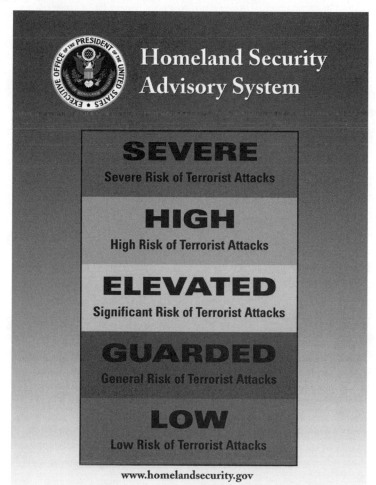

(page 48.6)

Fill-in-the-Blank

1. Weapons of mass destruction/casualties (page 48.4)
2. Covert (page 48.6)
3. Secondary (page 48.8)
4. Route of exposure (page 48.8)
5. Nerve agents (page 48.10)
6. German (page 48.10)
7. Lymphatic (page 48.15)
8. Anthrax (page 48.15)
9. Castor bean (page 48.16)
10. Points of distribution (page 48.18)

Identify

1. Chief complaint: Trauma, organophosphate poisoning.
2. Vital signs: Alert to start, but loses consciousness as the poisoning progresses. Heart rate 50 beats/min, blood pressure is 98/66 mm Hg, oxygen saturation is 88%, respirations are 9 breaths/min.
3. Pertinent negatives: There are no pertinent negatives.
   Always look around before running into the scene. You never know what people are carrying in the truck. It is no fun to become a patient yourself!

Ambulance Calls

1. **a.** This train derailment could be a terrorist attack, and so you need to be thinking about what kind of attack it was and be prepared for the type of scene you will be entering.
   (1) Biological, probably not this scene, but you never know what the train is carrying.
   (2) Nuclear, no signs of radiation, and so you should be okay here.
   (3) Incendiary, possibly at this scene; better to get away and stay away. A fire could have started to cause an explosion to derail the train.
   (4) Chemical, once again not very likely at this scene.
   (5) Explosives, this is the best bet here; either the tracks were blown up or something inside the train blew to cause the derailment. Be careful because there may be some secondary explosions. (page 48.4)
   b. You can designate someone to walk toward the vehicles but have the person stay clear of the vehicles. A person that is wearing a bright color is a good idea because people will be able to see him or her. Appoint that person and tell the person he or she is the leader. Have the person remain standing so the walking wounded have someone to walk toward. If you have enough responders, you can designate one of them. They can wave a white towel or some type of flag; whatever your solution, get the walking wounded cleared out of the wreckage as soon as possible! (page 47.14)
2. **a.** Chlorine, which is used a lot in swimming pools, is what is leaking and causing the green haze. It will have the smell of bleach.
   b. Before getting out, you better be calling for help. First, you need a hazmat team or at least the fire department to go into the pool area with their self-contained breathing apparatus (SCBA) gear and bring out the missing lifeguards. Leave all your windows up and use your external public address (PA) system to direct the children standing around to walk upwind and away from the pool. Have them follow the ambulance until you are a safe distance away.
   c. With chlorine gas, complete airway obstruction can occur as a result of pulmonary edema. Be prepared to intubate if necessary. Oxygen is a must! (page 48.10)

True/False

1. F (page 48.20)
2. T (page 48.19)
3. F (page 48.15)
4. F (page 48.14)
5. T (page 48.14)
6. T (page 48.14)
7. F (page 48.10)
8. F (page 48.4)
9. T (page 48.4)
10. T (page 48.7)

Short Answer

1. Three *reactions* sometimes seen in bystanders at a multiple-casualty incident (MCI) are the following:
   a. Overreaction
   b. Conversion hysteria
   c. Depression
      If you mentioned anxiety, that is also correct.

2. Triage tags are usually not very large and cannot accommodate a lot of information. But they should at least contain the most essential facts about the patient, especially if the person is unconscious or for any other reason is unable to provide information to the emergency department staff:
   a. Identifying information: name, age, address, next of kin's name and telephone number
   b. Information about the scene: anything that will help the emergency department staff understand the mechanisms of injury
   c. Pertinent (SAMPLE) medical history
   d. Physical findings: vital and neurologic signs, any positive findings on physical examination
   e. Any treatment given (if a drug, the dose given, the time it was given, and the route by which it was given)
   f. Priority (will usually be indicated by the color of the triage tag)

Word Find

```
A S N C H L O R I N E B T D E D
I A O S M G V S T C R F I T S I
D L I I D V U I Y O N R A I G S
R I T S C H E A N O T H S E Z S
A V A E G X N C I Y P O N I Y E
C A N M N I H T B S I I U U G M
Y T I E D O A O M P R K C X I
D I R E R M M H I O L L D H D N
A O U R I B P A R G N W T L X A
R N H R W O X T N H A T I O B T
B E C O N T A C T H A Z A R D I
A A J A N E G A T U M H I I M O
L F G P E V A P O R N W B D S N
X R E O Y C N E T S I S R E P W
O D E F E C A T I O N P Z R A T
T Y Z F T S E T O D I T N A Y Z
```

1. Persistency (page 48.8)
2. Vapor, contact hazard (page 48.8)
3. Mutagen (page 48.9)
4. Antidotes (page 48.9)
5. Chlorine (page 48.10)
6. Defecation, urination, miosis, bradycardia, bronchorrhea, emesis, lacrimation, salivation (page 48.11)
7. Atropine, chloride (page 48.12)
8. Organophosphate (page 48.10)
9. Cyanide (page 48.12)
10. Dissemination (page 48.13)
11. Dirty bomb (page 48.19)

Fill-in-the-Table

1. (page 48.12)

Nerve Agents						
Name	**Code Name**	**Odor**	**Special Features**	**Onset of Symptoms**	**Volatility**	**Route of Exposure**
Tabun	GA	Fruity	Easy to manufacture	Immediate	Low	Both contact and vapor hazard
Sarin	GB	None (if pure) or strong	Will off-gas while on victim's clothing	Immediate	High	Primarily respiratory vapor hazard; extremely lethal if skin contact is made
Soman	GD	Fruity	Ages rapidly, making it difficult to treat	Immediate	Moderate	Contact with skin; minimal vapor hazard
V agent	VX	None	Most lethal chemical agent; difficult to decontaminate	Immediate	Very low	Contact with skin; no vapor hazard (unless aerosolized)

2. (page 48.13)

Chemical Agents						
Class	**Military Designations**	**Odor**	**Lethality**	**Onset of Symptoms**	**Volatility**	**Primary Route of Exposure**
Nerve agents	Tabun (GA) Sarin (GB) Soman (GD) VX	Fruity or none	Most lethal chemical agents can kill within minutes; effects are reversible with antidotes	Immediate	Moderate (GA, GD) Very high (GB) Low (VX)	Vapor hazard (GB) Both vapor and contact hazard (GA, GD) Contact hazard (VX)
Vesicants	Mustard (H) Lewisite (L) Phosgene oxime (CX)	Garlic (H) Geranium (L)	Causes large blisters to form on victims; may severely damage upper airway if vapors are inhaled; severe intense pain and grayish skin discoloration (L, CX)	Delayed (H) Immediate (L, CX)	Very low (H, L) Moderate (CX)	Primarily contact; with some vapor hazard
Pulmonary agents	Chlorine (CL) Phosgene (CG)	Bleach (CL) Cut grass (CG)	Causes irritation; choking (CL); severe pulmonary edema (CG)	Immediate (CL) Delayed (CG)	Very high	Vapor hazard
Cyanide agents	Hydrogen cyanide (AC) Cyanogens chloride (CK)	Almonds (AC) Irritating (CK)	Highly lethal chemical gases; can kill within minutes; effects are reversible with antidotes	Immediate	Very high	Vapor hazard

Chapter 49: Rescue Awareness and Operations

Matching

1. E (page 49.27)
2. H (page 49.26)
3. A (page 49.22)
4. J (page 49.21)
5. D (page 49.21)

6. I (page 49.26)
7. B (page 49.24)
8. G (page 49.19)
9. F (page 49.24)
10. C (page 49.19)

Multiple Choice

1. B (page 49.4)
2. D (page 49.5)
3. A (page 49.6)
4. C (page 49.7)
5. A (page 49.9)

6. B (page 49.9)
7. B (page 49.11)
8. C (page 49.12)
9. D (page 49.12)
10. D (page 49.14)

Labeling

1. The anatomy of a vehicle (page 49.12)

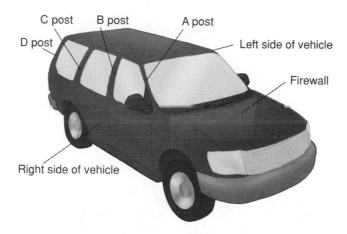

2. Stabilization techniques (page 49.13)

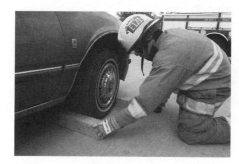
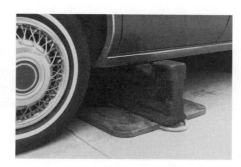
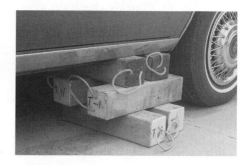

A. Step blocks

B. Box crib

C. Cribbing

Fill-in-the-Blank

1. Protect (page 49.17)
2. Hazard (page 49.18)
3. A (page 49.18)
4. Confined space (page 49.19)
5. Hydrogen sulfide (page 49.19)
6. Shoring (page 49.20)
7. Self-rescue position (page 49.21)
8. Reach out (page 49.22)
9. Recovery (page 49.23)
10. Low-angle (page 49.23)

Identify

1. Chief complaint: Decreased level of consciousness, trauma to left side region
2. Vital signs: Verbally responsive, blood pressure 102/68 mm Hg, pulse of 116 beats/min, sinus tachycardia, and thready at the wrist. Skin is pale and cool. Oxygen saturation is 96%. Respirations are 24 breaths/min and shallow with diminished lung sounds in left side. Pupils Equal And Round, Regular in size, but are slow to react to Light (PEARRL).
3. Pertinent negatives: Negative halo test

Ambulance Calls

1. To answer this question, you need to apply a lot of the information you have learned in the past chapters. How well did you do?
   a. The steps to take are as follows:
   (1) Assess the scene for
   (a) Hazards.
   (b) Missing patients. (Could a front-seat passenger who was not wearing a seat belt have been thrown through that shattered front windshield?)
   (2) Call for help. At the least, you're going to need the police, the fire department, and perhaps additional help in the extrication.
   (3) Once the hazards have been dealt with, gain access to the patient. Try all the doors first.
   (4) Enter the vehicle and start care, specifically:
   (a) Open the airway by lifting the head into neutral position; if possible, have one of your crew take up a position in the back seat where he or she can apply a cervical collar and hold the patient's head in neutral position.
   (b) Administer supplemental oxygen.
   (c) Quickly check the chest for signs of pneumothorax or sucking chest wound.
   (d) Control external hemorrhage by direct pressure.
   (e) Start a large-bore IV with lactated Ringer's.
   (f) Cover open wounds.
   (g) Splint fractures.
   (5) As soon as disentanglement is complete, remove the patient on a long backboard, and transfer the patient to the ambulance.
   (6) Notify the receiving hospital.
   (7) Transport. This is a "load-and-go" situation.
   (8) If possible, start another IV en route.
   b. (1) Once the patient has been transferred to the hospital, you have to clean up the ambulance and equipment.
   (2) Restock all kits used.

True/False

A lot of extrication is common sense.

1. F (page 49.8)   **4.** F (page 49.9)

2. F (page 49.13)   **5.** T (page 49.11)

3. T (page 49.15)   **6.** T (page 49.12)

Short Answer

1. **a.** Awareness: You need to be trained in recognizing hazards at the scene and being able to call for the appropriate assistance, such as the power company, or calling for the correct rescue team.

   b. Operations: You will be working in the area directly outside of the rescue zone. This area helps to assist the people working on the rescue. An example would be a rehab zone for a diving team.

   c. Technician: This is where you are directly involved in the rescue operation. It could be high-angle rappelling or swift-water rescue. You will be the person saving the patient from the incident. (pages 49.4, 49.5)

2. **a.** Be safe: Your safety and your team's safety should *always* be your number one priority. Check for hazards before entering the scene! Live to work another day!

   b. Follow orders: Don't do anything without checking for orders. Orders stop the duplication of work and provide for the most qualified personnel working in the right area.

   c. Work as a team: Team effort is essential, and it is the quickest way to get the job done. Every link of the chain is strong, but the chain is strongest when linked together.

   d. Think: You must have your head in the game. You should constantly be assessing and reassessing the scene safety. You should report anything that changes on the scene to the appropriate person.

   e. Follow the Golden Rule of public service: Keep your patient calm by letting the patient know what is going on around him or her and what you are trying to accomplish. There should be one person that is there for emotional support of the patient if possible. (pages 49.5, 49.6)

3. Gear that is standard for a water rescue is a personal floatation device, a lightweight helmet made for water rescue, a cutting device, a whistle, and some type of contamination protection. Remember you must be trained for the correct water rescue before attempting a rescue. (page 49.10)

4. Side glass vs. windshield. Tempered glass is used in the windows and the rear window. This glass will break in small pieces by using a spring-loaded punch in the corner. A windshield will not break because of the plastic that is between the layers of the glass, and it must be removed in one large piece. This is done by using an axe or a saw. The windshield will need to be removed before displacing the roof on a vehicle. Remember to always cover and tell your patient before attempting to remove or break glass around the patient. (page 49.17)

Word Find

1. In fact, this jumbled-up collection of rescue tools doesn't belong to a real paramedic because *real* paramedics keep all their gear neat, clean, and organized.

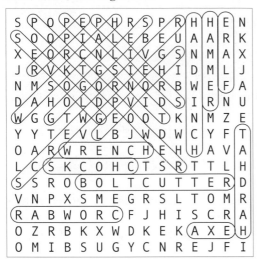

Item	Use in a Rescue Situation
1. flare	To demarcate a danger zone and caution oncoming traffic
2. wrench	Disassembly
3. screwdriver	Disassembly
4. hacksaw	Cutting through corner posts or steering wheel
5. pliers	Breaking away steering wheel covering
6. hammer	Making openings with cutting tools
7. axe	Cutting roof section
8. crowbar	Prying open a door
9. bolt cutter	Cutting padlocks, chains, fences
10. Portapower	Prying open doors, breaking seats loose
11. shovel	Removing debris
12. tin snip	Cutting seat belts
13. rope	Stabilizing a vehicle
14. hand winch	Displacing steering column, widening door opening, pulling seat back
15. chocks	Preventing motion
16. hard hat	Protects rescuer's head
17. gloves	Protect rescuer's hands
18. goggles	Protect rescuer's eyes

Fill-in-the-Table

1.

F: Failure to understand or underestimating the environment

A: Additional medical problems not considered

I: Inadequate rescue skills

L: Lack of teamwork or experience

U: Underestimating the logistics of the incident

R: Rescue versus recovery mode not considered

E: Equipment not mastered (page 49.6)

Skill Drills

1. *Stabilizing a Suspected Spinal Injury in the Water*

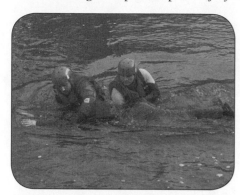

Step 1: Turn the patient to a supine position in the water by rotating the entire upper half of the body as a single unit.

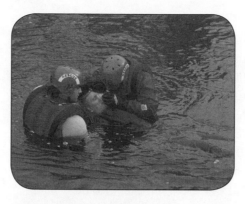

Step 2: As soon as the patient is turned, begin artificial ventilation using the mouth-to-mouth method or a pocket mask.

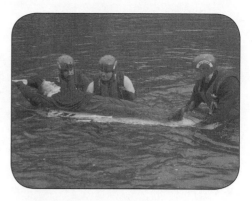

Step 3: Float a buoyant backboard under the patient.

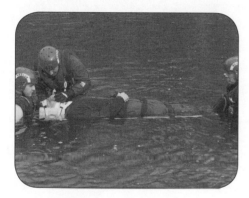

Step 4: Secure the patient to the backboard.

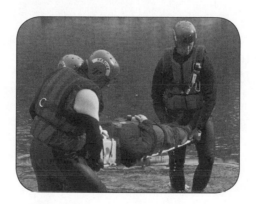

Step 5: Remove the patient from the water.

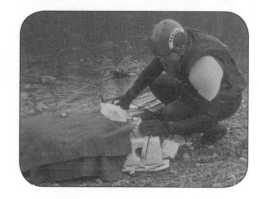

Step 6: Cover the patient with a blanket and apply oxygen if breathing. Begin cardiopulmonary resuscitation (CPR) if breathing and a pulse are still absent.

Chapter 50: Hazardous Materials Incidents

Matching

1. R (page 50.4)
2. O (page 50.4)
3. F (page 50.6)
4. T (page 50.6)
5. K (page 50.6)
6. Q (page 50.8)
7. A (page 50.9)
8. S (page 50.10)
9. G (page 50.13)
10. N (page 50.13)
11. L (page 50.10)
12. H (page 50.11)
13. C (page 50.11)
14. P (page 50.12)
15. J (page 50.7)
16. A (page 50.13)
17. M (page 50.9)
18. E (page 50.16)
19. D (page 50.12)
20. I (page 50.7)

Multiple Choice

1. D (page 50.12)
2. A (page 50.12)
3. D (page 50.13)
4. C (page 50.14)
5. D (page 50.16)
6. B (page 50.4)
7. C (page 50.7)
8. D (page 50.8)
9. A (page 50.10)
10. A (page 50.15)

Fill-in-the-Blank

1. Awareness level (page 50.4)
2. Hazardous material (page 50.5)
3. Dead heroes (page 50.4)
4. Information (page 50.6)
5. Commercial, train (page 50.6)
6. Bill of lading, waybill (page 50.7)
7. Primary, secondary (page 50.11)
8. Primary contamination (page 50.11)
9. Secondary contamination (page 50.11)

Identify

1. Based on the information provided in the *ERG*, this product is highly toxic and may be fatal if inhaled or absorbed through the skin.
2. Specialized protective clothing with SCBA is required. Structural fire fighter clothing will provide only a limited amount of protection. Most paramedics and ambulances don't carry the proper clothing unless it is a specialized unit with specially trained personnel.
3. Based on the information given, the ambulance and stopped nearby traffic are in immediate danger. It's important to relocate upwind and set up a staging area a safe distance as determined by Incident Command and the parameters of the guidebook. It's also advisable to begin requesting the allocation of additional resources and personnel based on the life-threatening nature of the incident.
4. The photos show the four levels of protection in the following order: level B, level A, level D, level C.

    Level A provides the greatest protection from exposure to hazardous substances. These suits look like an astronaut's suit because they are "fully encapsulating." These suits fully cover and protect the SCBA worn by hazardous materials technicians. The suits are rigorously tested by the manufacturers to determine resistance and permeability to many chemicals.

    Level B is called for when the technician needs protection from splashes and inhaled toxins. It is not fully encapsulating like Level A is, and it is worn with SCBA. B suits are typically worn by the hazardous materials decontamination team in the warm zone.

Level C is designed to protect against a known agent. The equipment provides splash protection and is worn with an air-purifying respirator that must have filters specifically chosen to provide protection against the known agent. Offering eye and hand protection and foot coverings, Level C protection could be used during transport of patients with the potential of secondary contamination.

Level D is the level of PPE offered by fire fighters' turnout gear. It is typically not worn in hazardous materials incidents but may be used by some personnel in the cold zone (page 50.11).

Ambulance Calls

1. a. What safety precautions are necessary in handling and decontaminating this patient? List three considerations. (page 50.13)

(1) Your safety comes first.

(2) You must work as part of a team to prevent more casualties.

(3) Use the incident command system, which permits only properly trained and equipped hazardous materials personnel to enter the hot zone.

2. a. Three potential sources of information regarding the nature of the train's cargo are the following:

(1) The USDOT placard on the side of each car

(2) The waybill and the consist carried by the conductor

(3) The conductor

b. Once you know that you are dealing with a hazardous cargo, you should radio your dispatcher with details of the accident and request help from the following sources:

(1) Hazmat team

(2) Fire department with heavy rescue gear

(3) Police for crowd and traffic control

(4) At least one ambulance for every two estimated casualties on the road

True/False

1 Transport accidents involving radioactive materials are likely to increase in frequency, so it is important to have a clear plan of action for such events and to know what you should and should not do at the scene.

a. T (page 50.8) **d.** T (page 50.12)

b. F (page 50.14) **e.** T (page 50.6)

c. F (page 50.16) **f.** T (page 50.19)

2. It is just as important to know what *not* to do at a hazmat incident as to know what *to* do.

a. F (page 50.6) **d.** F (page 50.10)

b. T (page 50.7) **e.** T (page 50.16)

c. F (page 50.13)

Short Answer

1. a. Name of substance

b. An emergency action guide

c. Evacuation and isolation information (50.18)

2. a. Chemtrec

b. Bill of lading

c. Waybill

d. EPA's Chemical Compatibility Chart

e. Material Safety Data Sheet (page 50.7)

3. The most important step in dealing with a hazmat incident is recognizing that a hazmat situation exists in the first place. If you have to wait until you start to feel sick from your own exposure to a poisonous material before you figure out that the situation might be dangerous, you've waited too long.

a. Two-car collision downtown: If either of those cars is on fire, you may be dealing with toxic products of the combustion of automobile upholstery, including phosgene, chlorine, and hydrogen chloride.

b. Apartment-house fire: Any fire produces toxic fumes, and at the least you need to think about carbon monoxide and cyanide.

c. Three municipal workers collapsed in a sewer: When three people get sick in the same place, you have to consider an environmental source; and when the place is a sewer, consider sewer gas, or hydrogen sulfide.

d. Two police officers injured in a riot: The tear gases used to quell urban violence may have toxic effects on a large number of exposed persons.

e. Fire in a garden supply store warehouse: The garden store is one of the places you are likely to find stocks of organophosphate pesticides, which are the very same compounds that have been used in wartime as nerve gases.

f. Semitrailer overturned on the interstate: A semitrailer might be carrying just about anything, and the chances are very high that the contents are toxic.

g. Two "men down" on the maintenance staff of the municipal swimming pool: Most large swimming pools are chlorinated using chlorine gas, and the use of chlorine gas for that purpose has led to numerous mass exposures at hotels and community recreation centers.

h. Freight train struck car on level crossing: Like the semitrailer, the freight train has to be regarded as suspect until proved otherwise; it could be carrying anything.

i. Fire in a furniture factory: Every fire is potentially dangerous. A fire in a furniture factory is likely to involve the toxic products of combustion from upholstery and wood, including ammonia, hydrogen cyanide, acrolein, acetaldehyde, acetic acid, and formic acid—at least six good reasons to don a self-contained breathing apparatus!

All of the calls listed, then, might involve hazardous materials. That is the whole message of this chapter.

Crossword Puzzle

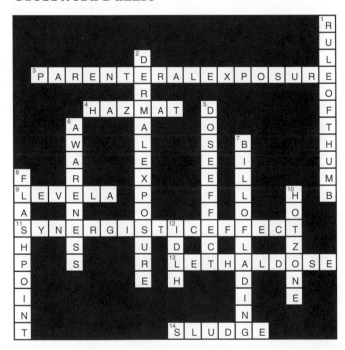

Chapter 51: Crime Scene Awareness

Matching

1. B (page 51.10)
2. F (page 51.14)
3. I (page 51.7)
4. D (page 51.10)
5. A (page 51.11)

6. H (page 51.6)
7. G (page 51.14)
8. E (page 51.4)
9. J (page 51.5)
10. C (page 51.5)

Multiple Choice

1. B (page 51.4)
2. C (page 51.5)
3. A (page 51.7)
4. C (page 51.7)
5. D (page 51.9)

6. B (page 51.7)
7. B (page 51.8)
8. C (page 51.10)
9. D (page 51.12)
10. A (page 51.14)

Fill-in-the-Blank

1. Tunnel vision (page 51.4)
2. 15, 10 (page 51.4)
3. Incident commander (IC) (page 51.5)
4. A (page 51.6)
5. Primary, secondary (page 51.7)
6. Contact, cover (page 51.8)
7. Surveillance (page 51.10)
   Capture
   Transport
   Holding
   Move
   Resolution

Identify

1. Possible errors in handling scene safety: Paramedics did not announce themselves at front, stood in front of door to knock, did not identify a secondary exit, did not look for visible weapons (drawers in tables can conceal weapons, and the poker in the fireplace stand is a potential weapon), and both approached the patient (should have considered using contact and cover technique).
2. Warning signs of danger: Loud conversation inside (possible domestic violence), the patient arguing with the other person, and the person getting between you and a means of egress.
3. Potential evidence: Ceramic object is possible evidence and should not be brushed away with shoe. Also, the patient's shirt is potential evidence that should not be cut or ripped unless absolutely necessary to provide care and no alternative is available to access injuries. (pages 51.7, 51.8, and 51.14)

Ambulance Calls

1. Listen for loud or threatening voices, glance through available windows for signs of a struggle, and look for visible weapons. Once at the door, stand to the doorknob side before knocking and announce yourself. Once inside, ask the person who answers to lead you to the patient. (page 51.7)
2. a. The ambulance should be positioned a minimum of 15 feet behind the car at a 10° angle to the driver's side facing the shoulder. (pages 51.5, 51.6)

    b. Before leaving the ambulance the license plate number and state-issued registration of the car should be recorded and left by the radio (some experts recommend giving it to the dispatcher). Also, notify the dispatcher of this information along with any additional information that might be helpful, such as the precise location.

    c. The incident commander, the person in the right front seat of the ambulance, should approach the rear passenger side of the car from the trunk to see that it is properly closed. Use a belly-in toward the motor vehicle and stop at the C column to look in the rear and side windows. Notice the number of people and pay close attention to their hands. Look for weapons. At any sign of a weapon or other danger, retreat immediately to a safe area. (pages 51.5, 51.6)

3. a. *Contact and cover* means you make contact with the patient to assess and provide care and your partner obtains patient information, gauges the level of tension, and warns you at the first sign of trouble.

    b. If you suspect that the location is a clandestine drug laboratory, immediately leave the house with the patient. Do not touch anything! Once clear of the lab, leave the area and notify the police as soon as possible without placing yourself in harm's way.

    c. Safety is a major issue for everyone because of the toxic nature of the material used, the highly flammable agents used, and the possibility of booby traps that are sometimes used to safeguard the illegal operations. (page 51.8)

4. Alter the scene as little as possible while providing care. Be mindful of physical evidence such as bullet casings, weapons, and blood. Do not move or pick up items that might be evidence. When you remove a patient's clothes to expose wounds, do not cut through bullet holes. Once you have removed the patient's clothes, do not shake the clothing because valuable evidence, including trace evidence, may fall off or from the pockets. (page 51.14)

True/False

1. F (page 51.14)   **6.** T (page 51.4)

2. T (page 51.10)   **7.** T (page 51.5)

3. F (page 51.7)   **8.** F (page 51.4)

4. F (page 51.7)   **9.** T (page 51.12)

5. F (page 51.5)   **10.** F (page 51.8)

Short Answer

1. a. Number of aggressors involved

    b. Number and type of injuries

    c. Number and type of weapons involved

    d. Make, color, body style, and license number of any vehicle involved

    e. Direction of travel if vehicle leaves scene (page 51.7)

2. a. Highly flammable properties of materials

    b. Toxic nature of chemicals and materials used

    c. Booby traps (fragmentation and incendiary devices) (page 51.8)

3. a. Glove box

    b. Top of sun visor

    c. Arm rest

    d. Under the seats

    e. In the center console

    f. Side door pocket

    g. Next to driver's right thigh (page 51.6)

4. A secondary exit could be used if the primary exit is blocked or an alternate means of egress is needed because of a threat or danger. A rear door or, in an emergency, a window can be used as a secondary exit. (page 51.7)

5. One paramedic makes contact with the patient to provide care. The second paramedic obtains patient information, gauges the level of tension, and warns his or her partner at the first sign of trouble. (page 51.8)

6. *Cover* includes objects that are usually impenetrable by bullets. *Concealment* includes objects that hide you until you can assess the situation and find cover. (page 51.9)

7. a. Cover

    (1) Trees

    (2) Mail collection boxes

    (3) Dumpsters

  b. Concealment

    (1) Tall grass

    (2) Shrubbery

    (3) Dark shadows (page 51.9)

8. At this stage, you are in grave danger. You must assume that the person on the other end of the gun will use violence if you do not follow instructions. (page 51.10)

9. a. Stand approximately an arm's length from the person.

  b. Stand at a 45° angle to the person.

  c. Keep feet shoulder width apart.

  d. Keep knees slightly bent.

  e. Keep hands relaxed. (page 51.12)

10. a. Testimonial evidence is oral documentation by a witness of the facts.

  b. Physical evidence ties a suspect to a crime and includes body materials, objects, and impressions. (page 51.14)

Word Find

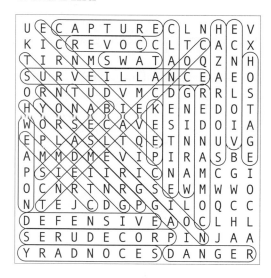

1. Aggressor (page 51.7)

2. Beams (page 51.4)

3. Capture (page 51.10)

4. Clandestine (page 51.8)

5. Commander (page 51.5)

6. Concealment (page 51.11)

7. Cover (page 51.11)

8. Crime (page 51.14)

9. Danger (page 51.4)

10. Defensive (page 51.12)

11. Evidence (page 51.14)

12. Hazardous (page 51.8)

13. Holding (page 51.10)

14. Hostage (page 51.9)

15. Peek (page 51.11)

16. Primary (page 51.7)

17. Procedures (page 51.4)

18. Secondary (page 51.7)

19. Surveillance (page 51.10)

20. SWAT (page 51.9)

21. Tactic (page 51.11)

22. Tunnel vision (page 51.4)

23. Violence (page 51.3)

24. Warning (page 51.7)

25. Weapon (page 51.7)

Section 7 Case Study: Answers and Summary

1. On the basis of your triage findings, how would you categorize these four patients?

During mass casualty situations, patients are rapidly triaged and then categorized based on the severity of their injuries or conditions **(Table 7-1)**. The *only* care provided during the triage process is immediate life-saving airway or hemorrhage management. Because the condition of patients may deteriorate, which would require recategorizing them to a different priority (usually higher); triage must be an ongoing process. On the basis of your rapid triage findings, the patients involved in this incident should be categorized as follows:

- **Critical (Red):** Patients 2 and 3
- **Urgent (Yellow):** Patients 1 and 4

Patient 2 (red) has signs of shock (ie, tachycardia, tachypnea, restlessness), abdominal pain that is suggestive of intraabdominal bleeding, and an underlying medical history of diabetes, which could exacerbate his condition.

Patient 3 (red) is demonstrating signs of severe head injury. He is unconscious, which places his airway in immediate jeopardy. Additionally, his respirations are 8 and shallow; therefore, he is breathing inadequately.

Patient 1 (yellow) appears hemodynamically stable at present; however, her inability to move her legs suggests a spinal injury. If the mechanism of injury was significant enough to cause spinal injury, she could have also sustained other injuries, which could result in deterioration of her hemodynamic status.

Patient 4 (yellow) is conscious with stable vital signs; however, she is complaining of hip pain, which could indicate a hip fracture. Like patient 1, a mechanism of injury significant enough to cause a high-energy hip fracture could also cause other potentially life-threatening injuries.

Because you and your partner are the only two paramedics at the scene, and the arrival of additional ambulances will be delayed, you should begin immediate treatment of the most critically injured patients (patients 2 and 3). Utilize fire personnel to tend to the lesser-injured patients (patients 1 and 4) until additional ambulances arrive.

Table 7-1   Triage Categories

Critical (Red)
- Patients who need immediate care and transport
  - Airway and breathing compromise
  - Uncontrolled or severe bleeding
  - Altered mental status
  - Severe underlying medical problems
  - Signs of shock (hypoperfusion)
  - Severe burns

Urgent (Yellow)
- Patients whose treatment and transport can be *temporarily* delayed
  - Burns without airway compromise
  - Major or multiple bone or joint injuries
  - Spinal injuries with or without spinal cord involvement

Delayed (Green)
- Patients whose treatment and transport can be delayed until last
  - Minor fractures
  - Minor soft-tissue injuries

Deceased (Black)
- Patients who are already dead or have little chance for survival
  - Cardiopulmonary arrest
  - Injuries that preclude survival (eg, head trauma with exposed brain matter)
  - Signs of obvious death (eg, decapitation, burned beyond recognition)

This incident is classified as a mass casualty incident (MCI). An MCI is defined as any situation that places a great demand on available resources. Clearly, as the sole ambulance at the scene, you and your partner cannot effectively care for all of the patients involved in this incident without assistance.

2. What are the components of the START triage system?

With the START (Simple Triage and Rapid Transport) triage system, a 60-second assessment of each patient is made that focuses on four areas: ability to walk, respiratory rate, pulses/perfusion, and mental status **(Table 7-2)**. The START triage system, which categorizes patients as being delayed (green), urgent (yellow), critical (red), or deceased (black), uses color-coded triage tags to identify the patient's triage category **(Figure 7-1)**.

Table 7-2 START Triage System

Able to walk?
- Yes – Delayed
- No – Assess respiratory rate
  - Apneic – Open airway
    - Remains apneic – Deceased
    - Respirations <10 or >30 breaths/min – Critical
    - Respirations >10 but <30 breaths/min – Assess Perfusion
      - Radial pulses absent – Critical
      - Radial pulses present – Assess mental status
        - Follows commands – Delayed
        - Can't follow commands – Critical

Several different types of triage tags can be used. However, a universally agreed upon color-coding system is used, regardless of the type of triage tag used.

Although there are several methods of triage, one commonality is that those who are pulseless or apneic (after opening the airway) are classified as being deceased. Because traumatic cardiac arrest patients rarely survive, focusing your resuscitative efforts on these patients will unnecessarily delay the care of other, potentially salvageable, patients, such as those with airway compromise or severe bleeding. Remember, the goal of triage is to provide the greatest good for the greatest number of patients.

The START triage system is typically used with large-scale mass casualty incidents; however, it can be a useful system if you are the first ambulance to arrive at the scene and the arrival of other ambulances at the scene will be delayed.

3. How would you justify the need for a third ambulance?

One ambulance and crew (two medics) can effectively care for only one critically injured patient at a time. Because you have two critical patients, you will need two ambulances. Although the two lesser-injured patients (patients 1 and 4) both have the potential for significant injuries (eg, spinal cord injury, hip fracture) and will require transport to a trauma center, they are hemodynamically stable at present and do not require immediate life-saving interventions. Therefore, they could both be transported in the same ambulance—one on the stretcher and the other on the bench seat. If necessary you can assign a firefighter to drive the ambulance, thus allowing both paramedics to tend to the patients.

Because of their significant mechanisms of injury, both patients require spinal immobilization and continuous monitoring for signs of deterioration.

Although the mechanisms of injury of patients 1 and 4 necessitate transport to a trauma center for evaluation, their present clinical conditions do not warrant taking a fourth ambulance out of service. It is important to follow locally established protocols regarding the most efficient use of ambulances and personnel during a mass casualty incident.

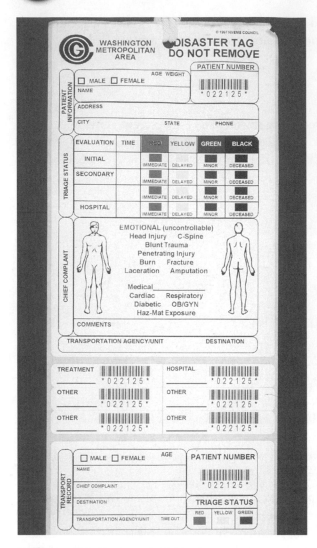
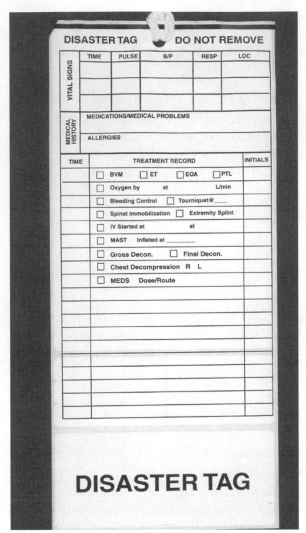

■ **Figure 7-1** A color-coded triage tag

Methods of transporting patients to the hospital are based on the size of the incident and the number of critical versus noncritical patients. Although ambulances are the typical method of transportation, buses may be used to transport large numbers of patients categorized as being delayed (green). Aeromedical services should be reserved for transporting critical patients or patients who require resources available only at a trauma center that is a great distance from the scene of the incident.

4. What areas are typically established during a mass-casualty incident?

During large-scale mass casualty incidents, responsibilities in eight different areas are assigned by the incident commander. These areas, or sectors, each have their own role in the overall management of the incident. The major areas of a mass-casualty incident are as follows:

■ **Command center**
  • The area where the incident commander oversees and coordinates the activities of the other areas.

■ **Staging area**
  • The holding area from where arriving ambulances and crews are assigned particular tasks.

■ **Operations/extrication area**
  • Where patients are disentangled and removed from a hazardous environment, allowing them to be moved to the triage area.

- **Triage area**
  - A sorting point, which is run by the triage officer. This is where patients are quickly assessed, categorized according to the severity of their injuries, and then, according to their assigned priority, directed to specific locations in the treatment area(s).
- **Treatment area**
  - Organized and managed by the treatment officer, this area is where a more thorough assessment is made and on-scene treatment is initiated while transport is being arranged.
- **Supply area**
  - Area where extra supplies and equipment are stored and distributed as needed.
- **Transportation area**
  - This area, which is managed by the transportation officer, is where ambulances and crews are organized to transport patients from the treatment area to area hospitals.
- **Rehabilitation area**
  - Provides protection and treatment to on-scene rescue personnel. As personnel enter and exit the scene, they are assessed and provided any needed medical care.

It is crucial that the incident command system remain intact at all times and that all personnel are able to effectively function in each of the eight different areas.

When you arrive at the scene of a mass-casualty incident, you will be assigned to a specific area by the incident commander. You should report immediately to that area's officer for further instructions. When you have completed the assigned task, report back to that same officer for another assignment. If your duties in that particular area are complete, you may be reassigned to a different area.

Summary

A mass-casualty incident is any situation that overwhelms the available resources of the EMS system, fire department, and area hospitals. Although the word "mass" implies many patients, two critical patients and one ambulance or four noncritical patients and two ambulances are just as much mass-casualty incidents as a situation involving 20 or more patients.

This case study presented a relatively small mass-casualty incident in which four patients, two of whom were critically injured, were effectively managed by three ambulances. Unfortunately, however, not all incidents are as limited in terms of numbers and criticality of patients.

In large-scale incidents, such as plane crashes, bus wrecks, and building collapses, an EMS system's resources are often quickly depleted and hospitals are quickly filled to capacity. This is when the incident management system is absolutely critical in order to effectively manage the incident and save as many lives as possible.

Once an incident command system has been established, all patients are rapidly triaged and, based on the severity of their injuries, are categorized with color-coded triage tags, which identifies their treatment and transport priority. During the triage process, the only care provided is immediate life-saving airway or hemorrhage management.

Because the patient's conditions may change, triage must be an ongoing process, recategorizing patients as needed. The goal of triage is to provide the greatest good for the greatest number of patients.

Once priority patients are identified, they are sent to the treatment area, where a more in-depth assessment is performed and emergency care is rendered. Following stabilization in the treatment area, patients are then directed by the transport officer to the appropriate medical facility.

The mass-casualty incident response that runs the smoothest is one that has been rehearsed. It is important for each EMS system to know its available resources (eg, mutual aid, trauma centers, HazMat teams) and to practice "mock" mass-casualty incidents.

Appendix A: Cardiac Life Support Fundamentals

Matching

1. D (page A.9)
2. A (page A.9)
3. E (page A.9)
4. B (page A.9)
5. C (page A.9)
6. D (page A.21)
7. C (page A.21)
8. A (page A.20)
9. E (page A.21)
10. B (page A.20)

Multiple Choice

1. C (page A.4)
2. A (page A.7)
3. D (page A.9)
4. C (page A.10)
5. B (page A.11)
6. B (page A.4)
7. B (page A.6)
8. C (page A.13)
9. C (page A.14)
10. A (page A.20)

Fill-in-the-Blank

1. 30, 2 (page A.7)
2. 2, 5 (page A.7)
3. 1, adolescence (page A.9)
4. Asynchronous, 100, without, 8, 10 (page A.11)
5. Ventricular fibrillation, pulseless ventricular tachycardia (page A.13)
6. Remove, dry (page A.14)
7. Epinephrine, vasopressin (page A.16)
8. Impedance threshold device (ITD) (page A.17)
9. Direct visualization (page A.18)
10. Teamwork (pages A.18, A.19)

Identify

1. (page A.4)

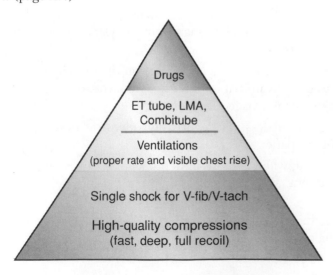

2. Techniques of verifying correct endotracheal tube placement. *Students will list seven of the following:*

   a. Direct visualization of the tube going through cords

   b. Physical exam of tube placement

   c. Use of esophageal detection device

   d. Bilateral chest expansion

   e. Five-point auscultation

   f. Tube condensation

   g. Exhaled CO_2 device (capnography)

   h. Clinical assessment (page A.18)

3. **a.** Compressor 1—BLS crew from Rescue 1

   b. Compressor 2—BLS crew from Rescue 1

   c. Ventilator—BLS crew from Rescue 1 and your partner

   d. Team leader—The paramedic

   e. Field supervisor—Captain from Rescue 1 (pages A.20, A.21)

Ambulance Calls

1.

H Hypovolemia	**T** Toxins
H Hypoxia	**T** Tamponade, cardiac
H Hydrogen ion (acidosis)	**T** Tension pneumothorax
H Hypokalemia/hyperkalemia	**T** Thrombosis (coronary or pulmonary)
H Hypoglycemia	**T** Trauma (page A.16)
H Hypothermia	

2. For advanced airway, consider using either an LMA or Combitube. Intraosseous (IO) cannulation is an alternative way to proceed to provide a route for drug administration. It is important to make sure that quality CPR continues with only minimal interruption as these interventions are performed. (page A.16)

3. **a.** Two mechanical devices can perform cardiac compressions: AutoPulse and Thumper. Both devices can provide compressions without interruption.

   b. The Thumper has an advantage over the AutoPulse because it is also equipped to provide ventilations in conjunction with the continuous compressions. (pages A.17, A.18)

True/False

1. F (page A.4)	**6.** F (page A.11)
2. F (page A.5)	**7.** T (page A.11)
3. T (page A.7)	**8.** F (page A.13)
4. T (page A.8)	**9.** F (page A.14)
5. T (page A.9)	**10.** T (page A.18)

Short Answer

1. **a.** Hard

   b. Fast

   c. Full recoil (page A.4)

2. **a.** Ventricular fibrillation

   b. Pulseless ventricular tachycardia (page A.13)

3. *Students will provide any three of the following:*

   a. Hairy chest

   b. Wet chest

   c. Pacemaker or automatic internal cardiac defibrillator (AICD)

   d. Transdermal medication patch (page A.14)

4. **a.** Direct visualization of tube going through the cords

   b. Bilateral chest expansion

   c. Five-point auscultation

   d. Physical examination of the tube placement

   e. Tube condensation (page A.18)

5. **a.** Obtaining patient history and performing physical exam

   b. Interpreting the echocardiogram (ECG)

   c. Keeping track of time

   d. Making medication decisions

   e. Clearly delegating tasks

   f. Providing documentation after the resuscitation

   g. Talking with Medical Control

   h. Controlling the scene (page A.20)

6. **a.** Both are advanced airway techniques that are inserted blindly.

   b. Both are placed orally and inserted past the hypopharyngeal space.

   c. Both are easy to use and do not require extensive training in laryngoscopy. (page A.16)

7. **a.** Load-distributing band CPR device (AutoPulse)

   b. Thumper device (page A.18)

Crossword Puzzle

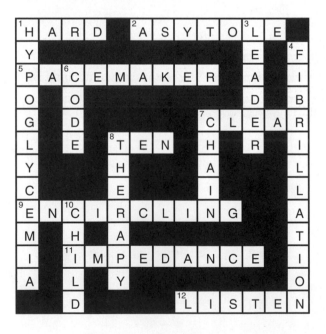

Rhythm Strips

1. B (page 27.59)

2. A (page 27.60)

3. D (page 27.48)

4. E (page 27.48)

5. C (page 27.48)

6. a. RHYTHM: _____ regular __X__ irregular

b. RATE: Cannot be calculated

c. P WAVES: _____ present __X__ absent

d. If present, is there a P before every QRS? _____ yes __X__ no

e. Is there a QRS after every P? _____ yes __X__ no

f. P–R INTERVAL: N/A

g. QRS complexes: N/A

h. Name of rhythm: **Ventricular fibrillation**

i. Treatment: Follow the pulseless arrest algorithm shown on page A.15.

(page 27.58)

Skill Drills

1. *Single-Rescuer Adult CPR* (page A.7)

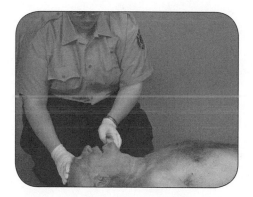

Step 1: Establish unresponsiveness. Open the airway.

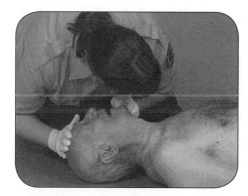

Step 2: Check for breathing (look, listen, and feel). If no breaths, administer two breaths, each 1 second, achieving visible chest rise.

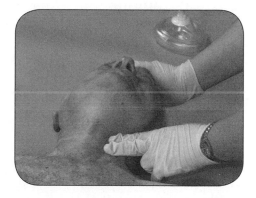

Step 3: Perform a carotid pulse check (maximum of 10 seconds each).

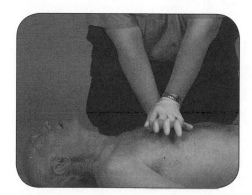

Step 4: Begin 30 compressions—center of the chest, push hard and fast (rate of 100/min), and allow full chest recoil.

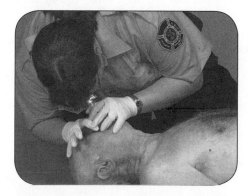

Step 5: Ventilate two times for 1 second each to achieve visible chest rise. Complete five cycles (approximately 2 minutes) and reassess the patient for a maximum of 10 seconds. If automated external defibrillator (AED) has arrived, attach it without interrupting compressions.

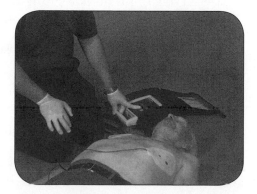

Step 6: Check the patient's rhythm. If it is shockable, administer a single shock, and then resume CPR immediately for five cycles. Reanalyze the rhythm. If it is not shockable, resume CPR immediately for five cycles.

Appendix B: Assessment-Based Management

Matching

a.

1. C (page B.4)   **4.** D (page B.4)

2. A (page B.4)   **5.** B (page B.4)

3. E (page B.4)

b.

1. D (page B.8)   **4.** E (page B.8)

2. B (page B.4)   **5.** C (page B.4)

3. A (page B.3)

Multiple Choice

1. B (page B.4)   **6.** B (page B.8)

2. D (page B.4)   **7.** A (page B.9)

3. C (page B.6)   **8.** D (page B.5)

4. A (page B.7)   **9.** D (page B.5)

5. D (page B.7)   **10.** C (page B.4)

Fill-in-the-Blank

1. History (page B.4)

2. "Vectored" (page B.4)

3. Subjective, objective (page B.4)

4. Attitude (page B.5)

5. Tunnel vision (myopia) (page B.5)

6. Environmental distracters (page B.5)

7. Team leader (page B.6)

8. Responsive, not responsive (page B.8)

9. Assessment, presentation skills (page B.9)

10. "Right stuff" (page B.7)

Identify

1. Chief complaint: Patient is only responsive to pain and has been involved in a motor vehicle crash.

2. Vital signs:
Pulse 90 beats/min and regular
Respirations 20 breaths/min and not labored
Blood pressure of 130/80 mm Hg
Oxygen saturation of 98%

3. Pertinent negatives:
Air is moving in all lung fields.
Vital signs are stable and within normal limits.
Abdomen is soft.
Pulses and motor responses are in all extremities.
ECG is normal sinus rhythm. (page B.4; B.8)

Ambulance Calls

1. a. Cardiopulmonary exam:

  (1) Assessment of the lungs and heart sounds

  (2) Assessment for jugular venous distention (JVD) and pedal edema

  (3) Obtain an ECG

  b. Subjective information:

  (1) OPQRST

  (2) SAMPLE history (page B.4)

2. The importance of a team leader choreographing the activities of the team at the scene of emergency cannot be overstated. The team leader and team members have specific roles that must be carried out to increase success, as in this case of a patient resuscitation. The role of the team leader is key to coordinating the efforts of the entire team. Clearly, the team gives and gets its best response when a leader manages and monitors an event with a clear understanding of the strategies, goals, and plans. (page B.6)

3. a. Unit identifier and level of training

  b. Patient identification information, such as age, gender, and degree of distress

  c. Chief complaint

  d. Present illness, including OPQRST

  e. Medical history (SAMPLE)

  f. Pertinent findings (positives and negatives)

  g. Treatment plan, including what has been done

  h. Request additional medical orders, if needed

  i. Estimated time of arrival (ETA) at the hospital (page B.9)

True/False

1. F (page B.4)   **6.** F (page B.8)

2. F (page B.4)   **7.** T (page B.8)

3. T (page B.8)   **8.** T (page B.7)

4. T (page B.5)   **9.** F (page B.8)

5. F (page B.7)   **10.** T (page B.6)

Short Answer

1. a. Crowds

  b. Unruly bystanders

  c. Potentially violent/dangerous situations

  d. High noise levels

  e. Excessive number of emergency medical services (EMS) providers on the scene (page B.5)

2. a. Dressings, bandages, and tape

  b. Sphygmomanometer, stethoscope

  c. Assessment card and pen

  d. Impedance threshold device (ITD) and cardiopulmonary resuscitation (CPR) prompt

  e. Automatic external defibrillator (AED) or manual defibrillator (page B.7)

3. a. Assess the cranial nerves

  b. Assess the Cincinnati Stroke Scale

  c. Assess sensory and motor functions in each extremity (page B.4)

4. a. Those with a significant mechanism of injury (MOI)

  b. Those without a significant mechanism of injury (MOI) (page B.8)

5. a. Hypoxia

  b. Hypovolemia

   c. Hypoglycemia

   d. Hypothermia

   e. Head injury (concussion) (page B.5)

Word Finds

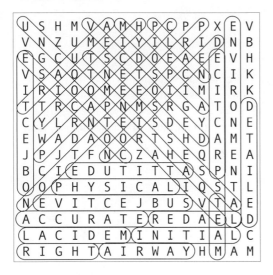

  1. Accurate (page B.3)

  2. Vectored (page B.4)

  3. History (page B.4)

  4. Detailed (page B.8)

  5. Subjective (page B.4)

  6. Decision (page B.4)

  7. Objective (page B.4)

  8. Plan (page B.4)

  9. Attitude (page B.5)

10. Myopia (page B.5)

11. Assessment (page B.5)

12. Uncooperative (page B.5)

13. Environmental (page B.5)

14. Leader (page B.6)

15. Team (page B.6)

16. Right stuff (page B.7)

17. Airway (page B.7)

18. Medical (page B.8)

19. Trauma (page B.8)

20. Concise (page B.9)

21. Presentation (page B.9)

22. Initial (page B.7)

23. Practice (page B.6)

24. Paramedic (page B.5)

25. Physical (page B.4)

Fill-in-the-Table

1.

Essential Equipment	
Function	**Essential Items**
Airway control	PPE (gloves, face shield, and HEPA or N-95 mask) Oral airways, nasal airways Suction unit (electric or manual) Rigid tip Yankauer and flexible suction catheters LMA, Combitube, ET tubes Laryngoscope and blades Tube check, tube restraint, tape, syringes, stylet End-tidal carbon dioxide device
Breathing	Pocket mask and one-way valve Bag-mask ventilation device(s) (adult and child), spare masks Oxygen-delivery devices (nonrebreathing mask, cannula, extension tubing) Oxygen tank, regulator, transport ventilator Occlusive dressings Large-bore IV catheter for thoracic decompression Pulse oximeter
Circulation	Dressings, bandages, and tape Sphygmomanometer, stethoscope Assessment card and pen Impedance threshold device (ITD) and CPR prompt AED or manual defibrillator Drug box Glucometer Venous access supplies (IV and IO)
Disability and dysrhythmia	Rigid collars Flashlight ECG monitor
Exposure	Space blanket to cover the patient Scissors

(page B.7)

Photo Credits

Chapter 7
pg 7.3 (pig) © Photos.com; pg 7.3 (calcium chloride) Courtesy of Yellowstone National Park; pg 7-3 (lab) Courtesy of Linda Bartlett/National Cancer Institute; pg 7-3 (foxglobe) © Stephen Aaron Rees/ShutterStock, Inc.

Case Study 2
pg S2.1 Arrhythmia Recognition: The Art of Interpretation, Courtesy of Tomas B. Garcia, MD.

Case Study 3
pg S3.0 Courtesy of Marilyn Westlake; pg S3.2 Arrhythmia Recognition: The Art of Interpretation, Courtesy of Tomas B. Garcia, MD.

Chapter 19
pg 19.2 (laceration) © English/Custom Medical Stock Photo; pg 19-3 (impaled object) © Custom Medical Stock Photo; pg 19-2 (thumb amputation) © E. M. Singletary, M.D. Used with permission.

Case Study 4
pg S4.0 © Eddie Sperling; pg S4.2 Arrhythmia Recognition: The Art of Interpretation, Courtesy of Tomas B. Garcia, MD.

Chapter 27
pgs 27.15–27.20 Arrhythmia Recognition: The Art of Interpretation, Courtesy of Tomas B. Garcia, MD.

Case Study 7
pg S7.0 © Keith Muratori/ShutterStock, Inc.

Appendix A
pg A.7–A.8 Arrhythmia Recognition: The Art of Interpretation, Courtesy of Tomas B. Garcia, MD.

Answer Key
pg K.61 Arrhythmia Recognition: The Art of Interpretation, Courtesy of Tomas B. Garcia, MD.; pg K.95 © Visuals Unlimited; K.234 Arrhythmia Recognition: The Art of Interpretation, Courtesy of Tomas B. Garcia, MD.; pg K.272 © Visuals Unlimited; K.273 (petechial rash) Courtesy of CDC

Unless otherwise indicated, photographs are under copyright of Jones and Bartlett Publishers and were photographed by the Maryland Institute of Emergency Medical Services Systems.

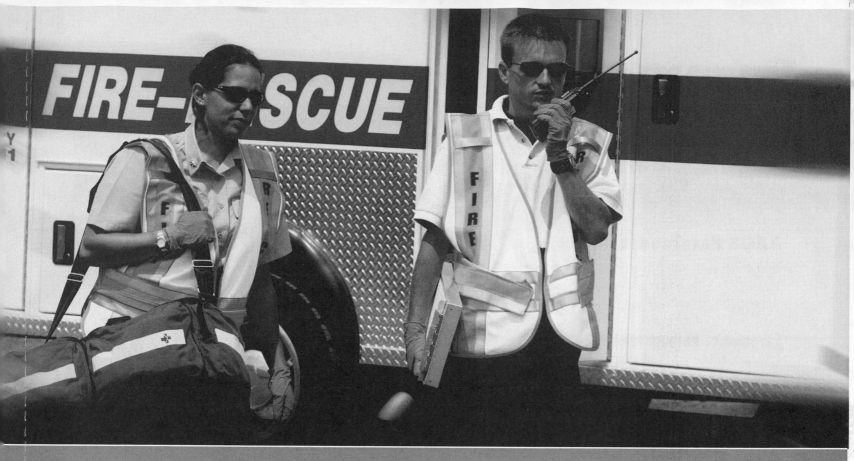

Essential Information in the **Palm of Your Hand!**

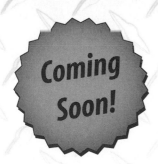
Coming Soon!

Paramedic Field Guide

American Academy of Orthopaedic Surgeons, **Bob Elling**, **Marilynn Jackson**, and **Lee Jackson**

ISBN-13: 978-0-7637-5122-7
ISBN-10: 0-7637-5122-7
$24.95* (Sugg. US List)
Spiral • 200 Pages • ©2008

This convenient field guide contains all the information that paramedics need at their fingertips in the field—instructions, conversion charts, assessment checklists, scales, tables, anatomies, lab tests, medication indications and administration, and other basic information for quick reference. The full-color, spiral-bound guide is divided into sections that follow the Paramedic National Standard Curriculum. Sections are divided by color-coded tabs to allow rapid retrieval of information when paramedics need it most.

Sections include:

1. Assessment
2. Airway and Respiratory Emergencies
3. Musculoskeletal and Soft-Tissue Injuries
4. Pharmacology
5. Neurological and Behavioral Emergencies
6. Cardiovascular Emergencies
7. Infectious Diseases, Environmental, Endocrine, and Allergy
8. GI, GU, and Hematologic Emergencies
9. OB/GYN and Neonatal Emergencies
10. Pediatrics
11. Special Operations
12. Communications and Documentation

Paramedics will be able to confirm appropriate pediatric ET tube sizes, emergency measures in the event of an infectious exposure, signs and symptoms of acute illnesses, conditions that warrant supplemental oxygen administration, fracture classifications based on displacement, and much more.

Take your paramedic training with you into the field with the most comprehensive field guide available!

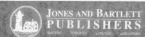

Paramedic Resources from

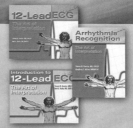
Image © Steve L. Smith

Jones and Bartlett Publishers

Case Studies for the Paramedic Series

Performing a systematic patient assessment and determining appropriate treatment is the most vital and complicated part of a paramedic's job. To help teach and refresh assessment and treatment decision-making principles, each book in this series provides 20 detailed scenarios to realistically test and refine paramedic assessment skills without actually being in the field.

Medical Case Studies for the Paramedic
American Academy of Orthopaedic Surgeons, Stephen J. Rahm, NREMT-P
ISBN-13: 978-0-7637-2581-5 • ISBN-10: 0-7637-2581-1 • $37.95* • Paperback • 196 Pages • © 2004

Pediatric Case Studies for the Paramedic
American Academy of Orthopaedic Surgeons, Stephen J. Rahm, NREMT-P
ISBN-13: 978-0-7637-2582-X • ISBN-10: 0-7637-2582-X • $37.95* • Paperback • 200 Pages • © 2006

Trauma Case Studies for the Paramedic
American Academy of Orthopaedic Surgeons, Stephen J. Rahm. NREMT-P
ISBN-13: 978-0-7637-2583-9 • ISBN-10: 0-7637-2583-8 • $37.95* • Paperback • 200 Pages • © 2005

Paramedic Review Manuals

Help students prepare for state and national exams with these review manuals. The *Paramedic Review Manual* includes the same types of skill-based and multiple choice questions they are likely to encounter on national exams, while *Pearls of Wisdom* is written in a rapid-fire question and answer format perfect for reviewing for any exam or simply brushing up on paramedic knowledge.

Paramedic Pearls of Wisdom, Second Edition
Guy Haskell, PhD, NREMT-P
ISBN-13: 978-0-7637-3870-9 • ISBN-10: 0-7637-3870-0 • $34.95* • Paperback • 520 Pages • © 2006

Paramedic Review Manual for National Certification
American Academy of Orthopaedic Surgeons, Stephen J. Rahm, NREMT-P
ISBN-13: 978-0-7637-4407-6 • ISBN-10: 0-7637-4407-7 • $29.95* • Paperback • 156 Pages • © 2004

*Suggested U.S. list price. Prices are subject to change. Shipping and sales tax will be applied to your order. If you are not completely satisfied with your purchase, please return it within 30 days for a full refund or replacement copy.

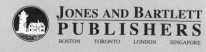

JONES AND BARTLETT
PUBLISHERS
BOSTON   TORONTO   LONDON   SINGAPORE

from first aid to CPR to paramedic, please visit www.EMSzone.com today!

MAXIMIZE YOUR TEST SCORES WITH OUR REVIEW MANUALS

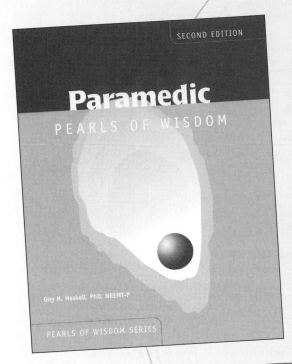

Guy Haskell, PhD, NREMT-P
ISBN-13: 978-0-7637-3870-9
ISBN-10: 0-7637-3870-0
$34.95*
Paperback • 520 pages • © 2006

Paramedic: Pearls of Wisdom, Second Edition is a review manual containing rapid-fire questions and answers to help students prepare for state and national certification and refresher exams. Designed to maximize test scores, the *Second Edition* prunes complex concepts down to the simplest kernel. The reader will receive immediate gratification with the correct answer. The manual is written in direct correlation to the U.S. Department of Transportation 1998 Paramedic National Standard Curriculum.

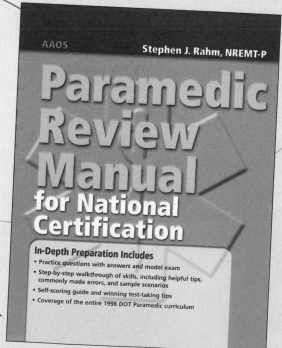

American Academy of Orthopaedic Surgeons
Stephen J. Rahm, NREMT-P
ISBN-13: 978-0-7637-4407-6
ISBN-10: 0-7637-4407-7
$29.95*
Paperback • 156 pages • © 2004

If you or your students need a traditional review manual for a state or national certification exam, the *Paramedic Review Manual for National Certification* is your answer! This manual consists of the same type of skill-based, multiple-choice questions used on the actual exams. It also includes a step-by-step walk-through of skills, including helpful tips, commonly made errors, and sample scenarios.

PLACE YOUR RISK-FREE ORDER TODAY!*

 Jones and Bartlett Publishers

Phone: 1-800-832-0034 | Web: www.jbpub.com

*Suggested U.S. list price. Prices are subject to change. Shipping and sales tax will be applied to your order. If you are not completely satisfied with your purchase, please return it within 30 days for a full refund or replacement copy.